INTERNAL MEDICINE

VOLUME 1
FOUNDATIONS OF ADULT CLINICAL PRACTICE

Dr. Ahmed Taha

ALLIED
HEALTH
PRESS

Internal Medicine

Volume 1: Foundations of Adult Clinical Practice

Author: **Dr. Ahmed Taha**

Allied Health Press
4164 Lakeshore Road
Burlington ON L7L 1A4
Canada
www.alliedhealthpress.com
Email: orders@arclereducation.com

ISBN: 978-1-77956-854-0

ABOUT THE AUTHOR

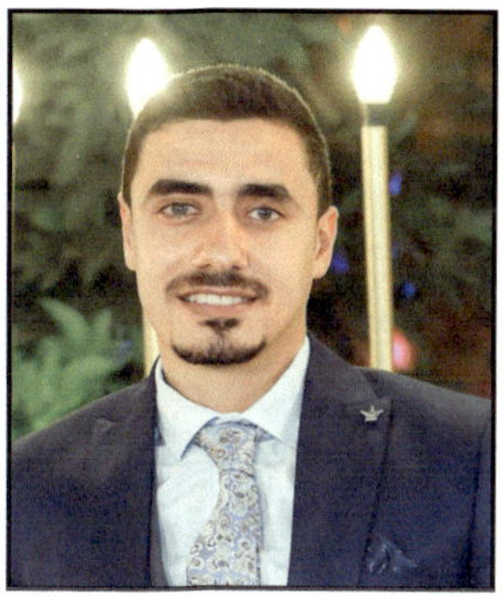

Dr. Ahmed Taha Abdel Sattar, MD, MBChB, is a distinguished graduate of Fayoum University with a GPA of 4 (Summa Cum Laude). Currently a Teaching Assistant in Ophthalmology at Fayoum University Hospital, he has over 14 peer-reviewed publications with 140+ citations and five years of experience in international medical publications. Committed to advancing medical knowledge and patient care, he mentors future healthcare professionals while providing compassionate care to patients.

Brief Table of Contents

1. Introduction to Internal Medicine	1
2. Cardiology	37
3. Respiratory Medicine	71
4. Gastroenterology	103
5. Nephrology	135
6. Endocrinology	171
7. Hematology	207
8. Infectious Diseases	241
9. Rheumatology	273
10. Neurology (Medical)	307
11. Clinical Pharmacology and Therapeutics	343
12. Environmental and Occupational Medicine	375
Index	405

Chapter Openers

A list of Chapter Outline is presented providing a brief Introduction to what will be covered in the chapter.

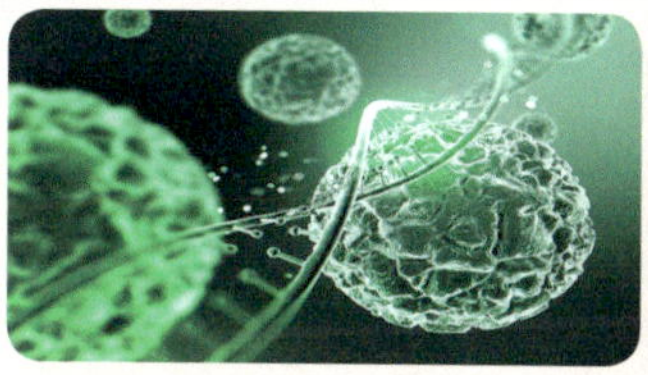

Introduction

Often referred to as the science of life, biology is a broad field of study aimed at comprehending the several kinds of life on Earth, from tiny creatures to sophisticated multicellular entities. Comprising several subfields, including molecular biology, ecology, and evolutionary biology, each of which advances our knowledge of living systems, this field clarifies the mechanisms controlling life events, including development, reproduction, and interaction with the surroundings, which is the central goal of biology. Moreover, biology fills in the void between the natural sciences and medicine by offering a necessary understanding of health, illness, and the interactions between organisms and their environments. Dealing with urgent global issues such as climate change, biodiversity loss, and new diseases depends on an awareness of these complex biological interactions, therefore highlighting the critical part biology plays in modern civilization. Fundamentally, biology explores and tests ideas about the living world using the scientific method. Through methodical observation and experimentation,

LEARNING OBJECTIVES

After studying this chapter, you will be able to:

1. Discuss the scientific method in biology;
2. Explain the cell theory;
3. Discuss the genetics and heredity;
4. Evolution and natural selection;
5. Focus on ecology and ecosystems;
6. Learn about human biology;
7. Evaluate the plant biology;
8. Explain the microbiology;
9. Focus on current trends in biology.

1.1. The Scientific Method in Biology

Learning Outcome

1. Describe the steps of the scientific method;
2. Focus on hypothesis formation;
3. Learn about experimental design.

Learning Outcomes

The beginning of each section of every chapter contains a set of Learning Outcomes that inform students of concepts they should understand. These outcomes help students understand what they should be able to do if they have mastered the material in that section.

Test Your Knowledge

Throughout each chapter, Test Your Knowledge cues you to note which topics have been covered and to self-test your understanding of the material presented.

Test Your Knowledge

1. Explain why correlation does not imply causation in scientific experiments.
2. How does the scientific method help reduce the influence of personal opinions in research?

Chapter Summary

The Summary Section appear at the end of each chapter and summarize main concepts covered throughout the chapter. These points provide key concepts in an engaging and meaningful way.

Summary

The investigation of biological principles highlights the importance of a comprehensive view of life by reflecting the intricate interactions that occur within living systems. The complexity of biology goes beyond individual species or systems, as this essay highlights; it also includes the interactions that mold ecosystems and affect biodiversity. Researchers can conduct in-depth analyses of metabolomic data using sophisticated technologies like MetaboAnalyst, which offer insights into the molecular mechanisms underlying these interactions. As demonstrated by the developments in MetaboAnalyst, for example, the integration of diverse omics data promotes a thorough understanding of metabolic pathways and helps identify important biological markers necessary for research on development and disease (Chong et al., 2018). Additionally, the phenomenon of ecological invasions is a key component of biological research and a vital field of study. The introduction of non-native species into unfamiliar habitats has significant ramifications and calls for multidisciplinary management strategies. Examining the origins and effects of these biological incursions, invasion science has become a crucial field that highlights the need to comprehend ecological dynamics and community interactions. As interest in biological invasions increases, new findings are emerging that put conventional ecological theories and practices to the test. The importance of incorporating various scientific viewpoints is shown by this developing discipline, which also highlights how invasive species shape ecosystems and advances our knowledge of ecological resilience (David et al., 2013). When taken as a whole, these discoveries from invasion science and metabolomics highlight the value of multidisciplinary biology research. Fostering cross-disciplinary collaboration and utilizing technological breakthroughs to improve our comprehension of intricate biological interactions are crucial as we look to the future of biological research. In addition to deepening our understanding of the complexities of life, this method lays the groundwork for tackling urgent environmental issues. Future studies can ensure the continued relevance of biology in a world that is constantly changing by acknowledging the interconnection of biological systems and opening the door to creative solutions that support sustainability and biodiversity conservation. We might imagine a thorough comprehension of life that serves both academia and society at large through ongoing investigation and integration of scientific knowledge.

Knowledge Assessment

The chapter includes material designed to review and reinforce each content. It includes Critical Thinking Questions to help test of your understanding of information presented in the chapter and Short answer Questions to review your understanding of the key concepts presented in the chapter.

Critical Thinking Questions

1. **Who is known as the "Father of Modern Biology"?**
   a. Aristotle
   b. Charles Darwin
   c. Gregor Mendel
   d. Louis Pasteur
2. **What is the basic unit of life?**
   a. Atom
   b. Molecule
   c. Cell
   d. Organism
3. **Which branch of biology studies the interaction of organisms with their environment?**
   a. Genetics
   b. Ecology
   c. Physiology
   d. Botany
4. **Which macromolecule is the main source of energy for living organisms?**
   a. Proteins
   b. Lipids
   c. Carbohydrates
   d. Nucleic acids
5. **DNA is primarily responsible for which function in living organisms?**
   a. Energy production
   b. Protein synthesis
   c. Storing genetic information
   d. Regulating body temperature

Short Answer Questions

1. What is biology, and why is it important to study biology?
2. What are the three main domains of life, and how are they different from one another?
3. Define homeostasis and give an example of how it works in living organisms.
4. What is the cell theory, and why is it fundamental to biology?
5. How do autotrophs and heterotrophs differ in the way they obtain energy?
6. What is the scientific method, and how is it applied in biological research?
7. Discuss how biology helps address global challenges such as climate change, disease, and food security.
8. Explain the levels of biological organization from the smallest unit to the largest. Provide examples at each level.
9. Describe the relationship between structure and function in biology, giving specific examples from cells or organs.
10. How has the discovery of genetics shaped our understanding of inheritance and variation among organisms?

Supplementary Materials

Key Terms: A list of key terms is given for quick reference

KEY TERMS FROM THIS CHAPTER

Annotation enrichment analysis	Biological structure	Cell
Cell theory	Cellular structure	Ecology
Ecosystems	Genetics	Human biology
Microbiology	Natural selection	Organism
Plant biology		

Further Resources: Recommendations for additional readings, websites, and multimedia resources.

References

1. Argelaguet, R., Velten, B., Arnol, D., Dietrich, S., Zenz, T., Marioni, J. C., Buettner, F., et al. (2018). Multi-omics factor analysis—A framework for unsupervised integration of multi-omics data sets. *Molecular Systems Biology, 14*. https://doi.org/10.15252/msb.20178124.
2. Bacher, S., Blackburn, T. M., Essl, F., & Genovesi, P. (2017). *Socio-Economic Impact Classification of Alien Taxa (SEICAT)*. https://core.ac.uk/download/286567949.pdf (accessed on 8th March 2025).
3. Barnett, R., Brace, S., Cucchi, T., & Dobney, K. (2013). *Divergent Evolutionary Processes Associated with Colonization of Offshore Islands*. https://core.ac.uk/download/20664364.pdf (accessed on 8th March 2025).

Detailed Table of Contents

List of Figures xv
Preface xxi

CHAPTER 1

Introduction to Internal Medicine 1

Introduction 1
1.1. History of Internal Medicine 5
1.1.1. Evolution of Internal Medicine Through the Centuries 6
1.1.2. Key Figures in the Development of Internal Medicine 7
1.1.3. Milestones in Internal Medicine Practices and Education 7
1.2. Core Principles of Internal Medicine 9
1.2.1. Patient-Centered Care and Holistic Approach 9
1.2.2. Emphasis on Diagnosis and Treatment of Adult Diseases 11
1.2.3. Role of Preventive Care in Internal Medicine 11
1.3. Common Conditions Treated in Internal Medicine 13
1.3.1. Chronic Diseases such as Diabetes and Hypertension 14
1.3.2. Infectious Diseases and Their Management 15
1.3.3. Cardiovascular Diseases (CVDs) and Their Implications 15
1.4. Diagnostic Techniques in Internal Medicine 17
1.4.1. Importance of Patient History and Physical Examination 18
1.4.2. Use of Laboratory Tests and Imaging Studies 18
1.4.3. Emerging Technologies in Diagnostics 19
1.5. Treatment Modalities in Internal Medicine 20
1.5.1. Pharmacological Interventions and Their Management 21
1.5.2. Lifestyle Modifications and Patient Education 22
1.5.3. Coordination of Care with Other Healthcare Providers 23
1.6. Challenges in Internal Medicine 24
1.6.1. Managing Complex and Comorbid Conditions 25
1.6.2. Navigating Healthcare Systems and Patient Access 26
1.6.3. Addressing the Physician Burnout Crisis 27
Summary 28
References 31

CHAPTER 2

Cardiology 37

Introduction 37
2.1. Role of Internal Medicine in Cardiology 40
2.1.1. Comprehensive Patient Assessment 41
2.1.2. Management of Comorbidities 42
2.1.3. Coordination of Care 43
2.2. Common Cardiovascular Diseases (CVDs) 44
2.2.1. Hypertension 45
2.2.2. Coronary Artery Disease (CAD) 46
2.2.3. Heart Failure 47
2.3. Diagnostic Tools in Cardiology 48

2.3.1. Electrocardiogram (ECG) 50
2.3.2. Echocardiography 50
2.3.3. Cardiac Catheterization 51
2.4. Treatment Modalities **52**
2.4.1. Pharmacological Interventions 53
2.4.2. Lifestyle Modifications 54
2.4.3. Surgical Options 55
2.5. Preventive Cardiology **56**
2.5.1. Risk Factor Identification 57
2.5.2. Patient Education and Counseling 58
2.5.3. Screening Guidelines 59
2.6. Challenges in Cardiology **60**
2.6.1. Access to Care 61
2.6.2. Patient Compliance 61
2.6.3. Advances in Technology 62
Summary **64**
References **67**

CHAPTER 3

Respiratory Medicine 71

Introduction **71**
3.1. Anatomy and Physiology of the Respiratory System **74**
3.1.1. Structure of the Respiratory System 74
3.1.2. Function of the Lungs and Airways 75
3.1.3. Mechanisms of Gas Exchange 77
3.2. Common Respiratory Diseases **78**
3.2.1. Asthma: Causes and Symptoms 79
3.2.2. Chronic Obstructive Pulmonary Disease (COPD) 80
3.2.3. Pneumonia: Types and Treatment Options 81
3.3. Diagnostic Techniques in Respiratory Medicine **82**
3.3.1. Pulmonary Function Tests (PFTs) 83
3.3.2. Imaging Studies: X-rays and Computed Tomography (CT) Scans 84
3.3.3. Bronchoscopy and Its Applications 85
3.4. Treatment Modalities **86**
3.4.1. Pharmacological Treatments: Inhalers and Medications 87
3.4.2. Non-Pharmacological Interventions: Pulmonary Rehabilitation 88
3.4.3. Surgical Options for Severe Cases 88
3.5. Public Health and Respiratory Medicine **90**
3.5.1. Impact of Air Quality on Respiratory Health 90
3.5.2. Preventive Measures and Health Education 91
3.5.3. Global Initiatives to Combat Respiratory Diseases 92
Summary **94**
References **97**

CHAPTER 4

Gastroenterology 103

Introduction **103**
4.1. Overview of Gastroenterology **105**
4.1.1. Definition and Focus of Gastroenterology 106
4.1.2. Common Conditions Treated in Gastroenterology 107
4.1.3. Role of Gastroenterologists in Patient Care 108
4.2. Diagnostic Techniques in Gastroenterology **109**
4.2.1. Endoscopy Procedures and Their Significance 110
4.2.2. Imaging Studies Used in Gastroenterology 111
4.2.3. Laboratory Tests and Their Role in Diagnosis 112
4.3. Treatment Modalities in Gastroenterology **113**
4.3.1. Pharmacological Treatments for Gastrointestinal Disorders 114
4.3.2. Surgical Interventions in Gastroenterology 115
4.3.3. Lifestyle Modifications and Their Impact on Treatment 116
4.4. Common Gastrointestinal Disorders **117**
4.4.1. Inflammatory Bowel Disease (IBD) 118
4.4.2. Gastroesophageal Reflux Disease (GERD) 119
4.4.3. Hepatic Disorders and Their Management 120
4.5. The Role of Nutrition in Gastroenterology **121**
4.5.1. Importance of Diet in Gastrointestinal Health 122
4.5.2. Nutritional Therapy for Specific Disorders 123
4.5.3. Role of Dietitians in Gastroenterology 124
4.6. Advances in Gastroenterology **125**
4.6.1. Emerging Technologies in Diagnosis and Treatment 125
4.6.2. Research Trends in Gastroenterology 126
4.6.3. Future Directions for the Field 127

Summary 128
References 131

CHAPTER 5

Nephrology 135

Introduction 135
5.1. Anatomy and Physiology of the Kidneys 138
5.1.1. Structure of the Kidneys 139
5.1.2. Functions of the Renal System 140
5.1.3. Regulation of Homeostasis by the Kidneys 141
5.2. Common Kidney Diseases 142
5.2.1. Chronic Kidney Disease (CKD) 143
5.2.2. Acute Kidney Injury (AKI) 144
5.2.3. Glomerulonephritis 145
5.3. Diagnostic Approaches in Nephrology 147
5.3.1. Laboratory Tests for Kidney Function 147
5.3.2. Imaging Techniques in Nephrology 148
5.3.3. Biopsy Procedures and Their Significance 149
5.4. Treatment Modalities in Nephrology 151
5.4.1. Pharmacological Interventions 151
5.4.2. Dialysis Options and Procedures 152
5.4.3. Kidney Transplantation 153
5.5. Role of Internal Medicine in Nephrology 155
5.5.1. Integration of Nephrology with Other Specialties 155
5.5.2. Management of Comorbid Conditions 156
5.5.3. Patient-Centered Care in Nephrology 157
5.6. Current Research and Advances in Nephrology 159
5.6.1. Innovations in Kidney Disease Treatment 159
5.6.2. Genetic Studies and Their Implications 160
5.6.3. Future Directions in Nephrology Research 161
Summary 163
References 166

CHAPTER 6

Endocrinology 171

Introduction 171
6.1. Fundamentals of Endocrinology 175
6.1.1. Definition and Significance of Endocrinology 176
6.1.2. Major Endocrine Glands and Their Functions 177
6.1.3. Hormonal Regulation and Feedback Mechanisms 178
6.2. Common Endocrine Disorders 179
6.2.1. Diabetes Mellitus: Types and Management 180
6.2.2. Thyroid Disorders: Hypothyroidism and Hyperthyroidism 180
6.2.3. Adrenal Disorders: Cushing's Syndrome and Addison's Disease 182
6.3. Diagnostic Approaches in Endocrinology 183
6.3.1. Laboratory Tests for Hormone Levels 184
6.3.2. Imaging Techniques for Endocrine Evaluation 185
6.3.3. Clinical Assessment and Patient History 185
6.4. Treatment Modalities in Endocrinology 187
6.4.1. Pharmacological Interventions 188
6.4.2. Lifestyle Modifications and Patient Education 188
6.4.3. Surgical Options for Endocrine Disorders 189
6.5. The Role of Technology in Endocrinology 190
6.5.1. Advancements in Diagnostic Tools 191
6.5.2. Telemedicine and Remote Patient Monitoring 192
6.5.3. Emerging Therapies and Research in Endocrinology 193
6.6. Challenges in Endocrinology 194
6.6.1. Managing Chronic Endocrine Diseases 195
6.6.2. Addressing Disparities in Healthcare Access 196
6.6.3. The Impact of Obesity and Lifestyle Factors on Endocrine Health 197
Summary 199
References 202

CHAPTER 7

Hematology 207

Introduction 207
7.1. Role of Internal Medicine in Hematology 211
7.1.1. Diagnosis of Hematological Disorders 211
7.1.2. Management of Chronic Blood Disorders 212

7.1.3. Coordination of Multidisciplinary Care 213
7.2. Common Hematological Conditions 214
7.2.1. Anemia: Types and Causes 215
7.2.2. Hemophilia: Genetic Considerations 216
7.2.3. Leukemia: Classification and Treatment 217
7.3. Diagnostic Techniques in Hematology 218
7.3.1. Complete Blood Count (CBC) 219
7.3.2. Bone Marrow Biopsy (BMB) 219
7.3.3. Coagulation Studies 220
7.4. Treatment Modalities in Hematology 221
7.4.1. Pharmacological Interventions 222
7.4.2. Blood Transfusion Therapy 223
7.4.3. Stem Cell Transplantation 224
7.5. Challenges in Hematological Care 225
7.5.1. Access to Specialized Care 226
7.5.2. Patient Compliance and Education 226
7.5.3. Emerging Resistance to Treatments 227
7.6. Future Directions in Hematology 228
7.6.1. Advances in Genetic Research 229
7.6.2. Innovations in Treatment Approaches 230
7.6.3. Role of Technology in Patient Monitoring 231
Summary 232
References 235

CHAPTER 8

Infectious Diseases 241

Introduction 241
8.1. Historical Context 245
8.1.1. Evolution of Infectious Disease Treatment 246
8.1.2. Key Figures in Internal Medicine 247
8.1.3. Milestones in Infectious Disease Research 247
8.2. Common Infectious Diseases 249
8.2.1. Bacterial Infections 249
8.2.2. Viral Infections 250
8.2.3. Fungal Infections 251
8.3. Diagnostic Techniques 252
8.3.1. Laboratory Testing 253
8.3.2. Imaging Studies 254
8.3.3. Clinical Evaluation 255
8.4. Treatment Modalities 256
8.4.1. Antibiotic Therapy 257
8.4.2. Antiviral Medications 257
8.4.3. Supportive Care 258
8.5. Challenges in Management 259
8.5.1. Antibiotic Resistance 260
8.5.2. Emerging Infectious Diseases 261
8.5.3. Socioeconomic Factors 262
8.6. Role of Preventive Medicine 263
8.6.1. Vaccination Strategies 264
8.6.2. Public Health Initiatives 265
8.6.3. Patient Education 265
Summary 267
References 270

CHAPTER 9

Rheumatology 273

Introduction 273
9.1. Common Rheumatological Conditions 277
9.1.1. Rheumatoid Arthritis 278
9.1.2. Systemic Lupus Erythematosus (SLE) 279
9.1.3. Osteoarthritis (OA) 280
9.2. Diagnostic Approaches in Rheumatology 282
9.2.1. Clinical Evaluation and History Taking 282
9.2.2. Laboratory Tests and Biomarkers 283
9.2.3. Imaging Techniques in Diagnosis 284
9.3. Treatment Modalities in Rheumatology 285
9.3.1. Pharmacological Treatments 286
9.3.2. Non-Pharmacological Interventions 287
9.3.3. Emerging Therapies and Research 288
9.4. Role of the Rheumatologist 289
9.4.1. Patient Management and Care Coordination 289
9.4.2. Interdisciplinary Collaboration 290
9.4.3. Patient Education and Support 291
9.5. Challenges in Rheumatology 292
9.5.1. Diagnostic Challenges 293
9.5.2. Treatment Adherence Issues 294
9.5.3. Access to Care and Health Disparities 294
9.6. Advances in Rheumatology 295
9.6.1. Innovations in Treatment Approaches 296

9.6.2. Research and Clinical Trials 297
9.6.3. Future Directions in Rheumatology 297
Summary 299
References 302

CHAPTER 10

Neurology (Medical) 307

Introduction 307
10.1. Anatomy of the Nervous System 311
10.1.1. Central Nervous System (CNS) 312
10.1.2. Peripheral Nervous System (PNS) 313
10.1.3. Functional Divisions of the Nervous System 314
10.2. Common Neurological Disorders 315
10.2.1. Stroke and Its Types 316
10.2.2. Neurodegenerative Diseases (e.g., Alzheimer's, Parkinson's) 317
10.2.3. Epilepsy and Seizure Disorders 318
10.3. Diagnostic Techniques in Neurology 320
10.3.1. Neuroimaging Methods (Magnetic Resonance Imaging (MRI), Computed Tomography (CT) Scans) 321
10.3.2. Electrophysiological Tests (Electroencephalography (EEG) and Electromyography (EMG)) 321
10.3.3. Lumbar Puncture (LP) and Cerebrospinal Fluid Analysis (CSF) 322
10.4. Treatment Approaches in Neurology 323
10.4.1. Pharmacological Treatments 324
10.4.2. Surgical Interventions 325
10.4.3. Rehabilitation Therapies 325
10.5. The Role of Neurologists 326
10.5.1. Education and Training Requirements 327
10.5.2. Specializations Within Neurology 328
10.5.3. Collaboration with Other Medical Professionals 329
10.6. Advances in Neurological Research 330
10.6.1. Emerging Technologies in Neurology 331
10.6.2. Genetic Research and its Implications 331
10.6.3. Future Directions in Neurological Studies 332
Summary 334
References 337

CHAPTER 11

Clinical Pharmacology and Therapeutics 343

Introduction 343
11.1. Pharmacokinetics 346
11.1.1. Absorption and Bioavailability 347
11.1.2. Distribution and Protein Binding 348
11.1.3. Metabolism and Excretion 349
11.2. Pharmacodynamics 350
11.2.1. Mechanisms of Drug Action 351
11.2.2. Dose-response Relationships 352
11.2.3. Therapeutic Index and Safety 353
11.3. Drug Development Process 354
11.3.1. Preclinical Research and Testing 355
11.3.2. Clinical Trial Phases 356
11.3.3. Regulatory Approval and Post-marketing Surveillance 356
11.4. Therapeutic Drug Monitoring (TDM) 357
11.4.1. Importance of Monitoring Drug Levels 359
11.4.2. Factors Affecting Drug Response 359
11.4.3. Case Studies in Therapeutic Drug Monitoring (TDM) 360
11.5. Adverse Drug Reactions (ADRs) 361
11.5.1. Types of Adverse Drug Reactions (ADRs) 362
11.5.2. Risk Factors and Patient Demographics 363
11.5.3. Strategies for Prevention and Management 364
11.6. Emerging Trends in Clinical Pharmacology 365
11.6.1. Personalized Medicine and Pharmacogenomics 366
11.6.2. Advances in Drug Delivery Systems 367
11.6.3. Role of Technology in Pharmacology 367
Summary 369
References 372

CHAPTER 12

Environmental and Occupational Medicine 375

Introduction 375

12.1. Historical Background **378**

12.1.1. Evolution of Environmental Medicine 379

12.1.2. Development of Occupational Medicine 380

12.1.3. Key Milestones in the Integration of Both Fields 381

12.2. Major Environmental Health Hazards **382**

12.2.1. Air Pollution and Its Effects 383

12.2.2. Water Contamination and Health Risks 384

12.2.3. Chemical Exposures in the Environment 384

12.3. Occupational Health Risks **386**

12.3.1. Common Workplace Hazards 387

12.3.2. Impact of Ergonomics on Worker Health 388

12.3.3. Role of Safety Regulations in Mitigating Risks 388

12.4. Assessment and Diagnosis **390**

12.4.1. Methods for Evaluating Environmental Exposures 390

12.4.2. Techniques for Assessing Occupational Health 391

12.4.3. Importance of Interdisciplinary Approaches 392

12.5. Prevention Strategies **393**

12.5.1. Public Health Initiatives for Environmental Protection 394

12.5.2. Workplace Safety Programs and Training 395

12.5.3. Role of Legislation in Promoting Health 396

Summary **398**

References **401**

INDEX **405**

LIST OF FIGURES

Figure 1.1. Internal medicine
Figure 1.2. Internal medicine and other specialties
Figure 1.3. General medical exam with internal medicine
Figure 1.4. World federation of hemophilia
Figure 1.5. Patient-centered care
Figure 1.6. The role of internal medicine in preventive health care
Figure 1.7. Common conditions treated by internal medicine
Figure 1.8. Diabetes is a chronic disease
Figure 1.9. HIV-associated neurocognitive disorder (HAND)
Figure 1.10. Diagnostic techniques in internal medicine
Figure 1.11. Complete blood count (CBC)
Figure 1.12. Sodium-glucose cotransporter 2 (SGLT2) inhibitors
Figure 1.13. Cognitive behavioral therapy (CBT)
Figure 1.14. An internal medicine doctor treats
Figure 1.15. Attitudes about complex therapy scale (ACTS
Figure 2.1. Cardiology: Life Medical Centre
Figure 2.2. Left ventricular assist devices (LVAD)
Figure 2.3. Role of internal medicine in cardiology
Figure 2.4. Comprehensive patient assessment
Figure 2.5. Atrial fibrillation (AF)
Figure 2.6. Coronary artery disease (CAD)
Figure 2.7. Hypertension
Figure 2.8. On the cutting edge of heart disease prevention and treatment
Figure 2.9. Medical tests to diagnose heart disease
Figure 2.10. Transesophageal echocardiogram (ECG)
Figure 2.11. Direct oral anticoagulants (DOACs)
Figure 2.12. Coronary artery bypass grafting (CABG)
Figure 2.13. Preventive cardiology
Figure 2.14. Patient education and counseling of cardiology

Figure 2.15. Challenges in cardiology

Figure 2.16. Cardiology and heart care

Figure 3.1. Respiratory system

Figure 3.2. Structure of the lungs

Figure 3.3. (a) Location of the respiratory structures in the body. (b) An enlarged view of the airways, alveoli (air sacs), and capillaries (tiny blood vessels). (c) A close-up view of gas exchange between the capillaries and alveoli. CO_2 is carbon dioxide, and O_2 is oxygen

Figure 3.4. Gas exchange in humans

Figure 3.5. Asthma disease

Figure 3.6. Chronic obstructive pulmonary disease (COPD)

Figure 3.7. Types of pneumonia

Figure 3.8. Pulmonary function test (PFTs)

Figure 3.9. Chest radiograph

Figure 3.10. Bronchoscopy

Figure 3.11. Pharmacological treatment of respiratory disorders

Figure 3.12. Lung surgery

Figure 3.13. The impact of air pollution on respiratory diseases in an era of climate change

Figure 4.1. Gastroenterology

Figure 4.2. Gastroesophageal reflux disease (GERD)

Figure 4.3. The role of gastroenterologists in patient care

Figure 4.4. Upper endoscopy

Figure 4.5. Diagnosis of inflammatory Crohn's disease with extraenteric complications by computed tomography enterography. (A) Multifocal segmental stricture showing wall thickening, mural hyperenhancement, and stratification shown by arrows and engorged vasa recta, the comb sign highlighted by a circle. (B) Arrowheads show mesenteric abscess. (C) Adjacent to the enteroenteric fistula shown by the arrow

Figure 4.6. Gastroenterology laboratory tests

Figure 4.7. Treatment modalities employed for various gastrointestinal disorders

Figure 4.8. Surgical gastroenterology

Figure 4.9. Inflammatory bowel disease (IBD)

Figure 4.10. The pathophysiology of gastroesophageal reflux disease (GERD)

Figure 4.11. Liver disease

Figure 4.12. Importance of diet in gastrointestinal health

Figure 5.1. Illustration of the kidney

Figure 5.2. Kidney structure

Figure 5.3. Functions of the kidney

Figure 5.4. A graphic representation of a chronically affected kidney

Figure 5.5. Stages of chronic kidney disease

Figure 5.6. Illustration of acute kidney injury (AKI)

Figure 5.7. Normal kidney vs. Glomerulonephritis

Figure 5.8. Glomerular filtration rate (GFR)

Figure 5.9. Imaging studies of the kidneys. Both kidneys contain multiple oval lesions, which are up to 20 mm in diameter, are hypoechoic, show low density on computed tomography (CT), and show high signal intensity in T2-weighted magnetic resonance imaging (MRI) (panel a: ultrasound image; panel b: CT image; panel c: T2-weighted MRI)

Figure 5.10. Kidney biopsy illustration

Figure 5.11. Pharmacological management of acute CRS (type 1). AKI = Acute kidney injury; AR = angiotensin receptor; CO = cardiac output

Figure 5.12. Patient receiving dialysis

Figure 5.13. Living donor kidney transplant recipients are treated with in vitro expanded polyclonal recipient Tregs, donor BM cells, and anti-IL6R mAb (tocilizumab)

Figure 5.14. Initiatives to be promoted by nephrologists and renal nurses to make true cardiorenal medicine for patients with chronic kidney disease (CKD) and heart failure (HF) (GPs, general practitioners; RRT, renal replacement therapy)

Figure 5.15. Interplay between acute kidney injury (AKI), acute kidney disease (AKD), and chronic kidney disease (CKD)

Figure 5.16. Patient-centric care in nephrology, enhancing engagement and outcomes

Figure 5.17. The future of nephrology research is focused on personalized medicine, advanced technologies, and novel therapies

Figure 6.1. Internal medicine

Figure 6.2. Importance of specialization in internal medicine

Figure 6.3. Fundamentals of endocrinology

Figure 6.4. Major endocrine glands and their functions

Figure 6.5. Common endocrine disorders

Figure 6.6. Thyroid Disorders: Hypothyroidism and Hyperthyroidism

Figure 6.7. Diagnostic approaches in endocrinology

Figure 6.8. Laboratory tests for hormone levels

Figure 6.9. Clinical assessment and patient history

Figure 6.10. Treatment modalities in endocrinology

Figure 6.11. Lifestyle modifications and patient education

Figure 6.12. Role of technology in endocrinology

Figure 6.13. Advancements in diagnostic tools

Figure 6.14. Emerging therapies and research in endocrinology

Figure 6.15. Managing chronic endocrine diseases

Figure 7.1. Internal medicine for hematology

Figure 7.2. Importance of internal medicine in hematology
Figure 7.3. Diagnosis of hematological disorders
Figure 7.4. Common hematological conditions
Figure 7.5. Diagnostic techniques in hematology
Figure 7.6. Complete blood count (CBC)
Figure 7.7. Treatment modalities in hematology
Figure 7.8. Stem cell transplantation
Figure 7.9. Patient compliance and education
Figure 7.10. Advances in genetic research
Figure 8.1. Internal medicine for infectious diseases
Figure 8.2. Overview of infectious diseases
Figure 8.3. Evolution of infectious disease treatment
Figure 8.4. Milestones in infectious disease research
Figure 8.5. Viral infections
Figure 8.6. Diagnostic techniques in internal medicine
Figure 8.7. Clinical evaluation in the realm of infectious diseases
Figure 8.8. Antibiotic therapy
Figure 8.9. Supportive care
Figure 8.10. Emerging infectious diseases
Figure 8.11. Role of preventive medicine
Figure 8.12. Public health initiatives
Figure 9.1. Internal medicine for rheumatology
Figure 9.2. Internal medicine
Figure 9.3. Rheumatology
Figure 9.4. Common conditions in rheumatology
Figure 9.5. Rheumatoid arthritis
Figure 9.6. Systemic lupus erythematosus (SLE)
Figure 9.7. Osteoarthritis (OA)
Figure 9.8. Blood tests are used to diagnose rheumatoid arthritis
Figure 9.9. Pharmacological treatments for rheumatoid arthritis
Figure 9.10. The role of physical therapy in rheumatoid arthritis management
Figure 9.11. Role of the rheumatologist
Figure 9.12. Challenges facing rheumatology
Figure 9.13. Advances in rheumatology
Figure 10.1. Neurology

Figure 10.2. Definition of neurology
Figure 10.3. Neurological disorders
Figure 10.4. The human nervous system
Figure 10.5. Central nervous system (CNS)
Figure 10.6. Peripheral nervous system (PNS)
Figure 10.7. Major subdivisions of the nervous system
Figure 10.8. Understanding neurological disorders
Figure 10.9. Types of strokes
Figure 10.10. Neurodegenerative diseases
Figure 10.11. Epilepsy
Figure 10.12. Understanding the diagnostic procedures neurologists use
Figure 10.13. Innovative approaches in treating neurological conditions
Figure 10.14. The role of neurologists
Figure 11.1. The field of clinical pharmacology encompasses the study of drugs and their clinical applications, focusing on understanding how these substances affect human physiology
Figure 11.2. Pharmacokinetics
Figure 11.3. Drug absorption is crucial for the effective design and administration of pharmaceuticals, as this process directly influences the therapeutic outcomes of medications
Figure 11.4. The phenomenon of first-pass metabolism plays a pivotal role in pharmacokinetics, primarily affecting the bioavailability of orally administered drugs
Figure 11.5. Pharmacodynamics
Figure 11.6. The therapeutic index (TI) serves as a crucial metric in evaluating the safety and efficacy of a drug
Figure 11.7. The stages of drug development are critical in ensuring the safety and efficacy of pharmaceutical interventions before they reach the market
Figure 11.8. Therapeutic drug monitoring (TDM)
Figure 11.9. A drug's therapeutic range is the concentration within which it yields the desired therapeutic effect without producing toxicity
Figure 11.10. Adverse drug reactions (ADRs)
Figure 11.11. Various types of adverse drug reactions (ADRs)
Figure 11.12. Advances such as high-throughput screening and computational drug design allow researchers to identify potential drug candidates more efficiently and accurately
Figure 12.1. Environmental medicine encompasses a multidisciplinary field that addresses the interactions between environmental factors and human health
Figure 12.2. The integration of occupational health into public health frameworks enhances the overall health of workers, which, in turn, contributes to improved community health outcomes
Figure 12.3. The evolution of occupational medicine has been significantly influenced by the growing

recognition of occupational health as a critical component of public health
Figure 12.4. Air pollution presents a significant challenge to public health, with its ramifications extending to various non-communicable diseases
Figure 12.5. Chemical exposures in the environment play a significant role in shaping public health and occupational safety, necessitating a robust understanding of their implications
Figure 12.6. Physical hazards encompass issues such as noise, radiation, and poor lighting, which can contribute to various health complications, including hearing loss and eye strain
Figure 12.7. Safety regulations play a pivotal role in mitigating risks associated with hazardous work environments
Figure 12.8. Assessing occupational health is crucial for maintaining a safe and productive work environment
Figure 12.9. Public health initiatives designed to protect the environment play a critical role in mitigating the adverse health outcomes associated with environmental degradation

PREFACE

The practice of caring for adult patients encompasses a vast array of clinical challenges, requiring a blend of scientific understanding, clinical judgment, and compassionate engagement. Physicians in this field must draw upon a broad knowledge base—ranging from common ailments to rare disorders—while remaining attentive to each individual's unique presentation. Knowledge of this specialty demands not only familiarity with diagnostic techniques and therapeutic modalities but also the finesse to recognize subtle cues, adapt as new information arises, and work effectively with other disciplines.

Over time, improvements in laboratory analysis, imaging methods, and pharmacology have vastly enhanced our capacity for disease diagnosis and treatment. Yet with each new technology comes an obligation to apply it responsibly, balancing benefits against costs and risks. At the same time, population aging has driven the epidemic curve of disease to chronic and multisystem conditions, again challenging clinicians to reconcile long-term management with prevention. The result is a changing practice setting that requires continuous learning and reflective practice.

Internal Medicine – Volume 1 is designed to serve as an introductory handbook and a comprehensive reference for clinicians, trainees, and other medical professionals who require a sound understanding of adult medicine. This volume integrates concise overviews, evidence-based guidelines, and practical recommendations into the major subspecialty areas that define modern internal medicine. Designed to facilitate sequential learning and intensive consultation, the book stresses key concepts, basic diagnostic algorithms, and up-to-date management principles to support clinical decision-making across a wide range of settings.

Chapter 1 presents the fundamental principles of adult medicine, which outline the historical evolution of the specialty, the structure of clinical thought, and the roles of preventive care and health promotion. Assessment techniques in patients—history taking, physical exam, and interpretation of imaging and laboratory findings—are adequately outlined as part of a systematic diagnostic process.

Chapter 2 deals with cardiac and vascular diseases. The chapter covers the pathophysiology, clinical presentation, and treatment of conditions such as ischemic heart disease, heart failure, valvular disease, and arrhythmias. Of special interest are the integration of noninvasive and invasive diagnostic and monitoring methods, and the tailoring of drug and device therapies to the individual patient profile.

Chapter 3 covers the spectrum of respiratory disorders, ranging from obstructive diseases of asthma and chronic obstructive pulmonary disease to restrictive processes of interstitial lung disease and pulmonary fibrosis. The chapter addresses indications for pulmonary function testing, radiographic assessment, and bronchoscopy, as well as modern practices in oxygen therapy and mechanical ventilation.

Chapter 4 addresses the digestive system and organs related to it. Chapter 4 guides readers through symptom assessment, such as abdominal pain, dysphagia, and gastrointestinal bleeding, and also discusses disorders such as peptic ulcer disease, inflammatory bowel disease, cirrhosis of the liver, and pancreatic insufficiency. Emphasized are key points about nutrition support, endoscopic methods, and hepatology consultation.

Chapter 5 discusses renal pathology and fluid-electrolyte balance. Topics include acute and chronic kidney injury, glomerular disease, tubular disease, and the management of electrolyte disturbances. The chapter also contains indications for renal replacement therapies, dialysis prescription principles, and pre- and post-transplantation management.

Chapter 6 consolidates endocrine illnesses of the system, with separate sections on thyroid, adrenal, pituitary axis, and metabolic disease. Clinical vignettes demonstrate the identification and treatment of diabetes mellitus, thyroid illness, adrenal insufficiency, and pituitary tumors by using both hormonal tests and imaging methods.

Chapter 7 covers blood and bone marrow disease conditions like anemias, coagulopathies, leukemias, lymphomas, and myeloproliferative neoplasms. Algorithmic strategies for diagnosing cytopenias and thrombotic syndromes are outlined, and issues related to transfusion, targeted therapy, and stem cell transplantation are updated.

Chapter 8 addresses identification and management of infectious syndromes by organ system. It emphasizes antibiotic stewardship, interpretation of microbiological cultures, and management of emerging pathogens. Discussion of sepsis protocols, prophylaxis in immunocompromised hosts, and hospital-acquired infections prepares readers for inpatient and outpatient environments.

Chapter 9 addresses rheumatologic and autoimmune illnesses. Comprehensive descriptions of presentations such as arthritis, vasculitis, connective tissue diseases, and systemic inflammatory diseases are paralleled by summaries of serologic evaluation and imaging. Therapeutic interventions involve classic immunosuppressants, biologic therapy, and monitoring regimens for prolonged treatment.

Chapter 10 addresses medical considerations of the nervous system. Clinical evaluation of headache, dizziness, seizure disorders, and neuropathies is detailed, including neuroimaging, electrodiagnostic tests, and lumbar puncture. Management includes prevention of stroke, management of seizures, and management of neurodegenerative diseases.

Chapter 11 provides the principles of pharmacology and safe use of medications in the adult patient. The topics covered are drug absorption and metabolism, dose adjustment in special populations, detection of adverse effects, and steps to minimize interactions. Guidelines on formulary management, patient education, and regulation enhance rational prescribing.

Chapter 12 presents the health dangers of environmental exposures and occupational risk. The chapter addresses chemical, physical, and biological agent assessment; occupational lung disease assessment; and management of acute and chronic toxic insults. Regulation and prevention recommendations are given to assist clinicians in counseling patients and advocating for community health.

This book is intended for medical students, residents, general practitioners, nurse practitioners, and physician assistants who need an easy-to-use yet reliable reference. Trainees will enjoy clearly written fundamental concepts and coherent frameworks for "think through" clinical challenges, while working physicians can look to specific sections for a rapid review or to refresh their knowledge. Both educators and allied health professionals will also benefit from the concise provision of evidence-based practice that informs outstanding patient care.

INTRODUCTION TO INTERNAL MEDICINE

1

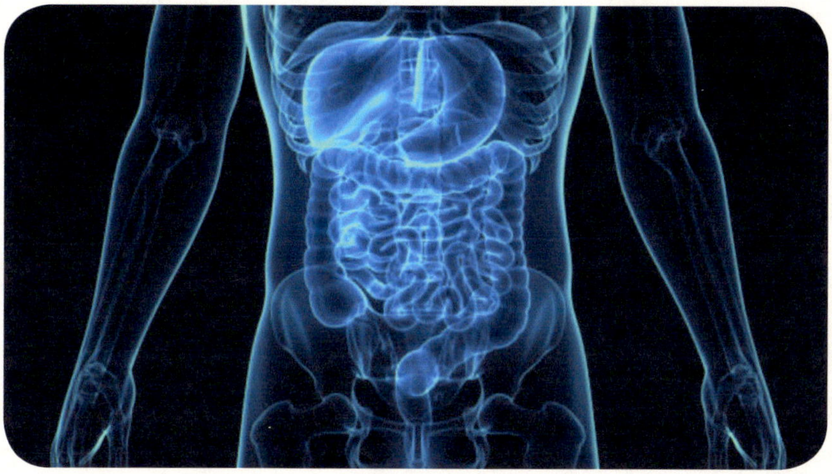

LEARNING OBJECTIVES

After studying this chapter, you will be able to:

1. Understand the history of internal medicine
2. Explain the core principles of internal medicine
3. Discuss the common conditions treated in internal medicine
4. Focus on diagnostic techniques in internal medicine
5. Learn about treatment modalities in internal medicine
6. Evaluate the challenges in internal medicine

Introduction

Internal medicine, alternatively referred to as the spirit of medicine, addresses a broad range of diseases that affect adults. The specialty not only addresses the diagnosis and management of various medical disorders but also provides comprehensive treatment for patients with long-standing diseases. Internal medicine doctors, or internists, specialise in treating complex patients with multisystem diseases and deliver an end-to-end healthcare approach. This specialty requires a profound understanding of processes of internal disease, methods of patient management, and satisfactory awareness of other subspecialties. In terms of scope, internal medicine is a foundational specialty for the creation of other specialties, as it is through fellowships in cardiology, gastroenterology, and endocrinology that most practitioners advance, thereby providing enhanced expertise and quality of care to patients (Hennus et al., 2022). Internal medicine is more than the treatment of the surface of illness; it's an integrative approach that includes preventive care, health promotion, and concern for overall patient welfare. Internists don't just treat acute disease; they also provide chronic disease care, often coordinating with several specialists to orchestrate overall treatment plans. This multidimensional approach implies that internal medicine is about comprehending the patient as a whole, taking into account psychological, social, and environmental factors that significantly impact health outcomes. This element of internal medicine is gaining prominence as necessary in today's healthcare practice, highlighting the importance of internists being adaptable and aware of the evolving landscape of medical knowledge and therapeutic innovation (Carney et al., 2016). In addition, the dynamic environment of healthcare requires a dynamic definition of internal medicine that includes evidence-based practices, especially in the management of chronic diseases prevalent among the adult population. The integration of evidence-based guidelines into clinical practice guides internists' decision-making, enhancing the quality and effectiveness of patient care. With technological innovations and research, the domain of internal medicine may now encompass telemedicine and personalized medicine, which have revolutionized patient interaction and treatment. As internists face this change, it becomes all the more critical for their role in promoting and effectuating evidence-based practice. Therefore, the boundaries and the definition of internal medicine are not defined; instead, they continue expanding so that the professionals can meet the different needs of patients effectively and compassionately (Carney et al., 2016; Hennus et al., 2022) (Figure 1.1).

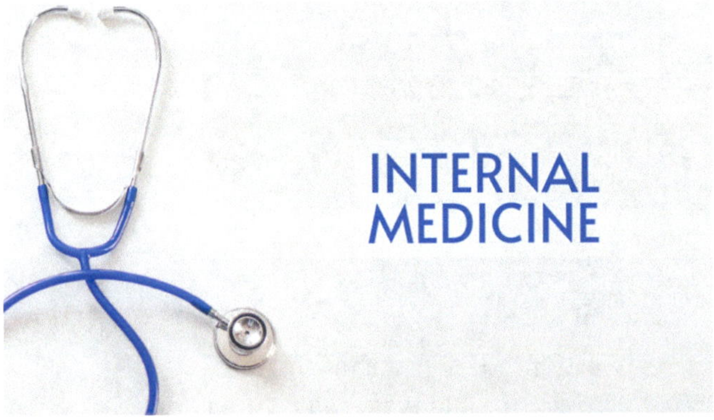

Figure 1.1. Internal medicine.

Source: https://haleclinics.com/wp-content/uploads/2023/12/Internal-medicine.webp.

Overview of Internal Medicine as a Medical Specialty

Internal medicine is a complex branch of medicine that deals with the prevention, diagnosis, and treatment of adult diseases. Internists or specialists in internal medicine are best positioned to manage complex, chronic diseases as well as acute illnesses that may happen to adult patients. The specialty also requires an integrated approach with a complete understanding of the physiological, psychological, and social factors of a person's health. In contrast to some specialties that may be devoted to specific organ systems, internal medicine doctors are often the first-line physicians who must also serve as a critical coordinating force for patient care, address many issues simultaneously, and be aware of the subtleties of healthcare organizations. This flexibility makes internal medicine a core and esteemed specialty that fills a critical niche in patient-care demand. To highlight the merits of ancient internal medicine in modern medicine, recent advances in ancient medical technologies and artificial intelligence have become frontline assets for bettering diagnostic procedures and treatment methodologies. Large language models like ChatGPT are best known for their phenomenal performance on medical knowledge assessments, achieving outstanding results on exams like the United States Medical Licensing Exam (USMLE) without specialized training. These models may help clinicians not only during training but also during the intricate decision-making steps that are integral to internal medicine (Kung et al., 2023). As internists increasingly face broad-scope clinical problems, the interface between healthcare professionals and sophisticated technology is becoming increasingly important, ensuring the place of internal medicine in today's era of modernizing patient care. Besides, with the paradigm shift in healthcare, integrative practice in internal medicine is becoming increasingly vital for addressing the multidimensional nature of patient care. Internal medicine doctors are often the first to treat chronic diseases, which have become more common among older patients. The difficulty of these conditions demands a special skill of an internist to synthesize data from multiple medical disciplines to foster a holistic treatment approach that prioritizes patients' overall well-being. Research underscores the continued need for robust evaluation of the framework for clinical decision-making and knowledge in the discipline (Singhal et al., 2023). Last but not least, internal medicine is a dynamic field that not only attends to immediate health issues but also addresses long-term health maintenance and disease prevention, thereby adding a valuable asset to the health care system.

Distinction Between Internal Medicine and Other Specialties

Internal medicine is a cornerstone of the medical profession that predominantly concerns itself with the prevention, diagnosis, and management of adult diseases. Unlike surgical specialties or those that deal with narrow organ systems, internal medicine treats a broad range of diseases that affect multiple body systems simultaneously. This allows internists to become deeply invested in complex cases where multiple comorbidities interact. By drawing on knowledge from the various disciplines of cardiology, endocrinology, and infectious diseases, internal medicine doctors can develop overall management plans. In comparison to these, specialties like pediatrics or surgery direct their practice and education toward specific procedural interventions or patient populations, which limits their practice scope less than internal medicine's wide ambit. So, the distinction is not merely one of practice emphasis but also one of implicit means of patient care. The internal medicine and other specialty educational pathways also highlight a radical distinction. Internal medicine residency is usually a three-year residency following medical school, giving a broad base in many medical sciences before specializing in subspecialty training, if at all. Such a system fosters a comprehensive appreciation of various internist pathologies encountered in clinics, thereby sharpening their diagnostic skills. Furthermore, as shown by more recent research, the incorporation of simulation-based instruction in internal medicine residency training programs has underscored the need to prepare residents for outside practices through hands-on, interactive approaches (Molik, 2024). Specialties, on the other hand, might utilize more specialized residency durations and curricula that emphasize procedural competency and respond to their limited scope of practice. So, then, the nature of training contributes to the differences between specialists and internists. Moreover, adaptability in internal medicine extends to the patient care philosophy, in which preventive and general health strategies are emphasized. Practice leads physicians to engage with patients on a personal basis, not only taking care of medical issues but spirituality and emotional status as well. Courses like cultural competence and spirituality education for residents are merely one more manifestation of the trend toward promoting a more intense relationship between patient and physician (Drumright et al., 2024). Specialties such as anesthesiology or radiology may not emphasize the interpersonal aspects of patient care as much. This multifaceted focus distinguishes internal medicine practitioners by their commitment to understanding and collaborating within the broader context of a patient's health. Therefore, the contrasts between internal medicine and the other specialties reflect the extent of knowledge required in practice as well as the philosophy underpinning patient interactions and the delivery of care (Figure 1.2).

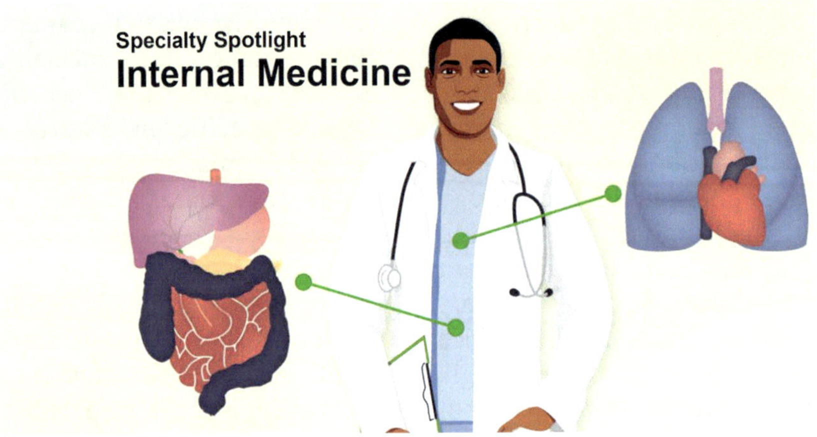

Figure 1.2. Internal medicine and other specialties.

Source: https://cdn.lecturio.com/assets/internal-medicine.jpg.

Importance of Internal Medicine in Healthcare

Internal medicine is a pillar of care that provides adult-oriented, multidisciplinary medical care for patients with a broad array of complex medical issues. Internists are more likely to be the first line of defense in the diagnosis and treatment of chronic diseases such as diabetes, hypertension, and heart disease that are prevalent across various populations. Their holistic understanding of disease mechanisms leads them to consider a comprehensive view of patient health, not only resolving immediate health issues but also addressing the causative factors most likely to give rise to these conditions. This broad strategy maximizes preventive and chronic disease care in patients, ultimately reducing the total health burden on the system and improving outcomes. Consequently, internal medicine is not merely essential to patient care at the individual level but also pivotal in maximizing community health and preventing diseases from advancing that could drain healthcare resources (Kutikov et al., 2020). The significance of internal medicine is also highlighted, especially during public health crises such as the COVID-19 pandemic, when internists' services have been invaluable. Internists are well-trained to spot the nuances of infectious diseases and to manage comorbid conditions that complicate management. For instance, patients with comorbidities, which are prevalent among COVID-19 patients, must be carefully monitored and administered individualized interventions in an effort to address the difficulties posed by such infections. The flexibility of internists enables timely triage and treatment of patients, thereby ensuring both personal and public safety. Without such a solid grounding in internal medicine in the daily delivery of healthcare, the healthcare system would perform much worse when facing the unprecedented challenges of history (Chopra et al., 2020). Internal medicine also emphasizes the need for coordination and communication among multidisciplinary teams, especially in complex cases involving multiple specialists. These internists are likely primary care physicians who oversee the nuances of patient care, navigating referrals and transitions between specialists. Their broad knowledge base across medical specialties enables them to synthesize information from disparate sources, thereby maximizing patient care and treatment continuity. This integrated model not only enhances the health outcomes but also enhances the education and training of medical specialists, inculcating in them the spirit of teamwork in healthcare delivery. With increasing specialization in the healthcare sector, the role of internal medicine in bridging gaps between specialties remains significant, leading to a scenario in which patients receive concurrent, coordinated care tailored to their specific health issues (Kutikov et al., 2020).

1.1. History of Internal Medicine

Learning Outcome

1. Discuss on evolution of internal medicine through the centuries
2. Define development of internal medicine
3. Explain the milestones in internal medicine practices and education

The history of internal medicine is deeply embedded in the history of medical progress, marked by grand milestones and paradigm shifts in understanding human disease. Its development began in ancient times, when early clinicians attempted to understand and manage diseases through observation and primitive methods. The Greeks and Romans, in particular, established fundamental principles, stressing reason and clinical observation as primary considerations. Men such as Hippocrates and Galen introduced concepts, including the humoral theory, which dominated medical thought for centuries. The Renaissance witnessed a turning point, as anatomy and physiology returned to focus, leading to a more scientific philosophy of disease and health. This period saw the introduction of milestone texts and pioneers who established the discipline and turned internal medicine into a specialty of adult primary care grounded in systemic knowledge and disease care. By the 17th and 18th centuries, the shift from speculative theory to experimental investigation began transforming the practice of internal medicine. Advances in anatomy, physiology, and pathology, spearheaded by William Harvey and Rudolf Virchow, enabled a more complex understanding of human health. The invention of the microscope further revolutionized the field, enabling clinicians to examine the microscopic world of cells and microorganisms and detect disease at the cellular level. This mass of growing knowledge facilitated the development of internal medicine into numerous sub-specialties, allowing practitioners to respond to the specific requirements of diseases and patient populations. With increasing maturity in internal medicine, the need for standardization of practice and greater rigor in treatment and diagnosis led to the development of several professional societies dedicated to improving the quality of care. In the 20th century, the history of internal medicine demonstrates a persistent commitment to integrating empirical evidence into clinical practice, characterized by techniques focused on patient care and research. The latter part of the 20th century saw a boom in medical knowledge, with advances in pharmacology, technology, and genetics reshaping the treatment landscape. These pioneering organizations, for example, the World Federation of Hemophilia (WFH), have updated their guidelines as new therapies are introduced, demonstrating the dynamic nature of internal medicine (Srivastava et al., 2020). In addition, the influence of the microbiota-gut-brain axis on disease conditions demonstrates the interconnectedness of biological systems and how this guides practice (Cryan et al., 2019). These innovations point to the necessity of recognizing that internal medicine is not a static science; rather, it is dynamic, with the latest evidence and new practices incorporated to enhance patient care and improve healthcare effectiveness (Figure 1.3).

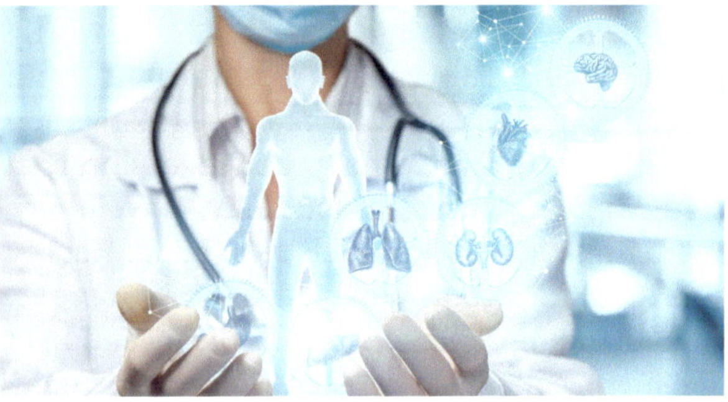

Figure 1.3. General medical exam with internal medicine.

Source: https://www.ttuhsc.edu/medicine/images/internal/divisions/im_divisionpage_image_0005.png.

1.1.1. Evolution of Internal Medicine Through the Centuries

Internal medicine's history is inextricably woven into the milieux in which practice evolved through the centuries. Ancient medicine in Egyptian and Greek settings was largely empirical, interwoven with religion, and focused on observing symptoms, as practitioners like Hippocrates attempted an integrated approach to patients. The establishment of the Hippocratic Corpus was significant in that it laid the foundations of clinical practice by promoting systematic observation and documentation of sickness, moving away from mysticism. The move away from mysticism was a turning point, forcing later generations to view medicine in more scientific terms. Increasingly, the Renaissance's anatomy and physiology studies further developed internal medicine into an evidence-based foundation, ultimately paving the way for more sophisticated diagnostic and treatment interventions that paved the way for modern practices in the field. As the centuries passed, internal medicine continued to change dramatically to reflect advancements in scientific knowledge and technology. The 19th century saw the genesis of the germ theory, which transformed the understanding of disease causation. Louis Pasteur and Robert Koch were pioneers who demonstrated the connection between microorganisms and human health, a connection that brought greater focus to infectious diseases. The period also saw the development of clinical practice guided by the principles of evidence-based medicine, an effort to standardize treatment procedures based on empirical evidence. In particular, the innovation of diagnostic devices, including the stethoscope and later radiological imaging, significantly enhanced doctors' ability to diagnose and manage a range of internal diseases. These innovations represented an evolutionary advance in the scientific principles of internal medicine, allowing doctors to address complex conditions hitherto beyond effective treatment. The 20th century brought an unprecedented array of advancements that further refined internal medicine, establishing it as a cornerstone of modern healthcare. Innovations in pharmacology, along with the advent of vaccines, transformed preventable diseases into manageable public health issues, significantly improving patient outcomes. Moreover, technologies such as medical imaging, laboratory testing, and data processing revolutionized disease management and enabled more nuanced understanding of chronic diseases. Here, the complexities of atherosclerotic cardiovascular disease demonstrate how an emerging scientific paradigm has further emphasized mechanisms such as endothelial cell dysfunction, which underpin the pathobiology of this prevalent disease (Gimbrone et al., 2016). Also, the application of advanced digital services for research, as illustrated by initiatives such as XSEDE, indicates the increased integration of medicine and technology, outlining how evolving practices continue to address issues introduced by modern society's diseases (Towns et al., 2014).

1.1.2. Key Figures in the Development of Internal Medicine

Internal Medicine has been shaped by primarily seminal individuals whose work radically transformed the practice of medicine. One such individual is Sir William Osler, known as the father of modern Internal Medicine. Oslers' belief in clinical practice and patient care led to bedside teaching that emphasized face-to-face interaction with patients and observation as fundamental components of medical education. His seminal work, The Principles and Practice of Medicine, published in 1892, served as a foundational text for medical students, integrating rigorous scientific knowledge with practical clinical expertise. Oslers' holistic approach to patient care resonated through his focus on understanding the person behind the illness, and he established principles that remain core to Internal Medicine today. Another prominent figure is Paul Ehrlich, whose work in the late 19th and early 20th centuries propelled the fields of bacteriology and immunology. His development of the first effective treatment for syphilis, known as Salvarsan, was groundbreaking, marking a pivotal moment in the treatment of infectious diseases. Ehrlich's emphasis on the pathogen-disease relationship formed rules for diagnostic and therapeutic processes in Internal Medicine. Further, his introduction of the concept of the magic bullet, targeting a specific pathogen without harming the host, not only defined the coming of pharmacology but also steered subsequent research into the realm of targeted therapy, mapping out the therapeutic landscape of Internal Medicine for centuries. Their legacy extends beyond their findings and techniques; they embody the relentless zeal for understanding and pursuit of excellence in patient care that is the hallmark of Internal Medicine. In addition to Osler and Ehrlich, modern advances in Internal Medicine owe much to multidisciplinary collaboration, as embodied by organizations such as the World Federation of Hemophilia (WFH), which continuously innovates in the management of bleeding disorders through evidence-based guidelines. The updated version of the WFH guidelines recognizes the value of systematic reviews and consensus guidance in improving treatment guidelines, emphasizing a significant aspect of Internal Medicine development: the incorporation of collaborative research and consensus into practice (Page et al., 2021; Srivastava et al., 2020). A commitment to high-quality care characterizes this legacy and strives to bridge the gap between changing science and practice in day-to-day clinical practice, keeping Internal Medicine at the forefront of medicine (Figure 1.4).

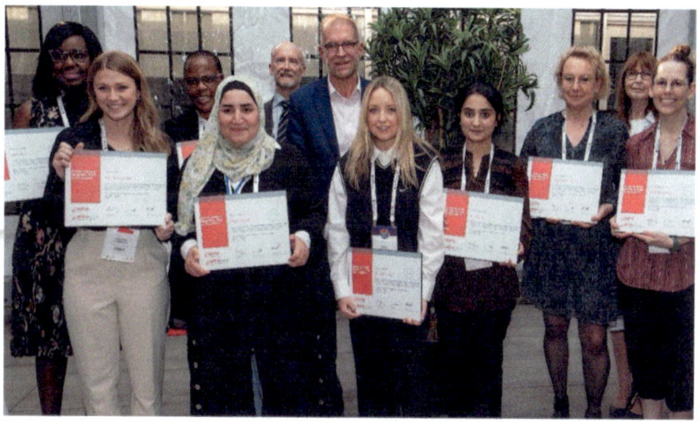

Figure 1.4. World federation of hemophilia.

Source: https://wfh.org/wp-content/uploads/2022/07/SSMF-header.jpg.

1.1.3. Milestones in Internal Medicine Practices and Education

Internal medicine practice milestones and education are critical markers of doctors' continuing career progression and of the quality of care to patients. ACGME developed a system with a mandate for milestones in medical fellows' career progression, based on delineated core competencies, such as Patient Care and Medical Knowledge. As with residency training programs in nephrology, completion of these milestones indicates that fellows are ready to practice independently. Such a methodical approach not only enhances the learning process for trainees but also aligns their training with quality improvement programs that are increasingly becoming crucial within healthcare institutions. Programs that explicitly engage fellows in quality improvement activities enable the application of medical expertise in practice, ultimately resulting in enhanced patient care and improved system efficiency in delivering health care services. Moreover, the adoption of competency-based curricula reflects a larger paradigm shift towards more systematic and standardized education in internal medicine. By integrating quality improvement principles into curricula, programs enable fellows to meet mandated skills and make contributions to related projects, demonstrating real-world problems. For instance, the ACGME mandates that fellows demonstrate concrete change across milestones in six broad competencies. Because of this, nephrology programs have established specific curricular milestones that are significantly intertangled with these general requirements. Such preparation ensures training that is pertinent and commensurate with the evolving field of internal medicine, which increasingly emphasizes evidence-based medicine and quality improvement. As medicine becomes increasingly advanced, the focus remains on building not only competent practitioners but also lifelong learners dedicated to improving clinical practice through ongoing education. A critical evaluation of the milestones of internal medicine training underscores the need for specialty-specific evaluations that account for each specialty's needs. Integrated nephrology-specific milestones into the broader ACGME framework suggests potential disparities in training effectiveness among subspecialties. Curriculum mapping to these milestones can assist program directors in identifying areas for improvement, thereby providing quality standards for training and patient care. Besides, Clinical Competency Committees play a crucial role in monitoring fellows' progress by assessing improvement and ensuring compliance with fixed competency levels. This cautious monitoring process decisively determines progression through training. With a culture of responsibility and ongoing improvement, the practice of internal medicine ensures the production of competent practitioners capable of meeting the complex demands of modern healthcare, ultimately transforming the profession as a whole (Yuan et al., 2015; Prince et al., 2017).

Test Your Knowledge

1. How does internal medicine approach the diagnosis and long-term management of chronic diseases such as diabetes mellitus and hypertension?
2. What role do internists play in coordinating care for patients with multiple coexisting conditions (multimorbidity)?

1.2. Core Principles of Internal Medicine

Learning Outcome

1. Discuss on patient-centered care and holistic approach
2. Understand the emphasis on diagnosis and treatment of adult diseases
3. Explain the role of preventive care in internal medicine

Internal medicine is built on a handful of fundamental principles, centered on a broad understanding of patient care. One of the foundations is the integration of sophisticated clinical acumen, encompassing a broad knowledge of disease mechanisms, diagnostic methods, and therapeutic approaches. Internal medicine physicians, also known as internists, consider not only the individual symptoms presented by patients but also the overall state of their health, including psychological, social, and economic factors. This comprehensive approach enables them to develop personalized management plans that take into account the details of each patient's case. The emphasis on continuous learning, particularly evidence-based practice, aligns directly with this principle, keeping clinicians current with the latest findings and enabling them to apply these results to improved patient outcomes. Along with this, one of the key issues in internal medicine is managing the usage and interpretation of enormous amounts of medical data. The progress of data-centric methods, particularly through applications of machine learning, offers promising potential for enhanced diagnostic accuracy and treatment efficacy. But genuine potential for such gains relies on overcoming impediments such as data silos and data privacy concerns that limit access to large medical datasets. Federated learning is a new method that can potentially facilitate collaborative data use without compromising patient confidentiality. Striving to address these challenges is central to bringing research breakthroughs into widespread clinical practice, ensuring that internists embrace new technologies while upholding ethical practices in patient care (Rieke et al., 2020). Lastly, collaborative care is yet another imperative principle of internal medicine that ensures interagency collaboration among healthcare providers to achieve optimal patient outcomes. Internists often work in coordination with specialists, nurses, and allied health providers to address complex health needs through multidisciplinary collaboration. Such collaboration is particularly applicable in new fields like microbiome science, which is linked to many health outcomes, ranging from autoimmune diseases to psychiatric disorders. Although there is some deficit in standardization and definition of microbiome studies, the recent workshops stressed the need for a clear definition of the term microbiome and related concepts. This will enable better integration of microbiome data into everyday clinical practice and empower internists to address the evolving challenges of patient care comprehensively (Berg et al., 2020).

1.2.1. Patient-Centered Care and Holistic Approach

The principle of patient-centered care is central to the practice of internal medicine, emphasizing that patients must be viewed as a whole rather than solely in terms of their medical conditions. This practice is intended to support greater understanding of patients' preferences, values, and social circumstances, thereby creating a more compassionate healthcare setting. By emphasizing the patient's role in decision-making and personalizing treatments to their life situation, satisfaction and outcomes may be greatly improved. This practice aligns with the Sustainable Development Goals (SDGs) guidelines, specifically SDG 3, which aims to ensure healthy lives and well-being for all people, underscoring the necessity of building inclusive healthcare systems that address various aspects of patients' health needs, as Ferrando et al. (2025) discuss. The intrinsic nature of patient-centered care is fundamentally inherent in the holistic approach, which necessitates collaboration between various healthcare specialties. Specifically, there is a need for convergence among internal medicine, anesthesiology, and surgical practices to offer comprehensive care along the patient continuum.

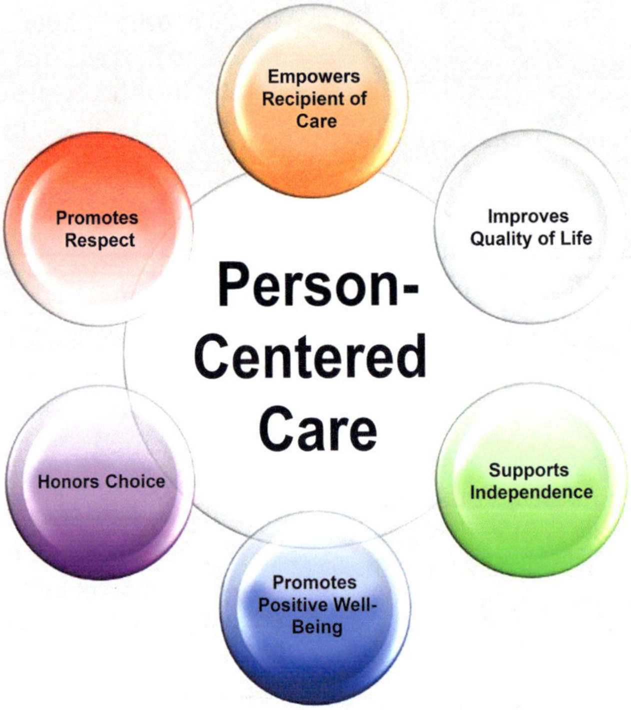

Figure 1.5. Patient centered care.

Source: https://www.aacnnursing.org/portals/0/images/5b/5B-Person-Centered-Care-Graph.png.

Interprofessional care fosters proper management of patient conditions pre-, intra-, and post-procedure to facilitate optimal preoperative risk assessment and individually tailored therapeutic interventions. The focus on comprehensive care not only improves clinical outcomes but also meets the patient's psychological and emotional needs, thereby promoting an equitable approach to health that considers all aspects of well-being. This harmony validates the need for a patient-centered approach, as recent studies show its effectiveness in patient recovery and well-being, as quoted in Jiménez Alemán et al. (2024). Furthermore, the application of patient-centered care from a holistic approach also influences systemic issues in healthcare delivery. By encouraging more integrated, linked systems of healthcare, we can offset the fragmentation that is typically present in medical settings. Ineffective resource allocation and prevalent medical errors can be signs of inadequacies in traditional models of care that do not engage patients fully and encourage team practice. This patient-focused, comprehensive approach not only involves providing care to every individual but also emphasizes considering broader social determinants of health, such as economic and environmental factors, that have a fundamental influence on shaping health outcomes. With intense concentration, as emphasized by Ferrando et al. (2025), adopting a syndemic perspective that recognizes this interdependence will be important for supporting sustainable healthcare systems that truly prioritize patient well-being (Figure 1.5).

1.2.2. Emphasis on Diagnosis and Treatment of Adult Diseases

Adult disease treatment and diagnosis form a cornerstone of internal medicine, reflecting the complexity and variability of adult health care needs. A strong emphasis on evidence-based practice ensures that clinicians have access to the most effective approaches for treating a wide range of health conditions. This system accommodates patient assessments that include chronic diseases, mental disease, and their interplay, reflecting the need for treatment under a comprehensive approach. As the number of patients looking for treatment of both medical and mental conditions increases, there is a need to be keenly aware of the impact of such comorbidities on overall health outcomes. As outlined below in recent literature, the influence of mortality, care quality, and cost burden is noteworthy in promoting the call for the implementation of treatment targeted to the unique patient's situation, particularly through support interventions for self-management (N/A, 2011). As internal medicine evolves as a science, it has increasingly been recognized that addressing cognitive health is crucial to managing adult disease, particularly in the elderly. The importance of cognitive impairment screening, particularly in acute illness settings, cannot be overemphasized, as cognitive impairment can significantly complicate disease care and result in adverse outcomes. The conversations at the National Academy of Neuropsychology's Summit on Population Health Solutions emphasized the key role of timely detection and intervention of cognitive impairment. All respondents emphasized the importance of uniform screening practices that account for multiple determinants, including level of education and culture, to ensure proper assessment. Being holistic in patient assessment is significant when creating effective care plans that consider the multifaceted needs of elderly patients with chronic diseases (Adler et al., 2018). Aside from this, the adoption of new technologies such as electronic health records (EHRs) offers new opportunities for enhancing adult disease diagnosis and treatment. EHRs facilitate comprehensive monitoring of patient data, including cognitive function, chronic disease, treatment response, and more, thereby improving continuity of care. Using EHRs, healthcare providers can also identify patient health trends over time, confirm adherence to treatment plans, and base decisions on evidence to enhance clinical outcomes. With advancing technology, so does the potential to generate more tailored and effective treatment plans based on a patient's individual profile. Last but not least, the emphasis on treatment and diagnosis in internal medicine is not just on treating existing health conditions but also on promoting long-term wellness and health among diverse adult populations.

1.2.3. Role of Preventive Care in Internal Medicine

Preventive care is the core of internal medicine, as it focuses on identifying and reducing health risks before they become full-blown diseases. The use of evidence-based preventive interventions not only enhances patient outcomes but also facilitates the generalizability of health systems' effectiveness. Internal medicine doctors are often leaders in the treatment of complex health issues, and incorporating preventive interventions—such as health education, routine screenings, and immunizations—can significantly reduce the incidence of chronic disease. For instance, a Midwestern internal medicine department recognized the need to increase age-related vaccinations and screenings for adults aged 50 and older. By using pre-visit planning checklists for vaccinations and cancer screening, the department increased the proportion of patients receiving preventive interventions, demonstrating how active methods can improve health outcomes (Rice et al., 2025). Furthermore, preventive care plays a crucial role in dealing with the appropriateness of medical interventions in most settings, including hospital settings. Despite existing guidelines that outline best practices for stress ulcer prophylaxis, many patients are treated unnecessarily without clear indications. This impacts not only patient health but also healthcare costs. An observational study revealed that there was a high prevalence of inappropriately administered stress ulcer prophylaxis among patients in internal medicine practice, which was causing avoidable morbidity and system cost. By adhering more systematically to preventive care, internists can minimize such practices so that interventions align with proven protocols and patient needs. This astute assessment of treatment need is a critical component of internal medicine, demonstrating the way preventive care must inform clinical decisions (Octavia et al., 2025). The wide-ranging efficacy of preventive care in internal medicine extends beyond patient-to-patient interactions to encompass population health management. As healthcare systems become increasingly value-based, the incorporation of preventive interventions remains critical to improving health outcomes at the population level. To illustrate, ensuring systematic screening for chronic disease—such as diabetes and high blood pressure—in primary care settings not only identifies those at risk but also ensures people adopt lifestyle modifications that can prevent illness progression. As demonstrated by current studies, pre-visit planning programs in internal medicine can anticipate gaps in preventive care delivery, thereby enhancing patient activation and responsibility for outcomes. This commitment to prevention not only establishes the therapeutic alliance among clinicians and patients but also promotes a healthier society by reducing the burden of treatable diseases (Octavia et al., 2025; Rice et al., 2025) (Figure 1.6).

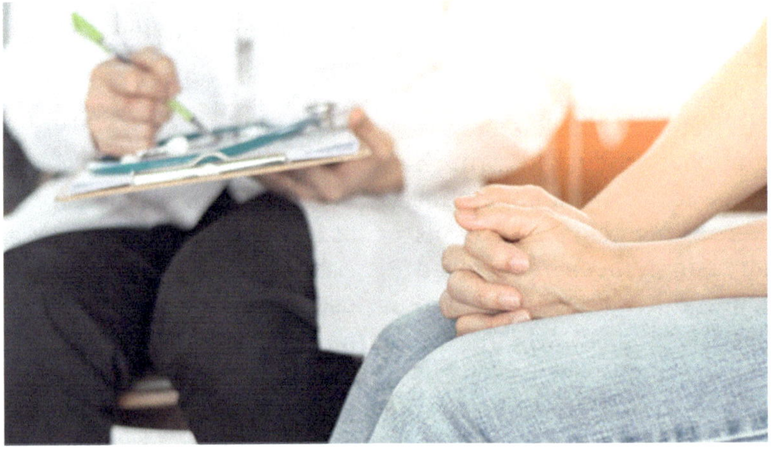

Figure 1.6. The role of internal medicine in preventive health care.

Source: https://campmedicine.org/wp-content/uploads/internal-medicine-2412.jpg.

Test Your Knowledge

1. What is the primary focus of internal medicine in patient care?
2. Why is a comprehensive patient history important in internal medicine?

1.3. Common Conditions Treated in Internal Medicine

Learning Outcome

1. Understand the chronic diseases such as diabetes and hypertension
2. Describe the infectious diseases and their management
3. Discuss the cardiovascular diseases (CVDs) and their implications

Internal medicine encompasses a broad spectrum of diseases that medical practitioners commonly encounter. One of the most prevalent conditions includes infectious diseases, such as pneumonia and sepsis, which are significant causes of morbidity and mortality, particularly in hospitalized patients. Not only must they be treated and diagnosed promptly, but they also highlight the importance of understanding patient demographics, as age, underlying disease, and socioeconomic status can significantly influence treatment outcomes. For instance, internal medicine doctors frequently use diagnostic tools such as imaging studies and lab tests to diagnose and treat infectious illnesses, thereby establishing a close relationship between patient care and clinical decision-making. Apart from contagious diseases, internal medicine frequently treats chronic conditions that demand continuous treatment, including diabetes mellitus, hypertension, and cardiovascular disease. These chronic illnesses not only affect the human body but also its psychological and social facets, requiring integrated management approaches. For example, control of hypertension demands lifestyle modification along with drug management, which are both components of the prevention of cardiovascular complications. Furthermore, as health disparities continue to influence the management of these chronic diseases, internal medicine clinicians are encouraged to examine the inequities identified in recent studies, which reveal how race and language proficiency can affect the fairness of care and access, with an emphasis on the need for culturally responsive care. Yet another universally widespread field of focus of internal medicine is the management of pain disorders, such as abdominal pain and those caused by trauma or chronic diseases. Treatment of pain is particularly tricky with mixed responses among diverse groups of patients. Findings suggest that there are vast differences in opioid prescribing among patients admitted with pain-related conditions, and the problem of unequal pain management across different racial and ethnic groups is an issue (Braun et al., 2024). As awareness of these disparities grows, internal medicine physicians are urged to develop and implement quality improvement programs to increase fairness in pain management. This integrated approach not only addresses immediate clinical needs but also supports broader health equity objectives, thereby maintaining the critical role that internal medicine plays in optimizing overall healthcare delivery (Braun et al., 2024) (Figure 1.7).

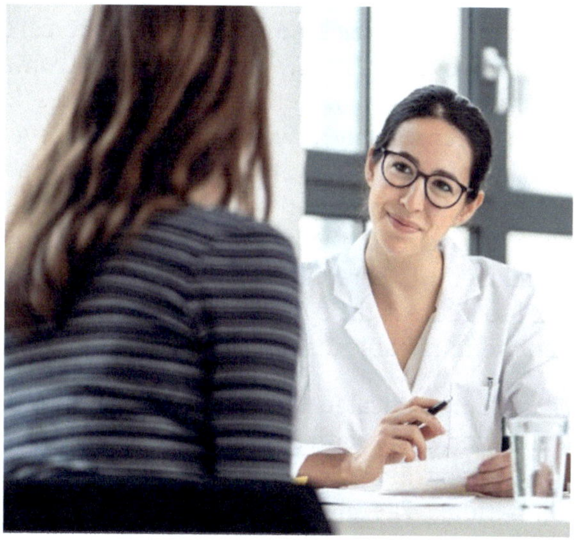

Figure 1.7. Common conditions treated by internal medicine.

Source: https://mosaicfamilycares.com/wp-content/uploads/internal-medicine-2302.jpg.

1.3.1. Chronic Diseases such as Diabetes and Hypertension

Chronic conditions like hypertension and diabetes are severe public health problems that need extensive management interventions in the practice of internal medicine. Diabetes, which is characterized by elevated blood glucose levels due to either insulin deficiency or resistance, affects millions of individuals around the world and is often associated with severe complications like cardiovascular disease, nephropathy, and neuropathy. Hypertension or high blood pressure is another prevalent condition that may accompany diabetes, thus adding further health risks. Both conditions are accounted for by lifestyle factors such as unhealthy eating, lack of physical exercise, and obesity, which need an integrative approach. Facts indicate that non-communicable diseases account for 70% of all deaths globally, and therefore, it is important to address these chronic diseases through specialized healthcare systems (Hout et al., 2024).

This needs innovative thinking in internal medicine that focuses on global patient care and improved results. The care of chronic conditions like hypertension and diabetes is moving increasingly towards community-level care interventions. In areas like Sub-Saharan Africa, the incorporation of healthcare services for these chronic conditions into already established HIV care models shows an emerging trend to address the syndemic of infectious and non-communicable diseases (Hout et al., 2024).

By utilizing educated lay staff and community health workers, health systems can decentralize care, thereby improving access for disadvantaged populations. The model also enhances patient monitoring and adherence to treatment, and emphasizes the importance of lifestyle modifications through dietary and physical exercise training. These multidisciplinary care methodologies are needed to counter the burden of comorbidity, ultimately improving the care and management of patients with chronic diseases. The interdependence between diabetes and hypertension calls for a stringent cross-examination of patient data and healthcare systems. Studies indicate that most patients with essential hypertension admitted to hospitals, particularly in older age groups, where optimal management involves knowledge of status playing a lesser role (Ndirahisha et al., 2024). This highlights the imperative need for enhanced education among healthcare workers and for patients to self-manage. In addition, trial results assessing community-based interventions indicate that comprehensive care models moderately promote health literacy and patient activation. By prioritizing the interaction between social determinants and healthcare access, future internal medicine practices can effectively address the challenges posed by chronic diseases, thereby building a healthy population able to maintain these lifelong conditions (Figure 1.8).

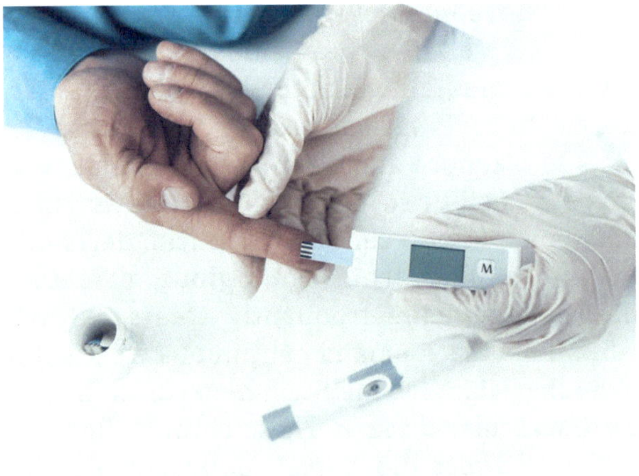

Figure 1.8. Diabetes is a chronic disease.

Source: https://static.wixstatic.com/media/9bc977_f780505c34fb4880bf5c0bb220143bf8~mv2.jpeg/v1/fill/w_1000,h_667,al_c,q_85,usm_0.66_1.00_0.01/9bc977_f780505c34fb4880bf5c0bb220143bf8~mv2.jpeg.

1.3.2. Infectious Diseases and Their Management

Infectious diseases are among the biggest challenges in internal medicine, and they require an in-depth understanding of the causative microorganisms, patterns of dissemination, and the complex interplay between host factors and pathogens. Management of infectious diseases also requires a multidisciplinary approach that includes prevention, early detection, and management. Recent technical advances in diagnostic imaging and the discovery of biomarkers for diseases, such as HIV-associated neurocognitive disorder (HAND), highlight the importance of comprehensive infectious disease care not only at the systemic level but also within closed organ systems, such as the central nervous system. The use of advanced techniques, including diffusion tensor imaging and resting-state functional MRI, has a decisive enhancing effect on the ability to monitor and quantify cognitive impairments associated with such infections, demonstrating a key point of intersection of infectious disease and brain health within internal medicine (Brew et al., 2017). Treatment of infectious diseases also increasingly leverages networks of collaborative relationships for disease surveillance and response. Initiatives like the Disease Surveillance Networks (DSN) encourage trans-boundary collaboration, enabling health systems to exchange information and resources and cross-match key data in real time. Such collaborations are needed for the detection and control of infectious disease outbreaks, particularly in the modern globalized world where pathogens flow freely across borders. The Rockefeller Foundation's evaluation of the DSN Initiative underscores the benefits of disease response strategies through such networks (Kimball et al., 2011). Through leveraging various expertise and resources, the networks not only enhance diagnostic accuracy but also ensure that therapeutic interventions are timely and contextually appropriate, ultimately leading to improved health outcomes among risk populations. In short, infectious disease practice in internal medicine is an evolving specialty that advances practice through research, technology, and global collaboration. As the infectious disease landscape continues to evolve due to antimicrobial resistance and new pathogens, it becomes necessary for clinicians to remain vigilant and responsive. Continuing education and training in the latest management strategies, combined with a commitment to interdisciplinarity, are essential for addressing the complexities attendant on such diseases. Through the intersection of state-of-the-art research evidence and interprofessional collaboration, the clinical practice of internal medicine can enhance its capacity to address infectious diseases effectively, creating healthier populations worldwide and establishing immunization programs for potential epidemic outbreaks (Figure 1.9).

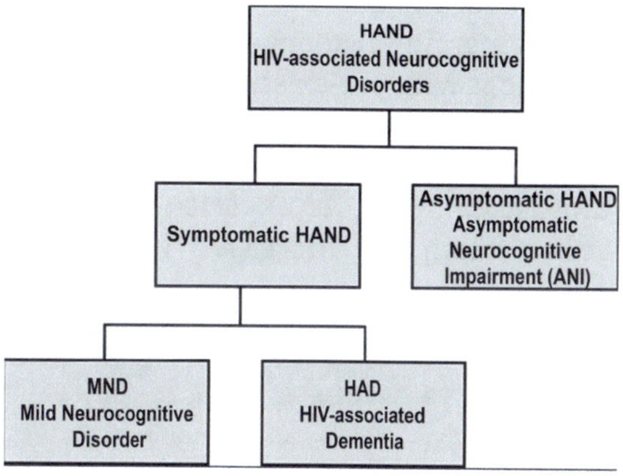

Figure 1.9. HIV-associated neurocognitive disorder (HAND).

Source: https://www.caregiver.org/uploads/legacy/hand_graphic.jpg.

1.3.3. Cardiovascular Diseases (CVDs) and Their Implications

CVDs are now a significant public health problem with increasing requirements for attention within the specialty of internal medicine. Characterized by cardiovascular disorders such as coronary artery disease, hypertension, heart failure, and arrhythmias, CVDs account for a high proportion of morbidity and mortality worldwide. As per the Global Burden of Diseases, Injuries, and Risk Factors Study 2017, the burden of disease due to CVD was considerable, with an estimated number of years lived with disability worldwide. The impact of these diseases extends beyond the individual level to the healthcare system as well. CVD therapies are mostly prolonged and chronic, hence the need for new solutions in prevention and management, which are fundamental to reducing the incidence and impact of such diseases on society (Campbell et al., 2020). Existing knowledge of cardiovascular disease pathophysiology suggests a convergence of determinants of disease progression, including lifestyle, genetics, and environment. There has been a paradigm shift in the strategy towards CVD, with an emphasis on prevention of early risk factors such as obesity, diabetes, and hypertension. The COVID-19 pandemic has also unveiled emerging challenges in cardiovascular management with pre-existing conditions, with such patients at higher risk of severe disease and complications. Research indicates that comorbid cardiovascular patients experience increased mortality alongside increased likelihood of experiencing systemic inflammation and coagulopathy throughout the processes of viral infections, indicative of the intricate dynamic relationship between infectious diseases and comorbid cardiovascular conditions (Campbell et al., 2020). Therefore, increased screening, patient education, and community health programs are essential to prevent cardiovascular complications resulting from both chronic and acute infectious diseases. The consequences of cardiovascular diseases echo in the lives of individuals, families, and communities, necessitating a multidisciplinary approach in internal medicine. Being aware of such diseases helps develop treatment plans tailored to the individual, including pharmacological therapy, lifestyle changes, and rehabilitation programs. Furthermore, closing cardiovascular health gaps among populations can yield improved outcomes. As physicians improve internal medicine skills, they must emphasize research, patient education, and advocacy for policies that promote cardiovascular health. Future reforms in cardiovascular disease management are necessary to develop targeted interventions capable of reversing the tide of CVDs, thereby improving overall public health and quality of life across diverse populations (James et al., 2018).

Test Your Knowledge

1. Which chronic diseases are most commonly managed by internists?
2. How do internists manage patients with both acute and chronic medical conditions?

1.4. Diagnostic Techniques in Internal Medicine

Learning Outcome

1. Explain the importance of patient history and physical examination
2. Describe use of laboratory tests and imaging studies
3. Identify the emerging technologies in diagnostics

The diagnostic practice of internal medicine has undergone a complete transformation, thanks to technological advances and improved understanding of diseases. The traditional diagnostic practice, comprising physical examinations and routine laboratory tests, has been the backbone of internal medicine. But the addition of newer imaging modalities such as magnetic resonance imaging (MRI) and computed tomography (CT) allows physicians to visualize internal structures better than ever. These tools not only enhance diagnostic accuracy but also facilitate early detection of disease conditions, thereby significantly improving patient outcomes. Furthermore, point-of-care testing has revolutionized the speed and accuracy with which a correct diagnosis is obtained, meeting urgent medical needs on time. These advancements highlight the imperative need to stay abreast of technological advances to optimize diagnostic capabilities in clinical practice, ultimately leading to improved patient care. Moreover, the application of artificial intelligence (AI) in diagnosis has opened up new vistas for internal medicine. AI tools, particularly those that rely on machine learning and deep learning algorithms, enhance diagnostic precision by exhaustively analyzing vast volumes of information, e.g., imaging reports, electronic health records, and laboratory tests. Such intelligent systems identify patterns and likely health threats that may escape human eyes at first glance. For instance, AI image analysis using convolutional neural networks has been shown to enable faster, more accurate radiological diagnoses. Such enhancements point to the potential of AI to revolutionize diagnostic procedures and improve the efficiency of clinical decision-making. Healthcare professionals can deploy such technologies and ensure that they embrace best practices, aligning diagnostic procedures with the evolving face of medicine (Kerna et al., 2025).

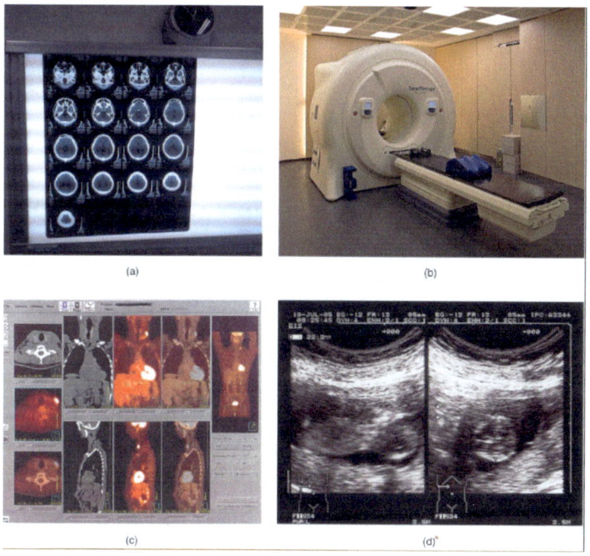

Figure 1.10. Diagnostic techniques in internal medicine.

Source: https://open.oregonstate.education/app/uploads/sites/157/2021/02/113abcd_Medical_Imaging_Techniques.jpg.

Furthermore, with the progress in the science of internal medicine, emphasis on personalized medicine and risk stratification has picked up pace. The use of predictive analytics enables the identification of patients at risk for the development of disease symptoms, enabling proactive intervention. Diagnostic methods are increasingly tailored to the patient's profile based on genetic, environmental, and lifestyle factors. This individualized strategy is supplemented by AI technology in clinical decision support systems that can drive the formulation of individualized treatment plans based on real-time data analysis. Such technologies present challenges regarding data privacy and algorithmic bias, and these must be negotiated judiciously to uphold ethical standards of practice. An intelligent integration of personalization in the diagnostic practice can produce more targeted interventions, ultimately resulting in better patient outcomes and satisfaction in internal medicine (Bashizadeh et al., 2024) (Figure 1.10).

1.4.1. Importance of Patient History and Physical Examination

In internal medicine, the importance of having a proper patient history and physical examination cannot be overemphasized. These fundamental components provide the foundation for acquiring essential diagnostic data, guiding medical practitioners to accurate conclusions and optimal management plans. Taking a thorough history from patients allows clinicians to identify potential risk factors, place symptoms in context, and establish a relationship with patients. This combined system encourages more patient-focused care, creating a greater understanding of the patient's health issues, previous treatments, and individual health choices that may affect outcomes. With proper communication at this juncture, this results in improved diagnosis and more suitable treatment, in keeping with the very essence of the physician-patient relationship that internal medicine entails. The physical examination complements the history-taking process, offering a valuable tool for clinicians to verify information collected and gain objective information regarding a patient's state of health. Through diligent assessment by inspection, palpation, percussion, and auscultation, physicians can uncover physiological dysfunction that cannot be easily diagnosed from history alone. The tactile examination plays a vital role in diagnosing acute illness, diagnosing chronic disease, and ordering necessary diagnostic studies. Further, it helps establish trust because patients typically feel listened to and cared for by their doctors when an excellent examination is performed. The ability to blend these elements into practice demonstrates the value placed on thorough care in internal medicine. Research confirms the clinical efficacy of assessing both patient history and physical examination as an educational imperative for practitioners of internal medicine. A formal curriculum that heightens sensitivity to these practices can significantly increase a clinician's confidence and knowledge of disease presentation and patient management. Practical training modules being designed today specifically speak to the necessity of sensitivity in dealing with patients, as evident in strategies designed for different populations, such as LGBT individuals, which raise the need for an appreciation of their special health issues. Such initiatives demonstrate a commitment to improving health trajectories and outcomes through meticulous, informed clinical practice, foregrounding the necessity of incorporating good history-taking and examination skills into the very fabric of internal medicine (Lechien et al., 2020; Ufomata et al., 2020).

1.4.2. Use of Laboratory Tests and Imaging Studies

In internal medicine, imaging studies and laboratory testing are vital for accurate diagnosis and management of many conditions. Laboratory examinations provide quantifiable data required to evaluate organ function, identify infection, and determine metabolic derangements. To illustrate, blood work such as complete blood counts (CBC) and comprehensive metabolic panels are fundamental components of any workup. These tests can uncover underlying conditions that are not obvious on clinical presentation through physical examination, thus guiding clinicians in the management. The combination of laboratory results and clinical presentation enables healthcare professionals to make accurate diagnoses and formulate individualized therapeutic plans, ultimately improving patient outcomes. Imaging studies encompass X-rays, computed tomography (CT), and magnetic resonance imaging (MRI), which all play complementary roles in reaching the diagnosis. These modalities allow clinicians to view inside the human body and detect abnormalities that might otherwise be missed. For example, magnetic resonance imaging has been extremely sensitive in identifying complex brain abnormalities in human and veterinary medicine, illustrated by its significance in comprehensive diagnostics (Creighton et al., 2016).

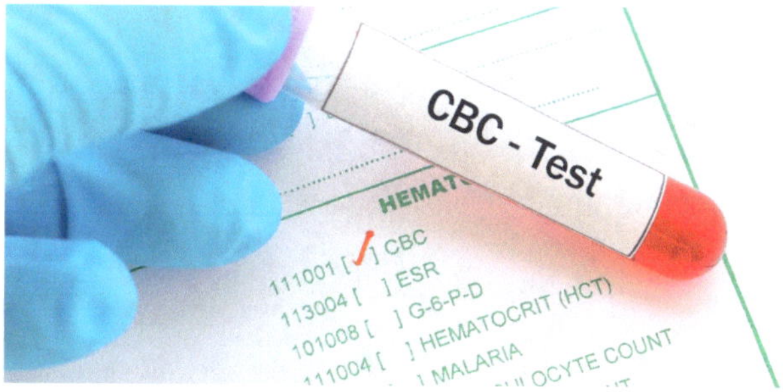

Figure 1.11. Complete-blood-count (CBC).

Source: https://cdn.dev.glasspress.io/info/cbc-blood-test-complete-blood-count-image-info-hero.jpg.

Specialized imaging techniques allow for the assessment of abnormalities that can complicate a patient's clinical presentation, making them valuable tools in the initial workup and ongoing management of complex medical issues. Imaging procedures of this nature not only contribute to the information available about a patient's illness but also inform decision-making for further diagnostic and therapeutic interventions. In addition, combining laboratory testing and imaging procedures offers a holistic outlook to patient evaluation, particularly in cases of neurological disorders. Research has established that abnormalities detected by abdominal ultrasound in canine neurologic conditions influence the decision to pursue advanced neurodiagnostics, suggesting the integrated nature of diagnostic modalities (Blair et al., 2015). This link underscores the importance of embracing a multidimensional paradigm in internal medicine, as it has a substantial impact on treatment pathways and patient outcomes. By developing an integrated diagnostic framework that combines laboratory and imaging information, clinicians can improve their diagnostic abilities, enhancing patient care and outcomes in internal medicine practice (Figure 1.11).

1.4.3. Emerging Technologies in Diagnostics

The field of internal medicine has been dominated by new technologies that enhance speed, accuracy, and access to disease detection. Possibly the most important among these is the integration of molecular diagnostics, which employs techniques such as next-generation sequencing (NGS) to diagnose genetic abnormalities that are associated with various diseases rapidly. This is particularly relevant in personalized medicine, where understanding a patient's unique genetic makeup enables customized therapeutic strategies. Furthermore, the development of point-of-care equipment has brought diagnostics to the patient's bedside, enabling real-time decision-making at the clinic and thereby improving outcomes. As these technologies advance, their potential to revolutionize standard diagnostic routines becomes increasingly clear, with more proactive patient management and care in internal medicine. At the same time, advances in imaging technology, such as high-end MRI and PET scans, have greatly enhanced diagnostic capabilities, particularly in detecting neurodegenerative diseases and cancers. These modalities leverage sophisticated algorithms and artificial intelligence to read imaging data, improving diagnostic precision and enabling earlier intervention. For instance, the use of machine learning models to analyze imaging biomarkers is enabling clinicians to differentiate among various forms of dementia and other forms of cognitive impairment with unprecedented accuracy. Besides, the inclusion of biomarkers within diagnostic criteria—such as those set by the National Institute on Aging and the Alzheimer's Association Research Framework—is also reflective of a trend toward symptomatically less-reliant diagnostic practices that rely on underlying biological processes (Jack et al., 2018). This indicates a shift away from syndromal traditional diagnoses toward a biological understanding of disease. Lastly, the incorporation of digital health technologies, such as telemedicine and wearables, is revolutionizing the clinical diagnostic framework. These technologies not only enable ongoing monitoring of patients' health conditions but also enable the accumulation of large health data over time, which can be used to detect patterns and forecast the onset of disease. For example, wearables can track vital signs or monitor markers of chronic conditions, enabling clinicians to intervene promptly. Also, data collected by such devices can help improve diagnostic accuracy by providing a complete picture of a patient's health. As we welcome the shift towards a more comprehensive understanding of illness and health, these technologies have the potential to bridge gaps where diagnosis has not helped us in the past, resulting in better patient outcomes in internal medicine (Srivastava et al., 2020).

Test Your Knowledge

1. What diagnostic tests are commonly used in internal medicine to identify systemic diseases?
2. Why is imaging important in the diagnostic process of internal medicine?

1.5. Treatment Modalities in Internal Medicine

Learning Outcome

1. Explain the pharmacological interventions and their management
2. Discuss the lifestyle modifications and patient education
3. Describe the coordination of care with other healthcare providers

In internal medicine, treatment options are broad, varying with the diversity and specificity of patient needs and illnesses. The field focuses on a patient-oriented, holistic approach that responds not only to the immediate medical issues but also prioritizes prevention and ultimate health outcomes. Improvements in recent diagnostic technology, such as the ankle-brachial index (ABI) for peripheral arterial disease assessment, have completely transformed the practice of internal medicine management. The application of non-invasive equipment such as this for early detection can lead to early treatment and, in turn, improved prognosis and quality of life for patients at risk for cardiovascular events. Continuing development of evidence-based recommendations is a cornerstone for practitioners to develop improved treatment plans that are sensitive to individualized patient needs and the underlying causal health conditions (Nordanstig et al., 2023). Pharmacologic treatment is an anchor of treatment in internal medicine, especially in long-term conditions such as diabetes, hypertension, and hyperlipidemia. The creation of new drug classes, such as the sodium-glucose cotransporter 2 (SGLT2) inhibitors and proprotein convertase subtilisin/kexin type 9 (PCSK9) inhibitors, demonstrates the tides of pharmacotherapy shifting towards optimizing patient outcomes. These medications have been found not only to best treat the principal disease but also to yield significant cardiovascular benefits. For instance, SGLT2 inhibitors, initially designed for the treatment of diabetes, have been found to prevent hospitalization for heart failure in patients with cardiovascular disease. Such a paradigm shift towards multifunctional drugs is the result of growing insight into the intertwined nature of chronic diseases in the discipline of internal medicine (Zhu et al., 2020). In addition to pharmacologic treatments, non-pharmacologic interventions, such as lifestyle modification and exercise therapy, have become more prominent in internal medicine treatment protocols. Physicians are writing more orders for supervised exercise therapy for conditions such as intermittent claudication, in line with findings of enhanced functional capacity and improved quality of life. The European Society for Vascular Surgery emphasizes the value of non-invasive management of peripheral arterial disease, which can be used in conjunction with, or in some cases instead of, invasive management. Lifestyle intervention, including diet modification and quitting smoking, also has a significant role in the prevention of disease worsening as well as overall improvement. The merging of these modalities represents an integrative internal medicine paradigm that recognizes the vital place that patient participation and self-management hold in achieving the optimal degree of health outcome (Nordanstig et al., 2023) (Figure 1.12).

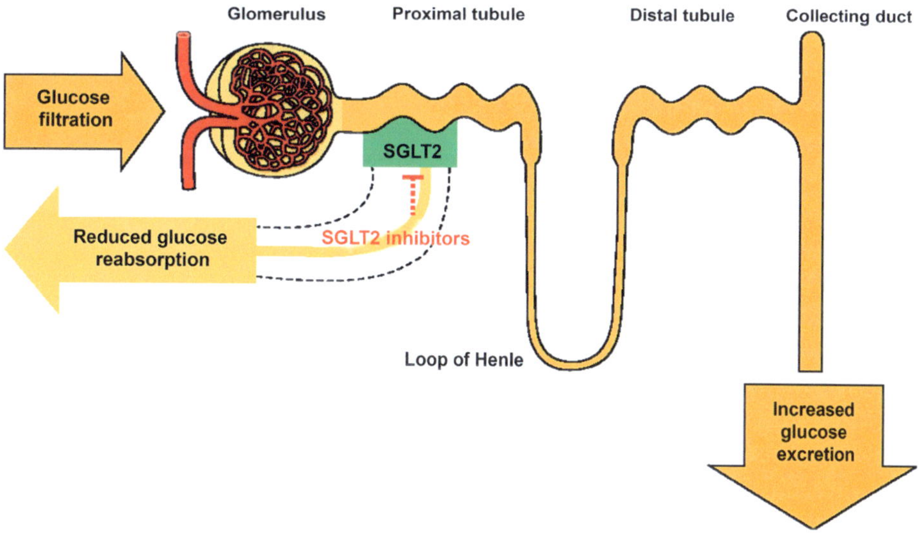

Figure 1.12. Sodium-glucose cotransporter 2 (SGLT2) inhibitors.

Source: https://external-content.duckduckgo.com/iu/?u=https%3A%2F%2Fd3i71xaburhd42.cloudfront.net%2F184e836ab98d09870ce2eb04753cac9a061075cd%2F4-Figure1-1.png&f=1&nofb=1&ipt=5992e1d79d1723b12b0e3c3df574306b80ad043a9518f70cd0c4547e82723ac9.

1.5.1. Pharmacological Interventions and Their Management

The contribution of pharmacological treatments cannot be overstated in internal medicine, particularly in the management of chronic illnesses such as multiple sclerosis (MS). They are most commonly primary therapy regimens used to relieve symptoms and improve patients' quality of life. The complexity of pharmacological management requires extensive knowledge of both the effectiveness and potential side effects of the drugs used. For instance, while pharmacological interventions can overcome pain, complications that also arise are complications that need their treatment, thus illustrating the thin line in treatment management. Secondly, since chronic pain in MS correlates with heightened anxiety as well as depression, targeted treatment is needed to control the holistic features of the disease. These circumstances highlight the importance of holistic approaches to the delivery of pharmacologic care, so that patients not only experience relief from symptoms but also receive treatment for their overall well-being. The inclusion of non-pharmacologic interventions within the pharmacologic management of conditions like MS has become more and more acceptable as an effective adjunct therapy. Cognitive Behavioral Therapy (CBT), for instance, has proven effective in supplementing treatment gains when used alongside pharmacologic interventions. In a study of patients with MS, subjects receiving CBT as an adjunct to standard care showed improved goal achievement and satisfaction, demonstrating the effectiveness of a multimodal pain management approach (Beauvais et al., 2019). This observation is consistent with the concept that, despite the important role pharmacologic drugs play in improving acute symptom control, psychological and educational elements can provide firmer support for patient care. Treatment of mental disorders associated with chronic pain should be considered an integral part of complex internal medicine treatment, enhancing the effectiveness of pharmacological treatment. While pharmacological and non-pharmacological interventions may complement each other, there are still issues in clinical trials regarding completeness and clarity. It has been supported by evidence that a significant number of non-pharmacological treatments are inadequately reported, which limits their replication and ease of implementation by other practitioners and researchers (Erueti et al., 2013). Poor reporting can lead to wastage of valuable resources in clinical research and inhibit maximal patient outcomes. To maximize the practice of pharmacological interventions and their corresponding management strategies, a combined effort is required from publishers, clinicians, and researchers. Through accurate reporting of all the therapeutic aspects, healthcare professionals can better work through and implement effective strategies within the complex arena of internal medicine and eventually improve patient care and treatment outcomes (Figure 1.13).

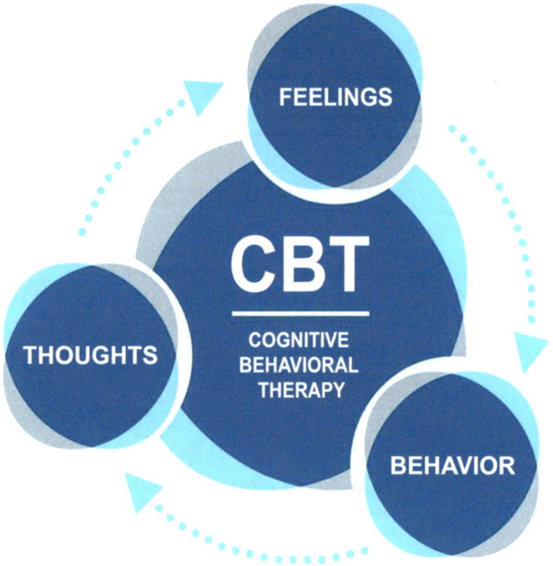

Figure 1.13. Cognitive behavioral therapy (CBT).

Source: https://www.milehighpsychology.com/wp-content/uploads/2023/09/CBT-infographic-1366x1330.jpg.

1.5.2. Lifestyle Modifications and Patient Education

In the practice of internal medicine, the use of patient education and lifestyle changes together is a powerful intervention for enhanced outcomes. Transcending reliance on pharmacologic intervention to an integrative model of lifestyle changes is not only a method for managing patients' immediate clinical problems, but also modulates long-term risks for chronic disease. Effective patient education is the cornerstone of this paradigm, empowering people with information and skills to make informed decisions about their own health. According to a study, high-performing health systems that deliver patient-centered care have a significant influence on improving health outcomes through lifestyle interventions, thereby emphasizing education as a determinant of healthier populations (Kruk et al., 2018). Secondarily, implementing educational structures is the solution, as they guide patients toward sustainable, health-promoting behaviors. Patient-led care, such as shared decision-making, supports individualized lifestyle changes tailored to each patient's needs. An example is presented in a case study that follows the experience of a patient named Rosa and describes the potential for lifestyle medicine to reorganize standard care. Rosas's case illustrates how the implementation of individualized action plans led to significant weight loss and improvements in her overall well-being. Involving patients in care enables health practitioners to engage them in discussions about feasible, culturally appropriate lifestyle adjustments. Not only is this measure efficient at handling medical issues, but it also promotes adherence and trust among patients, making them part of their healthcare process (Clarke et al., 2016). Thus, developing a culture in which patient education and lifestyle changes coexist is crucial to optimal health outcomes. Further, the importance of addressing avoidable chronic diseases makes it imperative to approach lifestyle medicine training in healthcare systems holistically. In light of increasing chronic diseases such as diabetes, hypertension, and obesity, it is essential to equip healthcare professionals with the requisite knowledge and skills to counsel patients regarding lifestyle changes. Current medical curricula are not schooled adequately in lifestyle medicine, thus limiting the ability of physicians to implement effective interventions. Hence, internal medicine physicians must urge extended education programs with nutritional counseling, physical activity, and behavioral modification techniques. By prioritizing lifestyle medicine in medical education, health systems are better positioned to train professionals to provide integrated care, thereby addressing the root causes of chronic diseases and responding to the emerging health needs of the population (Kruk et al., 2018). This proactive orientation marks a move towards a responsive, fair, and efficient healthcare system.

1.5.3. Coordination of Care with Other Healthcare Providers

Effective care coordination among medical professionals in the practice of internal medicine is an essential cornerstone because it directly influences patient outcomes and the efficiency of health systems. Patients typically progress through multiple layers of specialists and general practitioners, and this needs seamless transfer of medical information and cooperative decision-making regarding treatment plans. This collaborative approach minimizes the risk of fragmented care, which may lead to redundancies, medication mishandling, or incompatible diagnoses. The ability of the providers, thus, to communicate and coordinate their efforts is critical. An integrated care model not only maximizes the patient experience but also facilitates compliance with clinical guidelines, ultimately delivering on the vision of the healthcare system to provide high-quality care to evolving patient needs. Integrating big data in healthcare presents a big opportunity for enhancing coordination among providers of internal medicine. With enormous amounts of data generated from sources such as electronic health records and patient monitoring systems, healthcare providers can leverage this data to support their clinical practice and enable real-time decision-making. For instance, analyzing big data can detect trends in treatment outcomes and effectiveness, allowing providers to rapidly adjust treatment protocols. Further, this form of data can facilitate interprofessional collaboration by providing an integrated overview of a patient's medical history and current treatments, which is invaluable for effective care management. As one has seen in recent debates surrounding big data, healthcare organizations are increasingly realizing that they must equip themselves with the appropriate infrastructure to effectively use this data to better coordinate specialties (Dash et al., 2019). Proper quality health systems must pay attention not only to making health services accessible, but also to the efficiency and quality of care delivered through provider coordination. As highlighted in critical reviews of health systems, there are common gaps in the quality of care that particularly affect vulnerable populations in low and middle-income countries (Kruk et al., 2018). Poor coordination is likely to result in missed opportunities for preventive services, widening existing health inequalities. To meet this need, health systems should aim to build alliances with diverse sectors and stakeholders and foster an organizational culture of continuous improvement in the processes of providing care. By emphasizing methods that involve interdisciplinary communication and collaborative decision-making, health professionals can significantly enhance the quality of care, enabling patients to receive the best, evidence-based therapy tailored to their individual needs.

Test Your Knowledge

1. What are the common pharmacological treatment approaches used in internal medicine?
2. How do lifestyle modifications support medical treatment in internal medicine?

1.6. Challenges in Internal Medicine

Learning Outcome

1. Explain the managing complex and comorbid conditions
2. Understand the navigating healthcare systems and patient access
3. Describe the addressing the physician burnout crisis

Internal medicine involves many challenges that tend to arise from complex interactions among infectious diseases, access to health care, and socioeconomic factors. Both in the developing world and the developed world, internal medicine clinicians are challenged by diseases that include malaria, tuberculosis, and HIV/AIDS, and require innovative approaches to management. Solving these endemic health problems requires not just high-level clinical knowledge but also dedication to systematic transformation in healthcare delivery. In Sierra Leone, for instance, the prevalence of infectious diseases strains the already frail healthcare system, prompting practitioners to resort to innovative ways to tackle disease. As Sankoh et al. (2024) opine, significant effort must be devoted to strengthening healthcare access and treatment practices to ultimately attack these diseases directly while simultaneously fostering socioeconomic development in the affected regions.

Also, internal medicine experts face the critical challenge of substandard palliative care facilities, particularly in low- and middle-income countries. In Brazil alone, for example, the lack of palliative care facilities has led to the development of innovative solutions within existing medical treatment. Having a specialized palliative care team in oncology facilities is an example of how integrated solutions can address the complex needs of terminal patients. This follows the data presented in Mendes et al. (2024), which highlights the importance of incorporating complete support systems into standard medical practice. Internal medicine has to, therefore, change so that practitioners can tackle not just the patients' acute health conditions but also the full requirement for support in end-of-life care, commonly overlooked in traditional models of healthcare. In addition, internal medicine remains confronted with inherent complexities in the integration with public health in practice.

Variation in healthcare education and facilities intensifies the challenges professionals face in handling these matters. For instance, in locations like Rio de Janeiro, the variation in available palliative care multiplies the complexity of handling complicated healthcare outcomes in metastatic cancer patients.

As noted by Mendes et al. (2024), an institutionalized system that emphasizes collaboration between internal medicine and palliative care can be a replicable model for effectively addressing patients. By emphasizing continuous education, interdisciplinarity, and patient-centeredness, the practice of internal medicine can significantly improve the quality of care, addressing immediate health concerns and promoting long-term patient well-being (Figure 1.14).

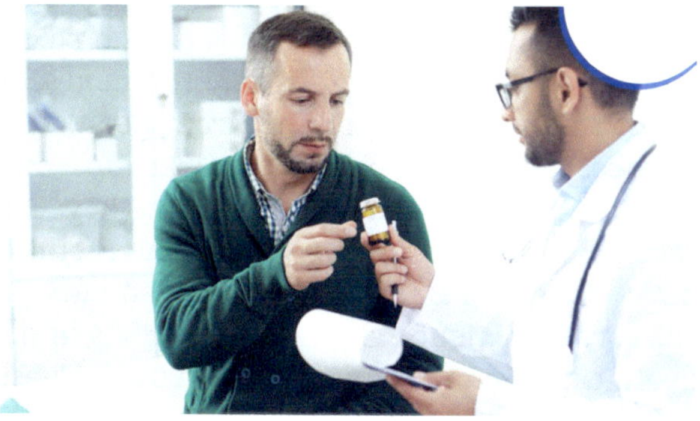

Figure 1.14. Internal medicine doctor treat.

Source: https://www.theaccesshealthcare.com/images/blog/what-does%20an-internal-medicine-doctor-treat.jpg.

1.6.1. Managing Complex and Comorbid Conditions

In internal medicine, treating complex, comorbid conditions involves understanding how various chronic diseases can interact and worsen one another. This complex interaction makes it difficult to treat, with a solution that demands a whole-person approach that takes into account the patient's complete health profile. For instance, CKD patients often have comorbid conditions like diabetes and hypertension, each of which has its own management requirements. PCPs face a range of barriers from regimen complexity to patient adherence problems. Research indicates that PCPs typically face access barriers, including limited resources, burdensome electronic medical records, and insufficient time, all of which interfere with their capacity to provide optimal CKD care. Addressing these problems is important for improving health outcomes in comorbid patients and for providing patient-centered, effective care (Abdel-Kader et al., 2019). The psychological aspect that accompanies long-term illness is another significant aspect of comorbid condition management. Patients with multiple conditions have higher levels of anxiety and depression, which negatively impact their compliance with treatment and health outcomes in general. As an example, patients with type 2 diabetes tend to develop cardiovascular complications and hence receive more complex medication therapy. Beyond attention to physiological symptoms, caring for such patients requires comprehension of their psychological status. Tools such as the Attitudes about Complex Therapy Scale (ACTS) were created to measure patients' attitudes and beliefs toward their medications and to identify patients who will knowingly not adhere to prescribed treatments. This not only aids in individualizing treatment plans but also improves patient education and support and creates a more effective way to manage comorbid conditions (Bundy et al., 2015). Controlling complicated and comorbid disorders effectively ultimately boils down to the collaboration between healthcare providers and patients. Interprofessional collaboration is central to the organization of complete care that considers the multifactorial disorders. The need for collaborative efforts becomes self-evident when one considers the variety of specialties involved, such as endocrinology for diabetes management and nephrology for kidney disease. Such cooperation facilitates communication and shared decision-making, enabling patients to become more active participants in their own care. Educational programs that enable PCPs to stay up to date with the latest treatment guidelines can help break down barriers by building confidence in managing patients' complex needs. Developing a supportive healthcare environment that fosters patient-provider communication and minimizes systemic barriers will significantly improve the health outcomes of patients and enhance the quality of care offered in internal medicine (Abdel-Kader et al., 2019) (Figure 1.15).

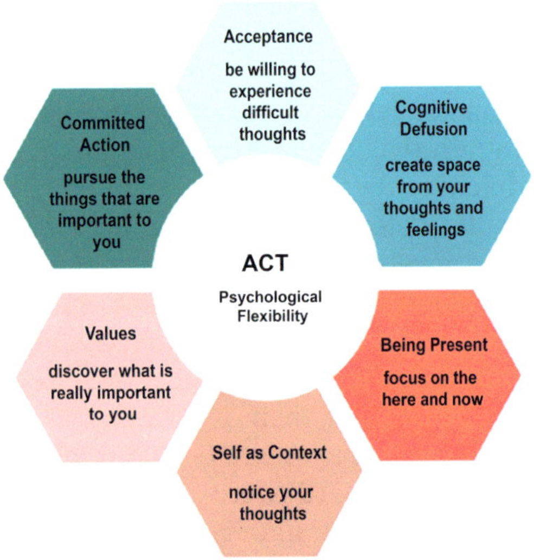

Figure 1.15. Attitudes about complex therapy scale (ACTS.

Source: https://www.healthandhealingtherapy.com/wp-content/uploads/2023/09/ACT-1024x1024.png.

1.6.2. Navigating Healthcare Systems and Patient Access

Guiding healthcare systems is a fundamental aspect of internal medicine, directly affecting patient access and overall health. The patient typically navigates a maze of services, from primary to specialty care. Internal medicine professionals possess the unique ability to guide patients through this maze, fostering integrated care and ensuring they receive appropriate interventions. Effective navigation involves an understanding of insurance, service coverage, and procedures for obtaining referrals and specialty care. Healthcare systems, according to researchers, are more likely to favor well-educated and active people; thus, physicians must educate their patients on available resources and support systems when offering access to care in the systems (Famouri et al., 2022). Another aspect of working within healthcare systems is overcoming the barriers that systematically prevent patient access, particularly in marginalized communities. Microaggressions—those ubiquitous yet insidious instances of bias that are experienced in interactions with patients—add up to disparities in healthcare access and quality. Health care professionals must understand how these biases impact patient care and adapt their approach to ensure that all patients feel seen, heard, and understood. Besides, fostering an open environment can enable all patients to benefit from healthcare services effectively. Training workshops that inform medical residents on how they can recognize and respond to these interactions have yielded remarkable improvements in supporting patients' rights and interests in the healthcare sector (Sukumar et al., 2021). These are required in designing a more equitable healthcare system. Even with the advancements in technology in healthcare delivery, the issue of fair access to healthcare remains. Telehealth has been a valuable tool, particularly during the COVID-19 pandemic, for conducting remote consultations and minimizing logistical barriers to treatment. It should be noted, however, that not all patients have equal access to the internet or technology, creating a digital divide that may limit the full utility of telehealth services. Internal medicine doctors must proactively close this gap by exploring alternative avenues of communication and support for those who may not be able to reach them via digital means. Investing in patient education on how to interact with new technologies and advocating for systemic reform to mitigate disparities in access will give patients the tools they need to effectively engage with evolving healthcare systems (Famouri et al., 2022). By focusing on widespread patient access, internal medicine can significantly improve health outcomes among diverse populations.

1.6.3. Addressing the Physician Burnout Crisis

Physician burnout has become a top-priority problem throughout the field of internal medicine, highlighting the multifaceted challenge facing healthcare providers. Burnout, as characterized by emotional exhaustion, depersonalization, and reduced personal accomplishment, can have profound effects not only on physicians' health but also on patient care and organizational performance. The ongoing pressures of increasing patient volumes, bureaucratic tasks, and expectations amid crises such as the COVID-19 pandemic exacerbate this issue. Burnout is only addressed when an end-to-end examination of the many stressors healthcare workers experience, such as moral distress and potential moral harms, is conducted. This calls for a paradigm shift in how healthcare facilities approach clinician well-being, including preventive measures based on psychological resilience and facilitative organizational climates (Riedel et al., 2022). Moreover, interventions to reduce physician burnout must operate at multiple levels, from the individual to the organizational and cultural levels. Individual-level interventions, such as regularly promoting exercise, maintaining healthy dietary practices, and fostering strong, supportive relationships, can provide valuable coping mechanisms. The organizational level is crucial to establishing blame-free cultures where healthcare providers can express their experiences without fear of stigma. Multidisciplinary psychosocial support teams can further be utilized to facilitate a joint response to workplace stressors. Having doctors involved in management decision-making can empower them and enhance job satisfaction, reducing the helplessness that contributes to burnout (Leo et al., 2021). Culturally, medicine must provide a climate that resists stigma in seeking mental health support. Being a promoter of reforming systems and prioritizing the health and well-being of providers is central. Strategies to create long-term research and evidence-based practice use can facilitate this cultural shift. By addressing both the symptoms and the causes of burnout, the healthcare system can build resilience among physicians. This holistic approach is critical not only to retain seasoned experts but also to deliver quality patient care, ultimately fostering the practice of internal medicine and a healthier society overall (Leo et al., 2021).

Test Your Knowledge

1. What challenges do internists face in managing patients with multiple chronic conditions?
2. How do diagnostic uncertainty and overlapping symptoms complicate internal medicine practice?

SUMMARY

Internal medicine is a comprehensive overview of the multifaceted, multidisciplinary science essential to modern healthcare. By analyzing the fundamentals of internal medicine, we understand its pivotal role in diagnosing, preventing, and controlling disease. By thoroughly analyzing the varied internal systems and their pathologies, physicians can significantly improve patient outcomes. This presentation has highlighted the importance of clinical insight, but also the socio-cultural determinants of the provision of care. As practitioners themselves grow in an era increasingly influenced by technological innovation and socio-economic growth, the underlying principles governing internal medicine must remain omnipresent in medical training. Moreover, internal medicine demonstrates the union of science and humanism in clinical practice. The integration of evidence-based practice with patient-centered care forms the bedrock of competent internal medicine. Each patient encounter offers a unique opportunity to apply clinical judgment and compassionate communication, both of which are essential for building trust and engagement in the treatment process. Awareness of patients' psychosocial context enables more targeted interventions that address specific health problems in an integrated manner. The growing importance of resilience within the healthcare field, especially in the context of adversity like that experienced during the COVID-19 pandemic, underscores the necessity for internal medicine specialists to create healthy environments that enhance their patients' overall well-being, as indicated in existing research (Sharland et al., 2022). Finally, internal medicine's future is with continually maintaining education and flexibility among its professionals. With evolving healthcare settings, internal medicine must adjust to increasing challenges and opportunities, particularly in technology adoption and coordinated patient care. The assessment of innovative tools, like LLMs, presents new frontiers for enhancing clinical decision-making and patient engagement (Chang et al., 2024). Internal medicine physicians in the future must remain vigilant in gauging these innovations to develop a more effective and compassionate healthcare system. Commitment to continuous professional growth and interprofessional practice will enable internal medicine to face complexity on an ongoing basis while ever placing patient well-being as the top priority. Combined, these items will strengthen the discipline and make it better able to respond to the demands of an evolving health care environment.

Internal Medicine is critical within the broader healthcare landscape, having evolved to address the complexity of adult patient care. Internal Medicine doctors, or internists, specialize in the diagnosis, treatment, and prevention of a wide range of chronic diseases and conditions that typically have vague symptoms. This specialty is especially critical because patients usually have a mix of situations that require an integrated and multifaceted treatment strategy. Internists play a central role in the healthcare system by using their knowledge to care for both simple and complex disease processes, thereby improving overall patient outcomes. Their commitment to a holistic appreciation of the interrelationships among multiple health conditions promotes a patient-centered orientation central to modern medicine, where treatment plans tailored to the unique needs of each individual are increasingly emphasized. In addition, Internal Medicine stands out for its emphasis on preventive medicine and public health education. Internists are best suited not only to treat current illnesses but also to promote preventive measures to reduce the incidence of chronic diseases. This two-way orientation to treatment and prevention is a sign of a broader view of health, encompassing lifestyle management, early-stage disease detection, and follow-up. Thus, the field of Internal Medicine extends far beyond the individual patient to encompass community health and resource planning within the healthcare system. Including preventive practices in routine work reduces long-term care costs for chronic disease and improves the overall health of the population. Case studies also identify the importance of Internal Medicine in treating one condition at a time, which characterizes the complexity of patient care. For instance, in a sample population of two tetanus patients, there were significant variations in recovery, primarily due to socioeconomic status and the ability to receive timely treatment. The case focuses on the imperative that economic status has on health outcomes and how this underscores the need for internists to take into account social determinants of health when creating treatment plans. Another schistosomiasis study again illustrated the intricacies of diagnosing and treating an infection that varies widely across populations. These are just some examples of the requirements for an intern's ability to cope with the sophisticated aspects of patient treatment, ultimately reflecting the more critical role of Internal Medicine as a basis for the successful management of health care in society.

KEY TERMS FROM THIS CHAPTER

Anemia
Chronic kidney disease (CKD)
Diabetes mellitus
Heart failure
Hypertension
Liver cirrhosis
Pneumonia
Sepsis
Thyroid disorders
Asthma
Deep vein thrombosis (DVT)
Electrolyte imbalance
HIV/AIDS
Infective endocarditis
Peptic ulcer disease
Rheumatoid arthritis
Systemic lupus erythematosus (SLE)
Tuberculosis

CRITICAL THINKING QUESTIONS

1. **Which of the following is the first-line treatment for newly diagnosed essential hypertension in an otherwise healthy adult?**
   a. Beta-blockers
   b. ACE inhibitors
   c. Alpha-blockers
   d. Loop diuretics
2. **A 55-year-old man presents with fatigue and pallor. Labs show microcytic, hypochromic anemia. What is the most likely diagnosis?**
   a. Iron deficiency anemia
   b. Vitamin B12 deficiency
   c. Aplastic anemia
   d. Hemolytic anemia
3. **Which of the following is most characteristic of nephrotic syndrome?**
   a. Hematuria and hypertension
   b. Proteinuria >3.5 g/day and edema
   c. Elevated creatinine and oliguria
   d. Hyperkalemia and metabolic acidosis
4. **Which of the following organisms is the most common cause of community-acquired pneumonia in adults?**
   a. *Mycoplasma pneumoniae*
   b. *Streptococcus pneumoniae*
   c. *Haemophilus influenzae*
   d. *Klebsiella pneumoniae*
5. **Which of the following is considered a diagnostic feature of diabetic ketoacidosis (DKA)?**
   a. Hypernatremia
   b. Metabolic alkalosis
   c. High anion gap metabolic acidosis
   d. Low serum osmolality

Short Answer Questions

1. What are the common causes and clinical features of fever of unknown origin (FUO)?
2. How is type 2 diabetes mellitus diagnosed and monitored over time?
3. What are the diagnostic criteria for systemic lupus erythematosus (SLE)?
4. Describe the typical presentation and initial management of community-acquired pneumonia.
5. What is the pathophysiology and treatment approach to iron deficiency anemia?
6. What are the indications for initiating dialysis in chronic kidney disease (CKD)?
7. Describe the clinical features and management of hepatic encephalopathy.
8. What are the key differences between ulcerative colitis and Crohn's disease?

Answers to Critical Thinking Questions

1. (b); 2. (a) ; 3. (b) ; 4. (b) ; 5. (c)

REFERENCES

1. Sperati, C. J., Soman, S., Agrawal, V., Liu, Y., Abdel-Kader, K., Diamantidis, C. J., Estrella, M. M., Cavanaugh, K., Plantinga, L., Schell, J., Simon, J., Vassalotti, J. A., Choi, M. J., Jaar, B. G., & Greer, R. C. (2019). Primary care physicians' perceptions of barriers and facilitators to management of chronic kidney disease: A mixed methods study. *PLoS ONE, 14*(8), e0221325. https://doi.org/10.1371/journal.pone.0221325Bashizadeh, M., Soufizadeh, P., Zamiri, M., Lamei, A., Sotoudehnejad, M., Daneshmand, M., Ghodrati, M., et al. (2024). An overview of artificial intelligence applications in prediction and diagnosis of diseases occurrence in veterinary medicine: Challenges and techniques. *Eltiam*. https://www.semanticscholar.org/paper/a48783e16252e156f7468b709c59738fdbad7f14 (accessed on 16th July 2025).
2. Beauvais, J., Beenken, B., Czlapinski, R., Gromisch, M., et al. (2019). Cognitive behavioral therapy for the management of multiple sclerosis–related pain: A randomized clinical trial. https://open.bu.edu/bitstream/2144/34298/1/CBT%20for%20MS%20Pain%20Merged%20PDF.pdf (accessed on 16th July 2025).
3. Berg, G., Rybakova, D., Fischer, D., Cernava, T., Champomier Vergès, M. C., Charles, T. C., Chen, X., et al. (2020). Microbiome definition re-visited: Old concepts and new challenges. *Microbiome, 8*. https://doi.org/10.1186/s40168-020-00875-0 (accessed on 16th July 2025).
4. Blair, W. H., Chen, R. X., Sturges, B. K., Taylor, M. A., et al. (2015). Effect of screening abdominal ultrasound examination on the decision to pursue advanced diagnostic tests and treatment in dogs with neurologic disease. https://core.ac.uk/download/323069729.pdf (accessed on 16th July 2025).
5. Braun, V., & Clarke, V. (2024). Supporting best practice in reflexive thematic analysis reporting in *Palliative Medicine*: A review of published research and introduction to the Reflexive Thematic Analysis Reporting Guidelines (RTARG). *Palliative Medicine, 38*, 608–616. https://www.semanticscholar.org/paper/f50be995ae7bc8b5889df68be77bf89d1d253a50 (accessed on 16th July 2025).
6. Brew, B., Ellero, J., & Lubomski, M. (2017). Interventions for neurocognitive dysfunction. https://core.ac.uk/download/84111210.pdf (accessed on 16th July 2025).
7. Bundy, C., New, J. P., Gibson, M., Noyce, P. R., Elliott, R. A., & Stack, R. J. (2015). The Attitudes about Complex Therapy Scale (ACTS) in type 2 diabetes and cardiovascular disease: Development, validity and reliability. https://core.ac.uk/download/30650779.pdf (accessed on 16th July 2025).
8. Campbell, C., & Kahwash, R. (2020). Will complement inhibition be the new target in treating COVID-19–related systemic thrombosis? *Circulation, 141*, 1739–1741. https://doi.org/10.1161/circulationaha.120.047419 (accessed on 16th July 2025).
9. Carney, N., Totten, A. M., O'Reilly, C., Ullman, J. S., Hawryluk, G. W. J., Bell, M. J., Bratton, S. L., et al. (2016). Guidelines for the management of severe traumatic brain injury, fourth edition. *Neurosurgery, 80*, 6–15. https://doi.org/10.1227/neu.0000000000001432 (accessed on 16th July 2025).
10. Chang, Y., Wang, X., Wang, J., Wu, Y., Yang, L., Zhu, K., Chen, H., et al. (2024). A survey on evaluation of large language models. *ACM Transactions on Intelligent Systems and Technology, 15*, 1–45. https://doi.org/10.1145/3641289 (accessed on 16th July 2025).

11. Chopra, V., Toner, E., Waldhorn, R., & Washer, L. (2020). How should U.S. hospitals prepare for Coronavirus Disease 2019 (COVID-19)? *Annals of Internal Medicine, 172*, 621–622. https://doi.org/10.7326/m20-0907 (accessed on 16th July 2025).

12. Clarke, C., & Hauser, M. E. (2016). Lifestyle medicine: A primary care perspective. *Journal of Graduate Medical Education, 8*, 665–667. https://doi.org/10.4300/jgme-d-15-00804.1 (accessed on 16th July 2025).

13. Creighton, E. K., Keating, M. K., Lyons, L. A., Sisó, S., et al. (2016). Characterization of an inherited neurologic syndrome in Toyger cats with forebrain commissural malformations, ventriculomegaly and interhemispheric cysts. https://core.ac.uk/download/323069548.pdf (accessed on 16th July 2025).

14. Cryan, J. F., O'Riordan, K. J., Cowan, C. S. M., Sandhu, K. V., Bastiaanssen, T. F. S., Boehme, M., Codagnone, M. G., et al. (2019). The microbiota-gut-brain axis. *Physiological Reviews, 99*, 1877–2013. https://doi.org/10.1152/physrev.00018.2018 (accessed on 16th July 2025).

15. Dash, S., Shakyawar, S. K., Sharma, L., & Kaushik, S. (2019). Big data in healthcare: Management, analysis and future prospects. *Journal of Big Data, 6*. https://doi.org/10.1186/s40537-019-0217-0 (accessed on 16th July 2025).

16. Drumright, B., Sacro, Y., & Nussbaum, A. (2024). Enriching spiritual care in medical residents through cultural humility and courage. *MedEdPORTAL: The Journal of Teaching and Learning Resources, 20*. https://www.semanticscholar.org/paper/b6b17dedc45313f0fadd43a899d60b46f580f112 (accessed on 16th July 2025).

17. Erueti, C., Glasziou, P. P., & Hoffmann, T. C. (2013). Poor description of non-pharmacological interventions: Analysis of consecutive sample of randomized trials. https://core.ac.uk/download/196601048.pdf (accessed on 16th July 2025).

18. Famouri, M. L., Hernandez, S., Omlor, R. L., Lane-Brown, M., Evans, S. M., McIntosh, D., & Denizard-Thompson, N. (2022). Active bystander training: Using standardized patient methodology to teach residents to navigate microaggressions in patient encounters. *MedEdPORTAL*. https://doi.org/10.15766/mep_2374-8265.11298 (accessed on 16th July 2025).

19. Ferrando, M. R., Proietti, E., Demontis, M., Montecucco, F., & Pisciotta, L. (2025). Sustainable development goals: A call for future internal medicine. *Internal and Emergency Medicine*. https://www.semanticscholar.org/paper/578ef0a02774c8972cb975f6e2a2463f3b88e636 (accessed on 16th July 2025).

20. Gimbrone, M. A., & García-Cardeña, G. (2016). Endothelial cell dysfunction and the pathobiology of atherosclerosis. *Circulation Research, 118*, 620–636. https://doi.org/10.1161/circresaha.115.306301 (accessed on 16th July 2025).

21. Hennus, M. P., van Dam, M., Gauthier, S., Taylor, D., & ten Cate, O. (2022). The logic behind entrustable professional activity frameworks: A scoping review of the literature. *Medical Education, 56*, 881–891. https://doi.org/10.1111/medu.14806 (accessed on 16th July 2025).

22. Jack, C. R., Bennett, D. A., Blennow, K., Carrillo, M. C., Dunn, B., Budd Haeberlein, S., Holtzman, D. M., et al. (2018). NIA-AA research framework: Toward a biological definition of Alzheimer's disease. *Alzheimer's & Dementia, 14*, 535–562. https://doi.org/10.1016/j.jalz.2018.02.018 (accessed on 16th July 2025).

23. James, S. L., Abate, D., Abate, K. H., Abay, S. M., Abbafati, C., Abbasi, N., Abbastabar, H., et al. (2018). Global, regional, and national incidence, prevalence, and years lived with disability for 354 diseases and injuries for 195 countries and territories, 1990–2017: A systematic analysis for the Global Burden of Disease Study 2017. *The Lancet, 392*, 1789–1858. https://doi.org/10.1016/s0140-6736(18)32279-7 (accessed on 16th July 2025).

24. Jiménez Alemán, V. N., Astudillo Pinos, D. I., Desiderio León, K. M., Costales Vallejo, L. R., Gómez Troya, J. I., Rosas Cunyarache, M. A., Neira Borja, J. E., et al. (2024). Holistic patient care: A narrative review on the synergy of internal medicine, anesthesiology, and surgical practices. *Salud, Ciencia y Tecnología*. https://www.semanticscholar.org/paper/7c6a0748c332687cecd07a52d502c41253699bda (accessed on 16th July 2025).

25. Joshi, M., Prasad, P. A., Hubbard, C. C., Iverson, N., Manuel, S., Fang, M. C., & Rambachan, A. (2023). Racial, ethnic, and language-based inequities in inpatient opioid prescribing by diagnosis from internal medicine services, a retrospective cohort study. *Pain Research & Management, 2023*. https://www.semanticscholar.org/paper/0b02daa30cac780c8f5beecf0d77da8bda137e4b (accessed on 16th July 2025).

26. Kéïta, K., Djeugoue, S. L., Camara, B., Doumbia, A., Kamissoko, C. O., Sandji, O., Sinayoko, A., et al. (2025). A cross-sectional analysis of schistosomiasis case detection by rectal mucosal biopsy among patients attending the digestive endoscopy unit of the internal medicine department. *Journal of Interventional Epidemiology and Public Health*. https://www.semanticscholar.org/paper/da81654888aeb1aeaa776ec241edcc619cb11f6e (accessed on 16th July 2025).

27. Kerna, N. A., Olatokun, T. P., Keke, C. O., Okwuokei, E. C., Chigozie, I. K., Fide-Nwoko, F. U., David, C. O., et al. (2025). Current applications of artificial intelligence in internal medicine. *European Journal of Medical and Health Research*. https://www.semanticscholar.org/paper/5013b1eb682852a7df8e09aa12dc6f4ed54b50d2 (accessed on 16th July 2025).

28. Kimball, A. M., Gugerty, M. K., Abernethy, N., & Curran, S. (2011). Disease Surveillance Networks Initiative Global: Final evaluation. https://core.ac.uk/download/86445037.pdf (accessed on 16th July 2025).

29. Kruk, M. E., Gage, A., Arsenault, C., Jordan, K., Leslie, H. H., Roder-DeWan, S., Adeyi, O., et al. (2018). High-quality health systems in the Sustainable Development Goals era: Time for a revolution. *The Lancet Global Health, 6*, e1196–e1252. https://doi.org/10.1016/s2214-109x(18)30386-3 (accessed on 16th July 2025).

30. Kung, T. H., Cheatham, M., Medenilla, A., Sillos, C., De Leon, L., Elepaño, C., Madriaga, M., et al. (2023). Performance of ChatGPT on USMLE: Potential for AI-assisted medical education using large language models. *PLOS Digital Health, 2*, e0000198–e0000198. https://doi.org/10.1371/journal.pdig.0000198 (accessed on 16th July 2025).

31. Kutikov, A., Weinberg, D. S., Edelman, M. J., Horwitz, E. M., Uzzo, R. G., & Fisher, R. I. (2020). A war on two fronts: Cancer care in the time of COVID-19. *Annals of Internal Medicine, 172*, 756–758. https://doi.org/10.7326/m20-1133 (accessed on 16th July 2025).

32. Lechien, J. R., Chiesa-Estomba, C. M., Hans, S., Barillari, M. R., Jouffe, L., & Saussez, S. (2020). Loss of smell and taste in 2013 European patients with mild to moderate COVID-19. *Annals of Internal Medicine, 173*, 672–675. https://doi.org/10.7326/m20-2428 (accessed on 16th July 2025).

33. Leo, C. G., Sabina, S., Tumolo, M. R., Bodini, A., Ponzini, G., Sabato, E., & Mincarone, P. (2021). Burnout among healthcare workers in the COVID-19 era: A review of the existing literature. *Frontiers in Public Health, 9*. https://doi.org/10.3389/fpubh.2021.750529 (accessed on 16th July 2025).

34. Mendes, C. E., Chimeli, D., Albuquerque, M., Ferreira, T., Carvalho, S., Ribeiro, C. A., & Gomes, S. A. A. (2024). Implementation of a palliative care service in a tertiary hospital in a developing country: Methods, strategies and results. *Journal of Clinical Oncology*. https://www.semanticscholar.org/paper/f795099ed5035bda573fdd7cf3b4d063f3b7ba99 (accessed on 16th July 2025).

35. Molik, M. (2024). Trainee's perceptions on simulation-based education and its impact on transitioning to the role of medical registrar: A qualitative study. *Cureus, 16*. https://www.semanticscholar.org/paper/c65c955598628cb75f97bc50b39d624df61dd625 (accessed on 16th July 2025).

36. Ndirahisha, E., Nyandwi, R., Nyandwi, J., Manirakiza, S., Barasukana, P., Sibomana, T., & Baransaka, E. (2024). Hypertension management among hospitalized patients at Kamenge University Hospital in Bujumbura. *The East African Health Research Journal, 8*, 20–24. https://www.semanticscholar.org/paper/3f998fe35a6af4bedfb0653eb329b5fa46b3af94 (accessed on 16th July 2025).

37. Nordanstig, J., Behrendt, C. A., Baumgärtner, I., Belch, J. J. F., Bäck, M., Fitridge, R., Hinchliffe, R. J., et al. (2023). Editor's choice–European Society for Vascular Surgery (ESVS) 2024 clinical practice guidelines on the management of asymptomatic lower limb peripheral arterial disease and intermittent claudication. *European Journal of Vascular and Endovascular Surgery, 67*, 9–96. https://doi.org/10.1016/j.ejvs.2023.08.067 (accessed on 16th July 2025).

38. Octavia, M., Firmansyah, A. A., & Hadning, I. (2025). Optimizing stress ulcer prophylaxis: A clinical and cost evaluation in RSUD Wates internal medicine ward. *Medical Sains: Jurnal Ilmiah Kefarmasian*. https://www.semanticscholar.org/paper/0d321076411ae758840c5a467e27497e10fb5512 (accessed on 16th July 2025).

39. Page, M. J., Moher, D., Bossuyt, P. M., Boutron, I., Hoffmann, T., Mulrow, C. D., Shamseer, L., et al. (2021). PRISMA 2020 explanation and elaboration: Updated guidance and exemplars for reporting systematic reviews. *BMJ*. https://doi.org/10.1136/bmj.n160 (accessed on 16th July 2025).

40. Prince, L., Little, D., Schexneider, K. I., & Yuan, C. (2017). Integrating quality improvement education into the nephrology curricular milestones framework and the clinical learning environment review. *Clinical Journal of the American Society of Nephrology: CJASN, 12*(2), 349–356. https://www.semanticscholar.org/paper/e33d8f7db03c97b1bf114c01068fffd0ec4f9939 (accessed on 16th July 2025).

41. Rice, D., & Callies, D. (2025). Enhancing preventive care for adults 50+ through pre-visit planning in primary care. *Journal of Nursing Care Quality, 40*, 272–278. https://www.semanticscholar.org/paper/2c0aac71dbdd4fd9b2403308faa5a536a8568645 (accessed on 16th July 2025).

42. Riedel, P. L., Kreh, A., Kulcar, V., Lieber, A. S., & Juen, B. (2022). A scoping review of moral stressors, moral distress and moral injury in healthcare workers during COVID-19. *International Journal of Environmental Research and Public Health, 19*, 1666–1666. https://doi.org/10.3390/ijerph19031666 (accessed on 16th July 2025).

43. Rieke, N., Hancox, J., Li, W., Milletarì, F., Roth, H. R., Albarqouni, S., Bakas, S., et al. (2020). The future of digital health with federated learning. *npj Digital Medicine, 3*. https://doi.org/10.1038/s41746-020-00323-1 (accessed on 16th July 2025).

44. Sankoh, M. A., Bangura, B. C. Y., Jalloh, M. J., Pambu, D. M., Turay, M. L., & Koroma, J. D. (2024). Challenges and opportunities in combating infectious diseases in Sierra Leone: A narrative review of the role of community health and internal medicine. *International Journal of Research and Scientific Innovation*. https://www.semanticscholar.org/paper/083973968f8ff8dfc76c0415305acec1b14ff367 (accessed on 16th July 2025).

45. Sharland, P. B., Haroun, J., & Saf, A. (2022). *Journal of Sports Medicine. Journal of Sports Medicine*. https://doi.org/10.1155/5363 (accessed on 16th July 2025).

46. Shrestha, B., Shrestha, P., Agrawal, G., Bastakoti, S., Gurmaita, R. K., & Khanal, S. (2025). Trauma-induced tetanus: Case series and an up-to-date pharmacoeconomic overview in Nepal. *Annals of Medicine and Surgery, 87*, 1808–1813. https://www.semanticscholar.org/paper/dd337bfbfc2751b01872e2fbe7386192510c3d3f (accessed on 16th July 2025).

47. Singhal, K., Azizi, S., Tu, T., Mahdavi, S. S., Lee, J., Chung, H. W., Scales, N., et al. (2023). Large language models encode clinical knowledge. *Nature, 620*, 172–180. https://doi.org/10.1038/s41586-023-06291-2 (accessed on 16th July 2025).

48. Srivastava, A., Santagostino, E., Dougall, A., Kitchen, S., Sutherland, M. L., Pipe, S. W., Carção, M., et al. (2020). WFH guidelines for the management of hemophilia, 3rd edition. *Haemophilia, 26*, 1–158. https://doi.org/10.1111/hae.14046 (accessed on 16th July 2025).

49. Sukumar, S., Zakaria, A., Lai, C. J., Sakumoto, M., Khanna, R., & Choi, N. (2021). Designing and implementing a novel virtual rounds curriculum for medical students' internal medicine clerkship during the COVID-19 pandemic. *MedEdPORTAL*. https://doi.org/10.15766/mep_2374-8265.11106 (accessed on 16th July 2025).

50. Towns, J., Cockerill, T. M., Dahan, M., Foster, I., Gaither, K., Grimshaw, A., Hazlewood, V., et al. (2014). XSEDE: Accelerating scientific discovery. *Computing in Science & Engineering, 16*, 62–74. https://doi.org/10.1109/mcse.2014.80 (accessed on 16th July 2025).

51. Ufomata, E., Eckstrand, K., Spagnoletti, C. L., Veet, C. A., Walk, T. J., Webb, C., Jiménez Gutiérrez, E., et al. (2020). Comprehensive curriculum for internal medicine residents on primary care of patients identifying as lesbian, gay, bisexual, or transgender. *MedEdPORTAL*. https://doi.org/10.15766/mep_2374-8265.10875 (accessed on 16th July 2025).

52. Van Hout, M., Akugizibwe, M., Shayo, E. H., Namulundu, M., Kasujja, F. X., Namakoola, I., Birungi, J., et al. (2024). Decentralizing chronic disease management in sub-Saharan Africa: A protocol for the qualitative process evaluation of community-based integrated management of HIV, diabetes and hypertension in Tanzania and Uganda. *BMJ Open, 14*. https://www.semanticscholar.org/paper/da5503502b6985965caa9022ba6de790445552f3 (accessed on 16th July 2025).

53. Yuan, C., Prince, L., Oliver, J. D., Abbott, K., & Nee, R. (2015). Implementation of nephrology subspecialty curricular milestones. *American Journal of Kidney Diseases: The Official Journal of the National Kidney Foundation, 66*(1), 15–22. https://www.semanticscholar.org/paper/f62ad25af59eab22bc773123349c7a969e22270e (accessed on 16th July 2025).

CARDIOLOGY

2

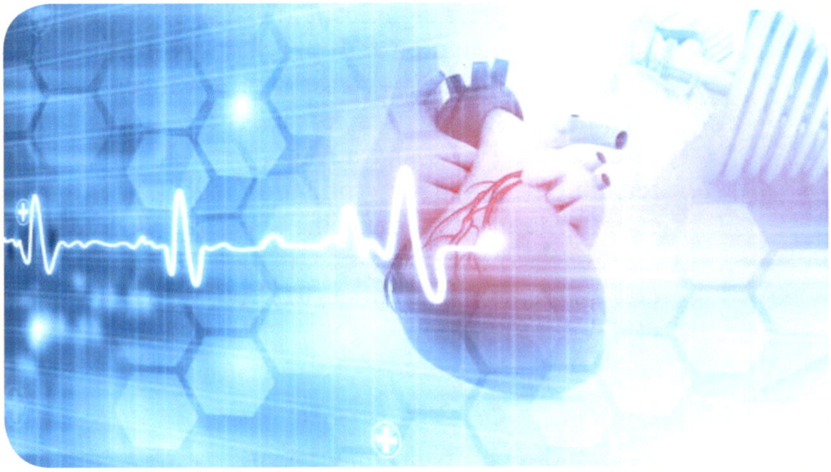

LEARNING OBJECTIVES

After studying this chapter, you will be able to:

1. Understand the role of internal medicine in cardiology
2. Explain the common cardiovascular diseases
3. Discuss the diagnostic tools in cardiology
4. Focus on treatment modalities in cardiology
5. Learn about preventive cardiology
6. Evaluate the challenges in cardiology

Introduction

The landscape of cardiology in internal medicine is changing rapidly due to advances in technology, shifts in patient demographics, and emerging health needs. With the world becoming increasingly older, the prevalence of cardiovascular illnesses is predicted to rise, resulting in an expanding reliance on advanced cardiology services. But this heightened demand stands in stark contrast to the current supply of the workforce, resulting in what has been termed a cardiology workforce crisis, as cited in a report by the American College of Cardiology. The shortage of cardiologists necessitates new strategies to ensure continued access to quality care. One of the proposed measures is expanded use of physician assistants (PAs) and nurse practitioners (NPs) in cardiovascular practice, particularly in echocardiography, an essential diagnostic test. This demands formal training programs to develop the skills of non-physician practitioners in cardiology to address workforce shortages (Moon et al., 2017). For smoother incorporation of PAs into the cardiology field, effective training curricula for skills such as echocardiographic procedures and interpretation are of paramount importance. Certain recent reports have discussed implementing pilot programs to design a uniform training process using Entrustable Professional Activities (EPA). Not only does this model offer a systematic approach to learning, but it also includes a procedure for assessing competence in essential clinical skills. By combining online didactic training with clinical practice education, these programs aim to train PAs to become competent in comprehensive cardiology positions, thereby alleviating the burden on cardiologists and even enhancing patient outcomes.

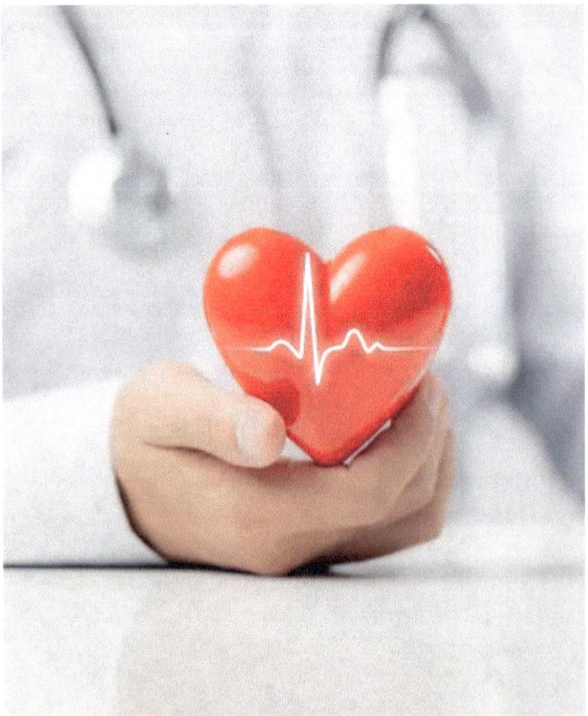

Figure 2.1. Cardiology: Life medical centre.

Furthermore, the proposed curriculum includes instruments for assessing graduates to ensure they have the requisite skills to practice independently, evidencing a proactive approach to addressing the manpower issue in cardiology (Moon et al., 2017). Parallel to the workforce strategic management, the emergence of deep learning in cardiology foretells a transition to more information-based, effective decision-making models. Traditional rule-based models have often struggled with the intricacies of cardiovascular care; however, deep learning technology offers a promising solution by allowing for more advanced analysis of medical data. These newer methodologies leverage massive electromagnetic datasets, such as structured data, signals, and imaging modalities, thus leading to increased diagnostic precision and predictive analytics. While deep learning integration offers significant advantages, it also raises implementation and applicability concerns in clinical settings. As research advances to examine these new uses, it is essential to tread through the limits and advantages well, while technology augments individualized patient care in the internal medicine specialty (Figure 2.1).*Source:* https://life-cdn.lifepharmacy.com/medical-centre/specialities/01J7AVQMHJR38FB00CFV2RF9P6.webp.

Overview of Cardiology

Cardiology, a vital subspecialty of internal medicine, involves the prevention, diagnosis, and management of cardiovascular disease. Cardiology has progressed significantly, with advances in technology and medical knowledge changing the way healthcare providers treat heart conditions. Cardiologists are experts at interpreting complex diagnostic tests, such as cardiac catheterizations, stress tests, and echocardiograms, which help detect heart disease even at its earliest stages and enable successful treatment. With heart failure and coronary artery disease remaining chief causes of morbidity, an awareness of their etiology and mechanisms is key. Perhaps the most significant aspect of cardiology is the development and modification of treatment regimens that not only address the acute presentation but also support long-term management plans to prevent cardiovascular disease. Current evidence underscores the importance of transitional care for patients transitioning from the hospital to home, particularly those with left ventricular assist devices (LVADs) (Hirschman et al., 2019). Such a patient group faces unique challenges that require targeted interventions and support to enhance their ability to manage complex medical needs. Improved transitional care has been proven to reduce hospital readmission rates, lower healthcare costs, and improve patients' quality of life, thereby strengthening cardiologists' role in whole-patient care. In such instances, nurse leadership becomes key to the process, facilitating patient and family education and support. By utilizing evidence-based transitional care, cardiologists can provide comprehensive care for heart failure and comorbid conditions.

This forward-looking approach has not only improved patient outcomes but also reflected the evolving nature of cardiology, advocating care models that emphasize teamwork. Parallel to these advances in patient care, deep learning technology is making a significant impact in cardiology. Such artificial intelligence technologies have the potential to continue enhancing diagnostic accuracy, risk stratification, and treatment decision-making using large, complex datasets (Bizopoulos et al., 2021). As cardiologists leverage the strength of deep learning, they will find themselves scanning imaging modalities and patient records for faint patterns that might otherwise go undetected. This shift toward data-driven approaches is but one part of a broader shift in medicine as traditional rule-based systems are being replaced by sophisticated algorithms capable of learning and adapting. However, the application of deep learning in cardiology also has benefits and challenges; effective utilization of these technologies in clinical practice will be the decisive factor in their success. Thus, as cardiology goes forward, synergy between traditional expertise and new technologies hopefully foretells a bright cardiovascular future (Figure 2.2).

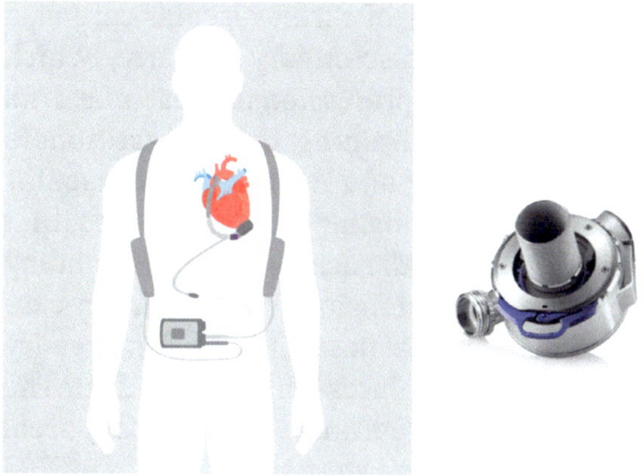

Figure 2.2. Left ventricular assist devices (LVAD).

Source: https://www.heartvascularcentre.com/wp-content/uploads/2019/08/HeartMate-3-LVAD-2.jpg.

Importance of Internal Medicine in Cardiology

Internal medicine becomes significant in cardiology due to its integrated approach to diagnosing and managing cardiovascular conditions. Internal medicine physicians play a pivotal role in evaluating patients presenting with nonspecific symptoms that may suggest coronary artery disease (CAD). For instance, women presenting with similar symptoms will likely have challenges in being diagnosed since clinical presentation is not as evident as that seen in men.

The inclusion of a blood-based precision medicine test, the age/sex/gene expression score (ASGES), was found to be clinically helpful for identifying obstructive CAD. The PRESET Registry showed that clinicians could personally tailor referrals for further cardiac assessment by ASGES and, in fact, enhance patient care and management strategy. This data shows how internal medicine effectively applies innovative testing in practice to improve patient outcomes by diagnosing those who will not benefit from aggressive cardiac interventions (Budoff et al., 2019). The growing complexity of cardiovascular care also necessitates multidisciplinary practice, which internal medicine professionals best perform. With the intensive training, these practitioners not only manage and treat cardiovascular diseases but also manage comorbidities that commonly occur with such conditions, including diabetes and hypertension. Whole-person care is particularly crucial in settings like emergency rooms, where early intervention is critical. The introduction of programs for extracorporeal cardiopulmonary resuscitation (eCPR) exemplifies this interprofessional collaboration.

By being aimed at cardiac arrest patients, such programs leverage the expertise of internal medicine, cardiothoracic surgery, and perfusion technology. The integration of eCPR's principles into practice illustrates the adaptability of internal medicine in new areas of cardiological practice, once more proving its pivotal role in the broader healthcare system (Becker et al., 2016). Additionally, preventive cardiology in internal medicine focuses on reducing the incidence of cardiovascular disease. Its reliance on lifestyle modification, risk factor identification, and early intervention makes internists responsible for guiding patients on heart health.

Proactive measures not only prevent the onset of coronary artery diseases but also reduce the severity of existing ones. Internal medicine physicians are often engaged in intensive risk assessment, which allows for expedient development of individualized care plans that foster patient involvement and compliance. Their role in ongoing patient follow-up and monitoring enhances the continuity of care required for long-term cardiovascular outcomes. The ability of internal medicine to integrate preventive interventions with specialized cardiological management is the essence of its role in optimizing health outcomes for affected and vulnerable patients with cardiac disease.

2.1. Role of Internal Medicine in Cardiology

Learning Outcome

1. Understand the comprehensive patient assessment
2. Describe the management of comorbidities
3. Identify the coordination of care

The integration of internal medicine with cardiology is imperative for managing the complex interactions among cardiovascular diseases and comorbidities. Internal medicine doctors are trained to address a broad spectrum of medical issues, which in cardiology is particularly useful because a majority of patients have multiple risk factors such as diabetes, hypertension, or renal impairment. All-around treatment allows internists to create well-rounded management protocols that are not only aimed at specific cardiac illnesses but also consider the patient's overall health condition. Research indicates that effective teamwork between primary care physicians and specialists can improve patient outcomes, particularly in chronic disease groups like heart failure, where collaborative interventions have achieved modest improvements in adherence to treatment guidelines (Forsyth et al., 2011). Thus, internal medicine's function is greater than mere diagnosis; it involves an integrated approach to patient care over the long term. Furthermore, internal medicine forms a foundation for preventive cardiology. Primary prevention is the focus of internal medicine professionals, who identify high-risk patients and implement early interventions to reduce risk factors for cardiac events. Preventive interventions are needed to create specific lifestyle changes, including diet and exercise programs, that have been established to lower the prevalence of cardiovascular disease significantly. Internists can collaborate with cardiologists to ensure that patients receive preventive and therapeutic interventions in accordance with current guidelines. The pharmacists' role in such a model, as supported by current clinical trials, is that when non-specialist pharmacists are involved in multidisciplinary care to optimize medical therapy, impressive gains in medication adherence are achieved (Forsyth et al., 2011). This model illustrates the synergy between cardiology and internal medicine in improving health outcomes. Apart from direct patient care, internal medicine plays a pivotal role in new pharmacological strategies into cardiology. The new drug listing process, for instance, as assessed by Hong Kong's Drug Advisory Committee (DAC), emphasizes the supremacy of evidence-based practice in cardiology. Internal medicine specialists conduct rigorous scrutiny of drugs, weighing their safety, efficacy, and economic value before endorsing their use. This scrutiny ensures therapeutic interventions offered to cardiologists are evidence-based, ultimately improving patient care. With the evolving situation in pharmaceuticals and treatment modalities, internal medicine-cardiology collaborations play an important role in adopting innovations that translate into patient care benefits, demonstrating how collaborative practice can lead to well-informed and effective clinical decisions (Figure 2.3).

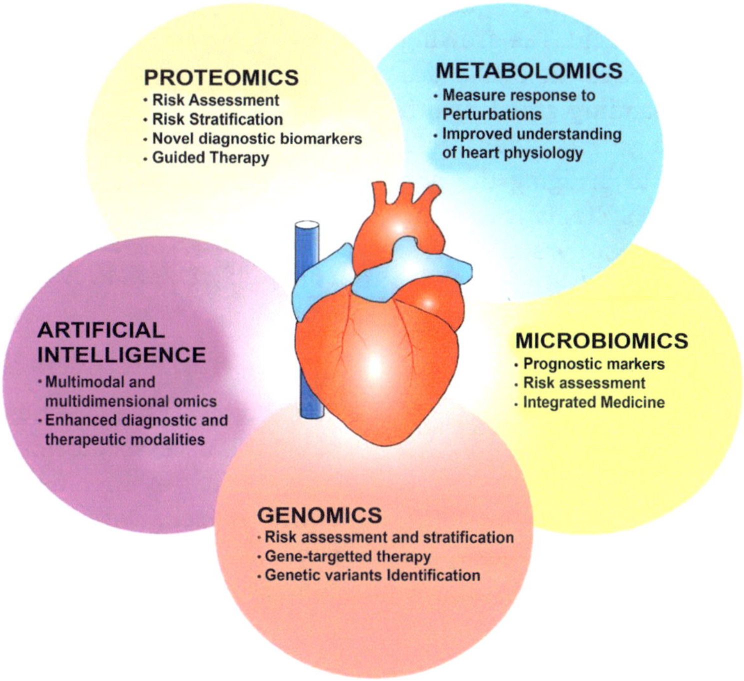

Figure 2.3. Role of internal medicine in cardiology.

Source: https://www.mdpi.com/jcm/jcm-12-01799/article_deploy/html/images/jcm-12-01799-g003.png.

2.1.1. Comprehensive Patient Assessment

A comprehensive patient workup is a key foundation in the practice of internal medicine, particularly in cardiology. The workup typically involves an in-depth understanding of the patient's history, a physical examination, and an evaluation of extensive pertinent diagnostic studies. In cardiology, the need for a methodical approach cannot be overstated, as cardiovascular disease often requires precise sensitivity to risk factors and symptomatology. To achieve this, medical professionals should tactfully elicit data about the patient's history, family history, and prior medical encounters. Such a multifaceted assessment enables clinicians to recognize subtle signs of cardiac disease that might otherwise go undetected, paving the way for timely interventions and better patient outcomes. Besides, the inclusion of specialized training programs for physician assistants (PAs) in cardiology, specifically in echocardiography, is necessary to address the need for high-quality tests for cardiac care (Moon et al., 2017). At a time when cardiovascular disease increases, particularly in the older population, the necessity of proper patient assessment becomes more evident. The growing consensus holds that, whereas cardiologists face a workforce shortage, expanding allied health practitioners' abilities, e.g., PAs and nurse practitioners, is essential to bridging the gap (Moon et al., 2017). By using systematic training processes designed for these practitioners, patient assessment quality and efficiency can be significantly improved. The proposed curriculum for teaching echocardiography to PAs meets this need, as it is designed to further enhance competence in cardiac imaging performance and interpretation. By providing solid foundation skills in echocardiography, PAs can play a primary role in the comprehensive assessment process, thereby improving healthcare practice in cardiology centers where specialty providers may be limited (Moon et al., 2017). Furthermore, the cycle of feedback created by continuous evaluation and training programs is essential to developing comprehensive patient assessments within cardiology. One step in establishing formal training, such as the pilot echocardiography curriculum, is to address individual areas of deficiency within PA training programs (Moon et al., 2017). Such programs not only equip PAs with the required competencies but also promote evidence-based practices in patient evaluation across various regions and health care settings. With the evolution of the profession, it becomes increasingly essential to develop evidence on the effectiveness of such training programs and ensure they meet the demands of both patients and providers. With broad, comprehensive patient assessment as a team-based effort among multidimensional healthcare providers, team-based care can deliver enhanced clinical outcomes and patient satisfaction in cardiology (Figure 2.4).

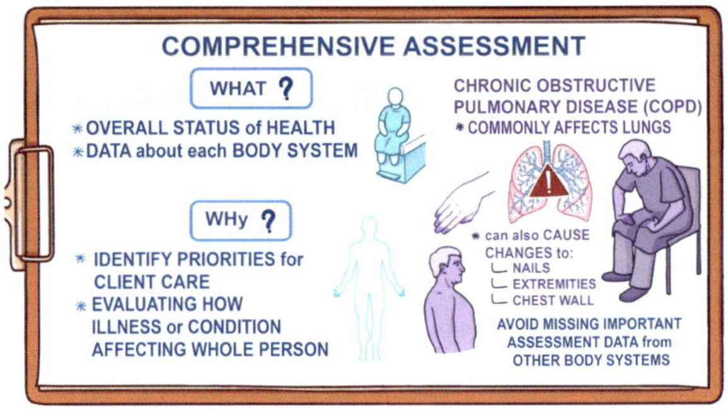

Figure 2.4. Comprehensive patient assessment.

Source: https://osmose-it.s3.amazonaws.com/Y6KvJJgjSyiIvZsKMOc9BqdLQd_uLVSR/_.jpg.

2.1.2. Management of Comorbidities

Comorbidities management for cardiovascular patients is necessary to improve patient outcomes and quality of life. Cardiovascular diseases typically occur with other chronic conditions, such as diabetes and hypertension, that complicate therapeutic regimens and aggravate the general health status of patients. It is imperative to apply a multidisciplinary approach that integrates evidence from specialties such as endocrinology, cardiology, and internal medicine to address the complexity of managing these interconnected health conditions. A recent article reached consensus among professionals, highlighting the need to address diabetes-related comorbidities, cardiovascular risk factors, and renal function management to develop effective management measures for patients with multicomorbidity (Campuzano-Ruiz et al., 2024). It can lead to individualized treatment approaches that not only manage the individual diseases but also address the risk generated by their comorbidity. Moreover, the intricacy of intertwined cardiovascular well-being with other comorbid diseases, such as atrial fibrillation (AF) and premature ventricular contractions (PVCs), necessitates vigilant monitoring and management. Atrial fibrillation is the most prevalent cardiac arrhythmia, and it is linked to numerous risk factors that may promote its occurrence and recurrence (Harvey et al., 2017). Evidence proves that patients who come in for catheter ablation of AF have a high likelihood of having PVCs, demonstrating the overlap of these arrhythmias. Treatment at this overlap is essential not only in the acute management of symptoms, but also long-term, especially in that those who come in with more than one condition will generally have a higher burden of mortality and morbidity.

Thus, ideal comorbid management must prioritize ongoing assessment and adjustment of treatment regimens to accommodate such complexities. Lastly, implementation of structured care plans involving lifestyle interventions remains a significant factor in managing comorbidities in the field of cardiology. Interventions like the cessation of smoking, dietary changes, and exercise can have significant impacts on cardiovascular status and also on other illnesses like diabetes. These interventions are supported by a growing body of evidence indicating that integrated lifestyle management can significantly reduce cardiovascular events and overall health outcomes in patients.

By educating and activating, healthcare professionals can empower patients to become contributing participants in managing their health. This method is aligned with evidence-based guidelines on diabetes management that emphasize lifestyle modification alongside medical treatment (Campuzano-Ruiz et al., 2024). Ultimately, efficient comorbid treatment in cardiovascular patients demands a holistic strategy that reconciles clinical expertise with patient participation in their own treatment (Figure 2.5).

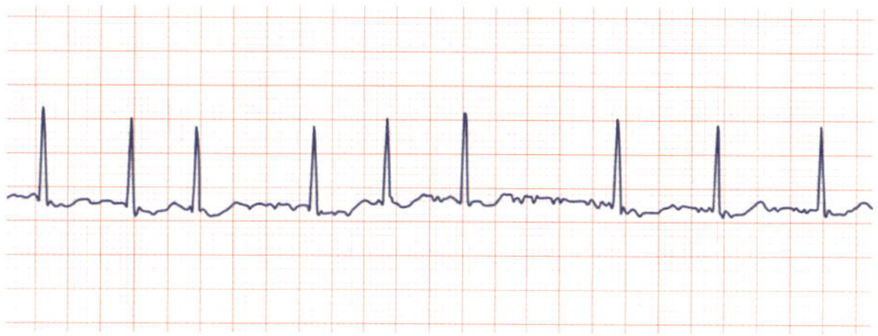

Figure 2.5. Atrial fibrillation (AF).

Source: https://www.aclsmedicaltraining.com/wp-content/uploads/2021/09/ACLS-Figure-30.jpg.

2.1.3. Coordination of Care

Efficient coordination of care is essential for the management of patients with complex cardiovascular conditions. This coordination is achieved with open communication among healthcare professionals, family, and patients to facilitate adherence to and knowledge of treatment regimens. For patients with chronic diseases like heart failure who might require sophisticated treatment such as left ventricular assist devices (LVADs), the nuances of LVAD care and lifestyle adjustments associated with it can be overwhelming. Implementing evidence-based transitional care interventions can reduce avoidable hospital rehospitalizations and improve overall quality of life (Hirschman et al., 2019). The interventions include proactive nurse engagement and protocol-following follow-up processes, which create a support system that enhances patient understanding and adherence. It then follows that effective organization and information transmission within interdisciplinary teams become critical because they have direct impacts on patient outcomes and transitions of care. Diagnostic errors are a significant problem in cardiology, highlighting the importance of care coordination. In intensive care environments like pediatric cardiac intensive care units, diagnostic collapse is caused by several factors, including inadequate appraisal of information and overload of clinician work (Aiyagari et al., 2018). Diagnostic errors may jeopardize patient safety and lead to disastrous complications or even death. The incorporation of coordinated, comprehensive care seeks to reduce these risks by ensuring that each team member is aligned on patient status, diagnostic interventions, and treatment regimens. Through teamwork and the implementation of standardized mechanisms for feedback, medical teams are more likely to recognize potential pitfalls in diagnosis and develop remedies to address them. Better communication encourages a culture of accountability and assists patient trust, which is essential for successful treatment outcomes. Finally, the application of advanced care coordination models in cardiology involves an integrated approach to enhancing patient management in healthcare environments. The models ensure a team-based process in which clinicians from various specialties interact to create harmoniously designed treatment plans tailored to each patient. For patients requiring advanced interventions, such as those with LVADs, this coordinated care model ensures continuity, facilitating improved transitions from inpatient to outpatient care (Hirschman et al., 2019). In addition, integrating technology, such as telehealth systems, can enable healthcare teams to monitor patients more effectively remotely, facilitating timely intervention and the modification of care plans. By continually improving these care coordination activities, the care system can better manage the complexity of cardiology and enhance the quality of care and patient outcomes. Thus, effective care coordination is a building block for quality in the ever-increasing complexity of cardiology within internal medicine.

Test Your Knowledge

1. How do internists contribute to the early detection of cardiovascular diseases?
2. What role does internal medicine play in managing cardiac risk factors such as hypertension and diabetes?

2.2. Common Cardiovascular Diseases (CVDs)

Learning Outcome

1. Define the hypertension
2. Describe the coronary artery disease (CAD)
3. Explain the heart failure

CVDs are a heavy public health toll and encompass diseases such as hypertension, coronary heart disease, heart failure, and arrhythmias. Of these, hypertension has become a significant cause of morbidity and mortality, particularly in the developing world. The implications of untreated hypertension are grim, as it is mainly found in young age groups in the sub-Saharan African region, resulting in sudden complications in the form of heart failure. The critical importance of early detection and management of hypertension in such low-resource settings cannot be overestimated. Preventive interventions, in combination with community-based treatment and screening models, have shown promise in blunting the burden of hypertension and improving cardiovascular well-being among vulnerable populations (Twagirumukiza et al., 2011). Successful control of hypertension is fundamental to the reduction of the incidence of cardiovascular disease, yet achievement of target blood pressures remains a challenge for the majority of health care systems. Despite advances in pharmacologic therapy, noncompliance with drug therapy and heterogeneity of patient response to treatment are determinants leading to failure in blood pressure control. The traditional management of hypertension, too often an oversimplified or hit-or-miss regimen, is not a sufficiently precise response to the multifactorial interaction between individual risk factors and genetic determinants that control treatment effectiveness. The illness needs a better understanding. This requires an interdisciplinary treatment strategy that encourages individualized management programs tailored to each patient's unique biological and psychosocial features to facilitate improved control of hypertension and protection against its complications (Borghi et al., 2017). In addition to hypertension, coronary heart disease represents another prevalent and deadly CVD that must be accorded intensive deliberation under internal medicine. Atherosclerosis, or the buildup of plaques in arterial walls, is the main cause of this condition. The risk factors for coronary artery disease include hypertension, diabetes mellitus, smoking, and dyslipidemia, which also tend to be present together in patients, increasing the difficulty of management. Lifestyle modification, including dietary changes, increased physical activity, and smoking cessation, cannot be overstressed in the treatment of these risk factors. Second, the position of pharmacotherapy, in particular with statins and antihypertensive agents, is imperative in managing high-risk patients for coronary events. To that end, an interlocked strategy comprising lifestyle interventions and appropriate medical treatment is called for to combat the increasing incidence of coronary artery disease and to improve overall cardiovascular well-being (Twagirumukiza et al., 2011) (Figure 2.6).

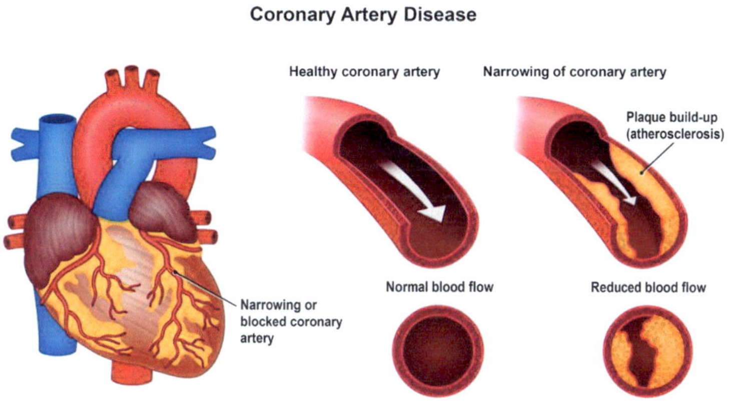

Figure 2.6. Coronary artery disease (CAD).

Source: https://cdn-assets-eu.frontify.com/s3/frontify-enterprise-files-eu/eyJwYXRoIjoiaWhoLWhlYWx0aGNhcmUtYmVyaGFkXC9hY2NvdW50c1wvYzNcLzQwMDA2MjRcL3Byb2plY3RzXC8yMDlcL2Fzc2V0c1wvZjJcL zM2MjIwXC80OTQ3YWY4YTQwZThhYWY0MjFjZTY4NjUwZDE2N DZmZC0xNjU2Mzg0MTAyLmpwZyJ9:ihh-healthcare-berhad:eR6HeX9v_KllIbbgX gvhWg kRyUy2f3FgFguRW9kQF40?format=webp.

2.2.1. Hypertension

Hypertension remains a significant public health problem around the world, particularly in the practice of internal medicine and cardiology, where its cardiovascular consequences are grave.

It is characterized by abnormally high blood pressure maintained over a long period of time, which increases the risk of potentially fatal complications like heart failure, stroke, and myocardial infarction. The epidemiology of hypertension is in line with an alarming trend, especially in developing nations where the disease is infecting young populations. The worst scenario is found in sub-Saharan Africa, with hypertension becoming the leading etiology of cardiovascular morbidity and mortality among young adults, posing an acute public health problem requiring swift response and intervention (Twagirumukiza et al., 2011). Effective control measures must prioritize early identification and treatment, since the condition of uncontrolled hypertension can lead to irreversible organ damage and drastically impaired quality of life. In the control of hypertension, the health system is tested in certain aspects, particularly in low-resource settings where medical treatment and selection of treatment are suboptimal. Socioeconomic constraints in the majority of developing countries make it impossible for patients to access needed medications and lifestyle interventions that would help mitigate the effects of hypertension. This reality necessitates implementing cost-reducing screening and management techniques at the community level. Standardized care protocols for the detection and treatment of hypertension can provide an organized approach that enables healthcare workers to allocate resources effectively and improve outcomes (Twagirumukiza et al., 2011). Further, population-level programs could also empower individuals by educating them and helping them adopt an active approach to health based on prevention and early intervention. Since the practice of internal medicine incorporates improved control mechanisms for hypertension, focus must also shift towards its correlation with other cardiovascular diseases, like atrial fibrillation. The co-occurrence of these two diseases makes it more difficult to develop treatment regimens and requires a holistic approach to understanding their interaction. Hypertensive individuals are at greater risk of developing atrial fibrillation due to long-standing high blood pressure's electrical and structural changes in the heart. In most cases, treatment of these comorbid conditions requires a careful balance between blood pressure control and anticoagulation therapy. Treatment innovations, such as the introduction of new oral anticoagulants (NOACs), hold promising alternatives that improve patient quality of life and reduce the need for intense monitoring. That said, the multifaceted interdependence among these cardiovascular risks underscores the utility of an integrative approach in internal medicine, with a focus on individualized therapies targeting hypertension and its potential sequelae (Figure 2.7).

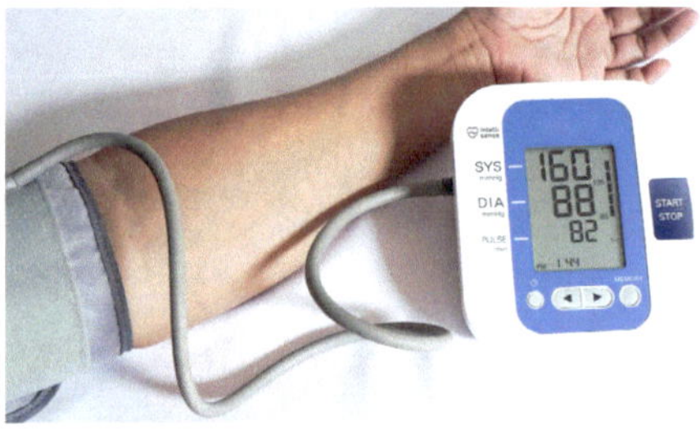

Figure 2.7. Hypertension.

Source: https://www.rafflesmedicalgroup.com/wp-content/uploads/2022/01/hypertension.jpg.

2.2.2. Coronary Artery Disease (CAD)

CAD remains a serious health problem, affecting millions and inflicting a tremendous burden of morbidity and mortality on the world. Its pathophysiology involves the insidious formation of atherosclerotic plaques in the coronary arteries, leading to reduced perfusion and potential myocardial ischemia. It is caused by hypertension, hyperlipidemia, diabetes, and lifestyle factors of smoking and physical inactivity. Most concerning, however, is the undertreatment of CAD in women diagnosed with atypical symptoms that fall outside normal diagnostic parameters. New technologies, particularly the use of techniques like the age/sex/gene expression score (ASGES), yield details on the diagnosis process and reveal that the inclusion of new biomarkers can enhance the sensitivity to diagnose obstructive CAD in women and thus ensure timely intervention and treatment (Budoff et al., 2019). The prognostic relevance of coronary artery disease extends beyond medical diagnosis and profoundly influences the lines of treatment. Accurate staging of CAD severity is a key factor in maximizing therapeutic interventions, including lifestyle modifications, pharmacological treatments, and interventional therapies. A new area of research integrates machine learning approaches with coronary computed tomography angiography to improve predictive value for rapid coronary plaque progression (RPP), which is also closely associated with adverse cardiovascular outcomes. By using quantitative measurements of plaque features alongside conventional clinical examinations, clinicians can more effectively stratify risk, ultimately leading to individualized treatment protocols that account for patient-specific profiles. The study presented in the PARADIGM registry demonstrates the ability of new imaging techniques and machine learning to identify patients at higher risk of coronary events, thereby improving overall CAD management (Al'Aref et al., 2020). In addition, the incorporation of several diagnostic instruments into routine clinical practice illustrates cardiology's evolving face in managing coronary artery disease. Physicians increasingly must contend with complex patient data, weighing older risk factors alongside more recent predictive analyses. Incorporation of ASGES scores has improved risk stratification in women, with those with low scores likely to have a lower need for further assessment and evaluation, and those with higher scores requiring aggressive management strategies. With the ongoing evolution of cardiology, ongoing education and interdisciplinary collaboration need to be emphasized to ensure that both existing and new techniques are appropriately applied in clinical practice. The newly emerging problems with CAD highlight the importance of integrated management strategies that include lifestyle interventions, drug therapy, and surveillance, all tailored to the individual, leading to improved patient outcomes in internal medicine and cardiology (Budoff et al., 2019; Al'Aref et al., 2020).

2.2.3. Heart Failure

Heart failure is a complex clinical syndrome characterized by the heart's inability to pump sufficient blood to maintain the metabolic demand of the body. It most often results from a range of primary diseases, the most significant being hypertension, which is now a major health issue globally, particularly in the developing world. As indicated in previous studies, hypertension in sub-Saharan Africa hits young adults hard, leading to severe complications such as heart failure. The interaction of socioeconomic determinants aggravates this situation, and optimal treatment approaches are inaccessible to most of the patients due to economic constraints. This situation points towards early identification of hypertensive patients and their management to prevent the occurrence of irreversible damage to the heart. Optimal community-level interventions focusing on both non-pharmacologic and pharmacologic care can significantly decrease the risk of hypertension complications and development into heart failure (Twagirumukiza et al., 2011). Moreover, heart failure treatment not only focuses on pharmacologic therapy but also on non-drug management practices such as patient self-management and lifestyle modification. Community education and awareness interventions in public health can empower patients to recognize symptoms early and adhere to prescribed management plans. Interventions such as care coordination and coordinated health services are needed; they facilitate comprehensive care that addresses not only the clinical but also the psychosocial aspects of heart failure.

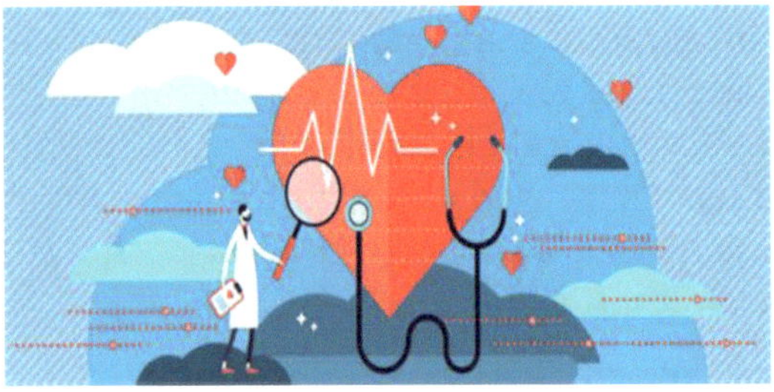

Figure 2.8. On the cutting edge of heart disease prevention and treatment.

Source: https://external-content.duckduckgo.com/iu/?u=https%3A%2F%2Ftse2.mm.bing.net%2Fth%2Fid%2FOIP.CU0099 OuJpGruhAaiPuWnQHaDA%3Fpid%3DApi&f=1&ipt=725463ad278f898b17bd2772a0a27 239ffab22f89f25b74c8e828d0fff0c3ac1.

Care continuity models supported by research evidence can lead to remarkable improvements in patients' outcomes. Encouraging patient self-management within the care system is crucial to enhancing quality of life, reducing hospitalizations, and ultimately improving survival in heart failure patients (Morton et al., 2015). Thus, developing standard algorithms for managing hypertension and heart failure in such environments has the potential to optimize resource use without compromising essential care for vulnerable populations. Stakeholder input, including that of healthcare professionals, policymakers, and community leaders, is critical for developing interventions that are specific and account for the challenges encountered by heart failure patients (Twagirumukiza et al., 2011) (Figure 2.8).

Interpreting policy and research knowledge into effective, practical, community-focused healthcare solutions remains a key element to successfully managing heart failure. As the literature has established, what is most needed in health care systems is to accord priority to access to affordable, appropriate treatment within the context of the populations they serve. Particularly so in low-resource environments where recommendations to traditional treatments may not be viable.

Test Your Knowledge

1. What are the most common types of cardiovascular diseases?
2. What are the major risk factors contributing to cardiovascular diseases?

2.3. Diagnostic Tools in Cardiology

Learning Outcome

1. Define electrocardiogram (ECG)
2. Discuss on echocardiography
3. Describe the cardiac catheterization

Cardiology evolves continuously, and the equipment used in diagnosis plays a leading role in enhancing patient care. Echocardiography is one such equipment that is a fundamental technique with the help of transmission and reflection of ultrasonic waves, to visualize cardiac structures and assess the function of the heart. Its non-invasive nature and ability to provide real-time data have made it essential for diagnosing several cardiovascular conditions, ranging from valvular heart disease to heart failure. However, the use of echocardiography is threatened by challenges, particularly the availability of experienced personnel. The

American College of Cardiology has documented a growing shortage of the cardiology workforce, which will likely be exacerbated by an aging population and the consequent increase in cardiovascular service needs (Moon et al., 2017). Thus, innovative training methods for physician assistants (PAs) and nurse practitioners (NPs) in echocardiography are required to address manpower shortages and improve patient outcomes. Besides echocardiography, other diagnostic modalities have become a cornerstone of cardiology. Electrocardiography (ECG) remains a valuable tool for diagnosing arrhythmias, myocardial ischemia, and other electrical heart diseases. Its simplicity and ease of access make patient monitoring both clinically efficient and accessible via remote ambulatory monitors. The integration of digital health technologies has also revolutionized ECG interpretation, enabling remote monitoring and intervention. In addition, advanced imaging modalities such as CMR and CT angiography can provide improved anatomical and functional information, facilitating the diagnosis of advanced cardiac disease. The integration of these modalities provides a comprehensive assessment and management of cardiovascular disease, enabling tailored treatment recommendations for patients. Moreover, the importance of continued education and standardized training for healthcare professionals cannot be overstated. Strong guidelines facilitate the establishment of echocardiography training programs to enhance PAs' and NPs' proficiency in this valuable diagnostic modality. The development of an echocardiography-specific, standardized curriculum, aligned with Entrustable Professional Activities (EPA) principles, provides an educational model for education providers to further develop expertise while easing workforce shortages (Moon et al., 2017). Such initiatives not only ensure that cardiology professionals remain up to date on emerging technologies but also encourage a culture of collaborative care, in which large numbers of healthcare professionals can be actively engaged in cardiac diagnostic practice. Lastly, these strides in training and the integration of technology support the significant role that diagnostic equipment plays in improving cardiovascular care in the practice of internal medicine for cardiology (Figure 2.9).

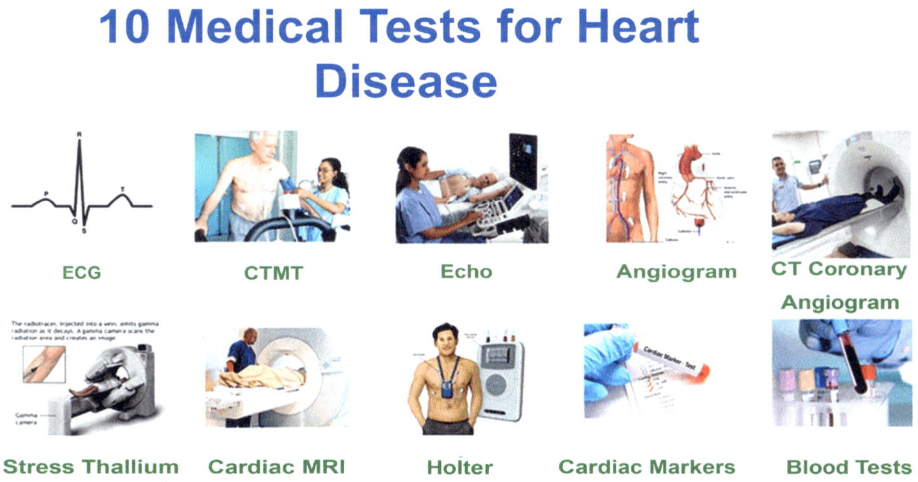

Figure 2.9. Medical tests to diagnose heart disease.

Source: https://www.peoplehearthealth.com/blog/wp-content/uploads/2021/03/10-Medical-Tests-for-Heart-Disease.png.

2.3.1. Electrocardiogram (ECG)

ECG is an important diagnostic tool in cardiology, providing a comprehensive view of cardiac function and rhythm. This process is non-invasive and measures the electrical activity of the heart by using electrodes on the skin to produce an ECG tracing. The widespread use of ECGs across clinical settings is a reminder of their value in diagnosing a wide range of cardiac diseases, including arrhythmias, ischemia, and structural heart disease. New advances in automated analysis have further enhanced the utility of ECGs, enabling doctors to receive quick interpretations to improve patient care. Although such innovation is promising, controversy remains over the limitations of automated systems and the need for trained human interpretation, particularly in complex cases where nuances are lost (Abächerli et al., 2017). Recent studies have highlighted the potential to apply machine learning techniques to enhance the capabilities of standard ECGs. By using large datasets, researchers have developed models that leverage convolutional neural networks and Hidden Markov Models to improve the accuracy of ECG results. For instance, computer processing of a large cohort has led to new methods for estimating key cardiac parameters, such as left ventricular mass and left atrial volume, derived from standard ECG recordings (Delling et al., 2018). Advanced models of this type have excellent performance in discriminating between various cardiac illnesses, potentially enabling earlier diagnosis and treatment. As machine learning continues to evolve, it will transform ECG interpretation, making it an even more powerful diagnostic tool for evaluating patients in cardiology. Incorporation of advanced algorithms and computer platforms into daily practice, however, requires careful balancing of their effects on interpretation. While machine learning models have remarkable predictive performance for cardiovascular endpoints, it is essential to preserve the transparency and interpretability of these analyses to support effective medical decision-making. Clinicians must remain engaged in the ECG interpretation process so they are aware of the context of the data observed and the assumptions made by automated systems. The optimal approach might involve a model of cooperation in which computerized testing is supplementary to professional human evaluation, providing diagnostic accuracy without sacrificing clinician involvement in patient management (Abächerli et al., 2017). The challenge is to balance innovation with pragmatism, drawing as much value as possible from ECG technology without undermining the value of cardiology consultations in internal medicine.

2.3.2. Echocardiography

Echocardiography is an important diagnostic modality in cardiology that provides vital information about cardiac anatomy and function through non-invasive imaging. Echocardiography employs ultrasound waves to generate accurate images of the heart and allows clinicians to assess various cardiac conditions such as valvular heart disease, heart failure, and congenital abnormalities. By visualizing live heart motion, echocardiography also provides for enhanced diagnosis and treatment planning, thereby becoming an integral component of outpatient and inpatient care. With advances in the field, the continuous development of echocardiographic technology, such as 3D imaging and sophisticated Doppler techniques, has transformed diagnostic accuracy and consistency. Also, the integration of point-of-care ultrasound (POCUS) into clinical practice underscores echocardiography's growing role in medical education and its utility in enhancing patient care, although the evidence base supporting some educational claims remains controversial (Dornan et al., 2017). In the field of internal medicine, echocardiography extends beyond diagnostic use; it significantly influences patient treatment and prognosis. Physicians can modify therapeutic maneuvers based on echocardiographic findings by assessing the severity of heart disease and its trend over time. In patients with suspected heart failure, for instance, echocardiography provides critical information on left ventricular function, which informs medical therapy and device-based interventions such as implantable cardioverter-defibrillators. Second, echocardiography facilitates risk stratification for surgery, such as valve replacement or repair, allowing clinicians to predict outcomes and make patient selection more individualized.

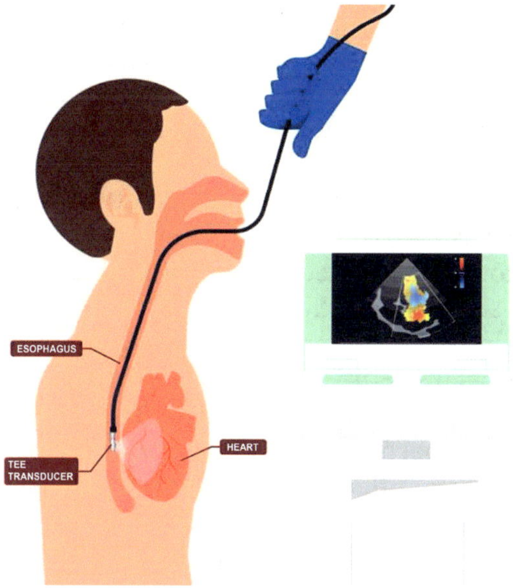

Figure 2.10. Transesophageal echocardiogram (ECG).

Source: https://www.ameliaheartcenter.com/wp-content/uploads/2021/12/TEE-768x768.jpg.

These applications illustrate echocardiography's contribution to personalized medicine in cardiology, further cementing its worth in developing holistic care plans (Biffi et al., 2019). The educational aspect of echocardiography is also essential, since students and residents are increasingly being instructed in this specialty to equip them with the skills needed for current clinical practice. As imaging becomes increasingly pertinent to patient assessment, the addition of echocardiography training to undergraduate medical education has become paramount. Despite this, recent concerns about the educational value of ultrasound in the teaching of anatomy and physical examination skills have arisen, with a need for more vigorous empirical justification for its use in teaching (Dornan et al., 2017). In light of these concerns, the medical community remains dedicated to equipping future healthcare professionals with the skills needed to use echocardiography effectively. Lastly, an appropriately established educational framework can foster the optimal utilization of echocardiography in internal medicine, enhancing the quality of overall patient care (Figure 2.10).

2.3.3. Cardiac Catheterization

Cardiac catheterization is a foundational diagnostic and therapeutic technique in cardiology that allows clinicians to visualize the inner workings of the heart and blood vessels. This minimally invasive technique involves placing a catheter into a blood vessel, typically in the arm or groin, and then threading it into the heart. Surgeons can measure pressures in the heart chambers, assess blood flow, and take fluoroscopic images. The data collected using catheterization is crucial for diagnosing several cardiac diseases, such as coronary artery disease, valve disease, and congenital heart defects. Its use is not only for diagnostic purposes; it is also employed in therapeutic interventions such as angioplasty and stenting, playing a critical role in the management of acute coronary syndromes. Within internal medicine, cardiac catheterization is the intersection of patient management and diagnostic technology. The process itself is most often an essential step toward informed treatment decision-making, serving as the foundation for tailored interventions based on each patient's unique cardiovascular condition. A greater emphasis on the importance of risk factor assessment, such as hypertension, diabetes, and family history, that may influence the success of the procedure has been laid. Also, advancements in catheter technologies and imaging modalities have greatly improved procedural efficacy and safety. For instance, newer catheters may reduce procedure-related complications, thereby reducing recovery times and overall patient outcomes. The continued evolution of these technologies underscores the field's commitment to improving patient care through enhanced procedural methods. Yet despite its benefits, cardiac catheterization carries risks and potential complications that must be weighed carefully by health professionals. Potential complications include bleeding at the site where the catheter has been inserted, infection, and even arrhythmias. All these dangers necessitate a thorough pre-procedure evaluation and informed patient consent. Guidelines from prominent cardiology societies recommend the use of a multi-disciplinary consensus in deciding which patients to catheterize based on the patient's symptoms, tests, and general health status. The controversy regarding the necessity and frequency of catheterization interventions among certain populations remains a pressing issue, requiring further investigation and revised clinical practices to ensure the risks are lower than the benefits of this precious diagnostic and therapeutic procedure in modern-day cardiology.

Test Your Knowledge

1. What is the role of an electrocardiogram (ECG) in diagnosing heart diseases?
2. Why is echocardiography important in cardiac assessment?

2.4. Treatment Modalities

Learning Outcome

1. Understand the pharmacological interventions
2. Define the lifestyle modifications
3. Discuss surgical options

Treatment modalities for many cardiovascular diseases are important considerations for maximizing patient outcomes and reducing morbidity. Treatment is most commonly multimodal, integrating lifestyle modification, pharmacologic treatment, and interventional therapies tailored to the patient's specific needs. For instance, hypertension treatment may involve dietary restrictions, increased physical activity, and medications such as ACE inhibitors or beta-blockers, targeting specific components of blood pressure regulation. Evidence-based guidelines often inform such treatments by targeting patient-centered care and shared decision-making strategies, which can enhance treatment adherence. Last but not least, effective cardiology interventions rely on a clear understanding of each patient's individualized clinical profile, thereby making treatment modalities both effective and feasible. The strongly rising prevalence of atrial fibrillation (AF) warrants an extensive scrutiny of treatment modalities against this complex arrhythmia. Several studies highlight catheter ablation as one of the most effective treatments for patients with symptomatic AF. Evidence presently indicates that a high percentage of patients undergoing pulmonary vein isolation ablation present with PVCs, and predictors for the development of new PVCs include a history of PVCs before ablation (Harvey et al., 2017). This finding underscores the importance of preoperative assessment and long-term follow-up after intervention to minimize the risk of complications. These observations inform cardiologists' practice in the management of AF, highlighting the active role of interprofessional collaboration in selecting effective interventions based on patient-specific variables. In addition to catheter-based treatments, medication remains a cornerstone of the treatment algorithm for the management of AF. Anticoagulants play a central role in mitigating stroke risk, a significant concern in patients diagnosed with the arrhythmia. The advent of direct oral anticoagulants (DOACs) has made pharmacologic management a piece of cake, with improved safety profiles compared with traditional vitamin K antagonists. Nonetheless, the choice among them should be carefully balanced against the patient's renal impairment, propensity for bleeding, and drug interactions. Owing to the dynamic nature of the treatment setting, ongoing research and clinical trials must be conducted to expand the understanding of pharmacotherapies' function in cardiology, as well as the identification of novel potential treatment modalities that can most effectively maximize patient management and results in heart disease (Kitsiou et al., 2013) (Figure 2.11).

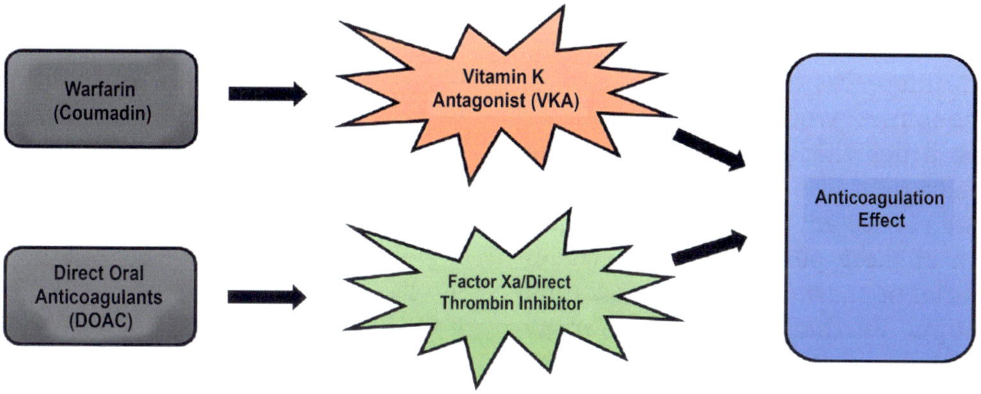

Figure 2.11. Direct oral anticoagulants (DOACs).

Source: https://health.ucdavis.edu/media-resources/pharmacy/images/Anticoag/DOAC-illustration.jpg.

2.4.1. Pharmacological Interventions

In the realm of internal medicine, pharmacological interventions play a pivotal role in the management of cardiovascular diseases. Through these interventions, a wide array of drugs specifically designed to counter risk factors, alleviate symptoms, and improve heart function are used. Among the most commonly employed agents are antihypertensives, statins, and antiplatelets that target specific parameters of cardiovascular health. Antihypertensive agents, for example, are crucial for regulating blood pressure, thereby preventing heart attacks and strokes. Statins are at the center of lipid management, effectively lowering low-density lipoprotein (LDL) cholesterol levels to help counter atherosclerosis. Another category of drugs, antiplatelet drugs such as aspirin, avoids clot formation, similarly safeguarding patients against acute coronary events. Thus, pharmacological management is central to the overall treatment practices employed in cardiology. Pharmacological interventions are usually patient-specific in their effectiveness, depending on age, sex, and comorbidities, so that ideally, pharmacological treatment would be patient-specific. In the case of cardiovascular diseases, pharmacology becomes particularly sophisticated, reflecting variability within risk categories, for example, in women and men. For instance, the prevalence of cardiovascular conditions, such as coronary heart disease, could be different in populations; in Saudi Arabia, for example, the burden of such diseases is exacerbated by risk factors like physical inactivity and obesity among women. Achieving the best therapeutic result requires taking such differences into account. Besides, pharmacogenomics would guide clinicians in selecting drugs that not only match the clinical scenario but also enhance therapeutic response and reduce adverse effects. A proper appreciation of these personal characteristics is hence crucial in pharmacologic optimization in cardiology. Further, pharmacotherapy remains subject to studies that direct the management of cardiovascular conditions. Recent advances have led to the development of novel agents and combination therapies that promise improved results in patients with heart disease. For example, the introduction of newer anticoagulants and new classes of antihypertensives has been demonstrated to be effective across different patient populations, with the promise of addressing unmet needs in the management of cardiovascular disease. In Saudi Arabia, where cultural factors and access to healthcare may influence medication adherence and outcomes, the inclusion of culturally acceptable medication management is all the more critical (Clark et al., 2012). As cardiology healthcare professionals face these challenges, the emphasis on pharmacologic interventions aims not just to inhibit disease progression but to enhance patients' quality of life. Such integrated interventions underscore the need for a dynamic model of therapy in cardiology.

2.4.2. Lifestyle Modifications

Lifestyle changes serve as an essential support in managing cardiovascular health, significantly lowering the risk of becoming a victim of conditions such as hypertension and heart disease. These tend to focus on changes in diet, exercise, and controlling stress. An appropriate diet rich in fruits, vegetables, whole grains, and lean protein not only supports weight maintenance but also lowers underlying risk factors. The Mediterranean diet, in particular, has shown promising results in clinical practice by promoting heart health through healthy fats and nutrient-dense foods, leading to better lipid levels and better control of blood pressure. Incorporating exercise into daily activity reinforces cardiovascular fitness by encouraging circulation, reducing blood pressure, and maintaining a healthy body weight. Overall, adherence to lifestyle modifications further maximizes existing health outcomes and encourages long-term cardiovascular health. While diet and exercise modification are crucial, reducing smoking and alcohol consumption, which are behavioral risk factors, are equally pivotal in the prevention of cardiovascular diseases. Smoking is the cause of atherosclerosis and has direct implications for heart function, thus emphasizing cessation services in at-risk subjects, particularly in low-resource environments. In addition to this, studies emphasize the need for alcohol restriction because excessive alcohol use can exacerbate hypertension and lead to heart failure. Additionally, stress-reducing interventions have implications for a good quality of life and enhanced cardiovascular outcomes. Lifestyle modification programs that include mindfulness interventions, cognitive-behavioral therapy, and support groups can help patients adopt long-term lifestyle changes. These holistic measures are needed to control cardiovascular health effectively because they address both physical and psychological factors contributing to lifestyle diseases. Combining these lifestyle modifications with the broad topic of internal medicine shows how they are used to enhance treatment regimens for patients with established cardiovascular disease. For instance, the prevention and management of hypertension at an early stage, particularly in resource-limited communities, needs community-oriented strategies emphasizing lifestyle changes as a first line of care. Research suggests that affordable non-pharmacologic interventions can have a significant impact on public health, ultimately reducing morbidity from hypertension and cardiovascular disease (Twagirumukiza et al., 2011). Further, among patients with complications such as erectile dysfunction, awareness of the interconnection between cardiovascular health and lifestyle elements can lead to individualized treatment that enhances health outcomes. Professionals should therefore place primary emphasis on lifestyle change in treatment strategies to offset the escalating cardiovascular epidemic across various socio-economic environments (Benea et al., 2016).

2.4.3. Surgical Options

The practice of surgical procedures in cardiology encompasses a wide variety of treatments aimed at the management of a range of cardiovascular conditions. Within these, traditional interventions such as CABG and repair or replacement surgeries for valves remain at the hub of ischemic heart disease and valvular disease control. CABG serves to divert occluded coronary arteries, essentially resuscitating myocardial tissues from blood and symptomatically alleviating angina. Conversely, valve procedures address structural heart disease, which, if left untreated, leads to heart failure. With ongoing advances in technology, the integration of minimally invasive techniques has revolutionized these surgical procedures, offering patients shorter recovery times and lower complication rates. The advent of three-dimensional (3D) printing technology in the last couple of years has significantly influenced surgical planning and patient outcomes in cardiology. By using patient-specific anatomical models, surgeons can perform meticulous preoperative planning, thereby improving surgical precision.

This new technique enables visualization of complex cardiac structures, facilitating individualized surgical strategies to address the anatomical challenges posed by unique patients. Besides serving as guides for simulated rehearsal during surgery, 3D-printed models also enable effective communication among multidisciplinary teams, facilitating enhanced collaborative decision-making in patient care. By effectively integrating technology into clinical practice, cardiovascular surgery is evolving toward a more personalized approach, thereby optimizing therapeutic outcomes for patients with diverse cardiac conditions (Anwar et al., 2018). Furthermore, research into minimally invasive cardiovascular surgical procedures, such as percutaneous interventions, has shown encouraging results as an alternative to traditional methods. Percutaneous coronary interventions (PCI), such as stenting and angioplasty, are a way of restoring patency of the coronary artery without open-heart surgery. It is especially useful for patients at high risk who might not be able to tolerate standard procedures. New advances in catheter-based therapies for heart valve diseases, like TAVR, are transforming the treatment of severe aortic stenosis to an outpatient procedure. As these less invasive techniques gain traction, they not only expand the range of surgical options but also improve patient outcomes and satisfaction. Ultimately, the continued innovation of surgical interventions in cardiology testifies to the field's commitment to advancing patient care through innovation (Al-Attar et al., 2017) (Figure 2.12).

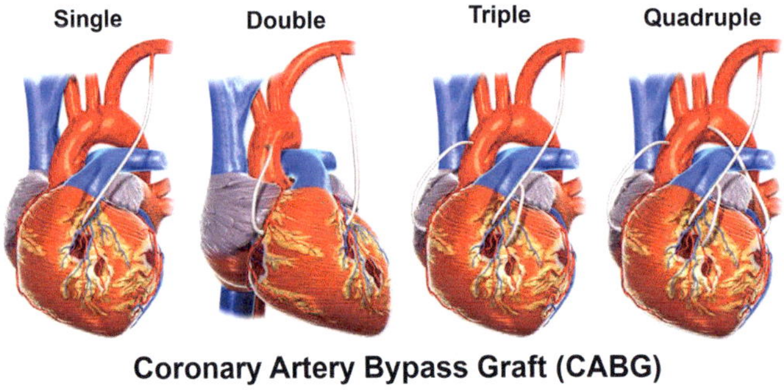

Figure 2.12. Coronary artery bypass grafting (CABG)

Source: https://www.akutkalpdamar.com/2018/07/picture4-1.png.

Test Your Knowledge

1. What are the common treatment options used to manage cardiovascular diseases?
2. How do medications and lifestyle changes work together in treating heart conditions?

2.5. Preventive Cardiology

Learning Outcome

1. Define risk factor identification in cardiology
2. Discuss the patient education and counseling
3. Understand the screening guidelines

Preventive cardiology plays an important role in enhancing cardiovascular health and preventing heart disease through early intervention and lifestyle modification. The process is concerned with the identification of risk factors such as hypertension, hyperlipidemia, and diabetes that are key causes of cardiovascular disease. Through efforts to adjust these risk factors by educating patients and providing individualized interventions, healthcare professionals can help reduce the occurrence of heart attacks and strokes substantially. Preventive methods that are successful include lifestyle modifications such as maintaining regular exercise, encouraging heart-healthy diets, and helping individuals quit smoking. The large-scale studies undertaken in preventive cardiology not only improve outcomes for individual patients but also advance the overall public health goal of reducing the social burden of cardiovascular illness. Preventive cardiology also integrates psychosocial aspects in its composition, as it is a recognition that mental health has a considerable influence on cardiovascular disease. Initiating cardiac rehabilitation programs can address patients' psychological needs while promoting physical recovery. Research has indicated that intense cardiac rehabilitation can effect profound changes in patients' attitudes toward their disease, as evidenced by the fact that the participants viewed their diseases as more chronic after being on the program (Caccamo et al., 2018). Affective and psychological interventions such as these can foster greater self-efficacy in coping with conditions, allowing individuals to take an active role in managing their care. The holistic approach of preventive cardiology that includes physical and psychological intervention enhances the overall quality of life in patients while lowering the threats of cardiovascular diseases. The economic aspects of preventive cardiology must also be questioned, particularly under high-deductible health plans (HDHPs) that have now gained prominence in the healthcare industry. Such strategies tend to restrict access to secondary prevention care, which can counteract effective management of chronic disease and perpetuate health inequities. There has to be a balance between cost containment and comprehensive care, as the care of chronic disease already represents a high percentage of U.S. health spending (Fendrick et al., 2014). Policies that allow first-dollar coverage for evidence-based preventive services can improve health outcomes by providing the necessary care to the population without significant financial barriers. Re-evaluating the policy infrastructure for health insurance coverage of preventive cardiology can make interventions more effective, which, in turn, will produce a better healthcare system and patient-centered outcomes (Figure 2.13).

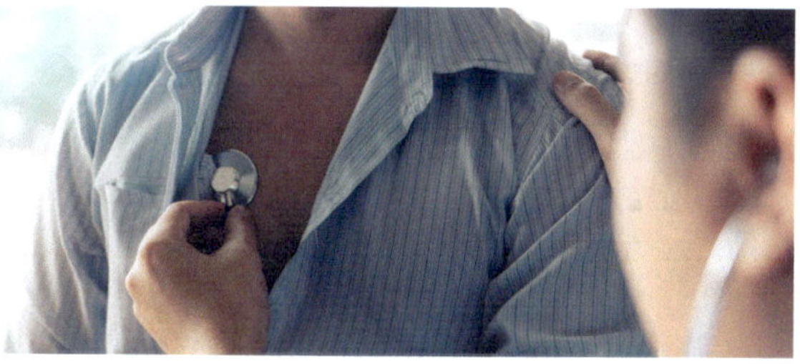

Figure 2.13. Preventive cardiology.

Source: https://www.augustahealth.org/images/cardio-preventive-hero-desktop.jpg.

2.5.1. Risk Factor Identification

The significance of identifying risk factors in cardiology cannot be overemphasized, as it remains the cornerstone of both preventive and therapeutic interventions in the management of cardiovascular disease (CVD). The recognized risk factors include hypertension, diabetes, dyslipidemia, and obesity as known causes of the development of heart disease. The National Cholesterol Education Program (NCEP) guidelines have addressed mainly these dichotomous risk factors to determine populations at risk. However, a recent study indicated that continuous measurement, for example, the MetS score derived from principal component analysis, could provide a better estimate of cardiovascular risk across diverse populations. Using a MetS-PC score, as shown in multiethnic cohort studies, clinicians can enhance risk stratification and tailor interventions to minimize CVD-related adverse events, thereby necessitating reassessment of traditional risk models (Agarwal et al., 2012). Further, the inclusion of multidimensional variables in patient care is critical for patients undergoing advanced cardiovascular interventions, such as left ventricular assist devices (LVADs). Transition home after LVAD implantation involves numerous lifestyle changes, including medication adherence and diet adaptation, that have the potential to impact risk factors related to heart failure profoundly. Proper identification of risk factors in this group is critical not only for ensuring optimal short-term outcomes but also for maximizing long-term quality of life at discharge. Evidence-based transitional care interventions have also been found to decrease avoidable rehospitalizations and enhance patient quality of life compared with standard care (Hirschman et al., 2019). Healthcare providers, therefore, must ensure risk factor identification gets the highest priority in an integrated cardiovascular patient management plan. Finally, emphasizing nurse leadership in transitional care interventions through closing patient outcome gaps and risk factor identification is a means of achieving desired outcomes. The tracking of clinical parameters and counseling patients on lifestyle changes necessary for cardiovascular risk management rest with nurses. Effective communication of tailored risk factors can be a strong tool for empowering patients to make independent health decisions. Transitional care interventions of moderate intensity have been reported to yield improved outcomes, making identification and reduction of risk factors more than an academic exercise, but an essential component of practice. By fostering a culture of cooperation among multidisciplinary teams, identifying risk factors can serve as a useful framework for reducing the burden of cardiovascular diseases across various populations (Hirschman et al., 2019).

2.5.2. Patient Education and Counseling

Patient counseling and education are vital approaches that enable patients to take charge of their cardiology care. Good patient-physician communication encourages greater understanding of cardiovascular disease, its treatment, and the benefits of lifestyle modification. For instance, encouraging exercise as a treatment component has been associated with significant patient gains. Acute care environments provide unique opportunities for this type of education, as they often require emergency lifestyle adaptations to manage or prevent chronic disease flare-ups. Studies show that although physical activity counseling is performed by the majority of nurses, it is rated lower in perceived usefulness than other patient care activities. Therefore, prioritizing this element of patient education can help promote healthy habits in patients, according to the new physical activity recommendations (Bayles et al., 2012). Moreover, patient self-management cannot be overstressed as an element of cardiology practice. Facilitating the patient's active engagement in their treatment regimens requires precise knowledge of their individual cardiovascular risks and the lifestyle changes they need to adopt to mitigate them. Evidence-based policies to enhance caregiving, prevention practices, and care coordination can significantly improve cardiovascular disease management. Of high interest is the efficacy of such policies, as demonstrated by their adoption and implementation in clinical settings, ensuring that providers are trained adequately in patient self-management and palliative care strategies. Addressing these issues, healthcare systems can meet individualized patient demand and address public health issues related to cardiovascular disease, advancing more effective healthcare delivery (Morton et al., 2015).

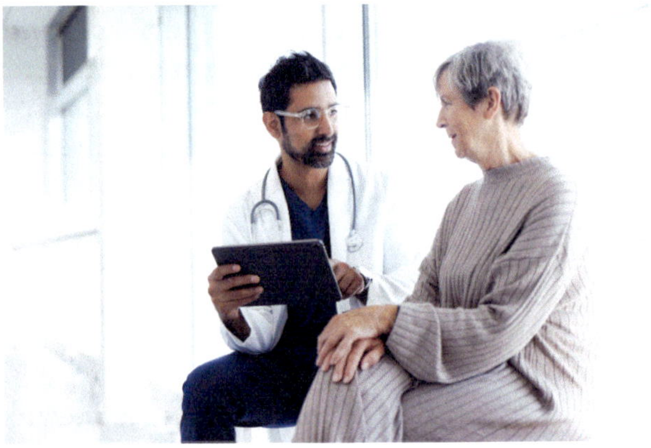

Figure 2.14. Patient education and counseling of cardiology.

Source: https://www.clinicaladvisor.com/wp-content/uploads/sites/11/2023/08/doctor-listening-older-woman-G-1365582872.jpg.

Lastly, the role of healthcare providers, particularly nurses, in transferring this information is of paramount significance. Nurses, as frontline providers, are the primary educators in most instances of patient care. They ought to be adequately trained and equipped to provide key information. There is evidence that nurses' self-efficacy in advising patients on physical exercise is highly dependent on their educational level and physical activity engagement. Thus, an investment in continuous professional development to enhance nurses' skills in patient education can yield substantial dividends in patient outcomes. By establishing a culture of learning and the importance of lifestyle intervention, nursing specialists can play a leading role in making patient education a central element of comprehensive cardiovascular care (Bayles et al., 2012) (Figure 2.14).

2.5.3. Screening Guidelines

In the field of cardiology, screening recommendations are significant for early detection and treatment of cardiovascular diseases, particularly hypertension. Recent European guidelines have placed greater importance on screening alcohol consumption as a key parameter in managing hypertension. Physicians are advised to use standard screening of alcohol consumption, which has been categorized as a class I, level of evidence A recommendation. However, a survey indicated that even though 81.9% of physicians generally quantify alcohol intake in hypertensive patients overall, only a minority, i.e., 28.6% and 14.5%, screen for alcohol intake in new-onset and treatment-resistant cases, respectively. This variation indicates a significant disparity in adherence to prescribed clinical practice guidelines and is a key area for improving treatment efficiency for hypertension and cardiovascular disease as a whole (Bolbrinker et al., 2018). In addition, screening competitive athletes presents unique challenges of screening that differentiate between physiological adaptation and pathological process, for which some guidelines need to be developed. Known as the Athlete's heart, the physiological changes typified by heavy training need to be carefully examined to rule out significant cardiac disease. Comprehensive screening should start with echocardiography to furnish measurements of left ventricular parameters. Separating an athlete's LV hypertrophy from HCM is particularly important. Because HCM can have morphologically equivalent features, a moderate appreciation of imaging findings is required. When echocardiographic results are indeterminate, cardiac magnetic resonance imaging (CMR) is a valuable asset for diagnosis, as it not only provides structural details but also tissue characterization necessary for accurate differentiation (Abergel et al., 2015). Proper use of screening guidelines plays a significant role in improving cardiovascular outcomes by enabling earlier diagnosis and intervention. For example, in patients presenting with symptoms of coronary artery disease, an exercise electrocardiogram (ECG) must be the first investigation. If the first screening is not conclusive, further investigation, such as exercise stress echocardiography or advanced imaging tests, such as coronary cardiac tomography (CCT) can be tried. Care is taken, however, especially in young athletic patients due to potential radiation exposure. Hence, judicious application of these newer imaging modalities, in accordance with consensus clinical guidelines, facilitates effective and safer cardiac screening across diverse patient populations, ultimately enhancing cardiology patient care (Abergel et al., 2015).

Test Your Knowledge

1. What are the primary strategies used in preventive cardiology to reduce cardiovascular risk?
2. How does early lifestyle intervention help prevent heart disease?

2.6. Challenges in Cardiology

Learning Outcome

1. Define the access to care in cardiology
2. Describe the patient compliance
3. Explain the advances in technology in cardiology

Cardiology faces numerous challenges that complicate diagnosis and treatment, particularly regarding the adoption of newer diagnostic technologies in clinical practice. A key problem is the exchange of best practices between doctors. Even if novel approaches, such as blood-based precision medicine tests, are highly promising for improving diagnostic accuracy, adoption may be slow due to a lack of awareness or implementation plans.

Quality improvement activities can smooth the diffusion of such best practices by placing them on the agenda of adopting organizations, providing practical tools and guidelines, and establishing networks that generate learning opportunities. Breaking down such barriers is a prerequisite for improving patient outcomes, since the adoption of evidence-based practice in cardiology holds the potential to trigger more effective treatments and better management of cardiovascular diseases, and ultimately bridge health gaps.

The second main challenge is the differential presentation of CAD symptoms, especially among women. Men tend to present with typical signs of heart disease, whereas women present with a greater variety of nonspecific signs that complicate the diagnostic process. Use of measures such as the age/sex/gene expression score (ASGES) could enhance clinical decision-making. Data from the PRESET Registry suggest that ASGES is effective at identifying women who are less likely to benefit from invasive cardiac assessment. In the population studied, a higher proportion of women with low ASGES scores were referred fewer times for further evaluation than those with higher scores. This stratification not only adds to better management but also fills a significant lacuna in cardiology—the under-detection of coronary artery disease among female patients, thereby leading to greater equity in care provision. Apart from the complicating factors in diagnosis and sexism, the care of patients with complex cardiac diseases poses additional challenges to cardiologists. Those with multiple comorbid conditions might require multidisciplinary treatment, but good communication and interprofessional collaborative practice among clinical teams are lacking. This can lead to ineffective, fragmented treatment plans that fail to address the patients' overall needs. Keeping current with evolving clinical guidelines and treatment algorithms while maintaining compatibility with the divergent expectations of care for each patient takes a lot of time and resources. The job is also made difficult by the rapid pace of innovations in medical technology and pharmacotherapy. Thus, continuing education and training in emergent therapy, as well as strategies to foster interdisciplinary cooperation, are crucial to cardiologists with a desire to provide comprehensive care and optimize outcomes for their patients, particularly those who have a complicated presentation (Figure 2.15).

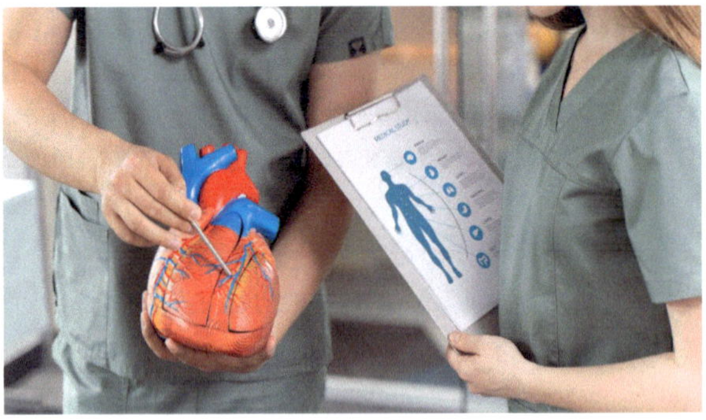

Figure 2.15. Challenges in cardiology.

Source: https://sunknowledge.com/wp-content/uploads/2024/05/cardiology-billing-services-1110x550.jpg.

2.6.1. Access to Care

Access to care is a determinant of health outcomes, and in cardiology, this cannot be emphasized enough. Systemic barriers such as socioeconomic status, geography, and racial/ethnic disparities tend to result in a lack of access. These systemic barriers will deter people from receiving cardiac care when they are in most need, and this is particularly concerning because heart disease is progressively more prevalent. Failure to seek timely access to the appropriate medical interventions may lead to patients developing worse health conditions with increased morbidity and mortality. Mitigating these barriers requires formulating targeted strategies to improve care accessibility, such as expanding insurance coverage, improving public transport to healthcare facilities, and strengthening community outreach initiatives to raise awareness of heart health. Efforts to improve access to cardiology care must be multifaceted and holistic, while remaining sensitive to the persistent inequalities in the health system. Evidence confirms that race and ethnicity have significant impacts not only on access to care but on the quality of care (N/A, 2002). Understanding these differences is crucial for health professionals who want to practice equity. Initiatives to eliminate disparities have gathered pace, most significantly in cardiology, where differences in outcomes of treatment among racial and ethnic minorities are widely documented. Doctors are ideally positioned as the most important decision-makers in eliminating disparities, with a need for ongoing education and sensitization initiatives that emphasize culturally competent care. Interventions to improve access to care need to align with organizational goals while providing valuable resources for healthcare providers (Stern et al., 2010). Quality improvement programs can take a leading role in this process by building environments that support best-practice sharing. Such programs can foster inter-professional collaboration among medical professionals, enabling them to share information and experience and enhance the collective knowledge of the problems faced by different patient groups. By developing tools for practical application, the medical fraternity can make its approach to the delivery of holistic, individually tailored care more robust, thereby facilitating equitable and effective access to the cardiovascular care required (Figure 2.16).

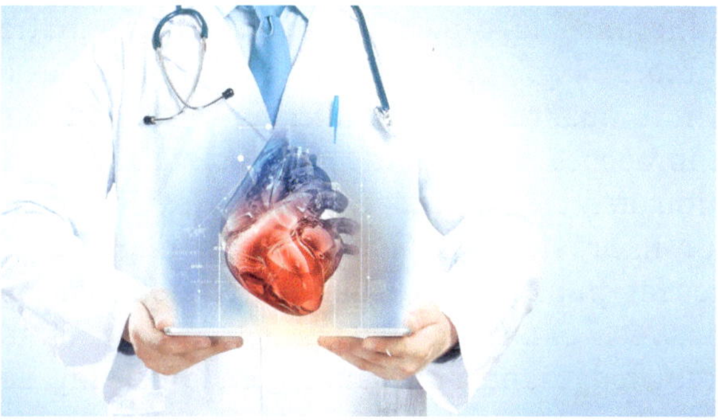

Figure 2.16. Cardiology and heart care.

Source: https://www.dashospital.com/myimages/services/cardiology-1.jpg.

2.6.2. Patient Compliance

In internal medicine, specifically cardiology, patient compliance has a direct impact on treatment. Effective control of cardiac conditions largely depends on patients adhering to drug therapy and lifestyle modifications. Patient non-compliance may lead to increased health risks, including frequent hospitalizations or worsening of existing cardiovascular conditions. Factors influencing adherence include the complexity of medication regimens, patients' knowledge of their disease, and social determinants such as economic stability and social support. Medical practitioners must also recognize the important role they can play in facilitating an environment that supports adherence. By focusing on the need for compliance, physicians can influence patients to recognize the importance of habitual medication use and a healthy lifestyle. An understanding of the specific types of non-adherence is of the utmost concern to healthcare practitioners in maintaining patient compliance. Non-adherence may be classified into intentional and unintentional actions, each with corresponding causes. Deliberate non-adherence is likely to result from patients' belief and perceptions of disease and treatment. This may be caused by misinformation or ignorance of the severity of the disease or the benefits of treatment. Conversely, unintentional non-adherence is typically driven by pragmatic factors, e.g., pill burden or forgetfulness. These nuances allow clinicians to tailor their approaches to patients' unique circumstances, ultimately creating a more favorable environment for improving compliance. As highlighted in recent publications, shared decision-making between clinicians and patients can promote knowledge and adherence, hence serving as an integral strategy in cardiology management (Banning et al., 2009). One of the principal ways to promote patient compliance in cardiology is to adopt a shared decision-making approach during consultations. The system focuses on integrating the patient's experience and conception of health into the management plan, thereby aligning medical guidance with the patient's principles and lifestyle. Discussing with patients the possibility of going beyond their impressions of sickness can be helpful in offering an extra participative setting where individuals feel empowered to engage actively in their health care choices. This interaction has a huge influence on how they comply with treatment regimens, especially when patients believe their intuition is respected and valued. Use of this model not only builds stronger patient-provider relationships but may also lead to improved health outcomes by reducing non-compliance-related complications. Therefore, maximizing patient compliance through efficient communication must be a priority in the practice of internal medicine, particularly cardiology (Banning et al., 2009).

2.6.3. Advances in Technology

The intersection of technology and cardiology has seen unprecedented advances that have transformed the way diagnoses and treatments in internal medicine are conducted. The widespread availability of telemedicine platforms enables patients to be monitored remotely, allowing medical professionals to assess heart conditions with unprecedented convenience. Wearable tech, such as smartwatches, now includes electrocardiogram (ECG) functionality, enabling patients to be more proactive in managing cardiovascular conditions and facilitating timely interventions. These advances signal a shift away from reactive toward proactive healthcare models, encouraging patient empowerment and preventing healthcare system overloads. As a whole, such technological progress underscores the pivotal role of innovation in providing comprehensive cardiology treatment and solving complex health problems through improved, timely understanding. Moreover, the development of artificial intelligence (AI) and machine learning in cardiology has triggered a change in clinicians' interpretation of cardiovascular information. AI programs equipped with advanced analytical capabilities can sort through large volumes of data, significantly enhancing the accuracy of cardiac diagnoses. For instance, convolutional neural networks (CNNs) have been successfully used to differentiate between myocardial infarction types and normal ECG signals with high accuracy and specificity, as shown in recent studies. The new application not only improves diagnostic accuracy but also helps predict patient outcomes, making patient-specific treatment plans feasible that respond to individual patients' needs. As they continue to evolve, they will be at the core of the cardiology practice and the outcome of the patient care revolution. Last but not least, cardiology technology incorporates not just diagnostic but also therapeutic elements, for example, with the introduction of sophisticated cardiac devices. Advanced implantable devices such as cardiac resynchronization therapy (CRT) and left ventricular assist devices (LVAD) are at the forefront of preventing heart failure symptoms and improving the quality of life of patients with advanced cardiovascular disease. They use the most advanced technology to continuously monitor and adjust cardiac function, ensuring appropriate medical treatment is provided in a timely manner. With ongoing research, the collaboration between technological innovation and cardiology is bound to yield further advances, making personalized, effective cardiovascular care a reality for an increasing number of patients, eventually altering the face of internal medicine for cardiology.

Test Your Knowledge

1. What challenges do cardiologists face in managing complex cardiovascular diseases?
2. How do lifestyle-related risk factors complicate the treatment of heart diseases?

SUMMARY

In the conversation on internal medicine's contribution to cardiology, it is therefore important to consider the key findings on the treatment of heart failure. Recent research indicates a striking disparity between formal guidelines and everyday practice in the treatment of heart failure. For instance, diuretics were prescribed to 86.9% of patients, while the rates for other important drugs, such as ACE inhibitors and beta-blockers, were extremely low, with only 61.8% and 36.9% of patients receiving them, respectively (Aguilar et al., 2003). Underutilization of guideline-recommended therapy not only weakens the potential clinical effect but also underscores the need for systemic change to improve guideline implementation. The identification of local variation in prescribing patterns underscores the difficulty of managing heart failure across varied healthcare settings. Age, presence of comorbidity, and some hospital factors had substantial impacts on drug prescribing. These findings highlight the need for treatment regimens tailored to the unique demographic profiles of patient cohorts. Notably, younger patients and patients on the cardiology ward showed better adherence to guideline-concordant care than elderly patients or patients with other respiratory diseases (Aguilar et al., 2003). This underscores the imperative of targeted educational interventions to equip healthcare professionals with optimal treatment guidelines and to optimize patient outcomes across various clinical practices. Lastly, evidence indicates that well-planned quality improvement interventions can ensure the implementation of cardiology best practices. By aligning campaigns with the goals of adopting organizations and providing practical implementation tools and guidelines, significant strides can be made to close the gap between guidelines and everyday clinical practice. Furthermore, establishing networks to promote learning opportunities for medical professionals might establish a culture of continuous improvement. This final layer of activity illustrates that cardiology transformation is not solely about following guidelines but also about creating an environment where best practices and knowledge sharing take place, ultimately enhancing patient care in heart failure treatment and other conditions.

Understanding the subtlety of heart failure is critical to improving patient outcomes in cardiology, particularly among older populations. Heart failure is predominantly a disease of elderly populations and therefore requires practical risk stratification tools in this population. The SENIORS risk model is a pertinent innovation in such a context. The model, developed from clinical trials in elderly patients with chronic heart failure, was found to be valid in an independent cohort of acute heart failure patients. Its use in the National Spanish Registry (RICA) is also indicative of its promise, as it effectively predicts composite outcomes such as all-cause mortality and cardiovascular hospitalizations in the elderly with high reliability, as shown by findings (Bettencourt et al., 2015). Also, the stable performance of the models is highlighted by their ability to discriminate between patient groups' risk levels. The experience of the RICA registry, with a mean age of patients of 78 years and a predominant distribution of patients in functional classes NYHA II and III, demonstrates that high percentages of these patients experienced adverse cardiovascular events. Although there is heterogeneity between predicted and actual risk outcomes, the SENIORS model provides a framework for clinical risk stratification that could lead to earlier intervention and more effective control of heart failure among the elderly. The model's validity lends credence to the need for continued work on the mechanisms of risk stratification in cardiology, which will ultimately lead to better patient care plans (Bettencourt et al., 2015). Beyond risk stratification, therapy refinements are the essence of optimizing outcomes in cardiac patients. New evidence from studies of branched-chain amino acid (BCAA) metabolism indicates a new direction for therapy. The small-molecule BT2 inhibitor has proven to have potential in preserving cardiac function and structure in mouse models of heart failure, thereby demonstrating the therapeutic promise of targeting metabolic pathways in the failing heart. Of specific significance, treatment with BT2 not only augmented cardiac contractile function but also augmented diastolic mechanics, effects that were independent of changes in left ventricular hypertrophy. This new evidence suggests that correcting BCAA catabolism could be a novel therapeutic option for heart failure. Treatment of metabolic derangement related to heart failure opens new lines of thinking in patient management, with the promise that clinicians may be able to supplement standard therapies with metabolic interventions.

KEY TERMS FROM THIS CHAPTER

- Angina pectoris
- Atherosclerosis
- Cardiac arrest
- Cardiomyopathy
- Coronary artery disease (CAD)
- Electrocardiogram (ECG/EKG)
- Heart failure
- Myocardial infarction (MI)
- Pericarditis
- Arrhythmia
- Atrial fibrillation
- Cardiac catheterization
- Congenital heart disease
- Echocardiography
- Endocarditis
- Hypertension
- Pacemaker
- Troponin

CRITICAL THINKING QUESTIONS

1. **Which of the following is the most specific biomarker for diagnosing acute myocardial infarction (MI)?**
   a. CK-MB
   b. Troponin I/T
   c. Myoglobin
   d. LDH
2. **A 60-year-old man presents with crushing chest pain radiating to his left arm. ECG shows ST-segment elevation in leads II, III, and aVF. Which artery is most likely occluded?**
   a. Left anterior descending artery
   b. Right coronary artery
   c. Circumflex artery
   d. Left main coronary artery
   2. Which antihypertensive is preferred in a patient with both hypertension and benign prostatic hyperplasia (BPH)?
   a. ACE inhibitor
   b. Beta-blocker
   c. Alpha-blocker (e.g., prazosin)
   d. Calcium channel blocker
3. **In atrial fibrillation, which of the following is the most important initial step in management in a hemodynamically unstable patient?**
   a. Rate control with beta-blockers
   b. Anticoagulation with warfarin
   c. Cardioversion
   d. Aspirin therapy
4. **Which heart sound is typically associated with heart failure and indicates a non-compliant left ventricle?**
   a. S1
   b. S2
   c. S3
   d. S4

Short Answer Questions

1. What are the diagnostic criteria for acute myocardial infarction (AMI)?
2. Explain the difference between stable and unstable angina.
3. What are the clinical features and ECG findings of atrial fibrillation?
4. List the causes and clinical signs of congestive heart failure (CHF).
5. How is hypertension classified and staged according to current guidelines?
6. Describe the indications for anticoagulation in patients with atrial fibrillation.
7. What are the hallmark features of pericarditis on ECG and physical examination?
8. How do you distinguish systolic from diastolic heart failure in clinical practice?

Answers to Critical Thinking Questions

1. (b); 2. (b) ; 3. (c) ; 4. (c) ; 5. (c)

REFERENCES

1. Macfarlane, P. W., Mason, J. W., Kligfield, P., Sommargren, C. E., Drew, B., Van Dam, P., Abächerli, R., Albert, D. E., & Hodges, M. (2017). Debatable issues in automated ECG reporting. *Journal of Electrocardiology*, *50*(6), 833–840. https://doi.org/10.1016/j.jelectrocard.2017.08.027A bergel, P., Abhayaratna, W. P., Andersson, C., Angell, P. J., Bartram, M. P., Basavarajaiah, S., Blair, E., et al. (2015). The multi-modality cardiac imaging approach to the athlete's heart: An expert consensus of the European Association of Cardiovascular Imaging. https://core.ac.uk/download/30698155.pdf (accessed on 16th July 2025).
2. Agarwal, S., Andrews, J. S., Chen, Y. D. I., Goodpaster, B. H., et al. (2012). Metabolic syndrome derived from principal component analysis and incident cardiovascular events: The Multi-Ethnic Study of Atherosclerosis (MESA) and Health, Aging, and Body Composition (Health ABC). https://core.ac.uk/download/323077353.pdf (accessed on 16th July 2025).
3. Aguilar, J. C., Cleland, J., Cohen-Solal, A., Dietz, R., et al. (2003). The EuroHeart Failure Survey Programmed—A survey on the quality of care among patients with heart failure in Europe. Part 2: Treatment. https://core.ac.uk/download/11855551.pdf (accessed on 16th July 2025).
4. Aiyagari, R., Algaze, C. A., Bhat, P. N., Costello, J. M., et al. (2018). Diagnostic errors in pediatric cardiac intensive care. https://core.ac.uk/download/212864670.pdf (accessed on 16th July 2025).
5. Akashi, Y. J., Bossone, E., Citro, R., Figtree, G. A., et al. (2015). Current state of knowledge on Takotsubo syndrome: A position statement from the Taskforce on Takotsubo Syndrome of the Heart Failure Association of the European Society of Cardiology. https://core.ac.uk/download/77004085.pdf (accessed on 16th July 2025).
6. Al-Attar, N., Coccia, R., Di Domenico, F., Nappi, F., et al. (2017). Introductory editorial: Drug-eluting stents or drug-eluting grafts? Insights from proteomic analysis. https://core.ac.uk/download/77601030.pdf (accessed on 16th July 2025).
7. Al'Aref, S. J., Andreini, D., Baskaran, L., Bax, J. J., et al. (2020). Machine learning framework to identify individuals at risk of rapid progression of coronary atherosclerosis: From the PARADIGM registry. https://core.ac.uk/download/288432787.pdf (accessed on 16th July 2025).
8. Anwar, S., Barach, P., Bhatla, P., Biglino, G., et al. (2018). 3D printing is a transformative technology in congenital heart disease. https://core.ac.uk/download/212858839.pdf (accessed on 16th July 2025).
9. Banning, M. (2009). Medication taking behavior and hypertension: A review of the literature. https://core.ac.uk/download/335817.pdf (accessed on 16th July 2025).
10. Bayles, C., Hoffman, L., Jakicic, J., Miketic, M., et al. (2012). Examination of acute care nurses' ability to engage in patient education related to physical activity as a health behavior. https://core.ac.uk/download/12212129.pdf (accessed on 16th July 2025).
11. Becker, L., Bellezo, J. M., Fair, J. F., Gaieski, D. F., et al. (2016). Practice characteristics of emergency department extracorporeal cardiopulmonary resuscitation (eCPR) programs in the United States: The current state of the art of emergency department extracorporeal membrane oxygenation (ED ECMO). https://core.ac.uk/download/299811653.pdf (accessed on 16th July 2025).

12. Benea, V., Georgescu, S. R., Mitran, C. I., Mitran, M., et al. (2016). The current treatment of erectile dysfunction. https://core.ac.uk/download/144552982.pdf (accessed on 16th July 2025).
13. Bettencourt, P., Coats, A., Diez-Manglano, J., Flather, M., et al. (2015). Utility of the SENIORS elderly heart failure risk model applied to the RICA registry of acute heart failure. https://core.ac.uk/download/41992549.pdf (accessed on 16th July 2025).
14. Biffi, A., D'Silva, A., Magalski, A., Malhotra, A., et al. (2019). Abnormal ECG findings in athletes: Clinical evaluation and considerations. https://core.ac.uk/download/286028675.pdf (accessed on 16th July 2025).
15. Bizopoulos, P., & Koutsouris, D. (2021). Deep learning in cardiology. http://arxiv.org/abs/1902.11122 (accessed on 16th July 2025).
16. Bodean, O., Diaconu, C. C., Laslo, C. L., Marcu, D., et al. (2018). New oral anticoagulants and their reversal agents. https://core.ac.uk/download/216809657.pdf (accessed on 16th July 2025).
17. Bolbrinker, J., Kreutz, R., Riemer, T. G., Zaidi Touis, M., et al. (2018). Moderation of alcohol consumption as a recommendation in European hypertension management guidelines: A survey on awareness, screening and implementation among European physicians. https://core.ac.uk/download/199424776.pdf (accessed on 16th July 2025).
18. Borghi, C., Grassi, G., Rosei, E. A., Savoia, C., et al. (2017). Personalized medicine—A modern approach for the diagnosis and management of hypertension. https://core.ac.uk/download/96884785.pdf (accessed on 16th July 2025).
19. Budoff, M. J., Gul, B., Herman, L., Huang, C., et al. (2019). The clinical utility of a precision medicine blood test incorporating age, sex, and gene expression for evaluating women with stable symptoms suggestive of obstructive coronary artery disease: Analysis from the PRESET Registry. https://core.ac.uk/download/323079913.pdf (accessed on 16th July 2025).
20. Caccamo, F., Carlon, R., Marogna, C., Pinton, G., et al. (2018). The perception of the illness and the self-efficacy in the management of emotions in cardiac patients. https://core.ac.uk/download/168406759.pdf (accessed on 16th July 2025).
21. Campuzano-Ruiz, R., Cebrián-Cuenca, A. M., García de Lucas, M. D., Moreno-Pérez, O., et al. (2024). Multidisciplinary panel consensus for the management of patients with type 2 diabetes: A Delphi study. https://core.ac.uk/download/617017981.pdf (accessed on 16th July 2025).
22. Chen, M., Chuang, D. T., Gao, C., Ren, B., et al. (2019). Therapeutic effect of targeting branched-chain amino acid catabolic flux in pressure-overload induced heart failure. https://core.ac.uk/download/323066857.pdf (accessed on 16th July 2025).
23. Cheung, B. M. Y., Wong, C. K. H., & Wu, O. (2017). Towards a transparent, credible, evidence-based decision-making process of new drug listing on the Hong Kong Hospital Authority Drug Formulary: Challenges and suggestions. https://core.ac.uk/download/84340532.pdf (accessed on 16th July 2025).
24. Clark, R., Rawas, H., Windsor, C., Yates, K., et al. (2012). Cultural challenges to secondary prevention: Implications for Saudi women. https://core.ac.uk/download/10909715.pdf (accessed on 16th July 2025).

25. Delling, F. N., Deo, R. C., Tison, G. H., Zhang, Y., et al. (2018). Automated and interpretable patient ECG profiles for disease detection, tracking, and discovery. http://arxiv.org/abs/1807.02569 (accessed on 16th July 2025).
26. Dornan, T., Feilchenfeld, Z., Kuper, A., Whitehead, C., et al. (2017). Ultrasound in undergraduate medical education: A systematic and critical review. https://core.ac.uk/download/74405617.pdf (accessed on 16th July 2025).
27. Fendrick, A. M., Cliff, E. Q., Milkovich, K., Spangler, K., McKellar, M. R., Chernew, M., & Parents, S. (2014). Health Savings Account-eligible high-deductible health plans: Updating the definition of prevention. https://core.ac.uk/download/75777849.pdf (accessed on 16th July 2025).
28. Forsyth, P., Greenlaw, N., Jhund, P. S., Lowrie, R., et al. (2011). Pharmacist intervention in primary care to improve outcomes in patients with left ventricular systolic dysfunction. https://core.ac.uk/download/110585.pdf (accessed on 16th July 2025).
29. Harvey, J. (2017). Incidence and predictors of premature ventricular complexes following catheter ablation for atrial fibrillation. https://open.bu.edu/bitstream/2144/23785/5/Harvey_bu_0017N_12743.pdf (accessed on 16th July 2025).
30. Hirschman, K., Iseler, J. I., Shaid, E. C., Wierenga, M., et al. (2019). Implications of transitional care interventions on hospital readmissions in patients with destination therapy left ventricular assist devices. https://core.ac.uk/download/299809046.pdf (accessed on 16th July 2025).
31. Kitsiou, A., Caforio, A. L. P., Porta-Sanchez, A., Vahanian, A., Iung, B., Carrera, C., Szymanski, C., et al. (2013). ESC core curriculum for the general cardiologist (2013). https://core.ac.uk/download/55756305.pdf (accessed on 16th July 2025).
32. Moon, S. (2017). Echocardiography curriculum development for physician assistants using entrustable professional activities. https://core.ac.uk/download/215924737.pdf (accessed on 16th July 2025).
33. Morton, S., & Dunn, W. (2015). Addressing the health needs of an aging America: New opportunities for evidence-based policy solutions. https://core.ac.uk/download/75783019.pdf (accessed on 16th July 2025).
34. Reasat, T., & Shahnaz, C. (2018). Detection of inferior myocardial infarction using shallow convolutional neural networks. http://arxiv.org/abs/1710.01115 (accessed on 16th July 2025).
35. Silva, A. M. R. da. (2019). Retrospective study of the association between neutering status and changes secondary to degenerative mitral valve disease. https://core.ac.uk/download/250589850.pdf (accessed on 16th July 2025).
36. Stern, A. F., Yuan, C. T., Bradley, E. H., Krumholz, H. M., Nembhard, I. M., & Brush, J. E. (2010). Blueprint for the dissemination of evidence-based practices in health care. https://core.ac.uk/download/71349600.pdf (accessed on 16th July 2025).
37. Twagirumukiza, M., & Van Bortel, L. (2011). Management of hypertension at the community level in Sub-Saharan Africa (SSA): Towards a rational use of available resources. https://core.ac.uk/download/55848620.pdf (accessed on 16th July 2025).

RESPIRATORY MEDICINE

3

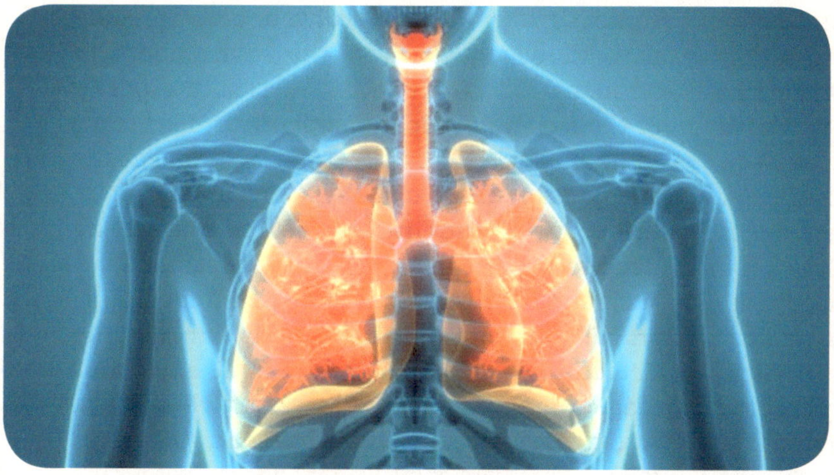

LEARNING OBJECTIVES

After studying this chapter, you will be able to:

1. Define anatomy and physiology of the respiratory system
2. Identify the common respiratory diseases
3. Understand the diagnostic techniques in respiratory medicine
4. Discuss the treatment modalities
5. Explain the advances in respiratory medicine
6. Define public health and respiratory medicine

Introduction

Respiratory medicine is concerned with a broad range of conditions affecting the lungs and respiratory tract, which are critical for maintaining overall health and well-being. It is essential to comprehend the intricate mechanics of breathing, as the respiratory system not only facilitates gas exchange but also plays a crucial role in maintaining homeostasis and adapting to environmental stress. Asthma, chronic obstructive pulmonary disease (COPD), pneumonia, and lung cancer all represent a sample of the numerous diseases that can be encountered in this system. A comprehensive introduction to respiratory medicine entails an exploration of these diseases, their related pathophysiology, and the socio-economic impacts they have on affected populations. Given the global rise in respiratory illnesses, it is important that healthcare providers are well aware of the complexities of respiratory medicine to provide effective diagnosis and treatment. Education and preventive care are important parts of respiratory medicine, particularly in culturally diverse settings such as university health services. According to studies, institutions of higher learning are essential stages where health consciousness among students is fostered, which can lead to particular health complications. The American College Health Association documents the need for health care to treat a variety of ailments, including respiratory illnesses compounded by environmental factors such as pollution and allergens. To this end, nurse practitioners play a crucial role in providing individualised care that meets the unique needs of the student population. By focusing on prevention and early-stage disease management through education and treatment, health care professionals can foster healthier lifestyles among students, whose implications ultimately affect their schoolwork and overall well-being (Gottlieb et al., 1979). Furthermore, the dangers of pandemics of infectious diseases and bioterrorism pose significant challenges to respiratory medicine. These conditions may cause fear and anxiety among the population, affecting both physical and mental health. Treating respiratory disease in such scenarios requires a good understanding of medical practice, as well as empathy for the psychological pressures patients may face. Research has suggested the implementation of a fear and resilience checklist to assist with the triage of patients presenting with respiratory symptoms during outbreaks. The device would enable prompt identification and treatment of patients experiencing higher levels of fear, thereby enhancing the capacity to deliver effective care during emergencies (Bracha et al., 2006). By addressing both the physical and emotional aspects of respiratory well-being, the field can more easily meet the challenges posed by rapid change in health environments.

Definition and Scope of Respiratory Medicine

Respiratory medicine is a clinical specialty dealing with the diagnosis, treatment, and management of diseases and conditions of the respiratory system, including the lungs, bronchial tubes, and other pertinent structures. The field of respiratory medicine encompasses a wide range of conditions, from common conditions like asthma and COPD to more complex illnesses such as pulmonary hypertension and lung cancer. The scope of respiratory medicine extends beyond direct clinical management; it also includes preventive interventions and public health strategies to reduce morbidity from respiratory disorders. As the pathophysiology of the respiratory system comes to be understood, so does the profession evolve to accommodate new knowledge on how the environment in its many forms affects us, such as the purity of the air and occupational hazards, necessary to finalize patient care. Advances in diagnostic and therapeutic techniques further expanded the scope of respiratory medicine, enabling doctors to better tailor care. New technologies such as high-resolution computed tomography (HRCT) and molecular diagnosis enhance the detection of respiratory illness at an earlier stage, which is crucial for effective control. Additionally, treatment has changed significantly, with a shift from conventional pharmacotherapy to the inclusion of newer modalities, such as biologics in asthma and pulmonary rehabilitation in COPD, thereby expanding therapeutic options. As outlined in the latest pulmonary hypertension guidelines, appropriate treatment hinges on accurate determination of the causes of respiratory disturbance, which can be highly diverse across cases and must be addressed with a multidisciplinary treatment and monitoring regimen (Abbott et al., 2020). All of this demonstrates the dynamic nature of respiratory medicine, where ongoing research continuously refines clinical practices. The role of respiratory medicine in public health cannot be overstressed, particularly against the backdrop of increasing respiratory disease burden worldwide. Factors that contribute to the burden include environmental pollution, smoking, and climate change, all of which directly affect the respiratory system. University health programs, as advocated by the American College Health

Association, emphasize having a comprehensive approach to managing such health problems across a variety of populations, like students and other vulnerable groups (Gottlieb et al., 1979). Awareness of prevention, screening, and early intervention educational programs is an essential component of respiratory care. By integrating respiratory medicine into broader health programs, practitioners can improve health outcomes, increase community awareness, and ultimately reduce the burden of respiratory disease, thereby securing its essential role in the continuum of care.

Importance of Respiratory Health

The significance of respiratory health cannot be overemphasized, particularly at a time when the prevalence of respiratory ailments such as asthma, COPD, and allergic diseases is increasing. These conditions not only affect individual well-being but also impose enormous burdens on healthcare systems worldwide. Rising levels of pollution and climate change globally further augment respiratory health issues, leading to greater numbers of respiratory infections and chronic disease exacerbations. Moreover, a complete understanding of respiratory health guides not only clinical practice but also public health policy for health promotion and disease prevention. The assessment of respiratory-related procedures has responded to these challenges by attaching heightened significance to appropriateness and efficiency in medical interventions, as highlighted by the latest health decrees that outline inappropriate allergological interventions, namely those for respiratory diseases (Lombardi et al., 2016).

Further, the intricate interdependence of respiratory health with general quality of life is testified to by the profound impacts that respiratory disease exerts on functional everyday living. Poor lung function leads to limitations in physical ability, increased healthcare costs, and even mental impacts such as depression and anxiety. These conditions highlight the value of early intervention and effective disease control. For instance, respiratory health has a unique interdependence with the environment in that conditions such as damp housing, exposure to tobacco smoke, and air quality have a direct influence over incidence rates of acute infection and chronic respiratory disease. In addition, the need for proper monitoring and appropriate treatment of respiratory diseases is underscored by evidence indicating that a significant proportion of affected individuals do not receive appropriate care (Lundborg et al., 2004). Hence, prioritizing respiratory health through well-informed healthcare decisions is paramount for minimizing the economic and social effects of these diseases.

Finally, advancing heightened awareness of respiratory health can lead to significant improvements in public health initiatives. Prevention-based educational programs, such as smoking cessation, improved indoor air quality, and immunization campaigns against respiratory pathogens, are highly effective in enhancing population-level health results. In addition, the emphasis on customized therapies, as discussed in the current healthcare debate, enables tailored interventions based on a patient's unique environmental exposures and health history.

This model of personalized medicine requires a shift from generalized treatment to one that respects the unique needs of individual patients, particularly in the areas of allergy and respiratory health. By combining evidence-based practice with appropriate medical procedures, healthcare systems can ensure the effective use of resources while maximizing patient outcomes in respiratory medicine (Lombardi et al., 2016). This precise concern for lung health not only benefits personal health but also the broader public health objectives.

3.1. Anatomy and Physiology of the Respiratory System

Learning Outcome

1. Understand the structure of the respiratory system
2. Define the function of the lungs and airways
3. Describe the mechanisms of gas exchange

The respiratory system's anatomy is incredibly intricate to facilitate efficient gas exchange, which is critical to supporting human life. Comprising the upper and lower respiratory tracts, the system begins in the nasal passages, which warm, humidify, and filter air. The passage proceeds through the larynx and pharynx to the trachea, which branches into the bronchi, which in turn divide into smaller bronchioles within the lungs. The alveoli, tiny air spaces at the terminal point, provide a huge surface area for oxygen and carbon dioxide exchange. Anatomy is vital in respiratory medicine, especially given the lungs' exposure to environmental toxins and pathogens. Chronic lower respiratory diseases, identified as the third leading cause of death in the United States, underscore the importance of comprehensive knowledge of respiratory anatomy and its role in achieving health (Miller et al., 2017). At the physiological level, respiration is conducted by the respiratory system through an extremely interdependent interaction between muscles and nerve impulses. Exhalation and inhalation are carried out by the intercostal muscles and diaphragm primarily because of changes in pressure within the thoracic cavity. The mechanical operation is intricately linked to the neural control centres in the brainstem, which respond to carbon dioxide levels and blood acidity to maintain homeostasis. Efficiency of gas exchange is also enhanced by the rich vascular network surrounding the alveoli, which enables rapid oxygenation and carbon dioxide elimination. Physiological principles that underlie breathing account for pathophysiological changes in respiratory diseases, requiring clinicians to understand these processes when diagnosing and treating respiratory disease (Miller et al., 2017). The interface between respiratory system anatomy and physiology is also evident in the immune system, which plays a central role in maintaining respiratory health. The respiratory tract has several immune components, including bronchus-associated lymphoid tissue (BALT), which orchestrates the immune response against pathogens. BALT develops an architecture that supports effective immunological function, thereby enabling an effective response to microbial invasion. In birds, for example, structural components of BALT exhibit clear compartmentalization that affects pathogen interactions and immune efficiency. This intricacy calls for an understanding not only of the structural and functional properties of the respiratory system in respiratory medicine but also of those employed in the design of therapeutic mechanisms to enhance host defense against respiratory infections. In conclusion, a thorough knowledge of respiratory physiology and anatomy is required to manage the intricacies of respiratory disease.

3.1.1. Structure of the Respiratory System

The respiratory system is a complex system that facilitates the vital process of gas exchange, which is necessary for the support of life. Its anatomy can be divided into two major categories: the upper respiratory system and the lower respiratory system. The upper respiratory tract includes the nasal cavity, pharynx, and larynx which filter, warm, and humidify air entering the body. These regions are lined with mucous membranes that trap pathogens and particulate matter, allowing only clean air to reach the lungs. The lower respiratory tract includes the trachea, bronchi, bronchioles, and alveoli, where gas exchange occurs. The extensive branching of the airways culminates in alveoli, tiny air sacs where oxygen diffuses into the bloodstream and carbon dioxide is eliminated, affirming the efficient structural organization of the respiratory system to support maximum breathing and metabolic functions required for homeostasis. Understanding the structural components of the respiratory system is of utmost significance in the clinical practice of respiratory medicine, especially in diagnosing and treating respiratory ailments. The interaction between structural elements and function becomes particularly relevant when the diverse pathology compromising ventilation is taken into account. Conditions such as COPD and asthma are associated with inflammatory processes that impair the normal structural integrity of airways, leading to airflow limitation. Furthermore, the alveolar architecture necessary for effective gas exchange may be destroyed in conditions such as emphysema. Understanding these structural shifts and their functional implications can guide treatment and enable targeted regimens that consider specific changes in the respiratory system (Wang et al., 2021). With advances in respiratory medicine, the addition of advanced diagnostic techniques illuminates the intricate structure of the respiratory system at the molecular and cellular levels. Technologies such as imaging modalities and spatiotemporal molecular medicine have enhanced the visualization of respiratory structures and the respiratory disease dynamics. For example, high-resolution imaging has enabled the study of lung architecture and the detection of real-time pathological changes, providing information about the disease process and therapeutic interventions. Such awareness underscores the importance of gaining a clear understanding of the anatomy of respiratory systems for diagnosis and treatment, as well as for the design of precision medicine approaches that individualize interventions based on specific patient needs to improve control of respiratory conditions (Guo et al., 2020) (Figure 3.1).

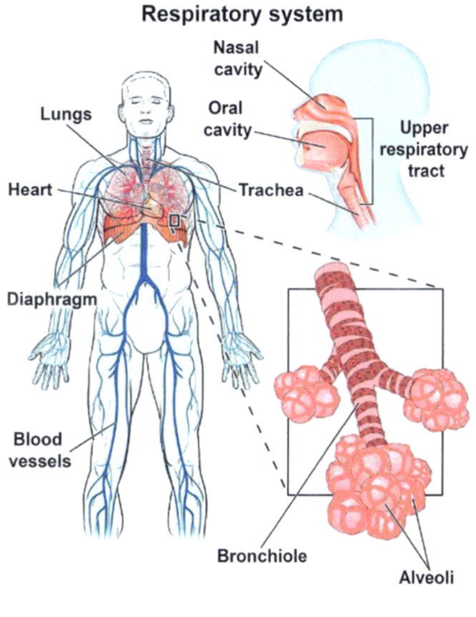

Figure 3.1. Respiratory system.

Source: https://my.clevelandclinic.org/-/scassets/images/org/health/articles/respiratory-system.

3.1.2. Function of the Lungs and Airways

The lungs and airways are the vital components of the respiratory system that serve the intricate function of gas exchange. The primary role of the lungs is to oxygenate blood and expel carbon dioxide, a metabolic waste product. This transfer occurs within the alveoli, minute air spaces that have an enormous surface area for diffusion due to their intricate vascular network. During every inhalation, fresh air oxygen enters the lungs via the airways, which consist of the nasal passages, the trachea, and the bronchi. This sequential chain optimizes airflow and filters, warms, and humidifies inspired air, thereby protecting the delicate lung tissue from external contaminants and disease-causing agents. Together, these roles emphasize the importance of healthy lungs, as an abnormal airway can lead to inefficient gas exchange and increased susceptibility to respiratory diseases that are highly prevalent across various groups (Miller et al., 2017). The airways also have a role beyond just being a conduit. They are lined by a mucosal membrane and cilia cover that work together to catch and clear away harmful particles and pathogens. It is most important for lung defense against inhaled pathogens and toxins, as evidenced by the role of clearance functions. Dysfunctions in this system, such as those due to chronic inflammation or infection, may lead to diseases such as asthma or COPD (Figure 3.2).

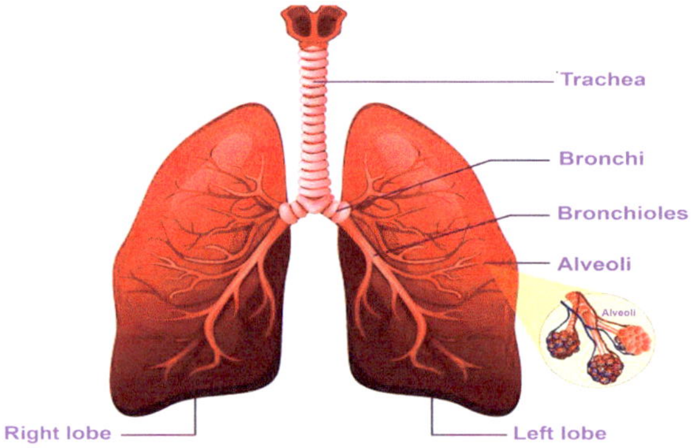

Figure 3.2. Structure of the lungs.

Source: https://cdn1.byjus.com/wp-content/uploads/2023/07/Lungs-Diagram-in-Human-Body.png.

Protective mechanisms are crucial to design preventive and therapeutic regimens in respiratory medicine. Non-invasive technologies, such as the forced oscillation technique (FOT), have expanded the ability to examine airway dynamics in both children and adults. These innovative technologies enable clinicians to assess lung function without invasive procedures, thereby maximizing diagnostic accuracy and patient satisfaction (Copot et al., 2019). Against these functions and the intricate airway and lung anatomy, respiratory medicine works toward insight into new strategies of treatment to support lung health. Progress in biomedical science highlights the interplay between environmental exposures, i.e., allergens and pollutants, and respiratory disease pathogenesis. Because of the lung's vulnerability to extrinsic factors, research using nonhuman primate models, for instance, has proven very useful in elucidating the mechanisms of these diseases. These models have yielded valuable insights into how inhaled substances affect lung function and immune responses. This information not only facilitates the identification of potential molecular targets for intervention but also enables the development of vaccines and other therapeutic agents. With advancing research in respiratory medicine, more information about lung function and airway health continues to be important for improving patient outcomes in respiratory disorders (Miller et al., 2017) (Figure 3.3).

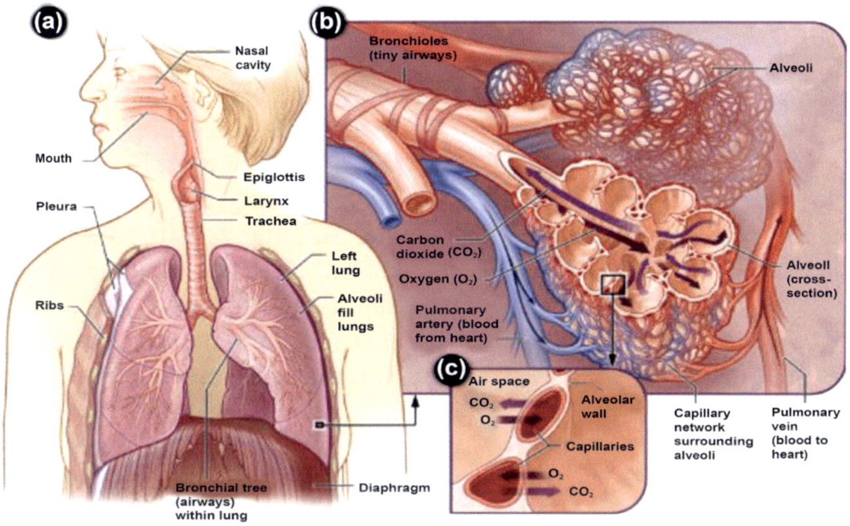

Figure 3.3. (a) Location of the respiratory structures in the body. (b) An enlarged view of the airways, alveoli (air sacs), and capillaries (tiny blood vessels). (c) A close-up view of gas exchange between the capillaries and alveoli. CO_2 is carbon dioxide, and O_2 is oxygen.

Source: https://ars.els-cdn.com/content/image/3-s2.0-B9780128029244000025-f02-18-9780128029244.jpg.

3.1.3. Mechanisms of Gas Exchange

Respiratory gas exchange processes are complex and vital. It primarily occurs within the alveoli and is diffusion-based, with oxygen in the incoming air in the lungs exchanged into the blood while carbon dioxide is moved in the opposite direction. The alveolar wall is thin, dividing these two halves and facilitating rapid gas transfer, leading to efficient equilibrium due to the humongous surface area provided by the alveolar structure. Alveoli are optimally designed to do this work, consisting of many small sacs each covered by an extensive network of capillaries. This structural modification highlights the biological evolution of the respiratory system, enabling increased efficiency in gas exchange, which is vital for supplying oxygen to tissues and removing metabolic waste, especially carbon dioxide, to maintain acid-base balance. Gas-exchange mechanisms in avian animals exhibit peculiar modifications that reflect their evolutionary demand for greater efficiency during flight. Birds possess a highly structured lung anatomy, very different from that of mammals, comprising a complex network of air sacs in communication with the thoracic parabronchi. The arrangement facilitates one-way flow, in which fresh air always flows over the respiratory surfaces, optimizing the oxygen for exchange. Bronchus-associated lymphoid tissue (BALT) is an important feature of the bird lung, comprising immune cells that protect against infection while continuing to perform gas exchange. The process of lymphoid development over time is indicative of the dynamic interaction between respiratory and immune function. It points out the evolutionary advancements that have occurred in response to environmental pressures. Understanding these mechanisms is significant as it can direct therapeutic management and interventions in animal and human respiratory medicine (Dalamani et al., 2006) (Figure 3.4).

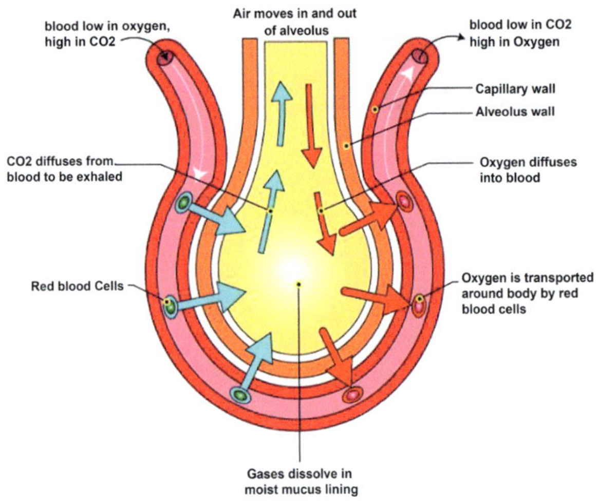

Figure 3.4. Gas exchange in humans.

Source: https://cdn1.byjus.com/wp-content/uploads/2018/11/exchange-regulation-of-gases.png.

Further, advances in non-invasive respiratory assistance have emerged to optimize gas exchange in patients with respiratory failure. High-flow nasal therapy (HFNT) represents a significant development in respiratory therapy, delivering heated, humidified gas to the patient at flow rates exceeding those of standard oxygen therapy. The physiology enhances oxygenation by increasing the fraction of inspired oxygen and simultaneously promoting carbon dioxide clearance. The efficacy of this method is most significant in the treatment of chronic lung disease and acute respiratory failure, as it minimizes the need for invasive procedures. As medical professionals increasingly adopt HFNT across various clinical settings, understanding the underlying pathophysiological mechanisms is significant. This enables health workers to make better decisions about patient management and ultimately improves outcomes by optimizing treatment for respiratory distress (Cortegiani et al., 2019).

Test Your Knowledge

1. What are the main organs involved in the human respiratory system?
2. How does gas exchange occur in the lungs?

3.2. Common Respiratory Diseases

Learning Outcome

1. Understand the asthma: causes and symptoms
2. Describe the chronic obstructive pulmonary disease (COPD)
3. Define the pneumonia: types and treatment options

There is no shortage of common respiratory diseases in respiratory medicine, each with its own unique set of issues for healthcare professionals. Among them, asthma stands out for its chronic nature and broad prevalence across age groups. Asthma is characterized by airway inflammation, hyperreactivity, and episodic airway obstruction, with associated symptoms of wheezing, breathlessness, and cough.

The pathophysiology involves intricate interactions between environmental triggers and genetic susceptibility, with the involvement of allergens and air pollution. In the last decade, research has shown the importance of individualized management, including inhaled corticosteroids and beta-agonists, for symptom treatment and the prevention of exacerbations. This latest research on asthma aims to clarify genetic determinants and environmental markers of disease severity with the ultimate aim of enhancing our capacity to tailor treatment modalities. Chronic obstructive pulmonary disease (COPD) is a highly prevalent condition with significant impacts on quality of life and still a dominant cause of morbidity and mortality across the world. COPD, caused primarily by smoking and air pollution, encompasses both chronic bronchitis and emphysema. Both of these cause airflow limitation, chronic cough, and sputum production. Airway inflammation and structural changes interact to cause progressive respiratory damage, often necessitating long-term therapy. Recent advances in COPD pathophysiology have highlighted the role of comorbidities and systemic inflammation in exacerbating symptoms (Zibrak et al., 2014).

Whole-person care approaches combining lung and patient wellness have thus gained popularity with renewed focus on smoking cessation, pulmonary rehabilitation, and pharmacotherapy to halt the progression of disease. Pneumonia, particularly bacterial pneumonia, remains a worthwhile area of research in respiratory medicine because it is common and potentially serious. Even though it is commonly diagnosed in most populations, some groups, such as the elderly and immunocompromised individuals, are at greater risk (Dear et al., 2020).

Bacterial pneumonia can result from various risk factors, such as viral infections, aspiration of foreign material, and defective mechanisms of clearance in the respiratory tract. Effective management is not just the use of targeted antibiotics to eliminate the responsible pathogens, but also the supportive treatment of the etiologic factors (Dear et al., 2020). With advancing knowledge of pneumonia, focus has shifted to prevention, such as vaccines and education about risk factors, to reduce incidence and improve patient outcomes in the setting of this ubiquitous respiratory infection.

3.2.1. Asthma: Causes and Symptoms

Asthma is a chronic respiratory illness characterized by inflammation of the airways, leading to recurring episodes of wheezing, breathlessness, chest tightness, and coughing. The etiology of asthma is multifactorial and complicated by interactions among genetic, environmental, and immunological factors. There is a significant genetic predisposition, as it usually runs in families with or without allergy. Environmental precipitants such as allergens (e.g., pollen, dust mite), industrial irritants, and cigarette smoke can trigger asthmatic attacks. Furthermore, viral respiratory infections during early childhood have been related to increased asthma development risk, suggesting a necessity for continuing research into the interrelationship between environmental exposure and genetic susceptibility. The symptoms and signs of asthma may vary in frequency and intensity and are usually triggered by irritants or allergens. Remarkably, asthma symptoms often correlate with the presence of co-existing allergic rhinitis, because both diseases share similar pathophysiology and inflammatory response (Figure 3.5).

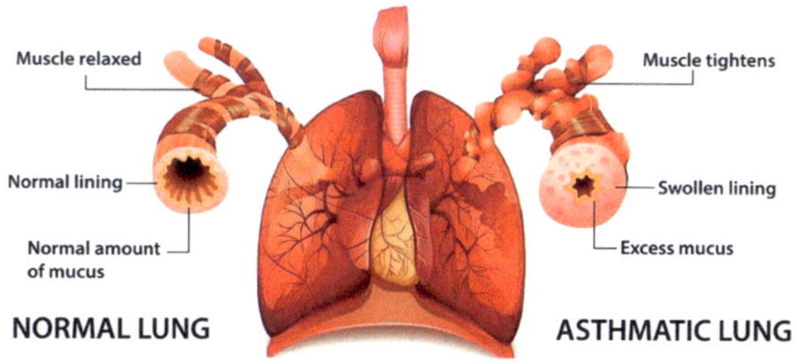

Figure 3.5. Asthma disease.

Source: https://cdn.shopify.com/s/files/1/0621/7062/8249/files/what-is-asthma-what-is-the-best-treatment-for-asthma_1_1024x1024.webp?v=1723716026.

During pollen season, for example, patients may present with increased respiratory distress due to seasonal pollen allergenicity, which triggers an intense immune response. Seasonal exacerbation is a sign of a more profound interaction between environmental allergens and basal immune mechanisms, namely Th2 cells, which play a significant role in orchestrating the allergic response (Czesnikiewicz-Guzik et al., 2016). In addition, combined conditions such as asthma-COPD may present with more severe symptomatology, leading to increased morbidity. Appreciation of the physiological aspects of asthma is required to individualize appropriate management. Severity of asthma has been found to correlate with respiratory muscle function and neuro-respiratory drive, particularly with combined conditions such as asthma-COPD. Severe asthma patients have weaker muscles, especially during exacerbations, which affect their ability to breathe effectively (Feschenko et al., 2017). Rehabilitation treatments that aim to enhance respiratory muscle endurance and strength can be beneficial for improving clinical outcomes. Thus, an effective asthma management plan should address both identifying the inciting agent and optimizing respiratory muscle function, offering a synergistic approach to the management of this complex respiratory disorder.

3.2.2. Chronic Obstructive Pulmonary Disease (COPD)

COPD is a global epidemic with a chronic respiratory symptom complex and airflow limitation. It is the most frequent chronic lung disease and is most often induced by prolonged exposure to toxic gases and particulates, particularly tobacco smoking. The multifactorial etiology of COPD underscores the importance of early diagnosis and effective management. Recent advances in understanding COPD have recognized its heterogeneity, as evidenced by its varied clinical presentations and treatment responses. The treatment regimens have therefore evolved from a generalized strategy to more specific interventions aimed at symptom relief and the reduction of exacerbations, thus improving quality of life. The integration of education and self-management interventions is also key to this process, by enhancing patients' compliance with treatment plans, which is crucial to long-term health outcomes as highlighted by evidence from patient education interventions (Pal et al., 2025) (Figure 3.6).

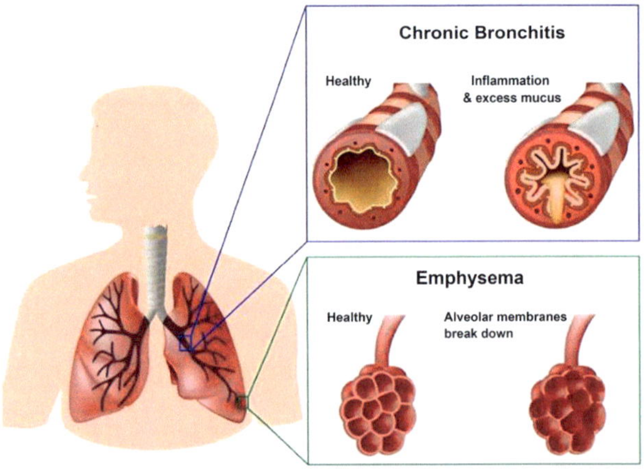

Figure 3.6. Chronic obstructive pulmonary disease (COPD).

Source: https://images.theconversation.com/files/51298/original/5vq77fd6-1402980783.jpg?ixlib=rb-4.1.0&q=45&auto=format&w=754&fit=clip.

Treatment for COPD will typically be a mix of pharmacological and non-pharmacological interventions tailored to the individual needs of different patients. Pharmacologic therapy generally is in the form of bronchodilators and corticosteroids for symptom relief and prevention of exacerbations. The role of global management strategies, however, such as lifestyle adjustment like smoking cessation and pulmonary rehabilitation, cannot be avoided. Pulmonary rehabilitation has indeed been shown to increase exercise tolerance and health-related quality of life in patients with COPD. Furthermore, growing evidence supports the use of complementary therapies, such as yoga and respiratory exercises, as adjuvants to conventional treatments. Integrative therapies do not only involve treating the pathophysiology of the disease but also enhance emotional well-being, thereby providing a holistic treatment approach that addresses the multidimensional needs of patients with COPD, as noted in Ayurvedic clinical research (Bhaskar et al., 2024). The integration of knowledge from traditional medical paradigms, such as Ayurveda, offers interesting possibilities for COPD treatment. Ayurvedic literature accounts for COPD in terms of a syndrome known as Tamaka Shwasa and emphasizes the disease's chronic and progressive course. This perspective inspires an exploration of various Ayurvedic treatment approaches, which may interact with conventional therapies. Systematic reviews of Ayurvedic practice have revealed that treatments and herbs applied in Ayurvedic medicine possess attributes that can prevent oxidative stress, a principal pathological feature of COPD. Also, the inclusion of Ayurveda in modern practice aims to verify and complement current treatment practices. As scientists continue to investigate such integrative paradigms, more and more therapeutic models—grounded in both modern and traditional roots—hold promise for optimizing patient outcomes for those afflicted with COPD (Bhaskar et al., 2024).

3.2.3. Pneumonia: Types and Treatment Options

Pneumonia, an acute respiratory illness characterized by inflammation of the lung parenchyma, presents in several forms, including community-acquired pneumonia (CAP), hospital-acquired pneumonia (HAP), and ventilator-associated pneumonia (VAP). CAP is most often caused by omnipresent pathogens such as Streptococcus pneumoniae and Haemophilus influenzae in individuals with standard immune systems. In contrast, HAP and VAP predominantly occur in hospitalized patients, with the outcome most often being multidrug-resistant organisms that have emerged in the context of healthcare. It is vital to be aware of these types to determine the most effective treatment modality, as the etiologic organisms typically dictate the use of antibiotics and other measures. Furthermore, comprehensive diagnosis using patient history, physical examination, and imaging has a significant impact on clinical outcomes by enabling early and appropriate treatment initiation (Figure 3.7).

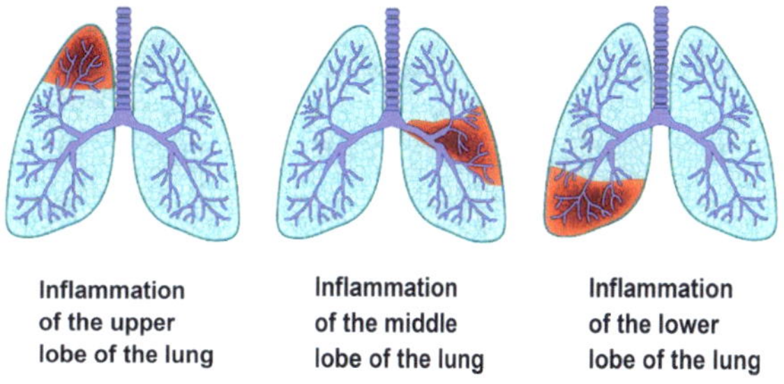

Figure 3.7. Types of pneumonia.

Source: https://www.pedilung.com/wp-content/uploads/2015/12/Dr-Schochet-Types-of-Pneumonia.png.

The treatment strategy for pneumonia depends on the type and severity of the illness, ranging from outpatient treatment to hospitalization in severe cases. In less severe infections, oral antibiotics such as amoxicillin or azithromycin are generally adequate, allowing patients to be treated in the outpatient setting. Intravenous antibiotics, hospitalization, or even intensive care support may be necessary in more severe infections, especially in those with respiratory failure. In addition to antimicrobial therapy, supportive interventions such as oxygen supplementation, bronchodilators, and corticosteroids may play important roles in recovery. Symptom management and the prevention of complications are critical; therefore, clinicians must implement a multidimensional treatment approach tailored to the patient's specific needs and state of health. Such interventions minimize morbidity, enhance recovery, and reduce hospitalization risk and progression to chronic respiratory disease. More literature is emphasizing the place of shared decision-making in pneumonia treatment, particularly in antibiotic treatment. The issue of antibiotic overuse is relevant, as it has promoted antibiotic resistance and complicated treatment outcomes. Some strategies employed to promote enhanced shared decision-making enable patients to learn about the possible advantages and disadvantages of antibiotics, enabling them to make well-informed decisions about their treatment. Research indicates that informed prescribing of antibiotics can reduce unnecessary prescriptions without affecting patient satisfaction or health. Thus, the use of shared decision-making not only synchronizes treatment with patient choice but also helps combat antibiotic resistance in the management of respiratory infections, e.g., pneumonia (Zibrak et al., 2014; Beller et al., 2015).

Test Your Knowledge

1. What are the most common respiratory diseases affecting adults?
2. How do respiratory infections differ from chronic respiratory disorders?

3.3. Diagnostic Techniques in Respiratory Medicine

Learning Outcome

1. Define the pulmonary function tests (PFTs)
2. Understand the imaging studies: x-rays and computed tomography (CT) scans
3. Describe the bronchoscopy and its applications

Respiratory medicine has made great strides with the advent of numerous diagnostic methods that improve the accuracy of patient diagnosis. Among these techniques, spirometry remains central, providing critical information on lung function by measuring airflow and lung volumes. Through this non-invasive method, health care providers can diagnose obstructive as well as restrictive lung diseases, including asthma and COPD. Furthermore, imaging modalities have evolved significantly, particularly HRCT, revolutionizing the depiction of lung architecture so that pulmonary pathologies can be identified early. The integration of such diagnostic instruments not only facilitates patient evaluation but also supports monitoring of disease status and response to therapy, thereby contributing to improved overall care in respiratory medicine. Improvements in laboratory techniques have also stimulated diagnostic precision in respiratory medicine. Among the foremost tools is clinical metagenomic next-generation sequencing (mNGS), which enables intensive analysis of microbial and host DNA and RNA in respiratory samples. The cutting-edge method has begun to move from research to clinical practice, providing data on infectious diseases like pneumonia that traditional methods may miss. mNGS can identify pathogens quickly and effectively, even those less familiar or resistant to conventional antibiotics. As this technology takes off in clinical labs, it has the potential to inform treatment plans holistically, allowing clinicians to prescribe treatments based on patient- and pathogen-specific profiles, thereby pre-empting the challenges of antimicrobial resistance and improving patient outcomes (Chiu et al., 2019). The application of high-tech diagnostic practices in respiratory medicine is inextricably interwoven with health equity, particularly as envisioned in the UN Sustainable Development Goals (SDGs). Access to advanced diagnostic modalities, such as those enabled by emerging 5G technologies, can help close healthcare gaps and ensure that larger populations receive timely and effective respiratory care. The convergence of high-speed data processing, artificial intelligence, and cloud computing offers the opportunity to democratize access to healthcare. Through these technologies, health systems can re-engineer current methodologies that often impede access due to geographical or socioeconomic barriers. This shift highlights that the future of respiratory medicine lies not only in clinical innovation but also in equitable healthcare delivery pathways that align with global health objectives. These developments can create a solid foundation for tackling respiratory disease worldwide (Farooq et al., 2017).

3.3.1. Pulmonary Function Tests (PFTs)

PFTs are critical diagnostic tools in respiratory health assessment, providing crucial information on lung function and guiding the diagnosis and treatment of numerous pulmonary disorders. The tests feature multiple techniques designed to measure airflow, lung volume, and gas exchange capacity. Among the most commonly used PFTs are spirometry, which assesses airflow rates, and plethysmography, which measures lung volumes. With this interpretation of these measurements, physicians can diagnose asthma, COPD, and restrictive lung diseases. In addition, the sensitivity and specificity of various PFTs allow precise discrimination between obstructive and restrictive patterns of ventilation, providing vital information to individualize treatment regimens effectively. Moreover, advances in imaging technologies, such as grating-based X-ray dark-field imaging, have enhanced the diagnostic profile of PFTs. This new method allows visualization of lung diseases like pulmonary emphysema in a way not possible with normal X-ray methods. For instance, studies have shown that normalized scatter signal imaging enhances discrimination between normal and emphysematous tissue, with significant increases in diagnostic accuracy when combined with standard PFT results. The cumulative data obtained through such imaging techniques augment those obtained with conventional PFTs, providing enhanced insight into pulmonary function and disease burden. With the integration of advanced imaging with routine PFTs, the evaluation process can be transformed and patient outcomes improved in respiratory diseases (Achterhold et al., 2013) (Figure 3.8).

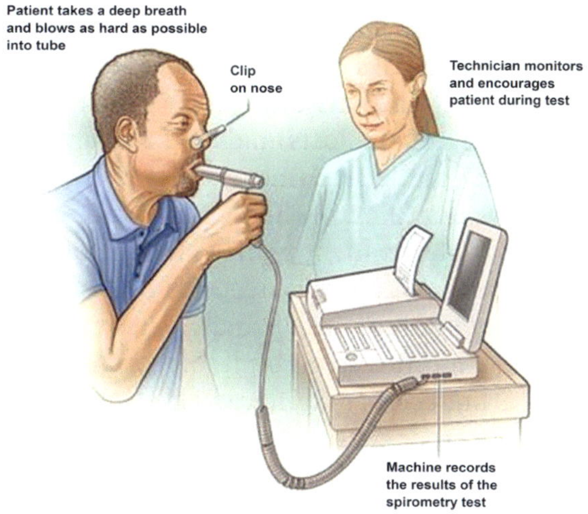

Figure 3.8. Pulmonary function test (PFTs).

Source: https://www.physio-pedia.com/images/thumb/a/a6/Spirometry1.jpg/399px-Spirometry1.jpg.

Further evidence also underscores the impact of body composition on lung function, underscoring the need for comprehensive assessments in respiratory medicine. More recent research has confirmed a strong correlation between body fat percentage and peak expiratory flow in children, further indicating that obesity can impair respiratory function. Specifically, when body fat accumulates, peak expiratory flow may decrease, an indicator of potential airway constriction. These findings confirm the need for comprehensive PFTs that consider not only lung function but also related factors, such as body composition. By incorporating measures of obesity and its impact on respiratory health, clinicians can improve management plans that ensure enhanced lung function and overall well-being for patients across various demographics (Indahswari et al., 2019).

3.3.2. Imaging Studies: X-rays and Computed Tomography (CT) Scans

Imaging studies such as X-rays and CT scans are central to practice in respiratory medicine, providing life-saving information on pulmonary pathologies. X-rays are the first evaluation of lung disease, and this aids in the diagnosis of pneumonia, tuberculosis, and lung cancer. Their availability and speed make them integral to acute care workflows, where immediate results are essential to patient management. However, the application of X-rays needs to be evaluated cautiously because, in a pediatric head trauma study, a significant amount of imaging was deemed unnecessary (Gharaibeh et al., 2025). This requires caution when evaluating by applying radiographic imaging to avoid excessive radiation exposure in subjects like children and potentially affect clinical decision-making in respiratory evaluation. CT scans offer the advantage of greater diagnostic potential than standard X-rays, enabling detailed cross-sectional images of the lung. This imaging modality has an upper hand in detecting subtle abnormalities like small lung nodules or complex structural change, which is extremely important for early cancer detection and staging, particularly in smokers or those with a high-risk background. One notable advancement in this field is the application of artificial intelligence (AI) to the analysis of chest X-rays and CT scans, with recent studies experimenting with AI systems to assess their performance in detecting lung nodules (Arzamasov et al., 2024) (Figure 3.9).

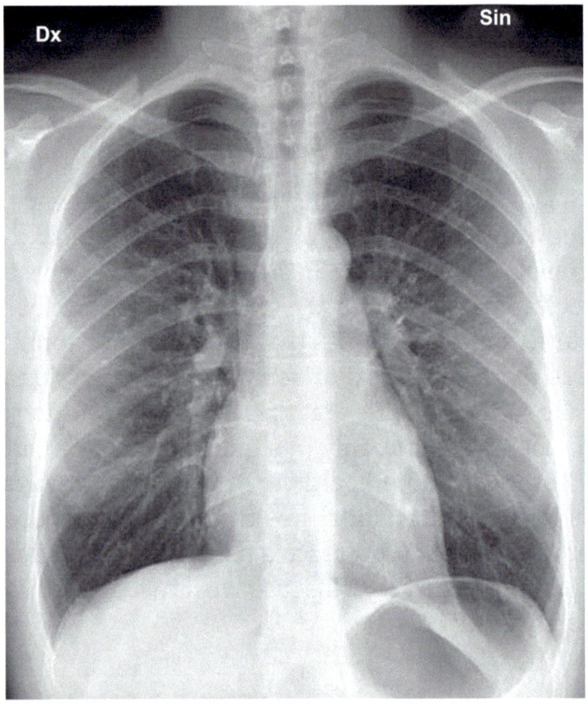

Figure 3.9. Chest radiograph.

Source: https://upload.wikimedia.org/wikipedia/commons/thumb/a/a1/Normal_posteroanterior_%28PA%29_chest_radiograph_%28X-ray%29.jpg/1200px-Normal_posteroanterior_%28PA%29_chest_radiograph_%28X-ray%29.jpg.

These technologies, as auspicious as they are, require careful testing to confirm that they meet clinical benchmarks for accuracy, testifying to the ongoing refinement of imaging strategies in respiratory medicine. The effectiveness of X-rays and CT scans in respiratory medicine also underscores the multifaceted equation between diagnostic imaging and the avoidance of unnecessary radiation exposure. As healthcare providers attempt to trade these factors off against each other, adherence to guidelines is necessary to achieve the best outcomes for patients. These research studies depict the overuse of imaging in clinical settings, where urgency and clinical necessity may not justify the need for imaging, leading to increased radiographic examinations among vulnerable populations (Gharaibeh et al., 2025). Additionally, ongoing technological innovation, including the development of AI applications, may yield advances in imaging studies, improving detection with reduced risk to imaging methodology. These advances ultimately aim to improve the diagnosis and treatment of respiratory disease, encouraging greater attention and patient-centered practice in respiratory medicine.

3.3.3. Bronchoscopy and Its Applications

Bronchoscopy has emerged as a standard practice in respiratory medicine, providing important diagnostic and therapeutic benefits for many pulmonary diseases. Equipped with a thin, flexible scope, a light source, and a camera, bronchoscopes allow physicians to visually inspect the airways and the lung interiors directly. This capability is translated into the retrieval and removal of tissue samples and the removal of obstructions, significantly enhancing diagnostic sensitivity. For instance, bronchoscopic biopsies can detect malignancy, infection, and inflammation that conventional imaging techniques would otherwise miss. Notably, the versatility of this technique extends to the management of acute respiratory diseases, where real-time intervention helps avoid complications. The breadth of possible applications underscores bronchoscopies' important role in modern respiratory care, allowing effective management plans to be tailored to individual patient needs and significantly improve outcomes. Advances in bronchoscopy technology have also broadened its use, addressing varied healthcare concerns related to respiratory illness. An example is the development of bronchial thermoplasty (BT), which illustrates how a new intervention can successfully treat severe asthma resistant to traditional treatment. This treatment, approved by the FDA, employs bronchoscopy to deliver thermal energy to smooth muscle within the airways, reducing its ability to constrict and, consequently, reducing asthma frequency and the severity of attacks (Figure 3.10).

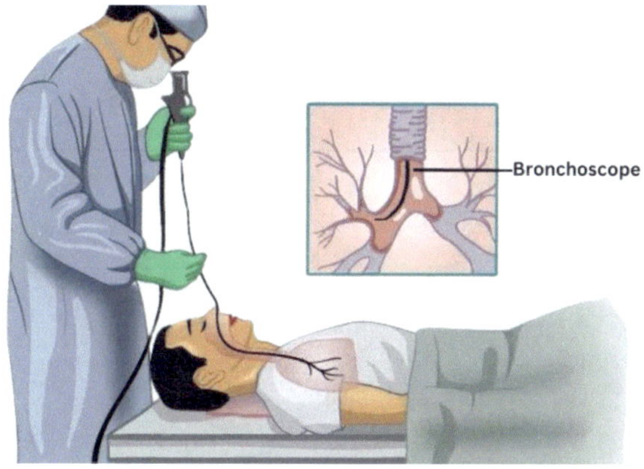

Figure 3.10. Bronchoscopy.

Source: https://www.universalhospitalsurat.com/wp-content/uploads/2023/11/Bronchoscope.png.

However, the addition of BT to clinical practice faces obstacles related to cost and accessibility. While promising emerging technologies are available, they also entail significant economic considerations relevant to health policy. Most prominently in environments of scarce resources, the meaning of such costs may restrict access to life-altering interventions, warranting strategic discourse on technology deployment in respiratory medicine, as suggested by problems with BT (Kenyon et al., 2017). The function of bronchoscopy is not confined to diagnosis and first-line treatments; it also identifies high-end viral pathogens, thereby contributing to enhanced clinical outcomes among respiratory patients.

The recent use of sophisticated technologies, such as the Virochip microarray, demonstrates that bronchoscopy can identify stealth viral infections that regular microbiologic testing may miss. In one instance, an adult with severe respiratory illness was diagnosed with human parainfluenzavirus 4 by bronchoscopy, when standard testing did not yield results (Blackburn et al., 2006). This case not only illustrates the usefulness of bronchoscopy in mass viral screening but also stresses the significance of research and development in respiratory medicine. By incorporating advanced diagnostic techniques into routine bronchoscopy, medical practitioners are best positioned to manage complex respiratory illnesses, enabling patients to be treated promptly and effectively as medical practice evolves.

Test Your Knowledge

1. What diagnostic tests are commonly used to assess lung function?
2. Why is chest imaging important in diagnosing respiratory diseases?

3.4. Treatment Modalities

Learning Outcome

1. Describe the pharmacological treatments: inhalers and medications
2. Discuss the non-pharmacological interventions: pulmonary rehabilitation
3. Identify the surgical options for severe cases

In respiratory medicine, the treatment landscape is always evolving, reflecting advances in technology and clinical practice. One of them is high-flow nasal cannula (HFNC) therapy, which has evolved into a significant intervention for patients with respiratory failure due to interstitial lung disease (ILD). The literature indicates that HFNC can significantly increase oxygen levels and alleviate dyspnea, thereby enhancing patient comfort and quality of life (Pagliaro et al., 2024). The systematic review of the application of HFNC across various clinical contexts underscores its suitability not just in acute care but also as a complementary intervention in palliative care. By understanding the complexities of ILD treatment, HFNC therapy is an established approach to the treatment of respiratory distress, suggesting the need for ongoing research to validate more rational protocols and ideal patient profiles. On further exploration of other treatment modalities, inhaled nanoparticle (NP) therapy emerges as a revolutionary approach in respiratory medicine. This new strategy leverages nanoparticles' ability to deliver drugs to targeted locations in the lungs, achieving optimized therapeutic activity while minimizing systemic side effects. Recent literature suggests that NP therapies, particularly those loaded with bronchodilators or anti-inflammatory agents, offer tailor-made solutions for long-term respiratory diseases such as COPD (Cojocaru et al., 2024). NP delivery precision ensures medication reaches the bronchial tree effectively, a radical departure from traditional systemic treatment approaches. Such an application not only addresses the limitations of existing therapy but also introduces new avenues for exploring nanoparticle technology that could ultimately reshape treatment concepts in respiratory health. In addition, the implementation of HFNC and NP therapies in practice highlights the growing emphasis on personalization in respiratory therapy. Both therapies indicate a transition towards personalized treatment approaches that take into account each patient's unique physiological response to heterogeneous respiratory conditions. HFNC therapies' non-invasiveness simplifies their use across settings, from acute care to terminal care, while NP therapies' targeted delivery system speaks to an intimate understanding of cellular disease processes (Cojocaru et al., 2024; Pagliaro et al., 2024). As each discipline advances, there is promise of better therapeutic and patient outcomes. Finally, the creation of novel modalities of care for respiratory illness marks a turning point in the evolution of patient-centered care, underscoring the need for ongoing innovation and rigorous clinical investigation.

3.4.1. Pharmacological Treatments: Inhalers and Medications

Treatment of respiratory conditions often depends on the use of inhalers and other pharmacologic treatments. Metered-dose inhalers (MDIs) and dry powder inhalers (DPIs) facilitate targeted drug delivery to the airways, lowering systemic side effects. These play a crucial role in managing conditions such as asthma and chronic obstructive pulmonary disease (COPD), where rapid relief of bronchoconstriction is needed to maintain patient health. Also, inhalers can carry several different types of medication, including bronchodilators, corticosteroids, or both, each targeting specific symptoms and disease progression. As technology in inhalers continues to improve, more effective formulations and user-friendly devices have become accessible, enhancing patient adherence to treatment and, consequently, patient outcomes in respiratory disease. The pharmacological treatment profile for respiratory illness also includes systemic agents that primarily regulate inflammation and mitigate exacerbations. In symptomatic patients with prolonged disease, suggesting severe forms of COPD, the addition of inhaled corticosteroids to bronchodilator therapy is standard. Double therapy not only aims at symptom relief but also attempts to reduce the frequency of exacerbations that contribute importantly to reduced quality of life. However, the efficacy of adding inhaled corticosteroids to long-acting bronchodilators, such as tiotropium, remains controversial among experts. More recent research shows that, in certain patients, adding inhaled corticosteroids to their therapy does not result in major benefits, further underscoring the need to adopt a personalized strategy for the treatment of respiratory disease (Aaron et al., 2011) (Figure 3.11).

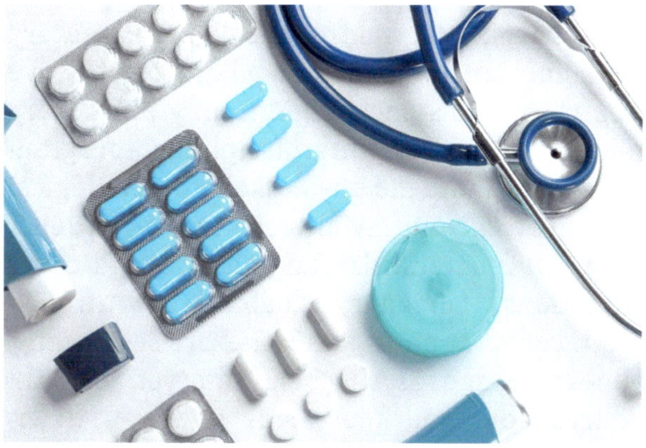

Figure 3.11. Pharmacological treatment of respiratory disorders.

Source: https://respiratory-therapy.com/wp-content/uploads/2019/03/inhaler-medications-healthcare-1500.jpg.

Besides, the balance between the benefits and risks of pharmacological treatment, particularly inhaled medications, requires patient observation under strict supervision. While inhalers are integral to managing chronic respiratory diseases, they also pose side effects, ranging from oral thrush and hoarseness to systemic effects from corticosteroid absorption. Patients should be instructed by clinicians on correct inhaler use and the importance of adhering to recommended therapies to achieve maximum effectiveness while minimizing unwanted effects. Additionally, it is critical to continuously monitor treatment effectiveness to modify therapy, especially when patients receive less-than-ideal outcomes or experience exacerbations. This prescient approach in respiratory medicine emphasizes the need for ongoing interaction between patients and clinicians (Amaducci et al., 2018), ensuring that treatment schedules remain effective and aligned with each patient's needs.

3.4.2. Non-Pharmacological Interventions: Pulmonary Rehabilitation

Non-pharmacological treatments in respiratory medicine are fundamental pillars of effective treatment plans, most significantly pulmonary rehabilitation. This interdisciplinary program aims to promote the physical and psychological health of chronically ill respiratory patients with COPD, interstitial lung disease, and other conditions. Pulmonary rehabilitation, through the incorporation of tailored exercise training, education, and psychosocial intervention, can address the multiple needs of the patients beyond symptom alleviation. It is shown that such interventions lead to enhanced exercise capacity, enhanced quality of life, and reduced dyspnea, highlighting the crucial function of non-pharmacological interventions in advanced care models. The use of pulmonary rehabilitation as a consequence not only alleviates physical symptoms but also fosters greater emotional resilience among patients with chronic lung diseases (Singanayagam et al., 2015).

Furthermore, mounting evidence of psychosocial determinants in the management of respiratory illness underscores the need for integration of psychological care within pulmonary rehabilitation programs. Patients tend to present with depression, anxiety, and loneliness as a direct consequence of their chronic illness, with a resultant effect on health status and compliance with treatment. Non-pharmacologic interventions, such as support groups and counseling, can reverse these effects by enhancing socialization and coping skills. The literature has established that these support interventions are important for optimizing the effectiveness of pulmonary rehabilitation by facilitating patients' active role in controlling their own health. Therefore, multidisciplinary interventions that combine physical and psychological components offer more complete benefits, thereby improving outcomes for patients in respiratory medicine (Boland et al., 2013). Regardless of the established efficacy of pulmonary rehabilitation, however, systemic barriers to delivery and access remain within health systems.

Restricted budgets, inadequate referral systems, and inadequate perception of its worth lead to underutilization by patients who would significantly benefit from such interventions. To address these challenges, healthcare providers must prioritize raising awareness and enhancing access to pulmonary rehabilitation services. Such a transition requires collaborative efforts among respiratory specialists, palliative care services, and general practitioners to develop comprehensive management guidelines for chronic lung diseases. By deconstructing existing obstacles and promoting a convergent focus on non-pharmacological treatment, healthcare professionals can significantly enhance the quality of life and treatment for respiratory patients, ultimately reconsidering respiratory medicine strategies (Singanayagam et al., 2015).

3.4.3. Surgical Options for Severe Cases

Treatment of respiratory diseases that become critical cases typically involves surgery, particularly when conservative treatment is insufficient for relief. In conditions such as severe pneumonia complicated by cardiac thrombosis, surgical options are considered. A case series of children pointed out the way in which, though anticoagulant treatments at first return good outcomes, some may not show improvement and thus require a more invasive intervention. Among those patients, surgical thrombectomy emerged as a helpful alternative, evidencing the necessity of multidisciplinary evaluation in intensive care departments. Such surgical procedures not only aim to minimize acute risks to survival in patients but also to optimize long-term respiratory performance, illustrating the interplay between pharmaceutical and surgical interventions in respiratory medicine (Yang et al., 2025). Surgical treatment is not merely mechanical management of the airway but rather a spectrum of interventions aiming at addressing underlying pathologies. In the given scenario of complicated pneumonia with an anatomical defect, procedures like lobectomy or decortication may be indicated. These procedures will remove infected or necrotic lung tissue, thereby significantly improving gas exchange and reducing systemic inflammation. A study examining cases of severe pneumonia in the Pediatric Intensive Care Units of Asia reported that 7.2% of patients admitted had such severe pneumonia that it necessitated intensive respiratory support, implying surgery in some conditions (Wong et al., 2024) (Figure 3.12).

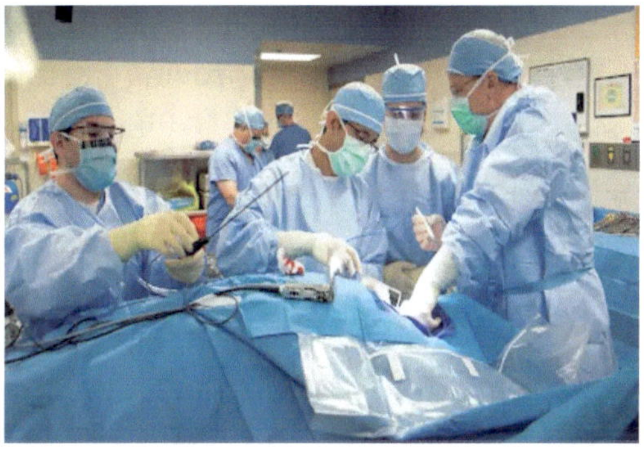

Figure 3.12. Lung surgery.

Source: https://stgaccinwbsdevlrs01.blob.core.windows.net/newcorporatewbsite/blogs/April2024/TaKCH7htHj4KIhORoI71.webp.

This illustration underscores the importance of evaluating each case for potential surgery after patients are unresponsive to standard treatment. Moreover, technological advancements in surgical mechanisms and procedures have significantly enhanced the versatility and safety of surgical interventions for complex respiratory disorders. Technologies such as video-assisted thoracoscopic surgery (VATS) have transformed severe pneumonia and its associated complication management through the promotion of minimally invasive interventions. These processes accelerate recovery and hospitalization and are particularly beneficial in the management of critically ill patients. Furthermore, the inclusion of multidisciplinary care teams comprising surgeons, pulmonologists, and intensivists ensures that surgical factors are addressed within a continuum of care, based on comprehensive assessments of patient-specific factors. Therefore, recognizing surgical interventions as a component of respiratory medicine helps bridge the gap between primary conservative treatment and the more severe treatments necessary for patient survival in critical situations (Yang et al., 2025).

Test Your Knowledge

1. What are the common treatment options used for respiratory diseases?
2. How do inhaled medications help in managing chronic respiratory conditions?

3.5. Public Health and Respiratory Medicine

Learning Outcome

1. Discuss how to impact of air quality on respiratory health
2. Define the preventive measures and health education
3. Explain the global initiatives to combat respiratory diseases

The intersection of public health and respiratory medicine brings significant challenges and opportunities to health systems worldwide. The burden of respiratory disease continues to increase, particularly in resource-poor environments. In Africa, for instance, the incidence of both transmissible diseases like pneumonia and tuberculosis, as well as the increasing frequency of non-transmissible respiratory diseases, underscores the general sophistication of addressing respiratory health. The recent COVID-19 pandemic has now also highlighted system vulnerabilities in health systems, presenting an opportune moment for actors in health to re-evaluate and further refine their approaches. Collaborative endeavors, including those by the Pan African Thoracic Society, are representative of the efforts to pool resources and capabilities in an aim to enhance respiratory health outcomes on the continent, setting the tone for an integrated regional response in the fight against these complex public health challenges (Erhabor et al., 2022). Antimicrobial resistance (AMR) adds an extra dimension of complexity to the field of respiratory medicine, affecting treatment effectiveness and influencing public health policy. The health problems posed by AMR require a comprehensive view of how it impacts different policy areas, including responsible use, surveillance, and infection prevention and control. As countries vary significantly in their financial strength and regulatory frameworks, many AMR control policies do not work. This reality calls for robust, evidence-based assessments of the existing intervention measures and making sure they can be locally fitted. The setting of a One Health priority can cut across sectors-humans and animals-and allow for policy-making taking into account the complicated issues of AMR and respiratory disease, especially among middle- and low-income nations (Aarestrup et al., 2015). Public health infrastructure development, particularly in respiratory medicine, is critical to improving overall health outcomes. To address the rising burden of respiratory disease, we need to strengthen preventive interventions, ensure equitable access to care, and encourage research and education. Social determinants of health also need to be addressed, as poverty, environmental exposures, and access to quality care affect the prevalence of respiratory illness. Altogether, government coordination, public health organizations, and community leaders can build resistance to respiratory diseases through rigorous health education, proactive interventions, and improved healthcare policies. Ultimately, a strong public health infrastructure dedicated to respiratory health will not only reduce personal suffering but also enhance community well-being and economic productivity, paving the way for a brighter future (Erhabor et al., 2022).

3.5.1. Impact of Air Quality on Respiratory Health

Respiratory health is highly influenced by air quality, and various toxins contribute to a range of lung conditions. Exposure to smog, particulate matter, and toxic gases correlates with chronic illnesses such as asthma and chronic obstructive pulmonary disease (COPD). Because respiratory systems interact closely with airborne substances, individuals exposed to poor air quality are at higher risk of exacerbation and worsening symptoms. Besides, acute exposure to high levels of air pollutants causes inflammation and acute respiratory distress, leading to hospitalization. Increasing urbanization and industrialization exacerbate these issues, creating a public health crisis that cannot be disregarded. A deep understanding of these interactions is essential to inform policies aimed at mitigating the adverse effects of air pollution on respiratory health and overall public health outcomes. Wildfires and the resulting smoke are exemplary illustrations of how air quality can deteriorate rapidly and pose severe health risks. As climate change increases the frequency and severity of wildfires, populations are increasingly exposed to hazardous smoke that can contain a wide range of chemicals. Emerging research is highlighting the reality that wildfire smoke can produce significant health consequences, including respiratory distress and chronic conditions, not only for humans but also for wildlife (Sanderfoot et al., 2021) (Figure 3.13).

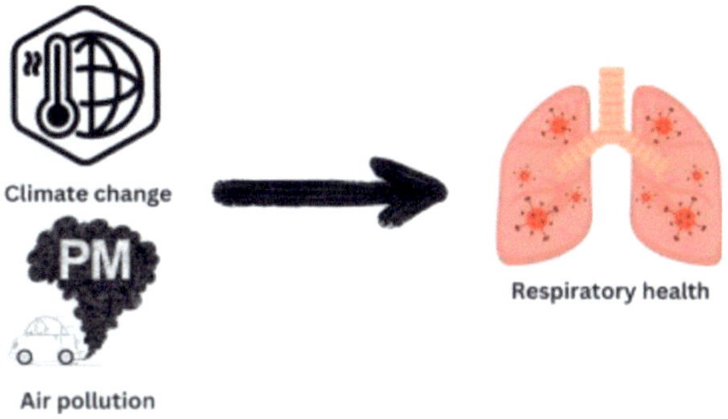

Figure 3.13. The impact of air pollution on respiratory diseases in an era of climate change.

Source: https://ars.els-cdn.com/content/image/1-s2.0-S0048969723049653-ga1.jpg.

The particulates emitted by such incidents penetrate deep into lung tissue, worsening preexisting conditions and causing new respiratory diseases. Secondly, shifts in species behavior caused by smoke exposure, such as retreating from smoke-impacted areas, accentuate the connectivity of air and breathing health across systems. This underscores the need for interdisciplinary approaches to address the implications of air quality. The global burden of cardiovascular disease (CVD) is also associated with air quality's impact on the respiratory system, reflecting the extensive effects of environmental pollutants. Studies have established that exposure to air pollution is not only harmful for the proper functioning of lungs but also poses an immense risk for cardiovascular disease (Roth et al., 2020). Pollutants such as particulate matter have been seen to cause systemic inflammatory reactions, thereby exacerbating the risk of heart attacks and stroke. The increasing number of CVD cases linked to poor air quality mean that interventions aimed at respiratory and cardiovascular health are urgently needed. As cities expand, so does the necessity for effective policies to improve air quality. Air pollution is associated with increased deaths worldwide. These interventions have the potential to reduce the healthcare load of chronic respiratory and cardiovascular illnesses, improve life expectancy, and quality of life in affected populations.

3.5.2. Preventive Measures and Health Education

Preventive interventions and health education are of utmost importance in respiratory medicine, particularly in preventing the onset and burden of respiratory diseases. Effective health education programs increase people's awareness of the risks of respiratory disorders, enabling them to make informed health choices. For instance, sensitizing the masses about the dangers of smoking and air contaminants can significantly decrease the number of cases of chronic obstructive pulmonary disease (COPD) and asthma. Furthermore, encouraging programs that promote physical activity can improve respiratory health, as organized interventions have been shown to increase physical activity and cardiorespiratory fitness in adults. These findings underpin the need for a comprehensive approach to health education that not only conveys information but also promotes favorable behavior change towards respiratory health (Foster et al., 2025). In addressing respiratory health, it is important to recognize that educational interventions must be integrated into overall public health policy. The Patient Protection and Affordable Care Act, although a milestone in healthcare access, underscores the importance of focusing on prevention and wellness to improve population health results. There needs to be a transition towards public health funding and investments in building robust health infrastructure with preventive programs.

This collaboration between public health and health care can facilitate an integrated approach to respiratory disease prevention, ensuring resources are allocated to both treatment and education. If health education is emphasized as a critical component of public health policy, researchers can effectively reduce health disparities in outcomes and enhance the quality of patient care (Gostin et al., 2011). Apart from this, conceptualizing a community-based intervention program on respiratory health can help make preventive interventions more impactful. Having local organizations and health care providers participate in promoting respiratory health services can lead to a program tailored to the community's specific needs. For example, smoking cessation seminars, asthma control training, and air quality education seminars can empower people and families to be their own "experts" of respiratory health. These interventions can simultaneously address environmental risk determinants and foster healthy lifestyle habits, with synergistic effects on population health. In effect, focusing on prevention through education and community involvement not only imposes personal responsibility for health but also leads to more robust, healthier communities, ultimately reducing the burden of respiratory disease (Gostin et al., 2011; Foster et al., 2025).

3.5.3. Global Initiatives to Combat Respiratory Diseases

In recent years, there has been tremendous momentum behind global action against respiratory diseases, reflecting the increasing burden of these diseases. Actions taken by agencies such as the World Health Organization (WHO) focus on developing an integrated response to treat both communicable and non-communicable respiratory diseases. Global action in this context seeks to enhance surveillance, improve access to health resources, and build community awareness on preventive measures. By developing guidelines and frameworks that emphasize good management practices, these global campaigns reduce morbidity and mortality of respiratory illnesses, particularly in low and middle-income nations where the impact is typically more widespread and aggravated by substandard healthcare infrastructure. A key feature of these programs is integrating a One Health approach, which recognizes the interconnectedness among human, animal, and environmental health. This integrated strategy is essential to create responsive policies that can respond to the evolving threats posed by respiratory diseases.

Effective policy development must consider the determinants of disease spread, including air quality, pollution, and the spread of infectious agents. Furthermore, the complexity of implementing such policies across various political and regulatory settings necessitates a rigorous evaluation of their impact as an imperative. A current study emphasizes the importance of intensive policy reviews, such as cost-effectiveness evaluations and generalizability to different socio-economic contexts, especially in low-income countries (Aarestrup et al., 2015). Global collaboration among international organizations, governments, and research organizations is also crucial in fostering research and development to combat respiratory diseases. Funding for innovative treatments, vaccination programs, and public health initiatives is highly important. As the Global IDEA Scientific Advisory Committee highlighted, there are immense economic and health benefits from accelerated research on global infectious illnesses, such as respiratory illnesses (Buxton et al., 2005). By drawing on current knowledge and focusing on cross-sector collaboration, the activities can significantly improve patient outcomes while building resilience against future health crises driven by respiratory diseases. Thus, commitment to a single, evidence-based process will become an integral part of the long-term global battle against respiratory disorders.

Test Your Knowledge

1. How does air pollution impact respiratory health at the population level?
2. What role do vaccination and smoking cessation play in preventing respiratory diseases?

SUMMARY

As a final note to this exploration of respiratory medicine, it is essential to recognize the profound changes occurring in the field through technological advances and shifting treatment methods. When new processes are introduced into practice, they not only enhance diagnostic testing but also improve patient outcomes. As research continues to advance our understanding of respiratory disease and therapy, the necessity of a multifaceted response becomes increasingly evident. By adopting an interdisciplinary approach and leveraging technological advances, respiratory medicine is better equipped to deliver improved patient care. This constantly shifting landscape highlights the importance of embracing change without compromising ethical standards and patient rights, so that any development does not undermine the dignity or safety of patients, as expounded in the health care literature on neurological interventions (Whitaker et al., 2018). Furthermore, the ethical dimensions of treatment modalities cannot be disregarded. With new developments in respiratory medicine, medical practitioners are compelled to walk that fine line between innovation and the ethical considerations that accompany it. This tightrope, of course, leads to dilemmas regarding how much technology should be employed in therapy. The implementation of new diagnostic technologies and intervention therapies, although lucrative, raises questions about patient autonomy and the acceptability of interventions (Whitaker et al., 2018). Healthcare workers must be diligent in addressing such matters while fostering a culture of transparency and open communication with patients. Such measures are crucial to facilitating trust in the patient-healthcare worker relationship, which is critical to achieving optimal medical care. Finally, addressing knowledge and resource shortages remains a priority in the specialty of respiratory medicine. As prior research has shown, vast disparities exist in access to advanced treatments and technologies, which greatly influence patient prognosis. The continued development of diagnostic criteria and treatment protocols necessitates commitment to ongoing education and training for healthcare professionals to ensure they can continue to provide the best possible care. Future research should strive to overcome these disparities, along with the challenges in efficient management of novel therapies. In the end, by placing the most significant emphasis on education, ethical issues, and equitable access to therapy, respiratory medicine can chart a visionary course, enhancing the quality of care for all suffering from respiratory disease.

The clinical investigation of respiratory medicine encompasses a range of diseases and syndromes with profound implications for patient health, especially chronic conditions like asthma. The understanding of the complexity of asthma is essential, as it is based on multiple immunologic and inflammatory mechanisms. Recent studies using transcriptomic profiling have delineated asthma phenotypes by carefully examining bronchial biopsies and epithelial brushings from patients. Surprisingly, studies identified two prominent subtypes characterized by high levels of T-helper type 2 (Th-2) cytokines and mixed corticosteroid responsiveness. Such stratification underscores the need for individualized therapeutic intervention, as patients with specific inflammatory profiles exhibit disparate clinical manifestations and drug responses, making precision medicine crucial for addressing respiratory disorders (Adcock et al., 2016). In addition to characterizing categorical asthma subtypes, new noninvasive techniques are critical to advancing respiratory medicine. Noninvasive medical testing, for instance, allows examination of an array of pathologies with less risk for invasive tests in patients. Although these tests may include enormous numbers of clinical parameters, embedded in the data is an intricacy of information processing that demands rigid statistical analysis to provide significant indicators of health. The research emphasizes the importance of establishing the correct correlations between these markers and patient health status to enable the assessment of respiratory function with greater confidence. Therefore, understanding the processing subtleties of noninvasive testing becomes key to streamlining patient care and providing appropriate treatment plans (Gulotta et al., 2000). The integration of machine-learning techniques into pulmonary medicine also reflects the paradigm shift in patient care. Applying sophisticated algorithms to assess inflammatory biomarkers such as sputum eosinophilia and exhaled nitric oxide levels, researchers can now predict asthma subtypes with excellent sensitivity and specificity. Not only does this new method shed more light on triggering disease mechanisms, but it also guides clinicians in selecting the appropriate therapeutic intervention for individual patient profiles. With treatment for asthma and other respiratory diseases becoming increasingly available, the merging of genetic, environmental, and clinical data through machine learning holds out a new era of respiratory medicine in which personalized medicine is no longer an illusion on the horizon but a practical reality within reach of every patient worldwide.

KEY TERMS FROM THIS CHAPTER

- Respiratory medicine
- Pneumonia
- High-resolution computed tomography (HRCT)
- Anxiety
- Bronchus-associated lymphoid tissue (BALT)
- Pulmonary Fibrosis
- Lung Cancer
- Spirometry
- Coug
- Chronic obstructive pulmonary disease
- Pathophysiology
- Depression
- Respiratory system
- Vascular network
- Tuberculosis
- Bronchoscopy
- Dyspnea

CRITICAL THINKING QUESTIONS

1. **Which of the following is the most common cause of community-acquired pneumonia?**
   a. Klebsiella pneumoniae
   b. Mycoplasma pneumoniae
   c. Streptococcus pneumoniae
   d. Haemophilus influenzae
2. **A 65-year-old man with a long smoking history presents with chronic cough and sputum production. The most likely diagnosis is:**
   a. Asthma
   b. Chronic bronchitis
   c. Emphysema
   d. Bronchiectasis
3. **Which of the following is a typical finding in a patient with asthma?**
   a. Decreased FEV1/FVC ratio
   b. Increased DLCO (diffusing capacity)
   c. Flattened diaphragm on chest X-ray
   d. Reduced total lung capacity
4. **Which investigation is most specific for diagnosing pulmonary embolism?**
   a. Chest X-ray
   b. D-dimer
   c. Ventilation-perfusion (V/Q) scan
   d. CT pulmonary angiography
5. **What is the first-line treatment for an acute asthma attack?**
   a. Oral corticosteroids
   b. Inhaled corticosteroids
   c. Inhaled short-acting beta-agonists (SABA)
   d. Leukotriene receptor antagonists

Short Answer Questions

1. What is the difference between the anatomy and physiology of the respiratory system?
2. Name three common respiratory diseases and briefly describe one.
3. What are two diagnostic techniques commonly used in respiratory medicine?
4. How does bronchodilator therapy help in managing respiratory conditions like asthma?
5. What role do imaging techniques such as CT scans play in diagnosing respiratory diseases?
6. Mention one recent advancement in respiratory medicine and its significance.

Answers to Critical Thinking Questions

1. (c); 2. (b) ; 3. (a); 4. (d); 5. (c)

REFERENCES

1. Dar, O. A., Hasan, R., Schlundt, J., Harbarth, S., Caleo, G., Dar, F. K., Littmann, J., Rweyemamu, M., Buckley, E. J., Shahid, M., Kock, R., Li, H. L., Giha, H., Khan, M., So, A. D., Bindayna, K. M., Kessel, A., Pedersen, H. B., Permanand, G., . . . Heymann, D. L. (2015c). Exploring the evidence base for national and regional policy interventions to combat resistance. *The Lancet, 387*(10015), 285–295. https://doi.org/10.1016/s0140-6736(15)00520-6Aaron, S. D., Agarwal, A., Akazawa, M., Appleton, S., Barr, R. G., Beeh, K. M., et al. (2011). The effect of adding inhaled corticosteroids to tiotropium and long-acting beta(2)-agonists for chronic obstructive pulmonary disease (Review). https://core.ac.uk/download/10674737.pdf (accessed on 16th July 2025).
2. Abbott, J., Borgarelli, M., Clercx, C., Kellihan, H. B., et al. (2020). ACVIM consensus statement guidelines for the diagnosis, classification, treatment, and monitoring of pulmonary hypertension in dogs. https://core.ac.uk/download/323070279.pdf (accessed on 16th July 2025).
3. Achterhold, K., Auweter, S., Bamberg, F., Bech, M., et al. (2013). Diagnosing and mapping pulmonary emphysema on X-ray projection images. https://core.ac.uk/download/12175665.pdf (accessed on 16th July 2025).
4. Adcock, I. M., Auffray, C., Baribaud, F., Chanez, P., et al. (2016). A transcriptome-driven analysis of epithelial brushings and bronchial biopsies to define asthma phenotypes in U-BIOPRED. https://core.ac.uk/download/77018710.pdf (accessed on 16th July 2025).
5. Al-Tawfiq, J. A., Benkouiten, S., & Memish, Z. A. (2018). A systematic review of emerging respiratory viruses at the Hajj and possible coinfection with *Streptococcus pneumoniae*. https://core.ac.uk/download/322846904.pdf (accessed on 16th July 2025).
6. Amaducci, S., Bacci, E., Baldacci, S., Bartoli, M., et al. (2018). Inhalation therapy in the next decade: Determinants of adherence to treatment in asthma and COPD. https://core.ac.uk/download/152415584.pdf (accessed on 16th July 2025).
7. Arzamasov, K., Vasilev, Y., Zelenova, M., Pestrenin, L., Busygina, Y., Bobrovskaya, T., Chetverikov, S., et al. (2024). Independent evaluation of the accuracy of 5 artificial intelligence software for detecting lung nodules on chest X-rays. *Quantitative Imaging in Medicine and Surgery, 14*, 5288–5303. https://www.semanticscholar.org/paper/3a1152462881f4da2497c8d705ef2dd8016f7aa2 (accessed on 16th July 2025).
8. Beller, E. M., Coxeter, P., Del Mar, C. B., Hoffmann, T., et al. (2015). Interventions to facilitate shared decision making to address antibiotic use for acute respiratory infections in primary care. https://core.ac.uk/download/196601007.pdf (accessed on 16th July 2025).
9. Bhaskar, A., Goyal, M., & Panara, K. (2024). Understanding chronic obstructive pulmonary disease and its management—Ayurvedic point of view: A scoping review. *AYU (An International Quarterly Journal of Research in Ayurveda)*. https://www.semanticscholar.org/paper/d2b592cd64b9f78f4d1e5fdabc2d5a1a264c3842 (accessed on 16th July 2025).
10. Blackburn, B. G., Chiu, C. Y., DeRisi, J. L., Eckburg, P. B., et al. (2006). Microarray detection of human parainfluenza virus 4 infection associated with respiratory failure in an immunocompetent adult. https://core.ac.uk/download/323072700.pdf (accessed on 16th July 2025).

11. Boland, J., Martin, J., Ross, J. R., Ross, C. M., et al. (2013). Palliative care for people with non-malignant lung disease: Summary of current evidence and future direction. https://core.ac.uk/download/151156967.pdf (accessed on 16th July 2025).

12. Bracha, H. S., & Burkle, F. M. (2006). Utility of fear severity and individual resilience scoring as a surge capacity, triage management tool during large-scale, bio-event disasters. https://core.ac.uk/download/pdf/86672.pdf (accessed on 16th July 2025).

13. Buxton, M. J., & Hanney, S. (2005). Global IDEA. https://core.ac.uk/download/333547.pdf (accessed on 16th July 2025).

14. Car, S., Padavic, I., & Velic, M. (2013). Computer-aided ECG analysis – State of the art and upcoming challenges. http://arxiv.org/abs/1306.5096 (accessed on 16th July 2025).

15. Chiu, C. Y., & Miller, S. A. (2019). Clinical metagenomics. https://core.ac.uk/download/323062552.pdf (accessed on 16th July 2025).

16. Chopra, V., Flanders, S. A., O'Malley, M., Malani, A. N., & Prescott, H. C. (2020). Sixty-day outcomes among patients hospitalized with COVID-19. *Annals of Internal Medicine, 174*, 576–578. https://doi.org/10.7326/m20-5661 (accessed on 16th July 2025).

17. Cojocaru, E., Petriș, O. R., & Cojocaru, C. (2024). Nanoparticle-based drug delivery systems in inhaled therapy: Improving respiratory medicine. *Pharmaceuticals, 17*. https://www.semanticscholar.org/paper/79f27cdcba510e41d7b40d33b1f2c92884761be9 (accessed on 16th July 2025).

18. Copot, D., Ghita, M., Ghita, M., Ionescu, C., et al. (2019). A medical information system for monitoring respiratory function and related nonlinear dynamics. https://core.ac.uk/download/322827882.pdf (accessed on 16th July 2025).

19. Cortegiani, A., Gregoretti, C., & Spoletini, G. (2019). Physio pathological rationale of using high-flow nasal therapy in the acute and chronic setting: A narrative review. https://core.ac.uk/download/224993362.pdf (accessed on 16th July 2025).

20. Czesnikiewicz-Guzik, M., Jasiewicz-Honkisz, B., Maciag, J., Matusik, P., et al. (2016). Th17 responses are not altered by natural exposure to seasonal allergens in pollen-sensitive patients. https://core.ac.uk/download/74230778.pdf (accessed on 16th July 2025).

21. Dalamani, G., Kaspers, B., & Reese, S. (2006). The avian lung-associated immune system. https://core.ac.uk/download/12174987.pdf (accessed on 16th July 2025).

22. Dear, J. D. (2020). Bacterial pneumonia in dogs and cats: An update. https://core.ac.uk/download/286361309.pdf (accessed on 16th July 2025).

23. Deary, I. J., Hart, C. L., Hole, D., Smith, G. D., et al. (2005). Childhood IQ and social factors on smoking behavior, lung function and smoking-related outcomes in adulthood: Linking the Scottish Mental Survey 1932 and the Midspan studies. https://core.ac.uk/download/1393705.pdf (accessed on 16th July 2025).

24. Du, L., Jiang, S., Ojcius, D. M., Pan, H., et al. (2020). Measures for diagnosing and treating infections by a novel coronavirus responsible for a pneumonia outbreak originating in Wuhan, China. https://core.ac.uk/download/323063844.pdf (accessed on 16th July 2025).

25. Erhabor, G. E. (2022). Respiratory health in Africa: Strides and challenges. https://core.ac.uk/download/552647920.pdf (accessed on 16th July 2025).

26. Farooq, S., Imran, M. A., Latif, S., Qadir, J., et al. (2017). How 5G wireless (and concomitant technologies) will revolutionize healthcare? https://core.ac.uk/download/143476480.pdf (accessed on 16th July 2025).

27. Feschenko, Y., & Nazarenko, K. (2017). Evaluation of functional condition of respiratory muscles of patients with a complicated bronchial asthma pathology and chronic obstructive pulmonary diseases. https://core.ac.uk/download/322516354.pdf (accessed on 16th July 2025).

28. Foster, C., Hillsdon, M., & Thorogood, M. (2025). Interventions for promoting physical activity (review). https://core.ac.uk/download/49216.pdf (accessed on 16th July 2025).

29. Gharaibeh, A., Lackova, A., Gharaibeh, M. M., Alwadiya, A., Čellár, R., Mitró, I., Filip, V., et al. (2025). Overuse of ionizing radiation imaging by skull X-ray scans for minor pediatric head trauma. *European Journal of Clinical and Experimental Medicine*. https://www.semanticscholar.org/paper/5cd1b5cd98f2aa51ef4b8b02eaed2cc74e0a117a (accessed on 16th July 2025).

30. Gostin, L. O., Hardcastle, L. E., Jacobson, P. D., Record, K. L., et al. (2011). Restoring health to health reform: Integrating medicine and public health to advance the population's wellbeing. https://core.ac.uk/download/70374138.pdf (accessed on 16th July 2025).

31. Gottlieb, M. L., & Moore, C. B. (1979). Activities of nurse practitioners as identified by medical directors of university student health services. https://core.ac.uk/download/215482198.pdf (accessed on 16th July 2025).

32. Gulotta, C., Parvis, M., & Torchio, R. (2000). Uncertainty analysis of feature extraction from expired gas traces. https://core.ac.uk/download/pdf/11373787.pdf (accessed on 16th July 2025).

33. Guo, Y. R., Cao, Q. D., Hong, Z. S., Tan, Y. Y., Chen, S. D., Jin, H. J., Tan, K. S., et al. (2020). The origin, transmission and clinical therapies on coronavirus disease 2019 (COVID-19) outbreak–An update on the status. *Military Medical Research, 7*. https://doi.org/10.1186/s40779-020-00240-0 (accessed on 16th July 2025).

34. Hasbe, P. B., Dhapke, P., & Baheti, J. R. (2025). Comprehensive narrative review on nanotechnology for the treatment of glaucoma. *Asian Journal of Pharmacy and Technology*. https://www.semanticscholar.org/paper/2c0937355005 85dd94e05f32cd398a338dd30951 (accessed on 16th July 2025).

35. Indahswari, N. W., Indrayani, A. W., Thanaya, S. A., Wibawa, I. D. M. A., et al. (2019). The correlation between body fat percentage and peak expiratory flow in children aged 10–12 years at SD Negeri 8 Dauh Puri. https://core.ac.uk/download/234033578.pdf (accessed on 16th July 2025).

36. Jarusevicius, L., Krilavicius, T., Simonavicius, H., Zliobaite, I., et al. (2015). Predicting respiratory motion for real-time tumor tracking in radiotherapy. http://arxiv.org/abs/1508.00749 (accessed on 16th July 2025).

37. Kenyon, N., Louie, S., Tan, L. D., Yoneda, K., et al. (2017). Bronchial thermoplasty: Implementing best practice in the era of cost containment. https://core.ac.uk/download/323071298.pdf (accessed on 16th July 2025).

38. Lombardi, C., Savi, E., Heffler, E., Canonica, G. W., Passalacqua, G., Milanese, M., Costantino, M. T., et al. (2016). Appropriateness in allergic respiratory diseases health care in Italy:

Definitions and organizational aspects. https://core.ac.uk/download/pdf/81832237.pdf (accessed on 16th July 2025).

39. Lundborg, K. (2004). Housing, management and health in Swedish dairy calves. https://core.ac.uk/download/11694701.pdf (accessed on 16th July 2025).

40. Miller, L., Pinkerton, K., Royer, C., Schelegle, E., et al. (2017). Nonhuman primate models of respiratory disease: Past, present, and future. https://core.ac.uk/download/323069778.pdf (accessed on 16th July 2025).

41. Pagliaro, R., Aronne, L., Fomez, R., Ferri, V., Montella, A., Sanduzzi Zamparelli, S., Bianco, A., et al. (2024). High-flow nasal cannula system in respiratory failure associated with interstitial lung diseases: A systematic review and narrative synthesis. *Journal of Clinical Medicine, 13*. https://www.semanticscholar.org/paper/a054b5278555663b0dd43f1d2ddd36a67d17d6e0 (accessed on 16th July 2025).

42. Pal, A., Munshi, S., & Tripathi, S. K. (2025). Impact of clinical pharmacological intervention on treatment adherence among adult patients with bronchial asthma and COPD: A randomized clinical study. *Journal of Clinical and Diagnostic Research*. https://www.semanticscholar.org/paper/f3fc3f4862d180cf7bf21e276946b07012105e0e (accessed on 16th July 2025).

43. Roth, G. A., Mensah, G. A., Johnson, C. O., Addolorato, G., Ammirati, E., Baddour, L. M., Barengo, N. C., et al. (2020). Global burden of cardiovascular diseases and risk factors, 1990–2019. *Journal of the American College of Cardiology, 76*, 2982–3021. https://doi.org/10.1016/j.jacc.2020.11.010 (accessed on 16th July 2025).

44. Sanderfoot, O. V., Bassing, S. B., Brusa, J. L., Emmet, R. L., Gillman, S. J., Swift, K., & Gardner, B. (2021). A review of the effects of wildfire smoke on the health and behavior of wildlife. *Environmental Research Letters, 16*, 123003–123003. https://doi.org/10.1088/1748-9326/ac30f6 (accessed on 16th July 2025).

45. Schultheis, W. W. F., Madeira, W. S., Narduci, J. C., Feitosa, T. E. C., Martins, K. S., Camara, L. O., Jeronimo, M. P. P., et al. (2025). 4D printed implants for the reconstruction of bone defects in craniomaxillofacial surgery: The evolution of regenerative bioengineering. *Revita CPAQV–Centro de Pesquisas Avançadas em Qualidade de Vida*. https://www.semanticscholar.org/paper/381817f4f5b308a836bf3fb1c86f41fa32f63275 (accessed on 16th July 2025).

46. Singanayagam, A., Crockett, A. J., Ries, A. L., Yohannes, A. M., Fletcher, C., Bucknall, C. E., Fletcher, C. M., et al. (2015). Four patients with a history of acute exacerbations of COPD: Implementing the CHEST/Canadian Thoracic Society guidelines for preventing exacerbations. https://core.ac.uk/download/30697683.pdf (accessed on 16th July 2025).

47. Tillotson, J. (2008). JENTIL: Responsive clothing that promotes a 'holistic approach to fashion' as a new vehicle to treat psychological conditions. http://ualresearchonline.arts.ac.uk/4907/1/Tillotson_Scent_IFFTI2008_doc_.pdf (accessed on 16th July 2025).

48. Wang, X., & Fan, J. (2021). Spatiotemporal molecular medicine: A new era of clinical and translational medicine. *Clinical and Translational Medicine, 11*. https://doi.org/10.1002/ctm2.294 (accessed on 16th July 2025).

49. Whitaker, H. N. (2018). Attitudes on medical ethics of criminal neurointerventional treatment. https://core.ac.uk/download/213462108.pdf (accessed on 16th July 2025).

50. Wong, J. J., Abbas, Q. E., Wang, J. Q. Y., Xu, W., Dang, H., Phan, P., Guo, L., et al. (2024). Severe pneumonia in PICU admissions: The Pediatric Acute and Critical Care Medicine Asian Network (PACCMAN) observational cohort study, 2020–2022. *Pediatric Critical Care Medicine, 25*, 1035–1044. https://www.semanticscholar.org/paper/e5e04d2fdf020cae1dc56187da207ff246fbd5a2 (accessed on 16th July 2025).

51. Wood, B. R., Young, J. D., Abdel-Massih, R., McCurdy, L., Vento, T. J., Dhanireddy, S., Moyer, K. J., et al. (2020). Advancing digital health equity: A policy paper of the Infectious Diseases Society of America and the HIV Medicine Association. *Clinical Infectious Diseases, 72*, 913–919. https://doi.org/10.1093/cid/ciaa1525 (accessed on 16th July 2025).

52. Yang, J., Liu, F., Chen, X., Guo, C. Y., Liang, Y., Dai, F., Ding, N., et al. (2025). [Clinical analysis of 15 cases of severe *Mycoplasma pneumoniae* pneumonia complicated by cardiac thrombosis in children]. *Zhonghua Er Ke Za Zhi = Chinese Journal of Pediatrics, 63*(5), 535–540. https://www.semanticscholar.org/paper/f30ab219eaeaa9e655de9208d742a2d563a63a70 (accessed on 16th July 2025).

53. Zibrak, J. D., & Price, D. (2014). Interstitial lung disease: Raising the index of suspicion in primary care. https://core.ac.uk/download/25497515.pdf (accessed on 16th July 2025).

GASTROENTEROLOGY

4

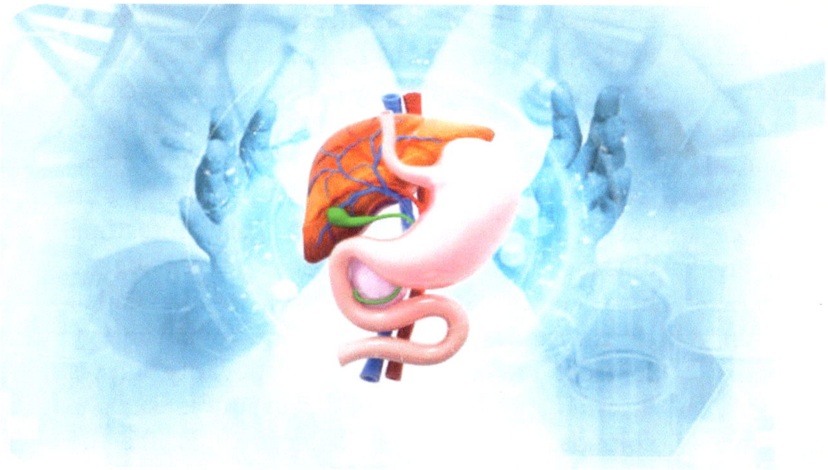

LEARNING OBJECTIVES

After studying this chapter, you will be able to:

1. Define an overview of gastroenterology
2. Explain the diagnostic techniques in gastroenterology
3. Discuss the treatment modalities in gastroenterology
4. Identify the common gastrointestinal disorders
5. Describe the role of nutrition in gastroenterology
6. Explain the advances in gastroenterology

Introduction

Internal medicine is the cornerstone of patient care, with a concentration on the comprehensive management of adult diseases. It includes an expansive range of disorders, particularly internal organ disorders, which are critical for gastroenterologists. Knowledge of the principles of internal medicine enables gastroenterologists to appreciate how systemic illnesses manifest as gastrointestinal symptoms. Moreover, internal medicine provides the mechanisms of differential diagnosis and clinical judgment required to treat complex cases. By integrating pathophysiology and pharmacology, internal medicine equips the gastroenterologist to develop effective treatment plans and tailor them to individual patient needs. A strong understanding of internal medicine is thus paramount to advancing patient care in gastroenterological practice. The need for broad patient assessment and intervention planning underscores the interfacing between gastroenterology and internal medicine. Gastroenterologists usually encounter patients with multiple comorbidities, and thus an internal medicine orientation is needed to control them best. This multidisciplinary approach provides a comprehensive understanding of the patient's health and addresses not only gastrointestinal diseases but also the interconnectedness of other organ systems. For instance, liver disease is more likely to be linked to metabolic syndromes, which are something that internal medicine physicians can manage. Moreover, best practice in internal medicine ensures that gastroenterologists are able to implement guidelines and evidence-based practice effectively. With ongoing awareness of the broader context of internal medicine, gastroenterologists can better encourage preventive care, thereby preventing the onset of chronic diseases that significantly affect the gastrointestinal system. Incorporating practical communication skills in the practice of internal medicine is important for enhancing rapport and patient trust. Gastroenterologists, as first-line providers, must be able to explain complex medical language in understandable terms for patients. Such communications allow for informed choices, making patients active participants in their health care. In addition, the ability to demonstrate empathy and sensitivity when discussing gastrointestinal diseases, such as colon cancer screening or inflammatory bowel disease, is an intrinsic part of the patient-provider relationship. Such soft skills are developed through internal medicine training in patient interaction, role-playing, and workshops so that practitioners can refine their styles. Thus, applying the principles of effective communication and internal medicine can lead to improved patient compliance and satisfaction and ultimately better health outcomes in gastroenterological situations.

Definition and Scope of Internal Medicine

Internal medicine is a medical specialty primarily concerned with the diagnosis, treatment, and prevention of adult diseases. Internists, being specifically qualified in internal medicine, are committed to understanding complex medical issues and applying scientific principles to clinical practice in ways that address complex patient needs. This medical specialty is not only critical for primary care but as a stepping-stone for subspecialties, such as gastroenterology. The richness of internal medicine lies in its in-depth knowledge of various body systems, pathophysiology, and disease interactions; hence, it is a critical category in managing chronic diseases and acute medical emergencies effectively. Internal medicine has its horizons overspilled into various subspecialties, so doctors can pursue extensive study in areas such as cardiology, endocrinology, and gastroenterology. Gastroenterology is particularly concerned with the digestive system, diagnosing and curing diseases ranging from gastrointestinal disease to liver disease. Gastroenterologists must have a solid foundation of knowledge in gastrointestinal anatomy and pathology to treat effectively. This subspecialty allows internists to perform vital procedures, such as colonoscopies, where advanced tools like the Endocuff have been shown to increase detection rates while simultaneously decreasing exam time, as measured in ongoing clinical trials (Garcia et al., 2019). Moreover, the practice of internal medicine extends beyond immediate care to include preventive interventions tailored to the patient's risk factors. For example, analysis of billing data in healthcare highlights the importance of accurate measurement of screening rates for diseases such as colorectal cancer (Avila et al., 2020). This meticulous process reflects a commitment to maximizing population health by thoroughly monitoring and evaluating preventive care. By using sound methodologies to track outcomes and improve quality measurement, internal medicine is an invaluable component of public health initiatives, underscoring its value in modern healthcare and reiterating its relevance in research and study fields such as gastroenterology, where prompt interventions can significantly influence patient outcomes.

Importance of Internal Medicine in Healthcare

Internal medicine plays a significant role in healthcare, particularly in its structure for managing complex medical conditions that require integrative, coordinated care. Physicians trained in internal medicine can diagnose and manage a broad range of diseases in adults. General knowledge is especially critical in gastroenterology, where patients present with complex symptoms that require sensitive evaluation and a tailored management plan. By being holistic in their approach, internal medicine practitioners can treat not only the gastrointestinal illness but also any potential comorbidities that may complicate the patient's overall health. For instance, the orderly management of illnesses like hypertension or diabetes can significantly influence treatment outcomes for gastrointestinal illnesses, underscoring how intertwined the body's systems can be in medicine. Practice of internal medicine also reinforces preventive care strategies, which is essential in the efficient management of chronic gastrointestinal disease. Internal medicine physicians generally anticipate the role of screening and early diagnosis. As observed in research on CRC screening uptake, multimodal interventions are more effective than single activities in enhancing early detection rates (Betlachin et al., 2018). Through activities that educate patients about screening modalities and support healthcare professionals, internal medicine contributes significantly to reducing disease incidence. Moreover, prioritization of preventive interventions allows patients to receive interventions promptly, which in turn may reduce the intensity of diseases, thereby improving health outcomes and limiting future health expenses. Besides, the relationship between infectious diseases and internal medicine underscores its pivotal role in the treatment of conditions in gastroenterology. With the rising rate of Clostridium Difficile infection (CDI) linked with prolonged hospital stays and compromised immune conditions for liver cirrhosis patients, internal medicine specialists are increasingly called in to address this issue. Understanding the pathophysiology of CDI in these patients is critical, as these infections are associated with morbidity and increased mortality (Dumitru et al., 2019). With their general training, internists can build comprehensive care plans that address gastrointestinal dysfunction and its resultant complications, including infection. This underscores the central role of internal medicine in solving the intricate problems faced in gastroenterology, further solidifying its role in the provision of healthcare.

4.1. Overview of Gastroenterology

Learning Outcome

1. Define the definition and focus of gastroenterology
2. Discuss on common conditions treated in gastroenterology
3. Understand the role of gastroenterologists in patient care

Gastroenterology is a broad branch of medicine that encompasses a range of disorders of the gastrointestinal (GI) tract, from the esophagus to the rectum. This specialty is central to the diagnosis, treatment, and management of gastroesophageal reflux disease (GERD), inflammatory bowel disease (IBD), and colorectal cancer (CRC). Preventive screening is particularly relevant, as CRC is a common but mostly preventable condition. Despite national guidelines that call for screening in persons aged 50-75 years, many remain unscreened. Evidence supports the idea that interventions beyond single-component interventions, such as multimodal interventions, are more efficient at improving screening rates—highlighting gastroenterology's pivotal role in enhancing patient compliance and healthcare outcomes (Betlachin et al., 2018). This combined process signifies the ever-evolving complexity of GI healthcare management, where prevention becomes the focal point. In the treatment of acute disorders, gastroenterology often has to deal with conditions such as acute pancreatitis, which has a rising incidence worldwide. Acute pancreatitis poses significant clinical challenges, as establishing the optimal therapeutic approaches is a major concern. About 25% of those cases diagnosed as acute pancreatitis have a potential of progressing to severe conditions, with necrotizing tissue changes and complications that significantly heighten mortality risk. Notably, treatment approaches for acute pancreatitis remain non-specific, hence underscoring the need for intensive research into its pathophysiology. Advances in the use of animal models now make it possible to gain clearer insight into the disease processes involved and to develop more focused treatments. These developments indicate optimism about creating more effective management regimens in gastroenterology, underscoring the importance of ongoing research in this long-established specialty (Tietz et al., 2005). Furthermore, gastroenterology is shifting towards an increasingly integrated paradigm, incorporating newer technologies and multi-professional interaction. The increasing prevalence of chronic gastrointestinal disease necessitates a holistic model of patient care that addresses not only the physical but also the psychological and social aspects of health. This change entails greater emphasis on lifestyle modification, nutritional advice, and mental health concerns, which are usually inexorably intertwined with gastrointestinal disease. In addition, telemedicine and digital health technologies provide new avenues for patient involvement and follow-up. Adopting a holistic understanding of patient well-being enables gastroenterologists to enhance the quality of care delivered significantly. An integral approach to this reflects the specialty's willingness to adapt as it addresses the complexities of patient needs in a changing healthcare landscape, ultimately manifesting in enhanced health outcomes for gastroenterology.

4.1.1. Definition and Focus of Gastroenterology

Gastroenterology is a branch of internal medicine focused on the diagnosis and treatment of diseases affecting the GI tract, including the esophagus, stomach, intestines, and organs near them, such as the liver and pancreas. The specialty traverses a wide range of conditions from minor conditions like gastroesophageal reflux disease (GERD) and irritable bowel syndrome (IBS) to more severe pathological conditions like inflammatory bowel disease (IBD) marked by Crohn's disease and ulcerative colitis. Gastroenterologists use various diagnostic techniques, including endoscopy and imaging, to assess the function and integrity of the gastrointestinal system. Through the identification of such conditions' etiologies, which may be multifactorial and complex, gastroenterology endeavors to provide specific treatment regimens that will alleviate both acute and chronic gastrointestinal illness, ultimately improving the patient's quality of life. The field of gastroenterology has expanded in recent years, reflecting advances in medical technology and a better understanding of gastrointestinal pathophysiology. The field not only addresses acute clinical symptoms but also addresses prevention and maintenance interventions for at-risk populations. Both medical and surgical therapies are complemented, as in the literature on the management of inflammatory bowel disease, by the development of guidelines and consensus recommendations from professional organizations such as the European Crohn's and Colitis Organisation. Such guidelines play a central role in the evolution of evidence-based practice in the management of conditions prevalent in gastroenterology, confirming the practice of clinical assessment and continuous training for healthcare professionals to keep pace with the field's evolving nature (Adamina et al., 2019) (Figure 4.1).

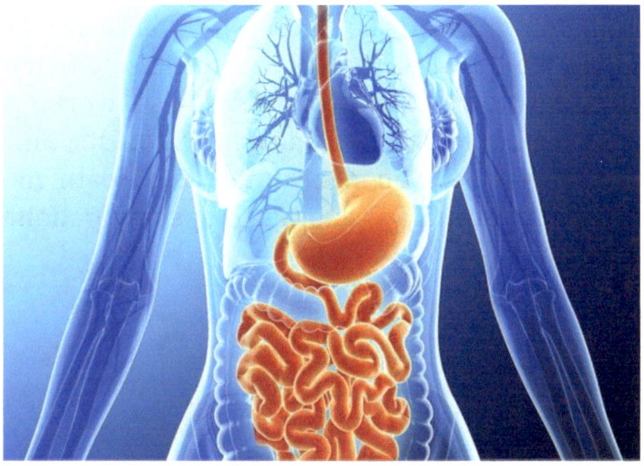

Figure 4.1. Gastroenterology.

Source: https://smb.ibsrv.net/imageresizer/image/article_manager/1200x1200/15634/344257/heroimage0.060560001634239371.jpg.

Furthermore, gastroenterology intersects with a variety of areas of care for patients, emphasizing an integrated approach that takes into account the psychosocial determinants of health outcomes. This interprofessional focus acknowledges the critical care transition from pediatric to adult care, particularly in the context of the special needs of young adults with chronic gastrointestinal illnesses. Up-to-date changes in clinical reports emphasize the need for holistic health care transition models that facilitate the transition from pediatric to adult-centered care. These are imperative in the demand for strong transition planning that acknowledges the complexity of managing GI disorders in young adults and adolescents (White et al., 2018). In conclusion, gastroenterology remains the backbone of internal medicine, both in identifying the biological and psychosocial dimensions of gastrointestinal health.

4.1.2. Common Conditions Treated in Gastroenterology

Gastroenterology, as a specialty, encompasses a broad spectrum of disorders, and gastroesophageal reflux disease (GERD) is among the most common. GERD occurs when acid from the stomach regularly backs up into the esophagus, leading to symptoms of heartburn and regurgitation. Treatment for GERD may involve lifestyle changes, medications, and, in some cases, surgery such as fundoplication.

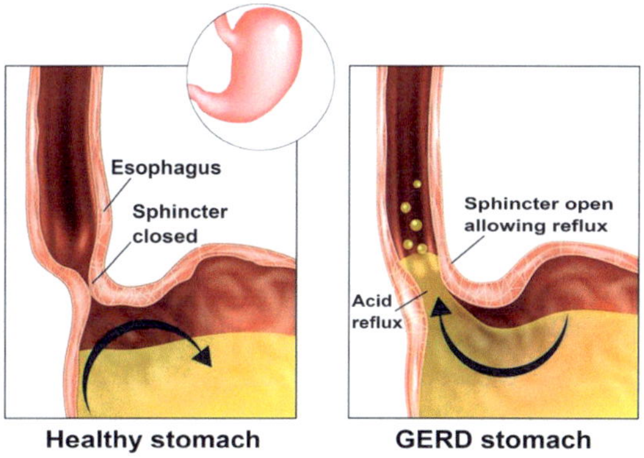

Figure 4.2. Gastroesophageal reflux disease (GERD).

Source: https://livgastro.in/wp-content/uploads/2023/01/Gastroesophageal-Reflux-Disease-feature.png.

Also, the condition impacts patients' quality of life considerably as a result of chronic symptoms that potentially lead to complications like Barrett's esophagus and esophagitis. Gastroenterologists need to understand the etiology and treatment of GERD, as these factors determine the treatment plan for other associated gastrointestinal disorders. With the prevalence of GERD continuing to rise globally, its management increasingly becomes a priority for gastroenterology clinicians. A further severe illness often treated in gastroenterology is peptic ulcer disease (PUD), most frequently associated with *Helicobacter pylori* infection and chronic non-steroidal anti-inflammatory drug

(NSAIDs) usage. PUD involves painful ulcers within the lining of the stomach or duodenum, and symptoms include abdominal pain, bloating, and nausea (Figure 4.2). The treatment of PUD is typically with *H. pylori* eradication by a combination of antibiotics and proton pump inhibitors, along with lifestyle modification to promote healing. Notably, gastroenterologists must also educate patients to adhere carefully to therapy since improper management may result in horrific complications in the form of bleeding or perforation. Given the frequency of PUD among gastrointestinal complaints, it is an essential consideration in the practice of outpatient and inpatient gastroenterologists (Canbaz et al., 2005). Irritable bowel syndrome (IBS) is another condition that occurs heavily in the practice of gastroenterology, where abdominal pain and bowel habits are changed with no organic explanation found. This functional gastrointestinal disorder has multifaceted symptoms that range from diarrhea, constipation, and bloating, and hence constitutes a complex clinical challenge both for diagnosis and treatment. Treatment options for IBS can vary from highly heterogeneous, involving dietary change, drug treatment, and psychotherapy to address the stress-related issues that often exacerbate the condition. A tailor-made therapy is required, given the heterogeneity in treatment response among individuals. Besides, as awareness of IBS's impact on a patient's functioning and productivity increases, gastroenterologists are tasked with long-term patient management and care in dealing with this mysterious illness (Roth et al., 2025).

4.1.3. Role of Gastroenterologists in Patient Care

The gastroenterologists' role in patient care is pivotal, as they are tasked with diagnosing and managing gastrointestinal (GI), liver, and pancreatic diseases. Their area of expertise is extensive, ranging from inflammatory bowel disease to liver cirrhosis. Clinically, gastroenterologists conduct comprehensive examinations, using endoscopy and colonoscopy to detect hidden issues such as cancer or polyps. The implications of their findings go far beyond immediate diagnosis; successful treatment of GI disorders often demands multidisciplinary collaboration, with gastroenterologists working with primary care clinicians, nutritionists, and surgeons to develop highly integrated treatment programs explicitly tailored to specific patient needs.

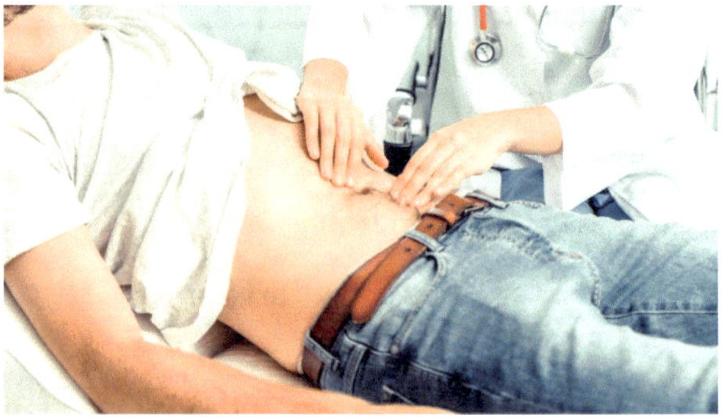

Figure 4.3. The role of gastroenterologists in patient care.

Source: https://cdn-prod.medicalnewstoday.com/content/images/articles/327/327441/a-gastroenterologists-feeling-a-persons-stomach.jpg.

This interdisciplinarity coordination is necessary to ensure integral care because it improves the results of the patient and creates a care continuum directed not only to the medical elements but also to the lifestyle factors that condition the gastrointestinal health. Additionally, the gastroenterologist's role includes an increasingly important aspect: managing the side effects of new, advanced therapies, such as checkpoint inhibitors used in cancer treatments. These therapies, while potentially curative, have the potential to induce major gastrointestinal, liver, and pancreatic complications for which they require early recognition and specialized treatment. Gastroenterologists are trained to recognize, evaluate, and treat these side effects and ensure that patients receive optimal therapy throughout their treatment. Their involvement in managing such side effects is crucial not only for patient compliance with cancer treatment but also for maximizing quality of life. Their expertise in sensing and acting on the impact of such therapies tells us volumes about their core contribution to medical practice today, preserving patient safety and enabling effective disease control (Ahmed et al., 2018) (Figure 4.3). An understanding of the complexities of healthcare delivery is also necessary for evaluating the gastroenterologist's role in patient care. Practice alterations in colonoscopy, which are influenced by non-clinical factors such as the organization of healthcare systems, have a substantial impact on patient outcomes. Empirical evidence shows that open-access colonoscopy units and high-volume centers are most likely to yield higher diagnostic yields, which eventually lead to earlier detection of significant lesions (Holly et al., 2025). This understanding necessitates refinement in gastroenterology models of healthcare delivery. It would mean that structuring specialist units to maximize performance and optimize diagnostic accuracy. Therefore, gastroenterologists should push for structural reform in health systems to facilitate access to high-quality diagnostic tests and define their pivotal role in optimizing the effectiveness of gastrointestinal care within a broader public health context.

Test Your Knowledge

1. What are the common disorders affecting the gastrointestinal tract?
2. How does diet influence digestive system health?

4.2. Diagnostic Techniques in Gastroenterology

Learning Outcome

1. Describe the endoscopy procedures and their significance
2. Define the imaging studies used in gastroenterology
3. Understand the laboratory tests and their role in diagnosis

The use of various diagnostic techniques in gastroenterology is central to the proper assessment and treatment of gastrointestinal conditions. Endoscopic tests, including upper and lower GI endoscopies, provide visualization of the gut, and clinicians can use them to diagnose conditions such as inflammatory bowel disease, polyps, and malignancy. The success of these exams depends on several factors, both clinical and non-clinical. Studies have revealed striking differences in colonoscopy performance across healthcare systems, and it should be noted that institutional attributes, such as the availability of open-access facilities and high-volume specialist facilities, are directly correlated with diagnostic yields. For instance, evidence indicates that high-volume facilities are more likely to detect larger lesions than low-volume facilities, underscoring the contribution of system design to achieving maximum diagnostic potential (Holly et al., 2025). Along with this, the need for new diagnostic equipment is also increasing in gastroenterology. Non-invasive tests, such as biomarkers and imaging studies, complement traditional endoscopic techniques by providing additional information on gastrointestinal pathology. Techniques such as magnetic resonance cholangiopancreatography (MRCP) and computed tomography enterography (CTE) have redefined the detection and characterization of diseases such as pancreatitis, cholangitis, and small bowel obstruction. These imaging technologies offer high-resolution information with low risk and discomfort to patients. In addition, advances in molecular diagnostics are enabling improved detection of infectious pathogens, such as soil-transmitted helminths, which carry a heavy burden in endemic settings. As infection awareness grows, effective diagnosis remains essential to guide treatment strategies (Addiss et al., 2018). The integration of state-of-the-art diagnostic techniques and the streamlining of existing protocols are essential to improving the quality of gastroenterological care. Continuous monitoring and adjustment of diagnostic practice are necessary to address the evolving epidemiology of gastroenterology. Integration of endoscopic skills, emerging non-invasive diagnostic tests, and understanding of the healthcare delivery system can enhance diagnostic accuracy and patient outcomes. Besides, addressing non-medical challenges, such as health care system design and provider education, appears crucial to minimizing disparities in diagnostic performance. As they tackle technological advances and system-level enhancements, gastroenterologists can significantly improve diagnostic performance, thereby enabling better management of severe gastrointestinal disease (Holly et al., 2025).

4.2.1. Endoscopy Procedures and Their Significance

Endoscopic procedures have evolved into pivotal tools in gastroenterology, facilitating both diagnostic and therapeutic modalities. These low-invasive techniques allow direct visualization of the upper and lower GI tracts and significantly enhance clinicians' diagnostic capabilities for a broad array of conditions, including cancers, ulcers, and inflammatory diseases. Diagnostic precision provided by endoscopy is particularly important in patients presenting with acute conditions such as upper GI bleeding, where timely intervention can radically change outcomes.

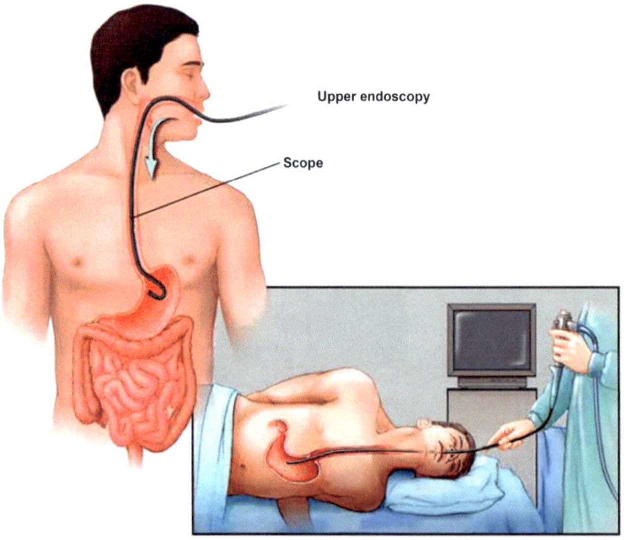

Figure 4.4. Upper endoscopy.

Source: https://www.mayoclinic.org/-/media/kcms/gbs/patient-consumer/images/2016/05/02/14/44/mcdc7_endoscopy-8col.jpg.

A study conducted at Bugando Medical Centre found that early fiberoptic upper GI endoscopy was able to diagnose bleeding sources with a diagnostic efficacy of 97.7%, further highlighting the procedures' central role in emergencies and their impact on patient morbidity and mortality rates (Elghuel et al., 2012). Additionally, endoscopy is not only diagnostic but also plays a highly vital therapeutic role.

Some examples are endoscopic band ligation and sclerotherapy for the management of variceal hemorrhage, one of the major complications of portal hypertension. TIPS and balloon-occluded retrograde transvenous obliteration (BRTO) are relevant examples of therapeutic endoscopy in patients with isolated gastric varices. Research indicates that even though TIPS and BRTO demonstrate similar re-bleeding rates, BRTO can lead to a lower rate of hepatic encephalopathy, thus enhancing patient outcomes and survival rates (Kim et al., 2017) (Figure 4.4). The above therapeutic applications demonstrate the dual potential of endoscopy in diagnosis and treatment in the gastroenterology specialty.

The significance of endoscopy transcends immediate clinical advantages, extending to influence the broader field of gastroenterological treatment. Aside from facilitating early diagnosis and treatment of severe conditions, these procedures are cost-effective in that they can avoid the need for more invasive procedures. They also enable doctors to deliver tailored treatment plans based on precise diagnostic information, thereby decreasing patient noncompliance and dissatisfaction. As technology advances further and increasingly maximizes the capabilities of endoscopic treatment, its role in gastroenterology will surely increase, increasingly streamlining the precision and speed of patient treatment. Pushing deeper into remote biopsies and therapeutic procedures, endoscopy is a mainstay in the preventative treatment of gastroenterological disease.

4.2.2. Imaging Studies Used in Gastroenterology

Imaging tests are also a significant part of gastroenterology, as they provide crucial information about the structure and function of the gastrointestinal organs. MRI is among the imaging modalities most frequently used for the evaluation of diseases that affect the liver. MRI offers high-quality images without ionizing radiation, thus making it more appropriate for repeated examinations. High-resolution hepatic MRI can define lesions and detect malignancies early, something essential for timely intervention. As of late, studies show that the majority of cited hepatic MRI articles appear in top-tier journals, demonstrating a robust body of literature on the topic. This also serves to emphasize its clinical relevance and to document innovation in imaging technologies that have increased diagnostic potential in gastroenterology (Abdullah et al., 2018).

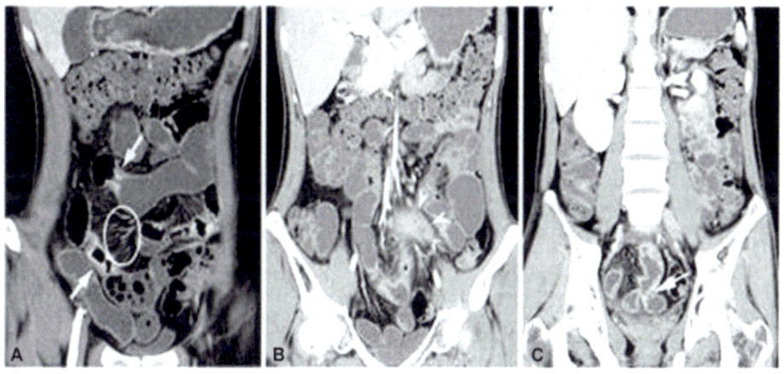

Figure 4.5. Diagnosis of inflammatory Crohn's disease with extraenteric complications by computed tomography enterography. (A) Multifocal segmental stricture showing wall thickening, mural hyperenhancement, and stratification shown by arrows and engorged vasa recta, comb sign highlighted by a circle. (B) Mesenteric abscess is shown by arrowheads. (C) Adjacent to the enteroenteric fistula shown by the arrow.

Source: https://www.mdpi.com/2313-433X/9/6/115.

Ultrasound imaging, or gastrointestinal ultrasound (GIUS), has also become increasingly accepted as a primary diagnostic tool in gastroenterology. GIUS was established by the European Federation of Societies for Ultrasound in Medicine and Biology and applies a variety of examination techniques to explore gastrointestinal anatomy and physiology. This painless method has the potential to allow clinicians to assess a wide range of conditions, including inflammatory bowel disease, liver cirrhosis, and pancreatic illness. Using ultrasound, clinicians can view pathological changes in real time and distinguish normal from abnormal results. In addition, evidence-based guidelines for the clinical application of GIUS further confirm its value in daily practice, highlighting its applicability across imaging investigations used in gastroenterology (Calabrese et al., 2016) (Figure 4.5). Computed tomography (CT) scans are also a foundation of gastrointestinal disease imaging, providing quick, high-resolution images that permit detailed examination. CT imaging has been of invaluable help in diagnosing acute appendicitis, diverticulitis, and abdominal cancer. Its ability to reveal cross-sectional pictures of the intra-abdominal organs enhances clinical decision-making by enabling accurate staging of malignancies and complications. Techniques such as contrast-enhanced CT have further improved diagnostic precision, enabling clinicians to visualize vascular structures and perfusion patterns. The universality and speed of CT render it an irreplaceable tool in emergency and outpatient medicine, solidifying its pivotal role in the range of imaging studies of concern to gastroenterology. With the ongoing advancements in imaging modalities, the collaboration among these modalities will undoubtedly shape the future of gastrointestinal diagnostics.

4.2.3. Laboratory Tests and Their Role in Diagnosis

Laboratory tests in gastroenterology practice are the most important diagnostic tools, allowing clinicians to identify various liver diseases. The use of new biomarkers has revolutionized the diagnosis of diseases such as cystic fibrosis-associated liver disease (CFLD). Traditional diagnostic approaches are generally insensitive, leading to the incorporation of serological tests capable of detecting subtle alterations in protein expression. Research indicates that specific serum proteins, such as TIMP-4 and Endoglin, are distinctly regulated in patients with CFLD and are potential biomarkers with increased diagnostic sensitivity. In addition, when combined with transient elastography, these markers enhance the sensitivity and specificity for diagnosing CFLD, enabling earlier intervention and management and halting disease progression (Hage et al., 2013).

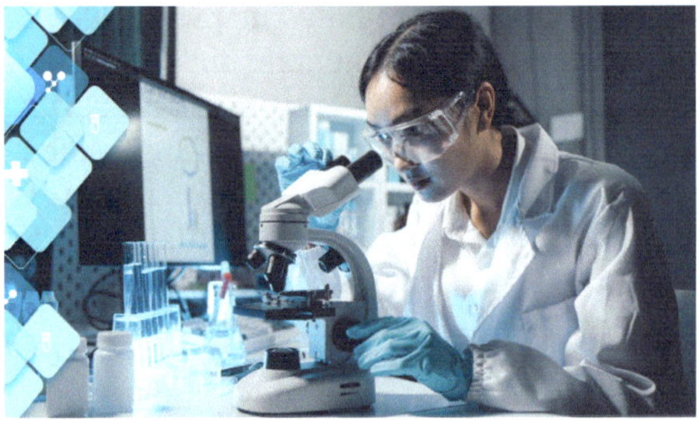

Figure 4.6. Gastroenterology laboratory tests.

Source: https://avignadiagnostics.com/creating-clarity/wp-content/uploads/2024/06/Types-of-gastroenterology-tests-that-are-conducted-in-labs-1600x900-px-01.jpg.

Laboratory testing not only diagnoses liver diseases but also sheds light on underlying metabolic conditions that affect liver health. Non-alcoholic fatty liver disease (NAFLD) is rapidly becoming a worrisome condition, particularly when the context is its prevalence among metabolic syndrome. Serum vitamin E level emerged as an issue of concern in the context of liver health, evidencing significantly low values in the context of simple steatosis (SS) and non-alcoholic steatohepatitis (NASH). The correlation between reduced vitamin E levels and fatty liver disease underscores the importance of comprehensive biochemical studies to elucidate the pathophysiologic mechanisms involved. This study supports further investigation of vitamin E supplementation in patients with SS, indicating that laboratory results can indeed influence therapeutic choices and improve patient outcomes (Angelico et al., 2015) (Figure 4.6). Furthermore, integrating laboratory tests into daily clinical practice elevates the level of care in internal medicine for gastroenterology. The data acquired from these studies not only aid in diagnosis but also support disease monitoring and assessment of treatment efficacy. By using an approach with multiple dimensions that includes biochemical tests, imaging studies, and the patient's history, clinicians can create a comprehensive clinical picture. This collaborative model ultimately improves patient communication, education, and treatment compliance. By leveraging information from laboratory testing, healthcare professionals are better equipped to individualize interventions, thereby personifying a patient-centered philosophy in the care of gastroenterological conditions. This changing environment reiterates the central position of laboratory diagnostics in ensuring optimal patient care in the specialty (Hage et al., 2013; Angelico et al., 2015).

Test Your Knowledge

1. What diagnostic tests are commonly used to evaluate gastrointestinal disorders?
2. Why is endoscopy important in diagnosing digestive system diseases?

4.3. Treatment Modalities in Gastroenterology

Learning Outcome

1. Describe the pharmacological treatments for gastrointestinal disorders
2. Discuss on surgical interventions in gastroenterology
3. Explain the lifestyle modifications and their impact on treatment

In gastroenterology, treatment modalities for various gastrointestinal disorders are of primary importance in controlling patient outcomes and enhancing quality of life. Colorectal cancer screening is one such area where recent data unequivocally demonstrate the efficacy of multifaceted interventions. Compared with single-component interventions, which have modest success, multifactorial interventions that include mailed educational letters, precolonoscopy counseling, and enhanced provider communication have achieved higher screening rates. Notably, research highlighted that screening uptake among a managed care population rose from 65.1% to 76.6% after the implementation of such a program, indicating that multi-faceted strategies to address patient and system-level barriers reap considerable rewards towards CRC early detection and ultimately toward better overall health outcomes (Betlachin et al., 2018). In addition, research into new biomarkers for diagnosing liver diseases such as cystic fibrosis-associated liver disease (CFLD) is an excellent illustration of the advancement in gastroenterology therapies. Current diagnostic methods are not sufficiently sensitive or specific, so new methods are required. Experiments identifying differential regulation of serum proteins have identified candidates such as TIMP-4 and Endoglin that have the potential for accurate diagnosis of CFLD. These biomarkers, when combined with transient elastography, are found to enhance diagnostic accuracy, providing avenues for early intervention among patients with the disease. The awareness of the relationship between these biomarkers and liver fibrosis staging is a significant advancement in non-invasive diagnostic technologies in gastroenterology and could transform patient treatment and outcomes in the context of chronic liver disease (Hage et al., 2013). It should also be noted that gastroenterological therapeutic modalities extend beyond diagnostic and screening procedures, with therapeutic interventions tailored to each patient. The pharmacologic treatment for inflammatory bowel disease (IBD) and the addition of dietary modifications are a case in point, and this emphasizes the diverse nature of the approaches adopted. The therapies are not only symptom-focused but also aim to achieve and maintain remission, further enhancing the role of personalized medicine in gastroenterology. Besides, improvements in access to multidisciplinary care, e.g., dietitians, psychologists, and gastroenterology specialists, improve the continuum of treatment, allowing holistic management of complex gastrointestinal disorders. By leveraging advanced diagnostic technology and customized therapeutic interventions, gastroenterology is continually improving, ultimately raising the level of care (Betlachin et al., 2018; Hage et al., 2013) (Figure 4.7).

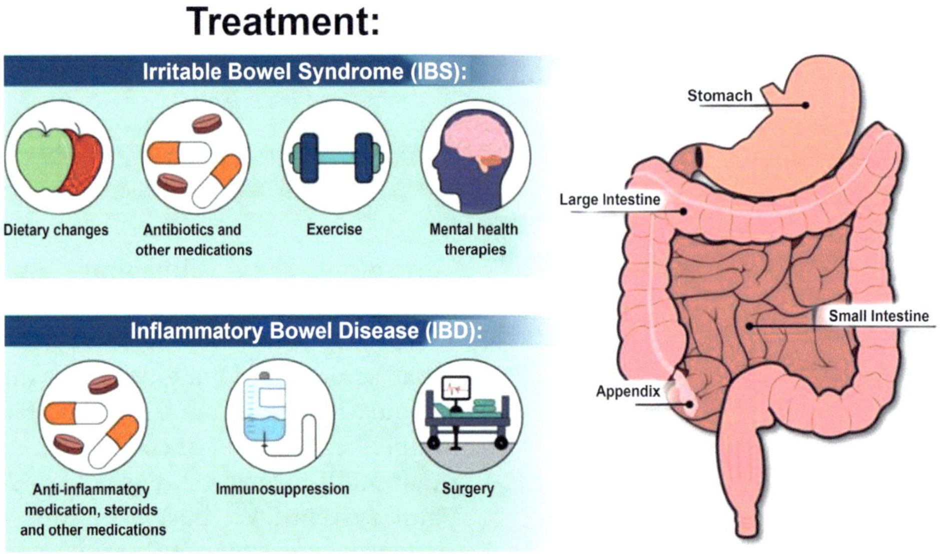

Figure 4.7. Treatment modalities employed for various gastrointestinal disorders.

Source: https://external-content.duckduckgo.com/iu/?u=https%3A%2F%2Fsurgery.wustl.edu%2Fwp-content%2Fuploads%2F2022%2F04%2FIBD-IBS-Treatment-graphic-1024x673.png&f=1&nofb=1&ipt=f319fae684bd4b4b180223806bd9c34b0fb8a89f7eeb3475a8a09e07ae073eb4.

4.3.1. Pharmacological Treatments for Gastrointestinal Disorders

Pharmacological therapy for gastrointestinal disease encompasses a broad array of medications designed to treat specific pathologies. Over-the-counter medicines like antacids and proton pump inhibitors (PPIs) are commonly prescribed for the management of gastroesophageal reflux disease (GERD) and peptic ulcers. These medications have a mechanism of action that involves decreasing gastric acidity, healing the mucosa, and curing pain. Further, prokinetic medications are typically prescribed to enhance gastrointestinal motility in functional dyspepsia and gastroparesis. Even though such medication treatment can significantly alter the status of patients, it is important to determine their potential side effects, such as Clostridioides difficile infection caused by prolonged intake of PPIs. The safety and effectiveness of such therapy are of primary importance to internists, especially when highlighting the need for individually adjusted therapy according to each patient's unique clinical presentation. In the treatment of inflammatory bowel disease (IBD), specifically Crohn's disease and ulcerative colitis, there is a more complex pharmacological strategy employed. Immunosuppressants such as azathioprine and biologic agents such as tumor necrosis factor (TNF) inhibitors form the foundation of managing remission and inflammation. These medications not only lower the risk for complications related to IBD but also reduce the severity of symptoms. Their administration must be accompanied by aggressive surveillance for side effects, such as increased susceptibility to infections and cancer. Moreover, whether to initiate such powerful medications must take into account the patient's history of treatment and response to previous therapies. With advancing pharmacotherapy, introducing multidisciplinary care is important for achieving maximal treatment in patients with IBD. For functional gastrointestinal disorders such as irritable bowel syndrome (IBS), drug treatments most often overlap with psychological interventions in managing the biopsychosocial component of the syndrome. Antidepressants, particularly tricyclic and selective serotonin reuptake inhibitors, have proved effective in treating IBS symptoms by affecting gut-brain interactions and reducing visceral hypersensitivity. Non-pharmacological interventions, including cognitive-behavioral therapy, also complement drug treatment so that patients learn to manage the affective and psychological dimensions of the disease. In general, the incorporation of pharmacologic treatments and psychosocial interventions emphasizes the need for a holistic treatment approach. As Alpers et al. (2007) argue, the heterogeneity of IBS necessitates specialized treatment regimens, since a single treatment is rarely sufficient. Thus, clinicians are called upon to adopt interdisciplinary treatment methods in the management of gastrointestinal diseases to provide integral patient care.

4.3.2. Surgical Interventions in Gastroenterology

Surgical procedures form a key aspect of the treatment of gastrointestinal diseases in gastroenterology. These operations may be as minimally invasive as perfections allow or more invasive operations, all aimed at curing specific pathological conditions. Surgical intervention is usually advised when other conservative measures have failed, e.g., in the case of colorectal cancer or inflammatory bowel disease. As has been mentioned, cancer of the colon and rectum is a worry, particularly in African American men who have increased incidence and mortality rates compared to White men. Early surgery and intervention can significantly improve outcomes, but disparities in screening do exist. This highlights the need to raise awareness and increase the availability of such interventions as part of gastroenterological services (Foster et al., 2014). Surgical management in gastroenterology is not just limited to cancers, but also functional disorders such as fecal incontinence and defecation disorders. Conservative management is essential, and conditions like fecal incontinence can have a major bearing on the quality of life of patients. Stepwise treatment is recommended for such situations, with conservative treatment like dietary changes and biofeedback initially, followed by surgery if initial management fails. Techniques such as sacral nerve stimulation and sphincter repair have increasingly been employed, reflecting a shift in operative procedure to restore function and alleviate symptoms in patients with severe to moderate disease. This innovative strategy highlights the importance of individualized therapy in achieving the optimal outcome for the patient (Bharucha et al., 2017) (Figure 4.8).

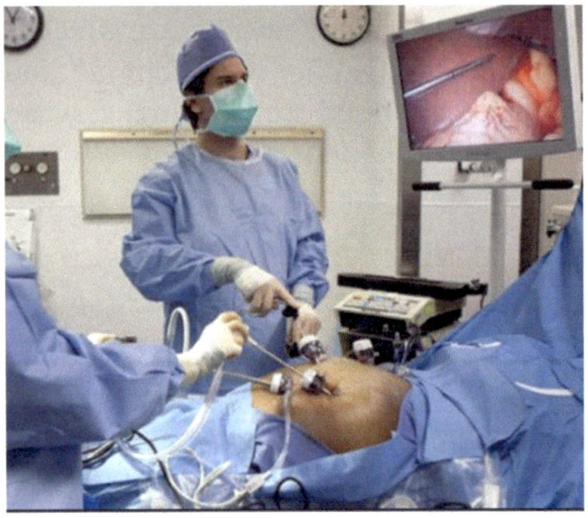

Figure 4.8. Surgical gastroenterology.

Source: https://external-content.duckduckgo.com/iu/?u=https%3A%2F%2Ftse4.mm.bing.net%2Fth%2Fid%2FOIP.xL1Qzq8MPy-3L3fY5rU-rwHaGL%3Fpid%3DApi&f=1&ipt=96ed8b75ff2ed156c1c182a5028f18820fa12afe1d32966a5fb290cdf6a73186.

In addition to correcting anatomical defects and maximizing functional capacity, surgery also includes the management of chronic gastrointestinal disease resistant to drug therapy. As a case in point, maximal care of severe fecal incontinence may involve pioneering surgery when conventional measures fail. Anal sphincter repair and magnetic anal sphincter implantation are being used with greater frequency in patients who have exhausted all other options. Further, the potential for colostomy can also be taken into account in refractory conditions, reflecting the utmost significance of surgery as a last resort in case conservative therapy is not enough. The integration of surgical procedures into the broader framework of gastroenterology is crucial for providing comprehensive treatment to patients with incapacitating gastrointestinal conditions (Bharucha et al., 2017).

4.3.3. Lifestyle Modifications and Their Impact on Treatment

Lifestyle modifications are a vital part of the therapy for gastrointestinal disease and are responsible for much of the treatment's success. In inflammatory bowel disease (IBD) patients, it has been shown that adherence to dietary restriction, exercise, and effective management of stress can enhance their response to drugs. In particular, there is evidence that lifestyle improvements can ameliorate disease activity and induce mucosal healing, and that treatment objectives could shift from simply controlling symptoms to attaining a state of disease freedom. This again highlights the value of an integrative approach that depends not only on drugs but also on patient education and behavior modification, thereby enhancing overall treatment outcomes. The interaction between lifestyle modification and conventional medical intervention urges physicians to personalize treatment protocols, adapting them to individual needs and conditions to achieve optimal therapeutic effects (Cai et al., 2021). In addition, removing weight bias remains essential in the context of lifestyle modification, particularly in patients with obesity and potentially gastrointestinal symptom presentation. Research indicates that weight bias can detrimentally affect physical and mental well-being, deterring individuals from taking advantage of timely medical intervention. Weight stigma initiates a cycle of avoidance that exacerbates illness and places patients at risk of undertreatment. By establishing a facilitative setting that embraces and responds to weight stigma, health professionals can support an inclusive model of care that encourages patients to adopt lifestyle changes. Significantly, learning about the adverse effects of discrimination by weight can initiate a more compassionate handling of obesity, allowing for higher levels of adherence to recommended lifestyle changes. Thus, addressing prejudices can lead to more effective therapies and improved general well-being among people with gastrointestinal diseases (Rubino et al., 2020). The role of lifestyle modifications in treatment programs not only empowers the patients but also serves as a prophylactic measure against most gastrointestinal disorders. Diet plays a pivotal role in conditions such as gastroesophageal reflux disease and irritable bowel syndrome, in which food irritants can provoke symptoms. The addition of specific dietary management, like fiber supplementation or avoidance of specific irritants, can lead to considerable symptom alleviation. In addition, modifying dietary habits and portion control help ensure better management of gastrointestinal health. By emphasizing this modification in addition to regular therapy, clinicians can empower patients to manage their health. Such an integrative methodology, by combining lifestyle modification and medical therapy, ultimately leads to better disease management and patient satisfaction, providing an improved, active approach to internal medicine and gastroenterology (Cai et al., 2021).

Test Your Knowledge

1. What are the common treatment approaches for gastrointestinal disorders?
2. How do dietary modifications support the treatment of digestive diseases?

4.4. Common Gastrointestinal Disorders

Learning Outcome

1. Understand the inflammatory bowel disease (IBD)
2. Define the gastroesophageal reflux disease (GERD)
3. Describe the hepatic disorders and their management

Gastrointestinal disorders represent a wide variety of conditions, among the most common of which are Irritable Bowel Syndrome (IBS) and IBD. Both of these conditions have a combination of symptoms, such as abdominal pain, bloating, and a change in bowel habits, that can necessitate an accurate diagnosis. IBS, as a functional gastrointestinal disorder, affects the majority of the population and typically involves a combination of abdominal components with psychological stressors. Conversely, IBD, which includes Crohn's disease and ulcerative colitis, involves more aggressive inflammatory pathways that can result in severe morbidity. These disorders are multifaceted and must be managed with an integrative approach that targets pathophysiology and optimal treatment planning, as reported in recent literature and clinical practice guidelines. The availability of advanced diagnostic modalities is solely imperative in the management of gastrointestinal disorders, particularly in the use of Gastrointestinal Ultrasound (GIUS). Commissioned under the patronage of the European Federation of Societies for Ultrasound in Medicine and Biology, GIUS is an innovative imaging modality that enables physicians to visualize structural and functional pathology in the gastrointestinal tract. Noninvasive, the technology surpasses traditional imaging modalities in its diagnostic accuracy and in reducing patient doses of ionizing radiation. The GIUS working group has recommended individual examination techniques for everyday practice, thereby promoting the broader use of this technology to facilitate early diagnosis and treatment of various gastrointestinal disorders (Calabrese et al., 2016). Furthermore, studying the hormonal regulation of gastrointestinal diseases adds another dimension to their etiology and symptomatology. Hormones estrogen and progesterone have been blamed for causing symptoms of IBS and IBD, providing insight into cyclic symptom patterns in affected people. Data show that alterations in progesterone levels may be to blame for causing IBS-like symptoms, providing new targets for therapy. By identifying hormonal pathways as potential mediators of gastrointestinal dysfunction, clinicians can more specifically target treatment not only to alleviate symptoms but to address the root causes of these disorders. This is the sort of reasoning that may revolutionize treatment modalities and ultimately improve the quality of life for patients suffering from these chronic gastrointestinal disorders (Linson et al., 2013).

4.4.1. Inflammatory Bowel Disease (IBD)

IBD, encompassing Crohn's disease and ulcerative colitis, is a chronic inflammation of the gastrointestinal tract. The pathogenesis of IBD remains complex, involving multifactorial interactions among genetic predisposition, environmental factors, and the gut microbiota. Recent studies highlight the significant role of food constituents as a potential cause and therapeutic measures for managing symptoms of IBD. The D-ECCO working group emphasized the need to establish dietary effects on disease initiation and progression. It proposed a framework for classifying evidence into three areas: dietary contribution towards the etiology of the diseases, its role in therapy, and measurement of nutritional status for adjunct treatment. This analysis of diet is not only theoretical but also clinically relevant for clinicians and patients alike interested in holistic disease management approaches (Allan et al., 2017). Management of IBD extends beyond drug use to include nutritional modalities that are critical owing to the prevalence of malnutrition among patients affected. Nutritional deficiencies, particularly iron deficiency, are common in IBD patients due to conditions like malabsorption, chronic inflammation, and medication side effects. Proper treatment of iron deficiency is essential, as untreated iron deficiency can lead to incapacitating anemia, significantly impairing patients' quality of life. Current evidence-based guidelines were developed through expert consensus in recent times, highlighting the importance of an individualized approach to treating iron deficiency in patients. Treatment ranges from dietary modifications and oral supplementation to intravenous high-dose iron, which is typically recommended for patients with anemia or non-responders to oral therapy (Chowers et al., 2013) (Figure 4.9).

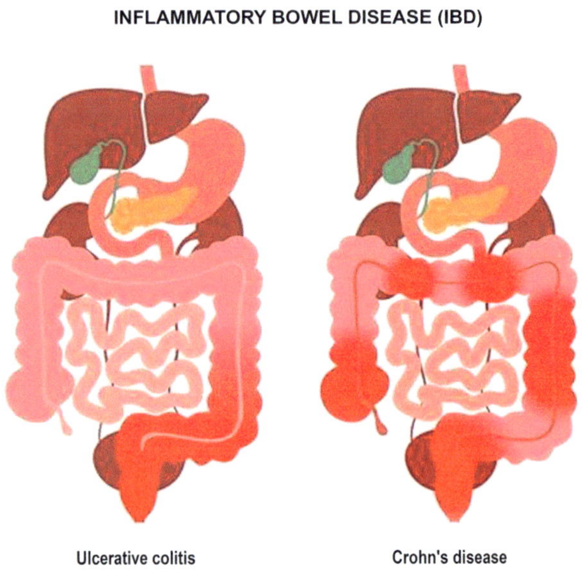

Figure 4.9. Inflammatory bowel disease (IBD).

Source: https://external-content.duckduckgo.com/iu/?u=https%3A%2F%2Ftse3.mm.bing.net%2Fth%2Fid%2FOIP.uUBOo7GlqMLJ1_lQzSOFfwHaHa%3Fr%3D0%26pid%3DApi&f=1&ipt=291da550ff8fa7542aa5b02fe6a94689e100da846e1f60688b0455afc441afbb.

This customized approach ensures utmost control over core nutrient-related problems alongside the primary IBD therapy. The multifaceted nature of IBD management necessitates a holistic approach involving both medication and nutritional therapies. Research advances indicate that personalized nutrition may positively influence clinical symptoms in IBD patients. Notably, the integration of evidence-based nutritional evaluation into clinical practice is emphasized to determine personal nutritional needs and deficiencies. As gastroenterology continues to develop, there is greater awareness of the potential for nutrition to assume an increasingly prominent role, and so the occasion arises for a paradigm shift toward greater emphasis on diet as an integral aspect of IBD management. As a result, greater research and clinical practice in nutritional interventions will be essential to improving the quality of care provided to IBD patients, facilitating better disease management and overall patient well-being (Allan et al., 2017).

4.4.2. Gastroesophageal Reflux Disease (GERD)

The pathophysiology of GERD is multidimensional, involving abnormalities in esophageal motility, the lower esophageal sphincter (LES), and gastric acid secretion. The LES, which guards against the regurgitation of gastric contents, can fail for several reasons, including obesity, medications, and food intake. Dysfunctional motility can lead to delayed gastric emptying as well as enhanced esophageal acid exposure, aggravating symptoms of GERD. In patients with GERD, heartburn and regurgitation symptoms can lead to significant morbidity, affecting daily life and sleep. Conventional therapy with lifestyle modification and proton pump inhibitor (PPI) usage is directed at symptom control and healing of the esophageal mucosa. However, a group of patients continues to experience intractable symptoms despite the best medical treatment, highlighting the need for further advanced diagnostic and therapeutic modalities in gastroenterology. Advanced diagnostic techniques have emerged as the primary means of accurately diagnosing refractory GERD. Combined multichannel intraluminal impedance (MII) and pH monitoring has played an essential role in making diagnoses more accurate for patients with persistent symptoms. Recent evidence suggests that standard diagnostic testing often cannot identify the underlying mechanisms of refractory GERD, such as weakly acidic reflux and prolonged bolus clearance time. Impedance-pH monitoring allows for a more comprehensive assessment of reflux events and their correlation with symptoms and thus a more precise esophageal reflux dynamic. It is particularly valuable in patients who are non-responsive to standard PPI therapy, as it defines the specific reflux features unique to these patients and guides individualized treatment modalities that can lead to better clinical outcomes in challenging GERD patients (Putri et al., 2025). In addition to typical GERD symptoms, chronic esophageal complications such as peptic stricture may be caused by long-term and uncontrolled reflux. Peptic esophageal strictures are a severe disease that seems to be a complication of GERD and presents with obstructive dysphagia. It is estimated that around 20% of untreated patients with GERD will develop this complication; thus, it is critical to treat and diagnose on time. Even though PPIs have reduced the incidence of such strictures, in the context of refractory GERD, they remain a problem. They are usually diagnosed by barium esophagography and esophagogastroduodenoscopy, both of which can provide valuable information about the esophagus. Treatment typically includes both acid-suppressive therapy and esophageal dilation, and, in exceptional cases such as those documented in clinical reports, esophagectomy may be necessary for the treatment of severe esophageal stricture (Abdullah et al., 2010). The approach is multidisciplinary and highlights the vitally important interaction between GERD treatment and the prevention of complications (Figure 4.10).

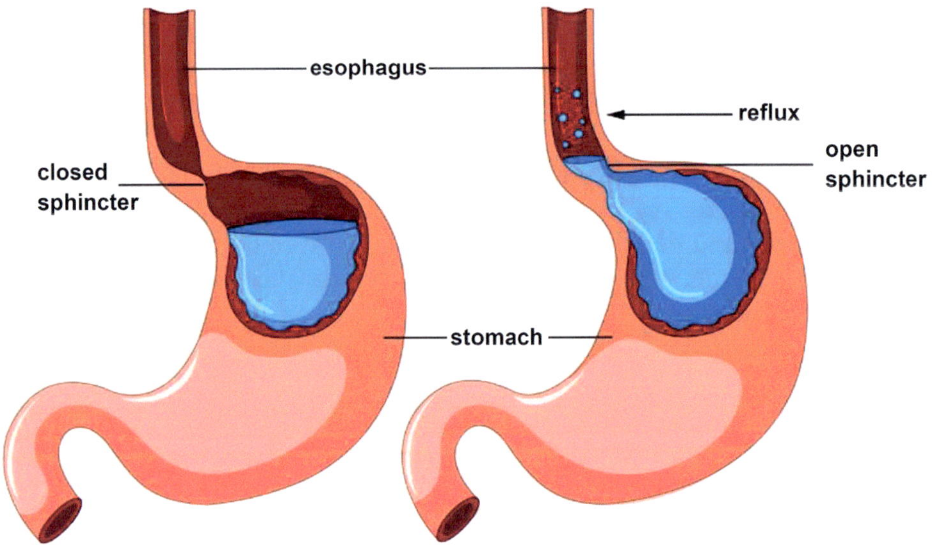

Figure 4.10. The pathophysiology of gastroesophageal reflux disease (GERD).

Source: https://external-content.duckduckgo.com/iu/?u=https%3A%2F%2Ftambarammedicalcenter.com%2Fwp-content%2Fuploads%2F2020%2F12%2FSDFSEF.jpg&f=1&nofb=1&ipt=cc694d90eb0e88386f4386d6a79a56563e2956e1a2e142d1c16fa92115fb7ed3.

4.4.3. Hepatic Disorders and Their Management

In internal medicine, liver disorders are treated from several directions owing to the liver's complex role in human anatomy. They comprise chronic infections, for instance, HCV infections, autoimmune diseases, and alcoholic liver diseases. Appropriate treatment is based on accurate diagnosis, which has improved incredibly with developments in non-invasive screening and diagnostic methods. Remarkably, the advent of all-oral antiviral treatment for HCV has transformed treatment options, superseding previous, less tolerable regimens. The new therapies not only provide improved efficacy and tolerability but also a less complex administration regimen. Furthermore, the Centres for Disease Control and Prevention (CDC) has established new programs to expand screening for HCV, particularly in individuals born between 1945 and 1965, that may enable prompt intervention of affected populations (Afdhal et al., 2013). Along with treatment for the infection, associated complications of hepatic disease need to be treated. Complications such as cirrhosis, liver failure, and hepatocellular carcinoma (HCC) require vigorous management, particularly as the patient transitions to end-stage liver disease. Transplantation becomes a part of routine consideration in these situations, along with careful candidate selection and customized management regimens. Specialist panels, such as the Italian Association for the Study of the Liver (AISF), have issued guidelines for the care of candidates with complex needs, particularly emphasizing early referral and nutritional assessment. As technology advances, the inclusion of direct-acting antiviral agents before and after transplantation is increasingly recognized as necessary to achieve optimized outcomes and reduce infection recurrence (Burra et al., 2018). Lastly, nevertheless, complete management of liver disease is entirely an interdisciplinary, team-oriented endeavor. Primary care clinicians, gastroenterologists, and hepatologists need to work together to ensure patients receive the level of care they require, particularly given the shifting paradigm of therapies. Coping with patient education and compliance remains fundamental, as increased awareness of hepatic health can spark interest in screening and therapy. Further, the incorporation of supportive systems and community resources will guarantee access, particularly for the underserved populations. Since administration is always on the move, keeping an eye on multidisciplinary care will enhance care delivery and patient outcomes and ultimately address the larger issues hepatic disease poses for the dynamic patterns of internal medicine (Afdhal et al., 2013; Burra et al., 2018) (Figure 4.11).

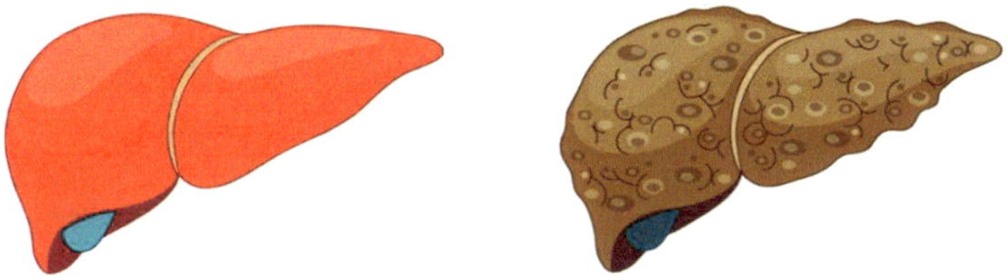

Figure 4.11. Liver disease.

Source: https://i0.wp.com/post.healthline.com/wp-content/uploads/2021/11/1684500-Liver-Problems-and-Their-Causes.png?w=1155&h=1436.

Test Your Knowledge

1. What are the most common gastrointestinal disorders seen in clinical practice?
2. How do symptoms of acute gastrointestinal disorders differ from chronic conditions?

4.5. The Role of Nutrition in Gastroenterology

Learning Outcome

1. Understand the importance of diet in gastrointestinal health
2. Define the nutritional therapy for specific disorders
3. Discuss the role of dietitians in gastroenterology

The interplay between nutrition and gastroenterology is a critical area of patient management and outcome. Nutrition is a key component in the maintenance of intestinal health, enabling the best recovery and the treatment of many gastrointestinal diseases. For instance, ALF patients require meticulous nutritional assessment and care since deficiencies may worsen their condition. Implementation of strict management guidelines, such as checklists, has been observed to yield promising results in streamlining the care processes in intensive care settings. This not only enhances patient safety but also enables healthcare personnel to make well-informed decisions when prescribing dietary guidance, thereby facilitating a holistic mode of treatment (Acute Liver Failure Study Group et al., 2016). Lastly, meeting the nutritional needs of gastroenterology patients alters the trajectory of recovery, highlighting the long-term importance of dietary management in this case. Nutritional therapies also play a significant role in controlling IBD, emphasizing the intricate relationship between diet and gastrointestinal illness. Research reveals that the rapid rise in IBD incidence is paralleled by changes in diet so that environmental factors, of which diet is the key, are responsible for the initiation and recurrence of the disease. The D-ECCO working group has taken into account comprehensive evidence on dietary determinants of IBD, structuring their findings into topical areas covering the contribution of diet to disease aetiology, induction therapy, and maintenance therapy (Allan et al., 2017).

By understanding these relationships, clinicians can customize dietary therapy to alleviate symptoms and promote remission, thereby reducing patient morbidity. Dietary control is therefore no longer ancillary but central to the therapeutic management of gastroenterological disease. It can be argued that nutritional treatment forms a pillar in the multidisciplinary management modality in gastroenterology. The profound implications of appropriate dietary interventions extend beyond symptom relief; they are a significant factor in disease management and overall health. While the understanding of nutrition's role in gut health continues to unfold, it is paramount that practitioners remain current with new research findings.

Furthermore, the delivery of nutrition-specific interventions necessitates multidisciplinary effort among gastroenterologists, dietitians, and other clinicians for the design of individualized care plans that acknowledge each patient's unique nutritional needs. Such co-management has ensured proper treatment in accordance with best practice, ultimately leading to better patient outcomes and greater overall effectiveness of internal medicine in gastroenterology.

4.5.1. Importance of Diet in Gastrointestinal Health

One of the most important factors in maintaining gastrointestinal health is incorporating an optimally balanced diet that meets the unique needs of the digestive system. Recent evidence has focused on the interaction between diet, gut microbiota, and the pathogenesis of various gastrointestinal diseases, including IBD. D-ECCO's working group summarized existing evidence on the role of diet in modulating IBD, highlighting that environmental exposures and dietary factors can have a significant impact on its development and course. This research highlights notable themes, including the role of diet in disease initiation and continuation therapies, suggesting that diet interventions could alter disease trajectories and improve clinical outcomes. With the shocking rise in the incidence of IBD as a marker, understanding the dietary determinants at play is paramount, thereby creating a platform for future research on optimizing nutritional strategies in gastroenterology (Allan et al., 2017). The quantity and quality of dietary fiber ingested also play an important role in managing gastrointestinal tract health. In particular, the impact of fiber ingestion on patients of pancreatic disease remains a matter of controversy even today. Findings show that an enriched prebiotic diet during acute pancreatitis is beneficial, leading to reduced infection rates and shorter hospitalization duration. This protective action is linked to the fiber's ability to reinforce intestinal barrier function, thereby preventing systemic inflammatory responses. However, in exocrine pancreatic insufficiency, excessive dietary fiber may disrupt pancreatic enzyme activity, leading to increased fecal fat excretion. This divide points to the complexity of nutritional advice, where one needs an individualized strategy based on the patient's state and disease states to yield positive results (Badiali et al., 2019) (Figure 4.12).

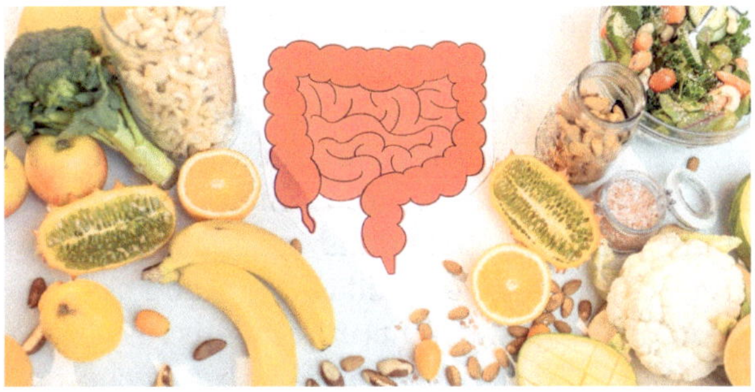

Figure 4.12. Importance of diet in gastrointestinal health.

Source: https://www.healixhospitals.com/tinyimages/Nutrition%20in%20Gastrointestinal%20Health%20-%20Healix%20Hospitals.jpg.

Further, diet and management of gastrointestinal disease interact beyond macronutrient sufficiency to encompass micronutrient status. Deficiencies in required vitamins and minerals may initiate or accelerate a number of gastrointestinal complications, rendering a complete nutrition assessment essential. If patients are deprived of essential nutrients, complications such as malnutrition, impaired wound healing, and changes in gut permeability may arise, aggravating their gastrointestinal disease. Well-crafted, evidence-based nutrition can potentially retard the progression of disease and support overall digestive function. Inclusion of dietary assessments in the treatment regimen for gastrointestinal disease may significantly improve patient outcomes. As such, further investigation into well-considered dietary interventions remains critical for those practising internal medicine in gastroenterology, with the potential to refine therapeutic models and improve long-term outcomes.

4.5.2. Nutritional Therapy for Specific Disorders

Nutritional therapy plays a critical role in the treatment of various gastrointestinal disorders, as evidenced by new evidence in inflammatory bowel disease (IBD). The interplay between environmental factors and the intestinal microbiota in genetically predisposed individuals underscores the importance of dietary exposure. This interaction has received increasing attention, particularly regarding the impact of diet on IBD pathogenesis. A systematic review by the D-ECCO working group highlights the role of diet, separating research into three categories: the role of diet in IBD pathogenesis, its application as induction and maintenance treatment, and the importance of measuring nutritional status as supportive treatment. Significantly, the review identifies deficiencies in existing research and recommends a future agenda for dietary management of IBD, thereby reflecting the role of nutrition therapy in improving patient outcomes and quality of life (Allan et al., 2017). For pancreatic conditions, the interaction between dietary fiber is more complicated, particularly in acute pancreatitis and exocrine pancreatic insufficiency. Research indicates that a prebiotic-supplemented diet reduces the incidence of complications, such as pancreatic necrosis, infection, and systemic inflammatory responses, thereby increasing recovery rates. The protective mechanism appears to be the fibers' ability to stabilize intestinal barrier function and reduce the risk of infection. But exocrine pancreatic insufficiency can be difficult to treat, as excessive fiber intake can increase fecal fat excretion by inhibiting pancreatic enzymes. Knowing these contrasting effects is important for personalizing dietary recommendations, since the polyvalent nature of fibers plays a determinant role in optimizing nutritional therapy for the treatment of pancreatic disease (Badiali et al., 2019). Combined, the data on IBD and pancreatic disease nutritional therapy illustrate the pivotal intersection of diet and gastroenterologic wellness. Effective nutritional therapy is increasingly recognized not only as an adjunct but also as an integral component of integrative treatment protocols. The addition of goal-directed dietary therapies can assist in achieving improved clinical outcomes, from reducing IBD flare severity to maximizing recovery with pancreatic disease. As studies continue to reveal the complexities of diet effects in gastrointestinal diseases, health care professionals must stay current to provide patient-focused nutritional guidance. Not only do these preventive interventions alleviate symptoms but also sustain long-term well-being, thereby justifying the primacy of nutritional therapy in gastroenterologic practice (Allan et al., 2017; Badiali et al., 2019).

4.5.3. Role of Dietitians in Gastroenterology

Dietitians are key to gastroenterology, particularly in the treatment of gastrointestinal disorders such as inflammatory bowel disease (IBD) and irritable bowel syndrome (IBS). With the increasing incidence of these diseases, patients' dietary decisions have immense potential to drive symptom management and overall health outcomes. Evidence has demonstrated that diet is an environmental determinant of the etiology of IBD, creating a pivotal link between nutrition and disease progression. Dietitians are well positioned to advise patients on the complex relationship between dietary intake and gastrointestinal function, and to provide tailored dietary management to promote healing and symptom control. Moreover, their expert advice enables nutritional evaluation to ensure patients are adequately fed while their illness is being managed. Such comprehensive food counseling is of extreme importance to patients managing the chronic long-term implications of such diseases (Allan et al., 2017). In the case of IBS, dietitians play a crucial role in navigating patients through the complexity of food triggers and sensitivities. One of the standard treatment interventions is the application of the low-FODMAP diet, demonstrated to alleviate symptoms in a high proportion of IBS patients. Dietitians assist patients by providing structured guidance on food choices, meal planning, and adherence to this restrictive diet. With their skills, dietitians can encourage people with IBS to reintroduce foods, thereby identify individual triggers and guide dietary interventions that enhance the quality of life. This is particularly important for some subtypes of IBS—IBS-D, IBS-C, and IBS-M—that respond uniquely to dietary intervention (Rentz et al., 2021). Hence, dietitians' personalized care is imperative to achieve maximum control of IBS symptoms. Dietitians' contributions to a gastroenterology multidisciplinary team also include collaborating with medical care teams to provide comprehensive patient care. Their ability to interpret dietary counseling in conjunction with prescribed medical management provides a cohesive plan addressing the body's physiological and nutritional components of gastrointestinal disease. This cooperative approach not only enhances patient compliance with treatment plans but also empowers patients to become engaged participants in their health. By staying abreast of new findings and evolving dietary advice, dietitians are well positioned to advocate for evidence-based practice that supports patients' nutritional well-being and improves their health outcomes. As gastroenterology continues to advance, the dietitian's role remains vital, further reinforcing the relationship between nutrition and intestinal health (Allan et al., 2017).

Test Your Knowledge

1. Why is proper nutrition important in the management of gastrointestinal diseases?
2. How do dietary fibers support digestive health?

4.6. Advances in Gastroenterology

Learning Outcome

1. Define the emerging technologies in diagnosis and treatment
2. Describe the research trends in gastroenterology
3. Understand the future directions for the field of gastroenterology

Advances in gastrointestinal research have continued to enhance our understanding of intricate diseases, particularly inflammatory and functional gastrointestinal disorders. For instance, the addition of newer imaging modalities, such as endoscopic ultrasonography and magnetic resonance enterography, has improved the accuracy of diagnosis and evaluation of conditions like Crohn's disease and ulcerative colitis. These advances are not only improving diagnostic accuracy but also facilitating the optimization of disease activity monitoring and treatment responsiveness. Besides, machine learning algorithms used in gastrointestinal imaging analysis have shown promise for early detection of pathological changes, enabling intervention at an earlier stage. Against this backdrop, clinicians should stay abreast of new diagnostic modalities to enhance patient outcomes in the management of gastrointestinal disorders. Furthermore, advances in treatment have transformed the management of a number of gastrointestinal diseases. The use of biologic therapies, particularly for inflammatory bowel disease, has been highly effective at reducing inflammation and increasing remission rates. The use of drugs that target specific cytokines, for example, TNF-alpha and interleukin-12/23, an ideal representation of this evolution in treatment modalities. The investigation into pharmacologic agents that target modification of the gut microbiota, such as rifaximin and probiotics, holds promise for controlling diseases like acute diverticulitis. However, the efficacy of these treatments in primary and secondary prevention remains under investigation, spurring ongoing clinical trials to understand better their potential impacts on disease recurrence and long-term control. The shifting treatment paradigm is therefore an indicator of the ongoing imperative for research and adjustment in therapeutic approaches in gastroenterology. The rising incidence of gastrointestinal diseases underscores the need to address their medical and socioeconomic aspects. Acute diverticulitis, for example, has shown a rising hospitalization trend, particularly among certain demographic groups, and necessitates effective, cost-effective management strategies that deliver maximum patient care. Outpatient innovations, in which uncomplicated cases can be treated with minimal supportive therapy, represent a significant practice change that can help minimize the economic burden of gastrointestinal disease. Furthermore, recognition of the multifactorial pathogenesis of diseases like diverticulitis encourages innovation in developing targeted approaches to individual patient risk factors, thereby enhancing prevention and treatment outcomes. Emphasizing the intersection between research and clinical practice will ensure that advances in gastroenterology are translated into improvements in healthcare delivery to patients.

4.6.1. Emerging Technologies in Diagnosis and Treatment

The introduction of novel technologies into gastroenterology is a revolutionary shift in diagnostic and treatment paradigms. Technologies such as next-generation sequencing and biomarker analyses are enhancing diagnostic accuracy in gastrointestinal disease. For example, the discovery of serum microRNAs as diagnostic biomarkers can help diagnose complex diseases such as primary sclerosing cholangitis (PSC) and its complications. As diagnosing PSC is difficult, the development of these biomarkers is a major breakthrough that can improve patient outcomes by enabling earlier diagnosis and treatment. As evidence continues to validate these biomarkers in the clinical setting, the promise of more uniform diagnostic tools becomes increasingly tangible, thereby changing the face of gastroenterological treatment (Alpini et al., 2016). In conjunction with diagnosis, new therapeutic opportunities are being explored, namely through recombinant peptide technology. This novel technique proposes the application of specific peptides that could treat many gastrointestinal disorders more effectively than traditional techniques. Research evidence indicates that these peptides have the potential to modulate growth factor receptor function and thereby offer new avenues for the treatment of inflammatory bowel diseases and certain cancers. While such preclinical trials appear highly promising, a transition towards their use in routine clinical practice has only just begun. Therefore, although there is such a vast scope for peptide therapies, determining their effectiveness and appropriate application in standard practice remains a persistent issue that must be addressed by both researchers and clinicians (Ghosh et al., 2004). In addition, the incorporation of artificial intelligence (AI) and machine learning into gastroenterological practice has promising fields for better patient care. AI-driven algorithms can analyze vast quantities of data from various diagnostic tools, including imaging and lab work, to uncover patterns that may not be immediately apparent to physicians. This predictive aspect would likely lead to earlier interventions and individually tailored treatment plans, essentially changing the way internal medicine approaches gastrointestinal disease. The validity and morality of AI in the clinical setting must be carefully considered as doctors attempt to deploy these technologies. As gastroenterology advances with technological development, the potential for increased diagnostic sensitivity and therapeutic efficacy is an exciting outlook for patient management in internal medicine (Ghosh et al., 2004; Alpini et al., 2016).

4.6.2. Research Trends in Gastroenterology

Gastroenterology has witnessed considerable research advances, particularly in closing gaps in colorectal cancer (CRC) research. Notably, colorectal cancer is among the leading cancer-causing deaths for African Americans, and both occurrence and mortality are decidedly higher in comparison with their White counterparts. The precarious situation calls for preventive measures such as colorectal cancer screening (CRCS), which is highly effective for early detection and improved outcomes. However, with these opportunities for screening, there are still significant gaps, particularly among young adult African American men, suggesting a field of study of utmost significance. Recent systematic analyses indicate that there is limited knowledge of the factors influencing these individuals' intention to undergo CRCS, and therefore an imperative for planned health education interventions to increase awareness and improve access to screening (Foster et al., 2014). In addition to alleviating disparities in CRC, the research climate in gastroenterology is increasingly dominated by translational research (TR), which seeks to bridge the gap between discovery and application. More attention to TR is a familiar longing for evidence that scientific progress translates into improved patient care in reality. TR holds vast promise but raises complex design issues regarding operational definitions and models. Recent analyses have indicated that the construction of TR may vary significantly across studies, reflecting both the complexity of translating science into practice and the importance of an accurate methodology. By breaking down the various dimensions of TR, researchers can better evaluate the barriers to the effective translation of knowledge into practice and thereby enhance patient outcomes in gastroenterology (Boenink et al., 2015). Furthermore, emerging gastroenterology research trends increasingly involve integrating technological advances, most importantly in artificial intelligence and genomics, that are revolutionizing diagnosis and treatment strategies. Machine learning is designed to scan vast databases, providing clinicians with data that traditional methods may miss. Genomic medicine is also transforming the landscape, offering individualized treatments tailored to patients' unique genetic profiles. By combining gastroenterology with technology, researchers can develop more targeted therapies that improve clinical outcomes without increasing the risks associated with various gastrointestinal diseases. As these advancements become operational, it is important that the discipline weaves technology integration with stringent clinical research so that progress gets adequately translated into practice and rewards the whole patient population.

4.6.3. Future Directions for the Field

In the evolving field of gastroenterology, one of the most pressing issues is advancing imaging technology, particularly hepatic magnetic resonance imaging (MRI). As noted in recent reviews, the existing body of research on hepatic MRI highlights its use in clinical practice; studies have shown that a large proportion of highly cited papers on the topic are published in top journals and provide insights into diagnostics and patient management (Abdullah et al., 2018). As the technology improves in resolution and capability, future studies can lead to more precise diagnosis and earlier detection of liver disease. Hence, the development and standardization of imaging protocols are important so that newer technologies can be made more widely available, thereby improving patient outcomes through better modalities and reducing healthcare costs through more targeted interventions. Another important area of future research in gastroenterology is the management of viral hepatitis-induced liver disease, particularly with the advent of DAAs. Recent evidence has revealed that there has been a remarkable decrease in registrations on liver transplantation waiting lists due to hepatitis C virus (HCV)-induced cirrhosis since the advent of DAAs in clinical practice. This paradigm shift emphasizes the potential of antiviral therapy not only to improve survival rates but also to minimize the burden on transplant systems, as patients achieve viral eradication more effectively than before (Angeli et al., 2018). Future research should focus on fine-tuning the treatment regimen and the long-term effects of DAAs on liver condition. By establishing comprehensive treatment protocols, gastroenterologists can tailor individual therapeutic plans to each patient, thereby enhancing the management of chronic liver diseases. With a focus on emerging technologies and therapeutic approaches, the future of gastroenterology will also necessitate an integrated framework. Multidisciplinary cooperation between gastroenterologists, hepatologists, radiologists, and primary care providers will be essential in developing integrated care pathways based on patient-centered outcomes. This collaborative environment can facilitate the sharing of knowledge and resources, wherein all aspects of gastroenterological well-being can be addressed through a balanced strategy. Further, encouraging research initiatives to address health disparities and improve access to care will create a more equal landscape for the healthcare system. Emphasizing such interdisciplinary methodologies will not only increase the scope of internal medicine for gastroenterology but also play an important role in better patient inclusion and healthcare models in the future.

Test Your Knowledge

1. What recent technological advances have improved the diagnosis of gastrointestinal diseases?
2. How have minimally invasive procedures transformed gastroenterological treatment?

SUMMARY

Given the context of internal medicine, there is a need to examine how various systemic factors influence the field's efficacy and trajectory. The history of gastroenterologists' labor markets, and in particular the role of centralized clearinghouses, has much to teach us about market dynamics. As indicated by the examination of the gastroenterology labor market, the implementation and subsequent withdrawal of a match program provided a valuable lens through which to examine market organization. The clearinghouse facilitated efficient coordination of timing, and the markets' thickness and scope were improved. This experience not only highlights the complexity of physician placement but also underscores the role of market forces in optimizing healthcare delivery. Thus, a review of centralized clearinghouses might be warranted to address current inefficiencies and build a more robust workforce to meet future patient demand (Roth et al., 2025). Moreover, familiarity with the subtleties of healthcare information, particularly medical billing information, is critical for accurate assessment of gastroenterological quality measures. The research indicates that while billing information is useful for considering trends in population health, it is susceptible to biases that distort findings. In a study assessing colorectal cancer screening rates, a discrepancy between computerized billing reports and manual review revealed widespread inaccuracies in the data. Whereas billing data suggested a robust screening rate, manual reviews revealed a different reality: high false negatives and positives. Such a finding underscores the need for caution when using billing data for inferential purposes in gastroenterological quality measures. An awareness of such limitations is central to taking the field forward and improving patient outcomes (Avila et al., 2020). In brief, the future of internal medicine gastroenterology must incorporate principles drawn from both the state of the labor market and best practices in data use. With better coordination of the gastroenterologist workforce and enhanced validity of health measurements, the field will be better positioned to serve its patients and populations. Centralized market mechanisms that engage in aggressive data analysis are essential for addressing current issues and encouraging sustainable growth in the field. In the days to come, attention should be directed toward creating policies that not only facilitate effective utilization of gastroenterologists but also more clearly define health data analysis practices. Such an integrated strategy can help elevate standards of care and patient outcomes, ultimately establishing gastroenterology's central position in internal medicine (Avila et al., 2020; Roth et al., 2025).

In exploring the complexities of internal medicine, particularly in gastroenterology, some pertinent points that emerge emphasize the field's multidisciplinary nature. Among the most dramatic is the role of microRNA in modulating gastrointestinal function, particularly smooth muscle contractility. Recent research has shown that specific microRNAs, such as rno-miR-133a, are increased in the senescent internal anal sphincter (IAS). This dysregulation underlies a decrease in IAS basal tone and may lead to diseases such as rectoanal incontinence. A description of these molecular bases is essential to the design of therapy-targeting strategies, demonstrating how advances in molecular biology can revolutionize our understanding of gastroenterological diseases and their treatment (Addya et al., 2016). Another cornerstone area of consideration is the dilemma of diagnosing conditions such as Gaucher disease (GD), which manifests itself within other gastrointestinal states. The Gaucher Early Diagnosis Consensus (GED-C) program has emphasized the importance of picking up early symptoms and signs of GD, such as splenomegaly and thrombocytopenia. These findings underscore the need for greater awareness among physicians, particularly non-specialist physicians, who may miss subtle signs of underlying pathologies. By identifying specific symptoms and co-variables for different types of GD, this project aims to reduce diagnostic delays and, subsequently, reduce the significant morbidity associated with the disease. Hence, enhancing clinical awareness is the secret to favorable patient outcomes in gastroenterology (Belmatoug et al., 2019). Moreover, the interplay between genetic susceptibilities and clinical expressions in gastroenterology further highlights the importance of more personalized approaches in internal medicine. Genetic factors, such as Ashkenazi Jewish ancestry in GD, are key to patient identification and care. The consensus among a global panel of experts emphasizes the integration of genetic risk markers into practice. Through this mechanism, healthcare professionals can better identify at-risk patients, illustrating the importance of personalized medicine in gastroenterology. As a result, the key issues discussed demonstrate a shift in internal medicine toward early diagnosis and targeted treatments, ultimately aimed at improving patient care in gastroenterology (Belmatoug et al., 2019).

KEY TERMS FROM THIS CHAPTER

- Comprehensive management
- Cardiology
- Liver disease
- Sound methodology
- Clostridium difficile infection (Cdi)
- Colorectal cancer (CRC)
- Irritable bowel syndrome (IBS)
- Peptic ulcer disease (PUD)
- Adult diseases
- Endocrinology
- Colorectal cancer
- Chronic gastrointestinal disease
- Gastroesophageal reflux disease (GERD)
- Gastroesophageal reflux disease (GERD)
- Inflammatory bowel disease (IBD)
- Computed tomography enterography

CRITICAL THINKING QUESTIONS

1. **A 45-year-old man presents with epigastric pain that improves with eating. What is the most likely diagnosis?**
   a. Gastric ulcer
   b. Duodenal ulcer
   c. Acute pancreatitis
   d. Gastroesophageal reflux disease (GERD)
2. **Which of the following is the most sensitive test for diagnosing acute pancreatitis?**
   a. Serum amylase
   b. Abdominal X-ray
   c. Serum lipase
   d. CT scan of the abdomen
3. **Which of the following conditions is associated with "skip lesions" in the gastrointestinal tract?**
   a. Ulcerative colitis
   b. Celiac disease
   c. Crohn's disease
   d. Irritable bowel syndrome
4. **A patient with chronic liver disease presents with confusion and asterixis. What is the most likely cause?**
   a. Hepatocellular carcinoma
   b. Hepatic encephalopathy
   c. Portal vein thrombosis
   d. Biliary obstruction
5. **Which of the following markers is most specific for the diagnosis of celiac disease?**
   a. Anti-nuclear antibody (ANA)
   b. Anti-smooth muscle antibody
   c. Anti-tissue transglutaminase (anti-tTG) antibody
   d. Anti-mitochondrial antibody

Short Answer Questions

1. What is the primary focus of the field of gastroenterology?
2. Name two standard diagnostic techniques used in gastroenterology.
3. List at least three common gastrointestinal (GI) disorders.
4. How does endoscopy assist in diagnosing gastrointestinal conditions?
5. What are two primary treatment modalities used in managing GI disorders?
6. Why is nutrition considered necessary in the management of gastrointestinal diseases?

Answers to Critical Thinking Questions

1. (b); 2. (c) ; 3. (c); 4. (b); 5. (c)

REFERENCES

1. Ullah, W., Abdullah, H. M. A., Ahmad, E., Rashid, M. U., Bashir, M., Rahman, A. U. U., Ahmad, A., & Hurairah, A. (2018). A bibliometric analysis of the top 100 cited articles on hepatic magnetic resonance imaging. *Cureus, 10*(6), e2733. https://doi.org/10.7759/cureus.2733Abdullah, H. M. A., Ali, N. S., Ilyas, G., Inayat, F., et al. (2018). Lafora disease masquerading as hepatic dysfunction. https://core.ac.uk/download/213441668.pdf (accessed on 16th July 2025).
2. Abdullah, M., Mulia, M., Simadibrata, M., Tenggara, I., et al. (2010). Complicated benign peptic stricture of the esophagus. https://media.neliti.com/media/publications/68270-EN-complicated-benign-peptic-stricture-of-t.pdf (accessed on 16th July 2025).
3. Acute Liver Failure Study Group, Boylan, A., Fix, O. K., Forde, K. A., et al. (2016). Development and pilot of a checklist for management of acute liver failure in the intensive care unit. https://core.ac.uk/download/79819898.pdf (accessed on 16th July 2025).
4. Adamina, M., Bonovas, S., Raine, T., Spinelli, A., Warusavitarne, J., Armuzzi, A., Bachmann, O., et al. (2019). ECCO guidelines on therapeutics in Crohn's disease: Surgical treatment. *Journal of Crohn's and Colitis, 14*, 155–168. https://doi.org/10.1093/ecco-jcc/jjz187 (accessed on 16th July 2025).
5. Addiss, D. G., Fenwick, A., Jourdan, P. M., Lamberton, P., et al. (2018). Soil-transmitted helminth infections. https://core.ac.uk/download/96884381.pdf (accessed on 16th July 2025).
6. Addya, S., Ettickan, B., Penn, R. B., Phillips, B. R., et al. (2016). Aging-associated changes in microRNA expression profile of internal anal sphincter smooth muscle: Role of microRNA-133a. https://core.ac.uk/download/83049401.pdf (accessed on 16th July 2025).
7. Afdhal, N. H., Castera, L., Church, D. R., Dee, A., et al. (2013). The new paradigm of hepatitis C therapy: Integration of oral therapies into best practices. https://core.ac.uk/download/323065592.pdf (accessed on 16th July 2025).
8. Ahmed, M. (2018). Checkpoint inhibitors: What gastroenterologists need to know. https://core.ac.uk/download/213444662.pdf (accessed on 16th July 2025).
9. Allan, P., Fiorino, G., Gatti, S., Gerasimidis, K., et al. (2017). Research gaps in diet and nutrition in inflammatory bowel disease: A topical review by D-ECCO Working Group (Dietitians of ECCO). https://core.ac.uk/download/84340703.pdf (accessed on 16th July 2025).
10. Alpers, D. H., Hong, B. A., & North, C. S. (2007). Relationship of functional gastrointestinal disorders and psychiatric disorders: Implications for treatment. https://core.ac.uk/download/70385399.pdf (accessed on 16th July 2025).
11. Alpini, G., Alvaro, D., Bernuzzi, F., Bowlus, C., et al. (2016). Serum microRNAs as novel biomarkers for primary sclerosing cholangitis and cholangiocarcinoma. https://core.ac.uk/download/54531174.pdf (accessed on 16th July 2025).
12. Angeli, P., Burra, P., Cillo, U., Ferrarese, A., et al. (2018). Hepatitis C virus-related cirrhosis decreased as indication to liver transplantation since the introduction of direct-acting antivirals: A single-center study. https://core.ac.uk/download/168405521.pdf (accessed on 16th July 2025).
13. Angelico, F., Baratta, F., Bucci, T., Cangemi, M., et al. (2015). Similar reduction of cholesterol-adjusted vitamin E serum levels in simple steatosis and non-alcoholic steatohepatitis. https://core.ac.uk/download/54525153.pdf (accessed on 16th July 2025).

14. Annibale, B., Carabotti, M., Cicenia, A., Pallotta, L., et al. (2018). Recent advances in understanding and managing diverticulitis. https://core.ac.uk/download/160052854.pdf (accessed on 16th July 2025).

15. Avila, P., Butte, A. J., Glicksberg, B. S., Harding-Theobald, E., et al. (2020). Accuracy of medical billing data against the electronic health record in the measurement of colorectal cancer screening rates. https://core.ac.uk/download/323062526.pdf (accessed on 16th July 2025).

16. Badiali, D., Bruno, G., Ribichini, E., Rossi, M., et al. (2019). Role of fiber in nutritional management of pancreatic diseases. https://core.ac.uk/download/231748461.pdf (accessed on 16th July 2025).

17. Belmatoug, N., Bembi, B., Bright, J., Deodato, F., et al. (2019). Presenting signs and patient co-variables in Gaucher disease: Outcome of the Gaucher Earlier Diagnosis Consensus (GED-C) Delphi initiative. https://core.ac.uk/download/287581712.pdf (accessed on 16th July 2025).

18. Betlachin, A., Esrailian, E., Garner, O. B., Grossman, M., et al. (2018). A multi-level FIT-based quality improvement initiative to improve colorectal cancer screening in a managed care population. https://core.ac.uk/download/323077113.pdf (accessed on 16th July 2025).

19. Bharucha, A. E., Rao, S. S. C., & Shin, A. (2017). Surgical interventions and the use of device-aided therapy for the treatment of fecal incontinence and defecatory disorders. https://core.ac.uk/download/129148926.pdf (accessed on 16th July 2025).

20. Boenink, M., & van der Laan, A. L. (2015). Beyond bench and bedside: Disentangling the concept of translational research. https://core.ac.uk/download/pdf/11486878.pdf (accessed on 16th July 2025).

21. Budhram, B., Deng, M., Elias, S., Endres, T., et al. (2020). Enrichissement et développement en médecine interne: Un programme d'exploration estivale pour les étudiants du pré-externat. https://core.ac.uk/download/328007498.pdf (accessed on 16th July 2025).

22. Burra, P., Caraceni, P., Ferri, F., Giannini, E., et al. (2018). Specific issues concerning the management of patients on the waiting list and after liver transplantation. https://core.ac.uk/download/159268374.pdf (accessed on 16th July 2025).

23. Cai, Z., Wang, S., & Li, J. (2021). Treatment of inflammatory bowel disease: A comprehensive review. *Frontiers in Medicine, 8*. https://doi.org/10.3389/fmed.2021.765474 (accessed on 16th July 2025).

24. Calabrese, E., Dietrich, C. F., Dirks, K., Gilja, O., et al. (2016). EFSUMB recommendations and guidelines for gastrointestinal ultrasound–Part 1: Examination techniques and normal findings (long version). https://core.ac.uk/download/74321241.pdf (accessed on 16th July 2025).

25. Canbaz, S., Leblebicioglu, H., Peksen, Y., Sunter, A., et al. (2005). Survey of general practitioners' knowledge about *Helicobacter pylori* infection. https://core.ac.uk/download/pdf/3561928.pdf (accessed on 16th July 2025).

26. Chowers, Y., Danese, S., Dignass, A., Gomollõn, F., et al. (2013). The management of iron deficiency in inflammatory bowel disease. https://core.ac.uk/download/19199342.pdf (accessed on 16th July 2025).

27. Dumitru, A. E., Popoiag, R., Micu, S. I., Moraru, C., et al. (2019). The burden of *Clostridium difficile* infection in patients with liver cirrhosis. https://core.ac.uk/download/232440323.pdf (accessed on 16th July 2025).

28. Elghuel, A., Timraz, A., Olokoba, A. B., Kankaria, A. G., Liwa, A., Meaden, C., Zaltman, C., et al. (2012). A fibreoptic endoscopic study of upper gastrointestinal bleeding at Bugando Medical Centre in Northwestern Tanzania: A retrospective review of 240 cases. https://core.ac.uk/download/pdf/11307794.pdf (accessed on 16th July 2025).

29. Foster, M., Goodson, P., & Rogers, C. R. (2014). Factors associated with colorectal cancer screening among younger African American men: A systematic review. https://core.ac.uk/download/186711270.pdf (accessed on 16th July 2025).

30. Garcia, J., Gross, S. A., Lahr, R., Rex, D. K., et al. (2019). Endocuff Vision reduces inspection time without decreasing lesion detection in a randomized colonoscopy trial. https://core.ac.uk/download/187423803.pdf (accessed on 16th July 2025).

31. Ghosh, S., Playford, R. J., & Wassan, H. (2004). Effects of growth factors and receptor blockade on gastrointestinal cancer. https://core.ac.uk/download/30694900.pdf (accessed on 16th July 2025).

32. Hage, L., Kügler, M., Menendez Menendez, K., Naehrlich, L., et al. (2013). Serum proteome profiling identifies novel and powerful markers of cystic fibrosis liver disease. https://core.ac.uk/download/12175519.pdf (accessed on 16th July 2025).

33. Holly, A., Burnand, B., Froehlich, F., Gonvers, J. J., Vader, J. P., Lamiraud, K., Juillerat, P., et al. (2025). The effect of non-medical factors on variations in the performance of colonoscopy among different health care settings. https://core.ac.uk/download/pdf/6617669.pdf (accessed on 16th July 2025).

34. Holtmann, G., & Talley, N. J. (2014). Herbal medicines for the treatment of functional and inflammatory bowel disorders. https://core.ac.uk/download/43355908.pdf (accessed on 16th July 2025).

35. Kim, S. K., Korenblat, K., Lee, K. A., Sauk, J. S., et al. (2017). Comparison of transjugular intrahepatic portosystemic shunt with covered stent and balloon-occluded retrograde transvenous obliteration in managing isolated gastric varices. https://core.ac.uk/download/83101055.pdf (accessed on 16th July 2025).

36. Linson, E. A. (2013). The interplay between hormones and irritable bowel disease. https://open.bu.edu/bitstream/2144/12149/6/Linson_Elyse_2013_nosig_nocv.pdf (accessed on 16th July 2025).

37. Putri, N. I., & Miftahussurur, M. (2025). The implication of multichannel intraluminal impedance and pH-monitoring in GERD patients. https://core.ac.uk/download/640070878.pdf (accessed on 16th July 2025).

38. Rentz, H. (2021). Assessing and comparing quality of life scores in patients with irritable bowel syndrome-diarrhea, irritable bowel syndrome-constipation, and irritable bowel syndrome-mixed. https://core.ac.uk/download/478599396.pdf (accessed on 16th July 2025).

39. Roth, A. E., & Niederle, M. (2025). The effects of a centralized clearinghouse on job placement, wages, and hiring practices. https://core.ac.uk/download/pdf/6501831.pdf (accessed on 16th July 2025).

40. Rubino, F., Puhl, R. M., Cummings, D. E., Eckel, R. H., Ryan, D. H., Mechanick, J. I., Nadglowski, J., et al. (2020). Joint international consensus statement for ending stigma of obesity. *Nature Medicine, 26*, 485–497. https://doi.org/10.1038/s41591-020-0803-x (accessed on 16th July 2025).

41. Tietz, A. B., Arnush, M., Bhagat, L., Bhatia, M., Bockman, D. E., Göke, B., et al. (2005). Pathophysiology of acute experimental pancreatitis: Lessons from genetically engineered animal models and new molecular approaches. https://core.ac.uk/download/16432751.pdf (accessed on 16th July 2025).

42. UNE Library Services. (2008). *E-books Acquisition 2007–2008*. https://core.ac.uk/download/146515833.pdf (accessed on 16th July 2025).

43. Virginia Commonwealth University. (2018). *Virginia Commonwealth University Professional Bulletin*. https://core.ac.uk/download/215485746.pdf (accessed on 16th July 2025).

44. White, P. H., & Cooley, W. C. (2018). Supporting the health care transition from adolescence to adulthood in the medical home. *Pediatrics, 142*. https://doi.org/10.1542/peds.2018-2587 (accessed on 16th July 2025).

NEPHROLOGY

5

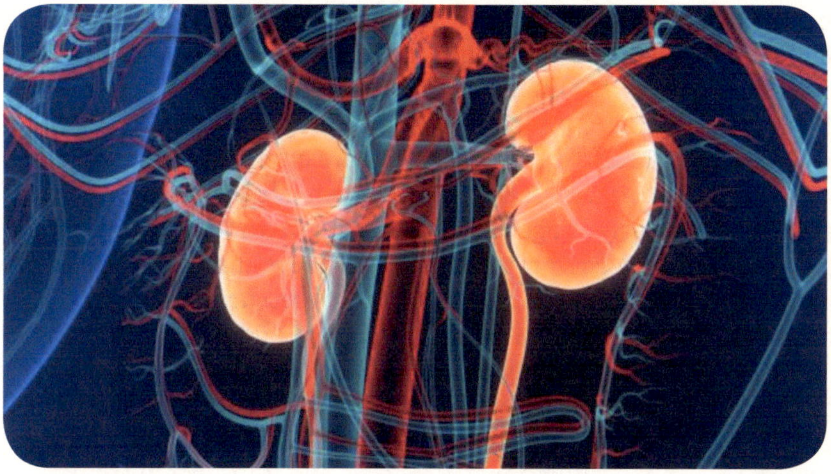

Introduction

Nephrology, the branch of medicine concerned with the health and disease of the kidneys, is a significant component of internal medicine. It is necessary to fully understand nephrology to diagnose and manage several kidney-related diseases, including acute kidney injury (AKI) and chronic kidney disease (CKD). The relationship between CKD and AKI is more and more recognized, with a recognition by clinicians that the two could be alternate stages of the same underlying disease process. The suggestion to use the term acute kidney disease (AKD) to describe the sustained pathophysiologic processes following an acute episode of AKI has been put forward to define the spectrum between acute and chronic renal impairment. Current classifications and policies for practice aim to maximize patient outcomes and keep practitioners current with the latest developments in kidney management (Chawla et al., 2017). Nephrology practice encompasses a wide range of diseases affecting kidney function, including those caused by systemic conditions such as diabetes, hypertension, or autoimmune disease. Within an

LEARNING OBJECTIVES

After studying this chapter, you will be able to:

1. Understand the anatomy and physiology of the kidneys
2. Describe common kidney diseases
3. Explain diagnostic approaches in nephrology
4. Discuss treatment modalities in nephrology
5. Define the role of internal medicine in nephrology
6. Focus on current research and advances in nephrology

evidence-based approach, nephrologists must be aware of current guidelines that mandate best practices for disease management. For instance, the European League Against Rheumatism (EULAR) guideline on the management of antineutrophil cytoplasmic antibody (ANCA)-associated vasculitis (AAV) provides insights into treatment strategies for conditions with a significant impact on renal health. This includes issues like immunosuppressive therapy, induction of remission, and clinician-patient shared decision-making, all of which are critical for optimal nephrological care. Adherence to guidelines that address overall treatment modalities and individual patient needs enables nephrologists to optimize patient outcomes and work within multidisciplinary teams of healthcare professionals (Yates et al., 2016). Nephrology education is imperative for creating a well-trained staff capable of handling the intricacies of kidney disease. As internal medicine increasingly overlaps with sub-specialties like nephrology, health practitioners must stay up to date with evolving treatments and diagnostic techniques. Continuing education can bridge knowledge gaps and stimulate research in areas such as AKI and AKD management, which remain under investigation for optimal therapeutic approaches. Consensus reports by organizations such as the Acute Disease Quality Initiative attempt to critically stage and define these conditions, paving the way for future clinical investigation and practice applications in nephrology. By fostering a culture of ongoing education and research inquiry in the subspecialty, specialists help promote patient care and deepen understanding of renal pathophysiology (Chawla et al., 2017).

Definition and Scope of Nephrology

Nephrology is a subspecialty of internal medicine specializing in the diagnosis and management of kidney disease and renal disorders. Kidneys, which are essential for maintaining electrolyte balance, fluid homeostasis, and waste removal, are central to health. Nephrology encompasses a wide range of pathologies, from chronic kidney disease (CKD) to glomerulonephritis and electrolyte disturbances. Also, nephrologists possess the ability to treat complicated renal replacement therapies such as kidney transplantation and dialysis. The field of nephrology also includes the clinical care of hypertension in patients with prior kidney disease, alluding to the intricate relationship between renal and cardiovascular health. The importance of nephrology is further underscored by the prevalence of kidney disease in the population and its status as an emerging public health problem worldwide. Because kidney diseases are often asymptomatic in their early stages, nephrologists focus on early diagnosis and the prevention of further disease progression. This prevention is crucial because most kidney diseases are associated with severe complications, including increased vulnerability to cardiovascular conditions and mortality. Nephrology also intersects with other medical specialties, such as endocrinology and infectious diseases, and thus requires a multidisciplinary, interdisciplinary approach to patient care. Recognition of the breadth and definition of nephrology not only vouches for the complexity of kidney disease but also emphasizes the necessity of continuous innovation in research and clinical endeavors in the discipline. Among the novel focuses of nephrology is the impact of systemic diseases, such as diabetes and hypertension, on the kidney. The interplay between these conditions and renal function necessitates holistic management strategies that address underlying risk factors and comorbidities. Given the economic and psychosocial burdens kidney diseases impose on patients and healthcare systems, nephrologists increasingly serve as key informants for patients about the importance of lifestyle changes and adherence to treatment plans. Besides, the global trend of rising healthcare demand, driven by factors such as a growing population and the COVID-19 pandemic, requires robust nephrology services to meet these needs. Understanding the scope of nephrology is central to developing effective healthcare policy and ensuring fair access to renal care for all populations, thereby highlighting nephrology's inherent role in improving overall health outcomes (Hert, 2020; Lechien et al., 2020) (Figure 5.1).

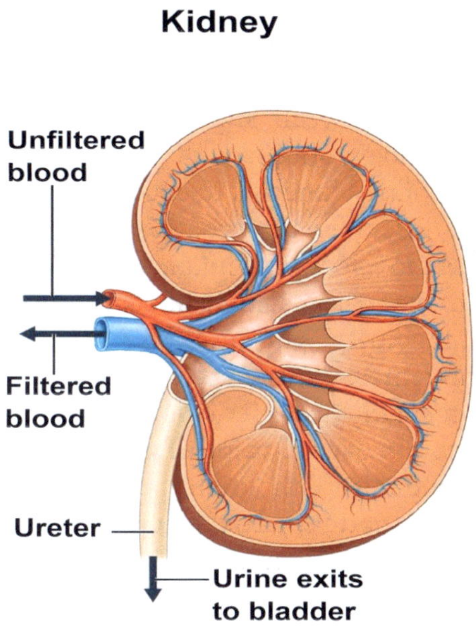

Figure 5.1. Illustration of kidney.

Source: https://www.niddk.nih.gov/-/media/Images/Health-Information/Kidney/Kidney_FINAL-Labels_1460x1623.jpg.

Importance of Nephrology in Internal Medicine

The role of nephrology in internal medicine cannot be overstated, especially as kidney-related diseases are increasing. Nephrologists deal with the diagnosis and management of conditions such as chronic kidney disease (CKD), a disease that occurs in association with other chronic diseases such as diabetes and hypertension. This crossing underscores the necessity of nephrology within the broader concept of internal medicine, as kidney function is central to cardiovascular health and overall systemic status. The problem is not merely that of curing kidney disease but also understanding how intricate renal function interacts with various comorbidities. Hence, nephrology is pivotal within the setting of internal medicine, both as a target of specialist intervention and as integral to holistic patient care. Additionally, the integration of nephrology into internal medicine contributes significantly to the outcome in patients, particularly where transplantation in the kidney is involved. The 2020 Kidney Disease: Improving Global Outcomes (KDIGO) Clinical Practice Guideline provides key assessment and management guidelines for prospective kidney transplant patients, focusing on the multifactorial variables that impact transplantation suitability, including psychosocial assessments and comorbidities (Chadban et al., 2020). It requires nephrologists to collaborate closely with other specialties to provide personalized treatment tailored to the prospective patient's medical history and overall health status.

By enhancing decision-making in transplantation, nephrology improves not only medical practice's ability to provide for individuals but also the standard practice of internal medicine as a whole. Additionally, physician burnout can significantly influence the practice of nephrology within internal medicine. Research shows that about one in three doctors suffers from burnout, which can affect the well-being of healthcare providers and the quality of care they provide to patients (Hert, 2020). In nephrology, with high-stress levels likely to arise from the complexity of patient management, identifying and addressing burnout are essential. Inclusion of measures to create a supportive work environment can enhance healthcare delivery and physician satisfaction. Lastly, integrating nephrology into internal medicine is not just about caring for patients but also about maintaining caregivers' health to create a healthier environment for both patients and caregivers.

Overview of Kidney Functions and Disorders

The kidney serves several vital roles in homeostasis, including filtration and elimination of waste products, regulation of electrolyte balance, acid-base balance, and regulation of blood pressure. Every kidney contains approximately 1 million nephrons, the functional components that filter blood and produce urine. Nephrons, through a complex process of filtration, reabsorption, and secretion, effectively remove toxins, excess salts, and metabolic waste such as urea and creatinine from the bloodstream. This balance prevents hypertension and fluid overload. Furthermore, the kidneys play a significant role in erythropoiesis by producing erythropoietin, a hormone that stimulates red blood cell production. These roles are crucial in nephrology because interruptions can lead to a range of disorders characterized by impaired renal function and systemic involvement, requiring delicate management and intervention. Kidney disease can manifest itself in several different forms, from acute kidney injury (AKI) to chronic kidney disease (CKD) and end-stage renal disease (ESRD). AKI is typically characterized by a rapid decline in kidney function, usually secondary to dehydration, infection, or nephrotoxic medication. CKD, however, occurs over time and can progress to ESRD, which would necessitate dialysis or transplant to maintain life. One of the well-known features of these conditions is uremic syndrome, which results as a consequence of the accumulation of waste products secondary to decreased kidney function. This phenomenon involves a range of symptoms affecting multiple organ systems, such as fatigue, anemia, and cardiovascular compromise. Also, systemic inflammation from ESRD is a vital concern as it accelerates mortality and accelerates the aging process on the body overall. For this reason, it is important to understand the etiology of kidney diseases, as this forms the basis for developing appropriate treatment strategies and improving outcomes of care in nephrology. The relationship between systemic inflammation and kidney diseases defines the complex interactions that modulate renal function. Patients with ESRD have an aging phenotype that involves wasting of muscles, vascular calcification, and enhanced frailty. Evidence indicates that uremic inflammation not only leads to such complications but also recapitulates the aging process of the population at large, termed "inflammaging." Such a connection underscores the necessity of an entire-systems approach to nephrology, one in which therapy extends beyond kidney function to encompass systemic health. Effective interventions will need to address the underlying inflammatory processes to overcome the harmful impact on mortality and morbidity potentially. Application of patient-centered strategies that incorporate the latest technological methods in healthcare can enhance the overall value of services provided to individuals with kidney disease, thereby improving patient satisfaction and outcomes in this high-risk population (Böbel et al., 2025; Schalkwijk et al., 2017).

5.1. Anatomy and Physiology of the Kidneys

Learning Outcome

1. Describe the structure of the kidneys
2. Define the functions of the renal system
3. Understand the regulation of homeostasis by the kidneys

The kidneys, which are essential organs of the urinary tract, are strategically positioned in the retroperitoneal space to filter blood and maintain homeostasis. One kidney has a complex structure with an outer cortex and an inner medulla. The nephron, the functional unit of the kidney, exists in approximately 1 million units per kidney, each performing filtration, reabsorption, and secretion. Anatomically, nephrons have a glomerulus that initiates the process of blood filtration and renal tubules that cause selective reabsorption of solute and water. Such a sophisticated organizational system is critical to fluid balance and electrolyte regulation, underlining the crucial role the kidneys play in the system's health. The physiological functions of the kidneys extend far beyond mere filtration; they also involve blood pressure regulation, electrolyte balance, and acid-base homeostasis. Within the nephron, glomerular filtration occurs when blood plasma is forced through the glomerular membrane by hydrostatic pressure, forming the renal filtrate. Subsequent processes within the renal tubules allow for reabsorption of essential nutrients such as glucose and amino acids as well as for the excretion of metabolic waste.

The kidneys also secrete hormones, such as erythropoietin, which stimulate the formation of red blood cells in response to hypoxia. Furthermore, the ability to concentrate or dilute urine adaptively in response to hydration requirements underscores the kidneys' significant integrative role in responding to the environment. Awareness of renal function disorders is essential in nephrology, particularly regarding conditions such as cystic kidney diseases (CKDs). These are conditions characterized by fluid-filled cysts in the kidneys, resulting from faulty cellular mechanisms that lead to malformation of nephric tubules. Alexander et al. (2015) note the maintenance of nephron structural integrity across species, illustrating the fundamental concepts that characterize kidney pathology. Further, historical contexts, as illustrated in Lameire et al. (2014), show how renal conditions have been understood as they are, particularly through acquired knowledge during wartime medical crises. With advances in nephrology, it is crucial to recognize these anatomical and physiological foundations to improve new treatment strategies and outcomes in kidney disease.

5.1.1. Structure of the Kidneys

Kidneys are crucial organs in the human body, with the primary tasks of filtering blood, removing waste, and maintaining electrolyte balance. There are approximately 1 million functioning nephrons in each kidney, the basic structural and functional units of the kidney. Each nephron has a glomerulus, a bed of capillaries where filtration begins, and the tubular system, which extends the processing of the filtrate. The complex structure of the nephrons allows for the regulation of water and solute reabsorption necessary to maintain homeostasis. This intricate organization not only facilitates efficient waste removal but also plays a vital role in blood pressure and volume control, representing the importance of the kidneys not only in excretory functions but in systemic health as well. The kidneys are organized into two main areas: the cortex and the medulla. The outer cortex contains the renal corpuscles and proximal convoluted tubules, which are involved in primary filtration and the reabsorption process. The renal medulla, conversely, contains the loops of Henle and collecting ducts, which contribute to urine concentration via the countercurrent mechanism. The anatomical design allows the kidneys to concentrate urine and maintain water loss and electrolyte balance effectively. In particular, their convergence serves to illustrate the dual role of the kidneys as regulatory and filtration organs. This is particularly relevant in the context of kidney disease, where disruption of these structures can lead to overt pathophysiologic sequelae, which further attests to the significance of a firm understanding of kidney anatomy in nephrology. Recent studies have identified the importance of maintaining nephron structural integrity with reference to a variety of kidney pathologies. A case in point is polycystic kidney disease, characterized by fluid-filled cysts within renal tubules, directly the result of defective cellular processes within the nephron structure (Alexander et al., 2015).

Furthermore, historical context for the development of traumatic outcomes, for instance, wars, has proven how particular kidney traumas were studied and managed, ultimately leading to the advancement of nephrology (Lameire et al., 2014). This awareness of the interactions between structure and pathology highlights the significance of the kidneys in disease and health, illustrating how a uniform understanding of kidney architecture lies at the heart of practice in internal medicine and nephrology (Figure 5.2).

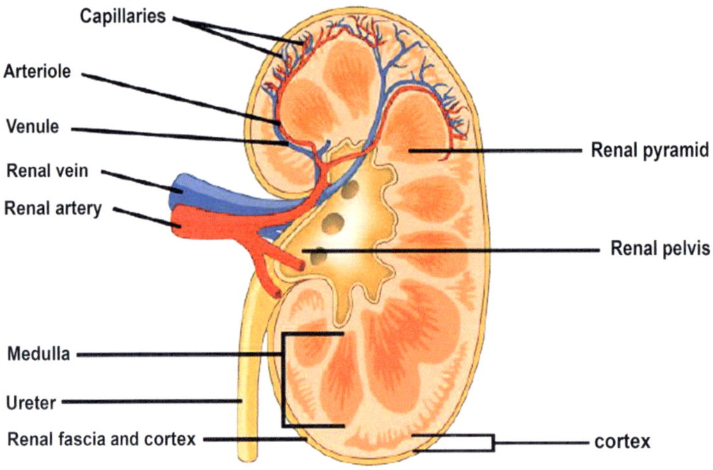

Figure 5.2. Kidney structure.

Source: https://s3-us-west-2.amazonaws.com/courses-images/wp-content/uploads/sites/1223/2017/02/09002541/Figure_41_06_02.png.

5.1.2. Functions of the Renal System

The renal system maintains the body's homeostasis through several functions, primarily regulating fluid and electrolyte balance. The kidneys remove waste products such as urea and creatinine from the blood and regulate the amount of water, sodium, and potassium lost. This is to prevent complications from dehydration and fluid overload. In addition, the kidneys assist with acid-base balance by secreting hydrogen ions and reabsorbing bicarbonate, and they greatly determine the body's pH level. A dysfunction of these filtering mechanisms can lead to serious conditions, underscoring the systemic importance of renal function in internal medicine, especially in nephrology (Borniche et al., 2010). An additional critical function served by the renal system is the regulation of blood pressure through the renin-angiotensin-aldosterone system (RAAS). The kidneys detect alterations in blood pressure and respond by releasing renin, an enzyme that catalyzes the conversion of angiotensinogen to angiotensin I, which is further converted to angiotensin II. This potent vasoconstrictor both raises blood pressure and increases secretion of aldosterone from the adrenal glands, promoting sodium reabsorption and stimulating water retention. This twofold mechanism of vascular and fluid regulation demonstrates the kidney's intricate role in cardiovascular homeostasis. Blood pressure control in nephrology is, however, a significant knowledge when working with CKD patients, where this mechanism will be dysregulated and result in increased hypertension as well as worsening of renal function (Elliott et al., 2015). Additionally, the kidney system is required for the production of hormones, such as erythropoietin and calcitriol, which have systemic effects on body physiology. Erythropoietin, secreted by the kidneys under hypoxic conditions, promotes red blood cell formation in the bone marrow and treats the anemia present in CKD patients. Simultaneously, calcitriol, the active metabolite of vitamin D, promotes calcium absorption in the gut and maintains phosphate balance, both of which are important for healthy bones. The interaction of these endocrine activities points to the multipurpose function of the kidneys beyond filtration; their roles in hematopoiesis and mineral regulation are fundamental to overall well-being. As nephrologists grapple with the complexity of renal pathology, the broader implications of renal activities are essential in devising holistic therapeutic approaches (Borniche et al., 2010) (Figure 5.3).

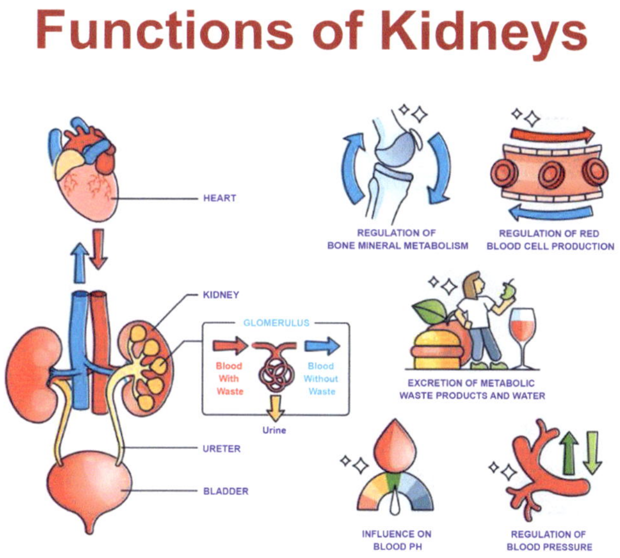

Figure 5.3. Function of kidney.

Source: https://assets.lybrate.com/imgs/tic/enadp/function-of-kidney.jpg.

5.1.3. Regulation of Homeostasis by the Kidneys

The kidneys play a pivotal role in homeostasis, an essential system that maintains fluid, electrolyte, and acid-base balance. They achieve this through a multifaceted process of filtration within the nephron, in which blood is filtered, reabsorbed, and excreted as urine. The filtration process allows the kidneys to remove waste products while conserving important substances such as glucose and amino acids. Moreover, the kidneys maintain excretion of sodium, potassium, and bicarbonate ions, which are essential for osmotic balance and body pH. During the progression of CKD, disturbances in these regulatory processes may lead to adverse systemic effects, underscoring the kidneys' significant role in overall physiological stability (Elliott et al., 2015). An understanding of the mechanisms by which the kidneys help achieve homeostasis is essential for the development of targeted therapy in nephrology. Besides their role in fluid and electrolyte balance, the kidneys also help regulate blood pressure through the renin-angiotensin-aldosterone system (RAAS). In response to decreased blood pressure, the kidneys harbor specific cells that sense the drop and subsequently secrete renin. This enzyme initiates a cascade of reactions that ultimately leads to the production of angiotensin II, a potent vasoconstrictor. Angiotensin II not only constricts vessels but also stimulates aldosterone release from the adrenal cortex, promoting sodium reabsorption in the kidneys. This maximizes water retention, effectively increasing blood volume and systemic pressure. RAAS is dysregulated in CKD patients, contributing to hypertension and further renal damage, and therefore, RAAS targeting is warranted in therapeutic strategies (Alexander et al., 2015). The kidneys also respond to physiological stress by modulating hormone secretion to maintain homeostasis. For instance, as a response to low oxygen tension, the kidneys release erythropoietin (EPO), a hormone that induces red blood cell production in the bone marrow. This is of paramount importance for ensuring adequate tissue oxygenation, especially when erythropoiesis is impaired. The kidneys also contribute to vitamin D activation, which is important for calcium absorption and bone mineral metabolism. Hormonal derangement in these processes may lead to anemia as well as bone metabolic disease in CKD patients. Hence, the regulatory roles of the kidneys extend beyond excretion alone, placing hormonal regulation under the umbrella of homeostatic regulation, highlighting their multifunctional nature within the internal medicine model (Elliott et al., 2015).

Test Your Knowledge

1. What are the primary structural components of the kidneys?
2. How do the kidneys maintain fluid and electrolyte balance in the body?

5.2. Common Kidney Diseases

Learning Outcome

1. Define the chronic kidney disease (CKD)
2. Discuss the acute kidney injury (AKI)
3. Explain the glomerulonephritis

Kidney disease is a significant global health issue and encompasses a continuum of disorders that can lead to either acute or chronic damage to the renal system. Of these, acute kidney injury (AKI) has gained more recognition in the past few years, particularly in intensive care units. In Mexico, for instance, the hospital incidence of AKI is typically described in conjunction with severe underlying illness, such as sepsis and preeclampsia during pregnancy. With a documented mortality of approximately 25% before the pandemic, there is evidence to show it can quickly escalate, particularly in vulnerable populations, i.e., children and patients with complex comorbidities, and it emphasizes a pressing necessity for improved diagnostic standardization and national registries to monitor the condition effectively (Chávez-Íñiguez et al., 2022). Chronic kidney disease (CKD) is another prevalent condition that has both clinical and societal implications. This chronic worsening of renal function with age is also widely associated with systemic diseases like diabetes and hypertension, which are both epidemic in the global population. Compounding the difficulty of managing CKD is not only the management of the renal damage itself but also the avoidance of attendant complications, such as cardiovascular disease, a leading cause of death among CKD patients. Renal function monitoring through regular screening and patient education on lifestyle intervention is also critical in restricting the progression of CKD. Besides, nephrology experts increasingly emphasize integrated management programs incorporating clinical and non-clinical interventions to enhance outcomes for patients in these populations (Ajaimy et al., 2020). Where common renal conditions overlap with emerging health conditions, including those introduced by the COVID-19 pandemic, management becomes significantly complex. Patients with underlying renal conditions, particularly those on dialysis or with compromised immunity following transplantation, are at increased risk of contracting severe SARS-CoV-2 infections. New findings indicate that atypical COVID-19 cases make diagnosis challenging for nephrologists, as classic symptoms such as fever are not expected to be prevalent in this group. Such intricacies require personalized screening procedures and aggressive monitoring to enable timely interventions. While nephrology moves beyond the conventional ways, knowledge about how common kidney diseases interact with outside environments, such as pandemics, will be essential to build an effective treatment plan in the future (Ajaimy et al., 2020; Chávez-Íñiguez et al., 2022).

5.2.1. Chronic Kidney Disease (CKD)

CKD is a major worldwide health problem that is faced by nearly 10% of the global population. The incidence of CKD is most marked in patients with comorbidities like type 2 diabetes and heart failure, where almost 50% of these patients suffer from some level of kidney impairment. CKD management needs to be multidisciplinary, involving the detection of risk factors and the implementation of treatment strategies in a more holistic manner. Recent research indicates that existing prescribing patterns in CKD do not follow evidence-based guidelines for its management, underscoring the critical need for greater cross-specialty collaboration among practitioners. International consensus has been reached among specialists such as nephrologists, endocrinologists, and family physicians to guide effective management practices, with emphasis on strict adherence to recommended clinical guidelines (Arici et al., 2024) (Figure 5.4).

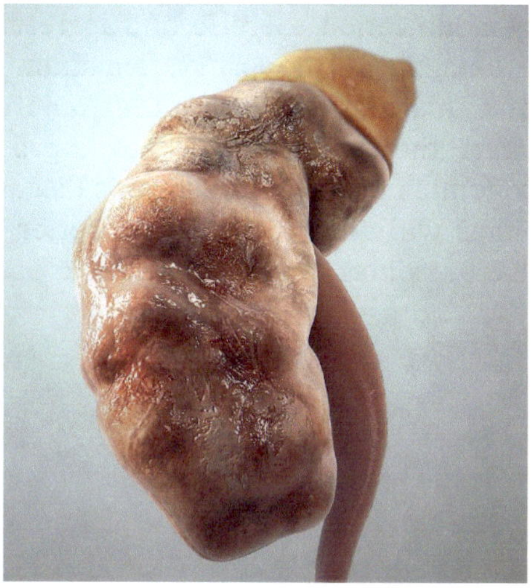

Figure 5.4. A graphic representation of a chronically affected kidney.

Source: https://upload.wikimedia.org/wikipedia/commons/thumb/0/0b/CKD_-_Chronic_kidney_disease.jpg/800px-CKD_-_Chronic_kidney_disease.jpg.

Nephroprotection is central to conservative CKD management, as it is a critical strategy for slowing disease progression. Evidence shows that the secret is to manage the underlying cause of CKD while addressing the concomitant biochemical derangement. A retrospective observational study has established the beneficial effect of supplementing the tricarboxylic acid (TCA) cycle intermediates with sodium bicarbonate and calcium carbonate, resulting in significant improvements in patients with end-stage CKD. It disclosed a substantial increase in estimated glomerular filtration rate (eGFR) and a decrease in serum creatinine levels, demonstrating that kidney function and overall well-being can be enhanced by adjuvant treatments—even among individuals who have not initiated renal replacement therapy (Hernández Miramontes et al., 2024). The results affirm the value of novel therapeutic interventions in nephrology for enhancing patient outcomes in the event of CKD. Management of CKD must also extend beyond the pharmacologic approach, incorporating lifestyle modification and patient education into treatment regimens. Engaging the patient in his/her own health care is essential to optimize adherence with lifestyle modifications that will slow the progression of renal disease. This includes dietary modification, exercise, and aggressive control of blood pressure and blood glucose. Moreover, institutionalizing a support system among healthcare providers can enable continuous monitoring and individualized care procedures tailored to each patient's profile. With coordinated effort from specialists, the ultimate goal is to improve the quality of care for CKD patients while mitigating the economic burden of the chronic disease. Greater communication and shared knowledge across disciplines will ultimately lead to better management practices in nephrology, resulting in more effective outcomes for this vulnerable patient population (Figure 5.5).

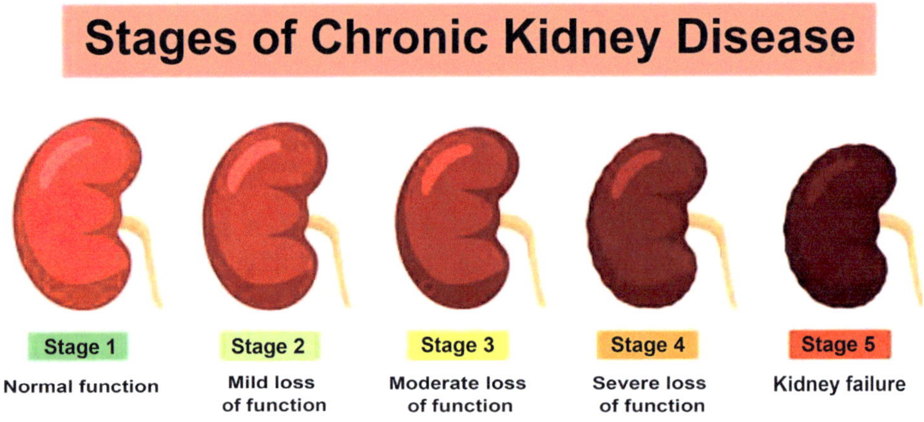

Figure 5.5. Stages of chronic kidney disease.

Source: https://www.carehospitals.com/ckfinder/userfiles/images/chronic-kidney-disease.webp.

5.2.2. Acute Kidney Injury (AKI)

AKI is a significant clinical problem in nephrology, where a sudden loss of renal function defines it. This syndrome can result from varied etiologies, including prerenal causes such as dehydration and renal hypoperfusion, or intrinsic causes such as acute glomerulonephritis or acute tubular necrosis. The consequences of AKI are severe, with potential long-term impact on renal injury and mortality. The significance of early intervention and treatment is to mitigate these risks, emphasizing the need for good monitoring methods. Early identification and appropriate management can significantly improve outcomes. The complex interaction between AKI and other systemic conditions necessitates an interdisciplinary approach, highlighting the pivotal role of nephrologists in treating engaged patients in an integrated manner. The interaction of AKI with malignancy renders cancer-associated AKI even more challenging to control in the clinic. Interestingly, patients with CKD are also at risk of developing malignancies, which will further exacerbate renal impairment by the tumor itself and its treatment. Patient management involves a nuanced understanding of the interfaces between nephrology and oncology. As newer cancer therapies evolve, nephrologists must stay up to date with the evolving evidence on the nephrotoxicity of the agents employed and develop commensurate strategies accordingly. Multidisciplinary teamwork becomes necessary to optimize both renal function and cancer treatment efficacy. Progress over recent years has raised controversy regarding the management of patients with kidney impairment in the context of malignancy, as emphasized by KDIGO's efforts to improve patient outcomes through greater multidisciplinary treatment (Bamias et al., 2020). During disasters, AKI incidence can skyrocket as a result of environmental stressors and disruption in medical infrastructure, as experienced in disaster-affected areas. Myoglobinuric acute renal failure is a classic example of the threats of acute events, with patients at times requiring urgent access to dialysis facilities. Nephrology societies have recognized the need to establish response teams and strategic protocols to meet these emergency demands. The concept of "austere" dialysis is now a significant issue, advocating for the accessibility of renal replacement therapy even in resource-poor settings. This approach not only addresses the acute health crisis but also seeks to restore the semblance of nephrological care after catastrophic disasters. Delivering these frameworks will likely to mitigate the long-term nephrological impacts in those populations of sudden and unforeseen catastrophes (Perkins et al., 2011) (Figure 5.6).

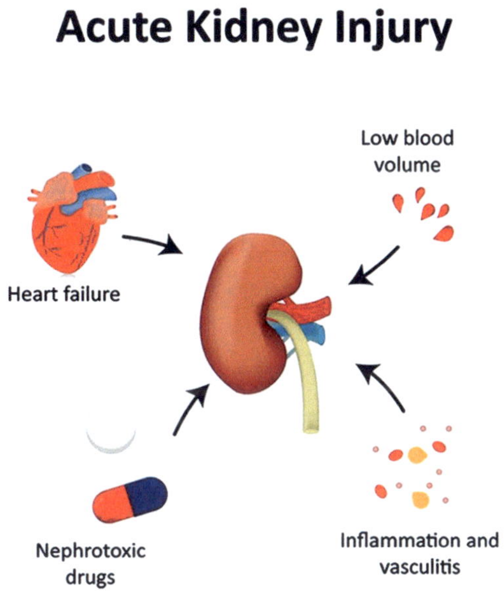

Figure 5.6. Illustration of acute kidney injury (AKI).

Source: https://dam.upmc.com/-/media/upmc/services/kidney-disease/images/conditions/aki.png?rev=9011c27bea344c06af3dfabbb989d118&hash=41D41F0CD4948A533E60EDF9F7F7D423.

5.2.3. Glomerulonephritis

Glomerulonephritis is a family of kidney diseases, primarily characterized by glomerulitis, that are critical for blood filtration. Glomerulonephritis can result from various reasons, such as infectious etiologies, autoimmune mechanisms, and toxin or drug exposure. With the damage to glomeruli, the patients can have hematuria, proteinuria, and hypertension, which together indicate a reduction in renal function. Among the infective causes, cryoglobulinaemia, often present in hepatitis C virus infection, has been a leading cause of glomerulonephritis. The mechanisms of pathogenesis involve the deposition of immune complexes within glomerular capillaries, with subsequent inflammatory damage that can accelerate the progression towards end-stage renal failure (Braun et al., 2007). Understanding these mechanisms of pathogenesis is necessary to devise effective treatment strategies that can prevent morbidity from glomerulonephritis. Therapy for glomerulonephritis is varied and depends largely on the etiology. For instance, in autoimmune disease-related ones such as lupus, the therapeutic approaches have been guided by extensive clinical trials. These have led to numerous clinical practice guidelines that outline optimal induction and maintenance therapies tailored to specific histological classes of lupus nephritis. Such regulations also highlight the importance of monitoring patients for potential relapse and deterioration of renal function, particularly in high-risk groups, including children and patients with associated vascular complications (Bajema et al., 2015). This multi-faceted approach not only aims to suppress the inflammatory process but also attempts to preserve kidney function, thereby improving long-term outcomes for patients with glomerulonephritis. Besides, the management of glomerulonephritis involves a multidimensional approach that integrates pharmacologic treatment with patient education and lifestyle modification. Pharmacologic treatments can include corticosteroids and immunosuppressants to influence the inflammatory process. However, it is equally crucial that healthcare providers collaborate more aggressively with their patients on treatment. By educating patients about their disease and the importance of medication adherence, healthcare providers can help improve health outcomes. Lifestyle modifications, such as a sodium- and protein-restricted diet and regular monitoring of blood pressure and kidney function, can go a long way in managing symptoms and slowing disease progression to chronic kidney disease. Thus, a multidisciplinary team approach combining medical and supportive care is necessary to manage the nuances of glomerulonephritis (Figure 5.7).

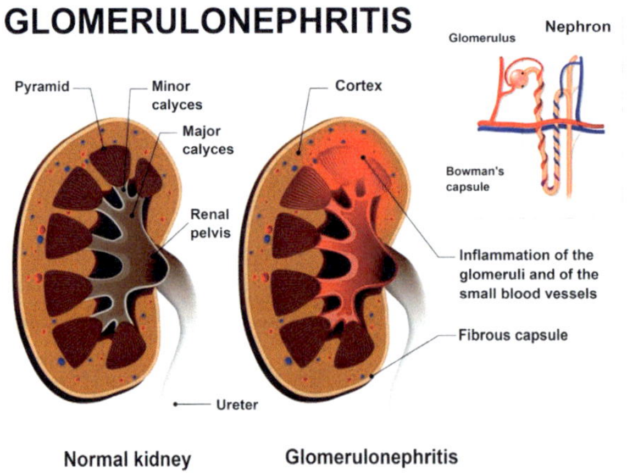

Figure 5.7. Normal kidney vs. Glomerulonephritis.

Source: https://kidneycareep.com/images/page/glomerulonephritis-elpaso.jpg.

Test Your Knowledge

1. What are the most common diseases affecting the kidneys?
2. How does chronic kidney disease differ from acute kidney injury?

5.3. Diagnostic Approaches in Nephrology

Learning Outcome

1. Describe the laboratory tests for kidney function
2. Understand the imaging techniques in nephrology
3. Explain the biopsy procedures and their significance

Diagnostic strategies in nephrology are a critical component of effective kidney disease management. Diagnostic strategies combine clinical examination, laboratory investigations, and imaging studies to assess the structure and function of the kidneys. Doctors commonly begin with a history and physical examination, which can identify familial patterns of disease or specific symptoms of renal insufficiency, such as edema or hypertension. Laboratory analysis, following this initial assessment, including urinalysis, blood urea nitrogen (BUN), and serum creatinine, is essential to identify alterations in renal function. These tests can also provide significant insight into acute conditions such as acute kidney injury and chronic conditions such as chronic kidney disease. Refinement of these diagnostic techniques ensures that nephrologists can tailor treatment protocols to individual patient needs, which is significant for maximizing patient outcomes and enhancing the quality of care delivered in this specialty (Berney et al., 2025). In addition to laboratory testing, imaging modalities have significantly transformed the practice of nephrology diagnostics. Ultrasound, though, remains a first-line imaging technique because it is non-invasive and can assess kidney shape and size, as well as any obstructions in the urinary system. Additional imaging techniques, including CT and MRI, may also be used to clarify complicated cases further or determine the presence of renal masses. These newer imaging methods enable nephrologists to detect abnormalities earlier in the disease process and to implement appropriate interventions. The advent of newer imaging equipment has also created opportunities for improved visualization, enabling enhanced examination of renal function and structure. This integration of imaging into diagnosis aligns with current standards that prioritize individualized care for patients and efficient diagnostic processes in nephrology (Miao et al., 2024). In summary, nephrology's diagnostic processes are crucial in the diagnosis and management of kidney diseases. By incorporating clinical evaluation, laboratory data, and advanced imaging techniques, clinicians can make accurate diagnoses that guide therapy regimens. Through the combined approach, there is a sophisticated understanding of the individual's kidney status that guides treatment decisions with tangible effects on long-term health outcomes. The integration of these diagnostics not only helps nephrologists make clinical decisions but also addresses broader healthcare objectives, including optimizing resource use and improving patient care pathways. Further, as nephrology practice continues to evolve with technological advancements and shifts in healthcare priorities, the relevance of these diagnostic methods will only increase, underscoring the necessity of continued education and research (Berney et al., 2025).

5.3.1. Laboratory Tests for Kidney Function

Laboratory investigation of kidney function is critical in the diagnosis and management of chronic kidney disease (CKD), a prevalent condition of significant morbidity and mortality. Measurement of serum creatinine is the most common laboratory test used to estimate glomerular filtration rate (GFR), a function of kidney function. There are various equations to estimate GFR, and the CKD-EPI equation is considered the gold standard because it is precise across a broad population. Various factors, though, may affect the estimation, such as age, sex, and muscle mass, thereby leading to misinterpretation of kidney function. The elimination of race-based adjustments from these equations marks a milestone towards more equitable healthcare practice, eschewing overestimates that can postpone treatments such as dialysis or transplantation (Kirsztajn et al., 2024). In addition to serum creatinine, the urine albumin-to-creatinine ratio (ACR) is a critical marker for kidney damage. The measurement quantifies albumin in urine, indicating kidney damage at an early stage. Clinical practice guidelines recommend that individuals with elevated creatinine also undergo ACR testing to allow for complete kidney evaluation. According to current research, however, many patients who are tested for serum creatinine are not followed with ACR testing, particularly in disadvantaged regions with fewer healthcare resources (Kirsztajn et al., 2024). This difference is a significant barrier to successful CKD management and underscores the need for health care systems to invest in systematic screening protocols that include both serum creatinine and ACR measurements, thereby improving patient outcomes. Integration of the laboratory tests within a multidisciplinary health strategy is pivotal for successful CKD management and prevention interventions. Nephrologists and other specialists must collaborate to ensure that the kidney function tests are performed well and interpreted correctly. Significantly, this occurs because the majority of kidney function tests are prescribed by non-nephrologist practitioners and, on occasion, this leads to delayed diagnosis and treatment of CKD (Guedes et al., 2024). Having established standardized testing protocols and educational campaigns about kidney health will enhance the quality of care across various medical practices. By continuing this progress in the realization of the importance of comprehensive kidney assessment, the health community can improve prevention of CKD progression and promote patients' quality of life (Figure 5.8).

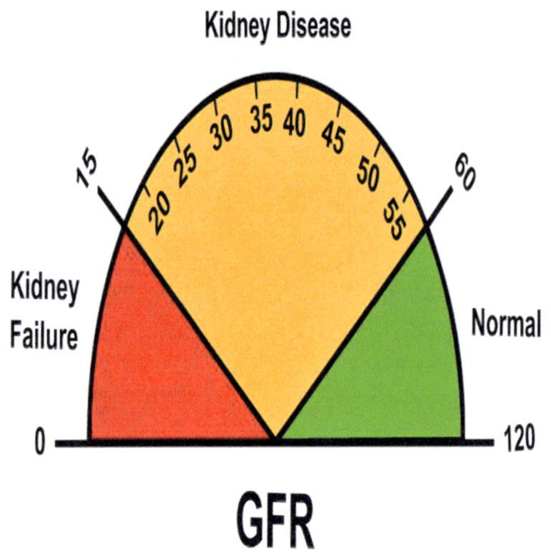

Figure 5.8. Glomerular filtration rate (GFR).

Source: https://www.niddk.nih.gov/-/media/Images/Nkdep/NKDEP_GFR_DIAL_953x573.JPG.

5.3.2. Imaging Techniques in Nephrology

Imaging techniques are significant in nephrology and facilitate the diagnosis and management of renal illness. Renal ultrasounds are usually the preferred option for diagnosis because they are noninvasive and provide real-time images of renal anatomy. The procedure is particularly effective for identifying obstructive uropathy and evaluating cystic kidney diseases. Computed tomography (CT) scans also give a good representation of the renal vasculature and aid in the identification of renal stones and tumors. The high-resolution images obtained from CT can assist in more accurate planning of treatment, especially in complex cases where anatomical features play a crucial role. As imaging modalities continue to be developed, their integration enhances clinicians' capacity to detect and follow up renal pathologies, thereby improving patient outcomes through personalized therapeutic measures. Renal scintigraphy is another integral part of nephrology imaging modalities. It provides functional renal perfusion and excretion evaluation, enabling nephrologists to assess renal artery stenosis and kidney transplant viability. It employs radiotracers injected intravenously to measure glomerular filtration rate and evaluate renal function throughout the kidneys. New imaging technologies, such as MRI, are also expanding the diagnostic options available to nephrologists. MRI provides exquisite soft-tissue contrast, which is beneficial for detecting renal masses that may be masked on other imaging modalities. Furthermore, new applications of advanced functional MRI techniques may yet improve assessment of renal perfusion and oxygenation kinetics, paving the way for improved management of a variety of renal diseases. Emerging imaging modalities, such as autofluorescence (AF) imaging, are beginning to find a place in nephrology, well beyond their renowned positions in ophthalmology. AF imaging capitalizes on the native fluorescence of endogenous biomolecules within renal tissue, enabling label-free imaging that may enhance pathology detection. Implementation of AF techniques in nephrology practice can facilitate real-time imaging during surgical interventions and thereby increase the accuracy of procedures such as nephrectomy or kidney biopsies. With expanding volumes of research, particularly in clinical applications, such advanced imaging technologies can potentially significantly increase diagnostic sensitivity and therapeutic outcomes in nephrology. But to achieve their maximum potential in real-world clinical application, AF techniques and others must have further studies to standardize imaging protocols as well as establish their effectiveness in diverse renal pathologies, and call for collaborative efforts in the medical community, as seen in previous studies Aigner et al. (2020) and Bartoletti et al. (2016) (Figure 5.9).

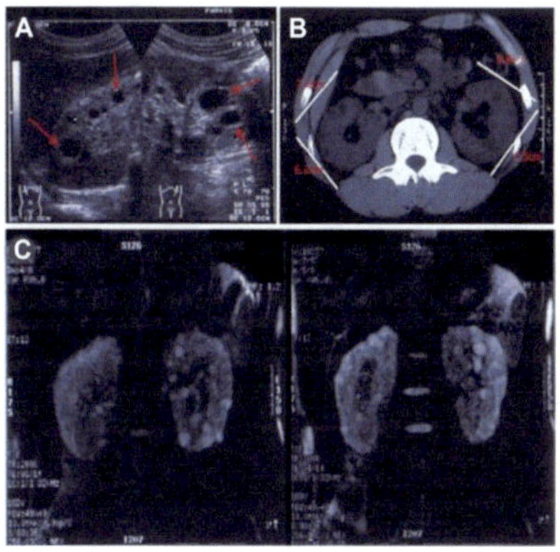

Figure 5.9. Imaging studies of the kidneys. Both kidneys contain multiple oval lesions, which are up to 20 mm in diameter, are hypoechoic, show low density on computed tomography (CT), and show high signal intensity in T2-weighted magnetic resonance imaging (MRI) (panel a: ultrasound image; panel b: CT image; panel c: T2-weighted MRI)

Source: https://www.researchgate.net/publication/335447802/figure/fig2/AS:796859375312902@1566997488239/maging-studies-of-the-kidneys-Both-kidneys-contain-multiple-oval-lesions-which-are-up.png.

5.3.3. Biopsy Procedures and Their Significance

Biopsy procedures are a significant aspect of nephrology, providing insight into the etiology of renal disease. The procedures, particularly renal biopsies, provide direct visualization of kidney tissue to identify pathological changes of many diseases, including glomerulonephritis and FSGS. Renal biopsies are significant because they can guide treatment strategy, monitor disease activity during follow-up, and assess prognosis in renal diseases. For instance, in FSGS patients, biopsies yield findings that guide clinicians to the precise nature of the injury and to responsiveness to treatments such as immunosuppressants or plasmapheresis (Fink et al., 2002). In the absence of such specificity, nephrologists would have to rely almost exclusively on clinical and biochemical markers, which can sometimes lead to misdiagnosis and inappropriate treatment regimens. In conditions such as autosomal dominant polycystic kidney disease (ADPKD), biopsy procedures aided by high-technology imaging techniques play an imperative role in estimating renal function. With advancing studies, greater emphasis has been placed on using new imaging technologies, such as 3 Tesla MRI, to identify renal fibrosis and correlate findings with renal function. This indicates the need for non-invasive yet efficient diagnostic tools in nephrology. The importance of monitoring parenchymal evolution by MRI should not be overstated, as these measurements enable clinicians to more accurately quantify disease progression and adapt therapeutic strategies accordingly. Blending of biopsy outcomes with imaging outcomes allows nephrologists to obtain a clear understanding of renal pathophysiology and to make more rational clinical decisions and manage patients in a better way (Ciccariello et al., 2018). In addition, biopsy results extend beyond diagnostic use; they are also crucial for fine-tuning our understanding of kidney disease at the cellular level. Biopsies provide tissue for histopathologic analysis, allowing researchers to explore the cellular mechanisms of potassium channels in podocytes or the effect of circulating factors in conditions like FSGS. Such exploration can reveal important correlations between specific pathologies and potential therapeutic interventions. For example, detection of kinin involvement in podocyte injury using immunoadsorption techniques underscores the utility of biopsy for distinguishing complex renal disease mechanisms (Fink et al., 2002). With ongoing advances in nephrology, correlating biopsy data with emerging studies aims to enhance current treatment regimens and pave the way for personalized medicine to address the unique requirements of individual patients (Figure 5.10).

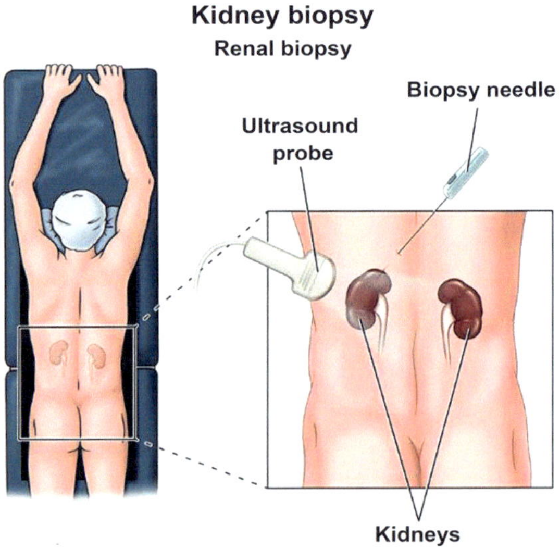

Figure 5.10. Kidney biopsy illustration.

Source: https://my.clevelandclinic.org/-/scassets/images/org/health/articles/kidney-biopsy.

Test Your Knowledge

1. What laboratory tests are commonly used to assess kidney function?
2. Why is urinalysis important in diagnosing kidney diseases?

5.4. Treatment Modalities in Nephrology

Learning Outcome

1. Discuss on pharmacological interventions
2. Describe the dialysis options and procedures
3. Focus on kidney transplantation

Treatment modalities in nephrology involve a complex interplay of therapeutic interventions aimed at treating kidney disease and its complications. Among the treatments necessary are dialysis and renal transplantation, both of which are lifelines for end-stage renal disease (ESRD) patients. Either hemodialysis or peritoneal dialysis is a dialysis that artificially removes waste products from the blood, keeping a patient alive when the kidneys can no longer perform their function. While helpful, they have their drawbacks; complications in the form of increased morbidity and mortality, along with their respective heavy economic burdens to healthcare systems, underscore the need for novel therapies. Additionally, the psychological weight carried by transplant patients is noteworthy, which underlines the importance of integrated care plans in the nephrology setting, such as patient education and mental health support. In recent years, scientific investigation has increasingly focused on the therapeutic potential of cell-based regenerative medicine therapies (RMTs) as adjuvant treatments to traditional modalities. Although in the early stages of development, RMTs hold promise for stimulating renal repair and restoring renal function, particularly in rodent models. Therapies could be active via paracrine actions, whereby cells secrete factors that enhance the regenerative potential of the available tissue and obviate the need for dialysis or transplantation. Further clarification of the precise mechanism involved in these therapies remains necessary before clinical application. As highlighted in recent studies, new imaging modalities are being developed to track the biodistribution and effects of these RMTs in preclinical models. The advancement of techniques such as bioluminescence and multispectral optoacoustic tomography could make personalized treatments for patients with kidney disease more possible, potentially transforming present practice norms in nephrology. Lastly, contemporary nephrology therapy encompasses not only physiological outcomes but also psychosocial factors that affect patients' quality of life (QoL). The C-DIRECT intervention, for instance, couples motivational interviewing and self-management interventions in patients with concomitant diabetes and ESRD. The trial results show that holistic treatments are effective in achieving improved glycemic control and fewer physical role limitations, empowering patients. While conventional remedies target symptoms, interventions that target behavioral and emotional aspects of patient care offer a more holistic approach to the issues related to kidney disease. By raising awareness and implementing such practices, nephrology can enhance not only clinical outcomes but also the patient experience as a whole, corroborating the relevance of holistic models of care in internal medicine to nephrology (Garcia-Finana et al., 2016; Jacobson et al., 2019).

5.4.1. Pharmacological Interventions

Pharmacologic interventions in nephrology are critical for the management of various renal diseases, such as acute kidney injury (AKI) and chronic renal fibrosis. AKI, a prevalent but complex condition, is most often the result of ischemic events that damage renal tissue. Heparanase inhibitors have been suggested as a potential therapy in recent research. Heparanase, a proteoglycanase involved in inflammation and kidney disease, was found to exacerbate AKI by upregulating injury and fibrosis markers, such as TGF-β and IL-6. PG545 treatment, a potent inhibitor of heparanase, demonstrated protective effects against kidney injury in preclinical models and suggested that targeting this pathway can yield significant therapeutic benefit in AKI and its outcome patients (Abassi et al., 2017). Chronic kidney disease (CKD) is another major field of nephrology that requires robust pharmacological approaches. One common pathway contributing to the development of CKD is the TGF-β signaling cascade, which is implicated in renal fibrosis. Specifically, FKBP12.6, a protein involved in TGF-β signaling, has been implicated in the deposition of extracellular matrix components. In animal models of renal fibrosis in conditions like pyelonephritis, androgen exposure has been shown to exacerbate the disease process by enhanced production of TGF-β1 and disruption in Smad protein balance mediating fibrotic responses. Pharmacological inhibition of the TGF-β pathway can halt renal fibrosis, as medications that target this pathway have been shown to downregulate myofibroblast activation and subsequent fibrosis, offering a therapeutic avenue for the treatment of CKD (Collins et al., 2020). Moreover, adding pharmacotherapy to lifestyle modification and education in patients can offer a synergistic effect in renal disease treatment. While pharmacotherapy targets the biochemical or pathophysiologic underpinnings of diseases such as AKI and CKD, integrated treatment includes dietary adjustments, fluid management, and strict adherence to prescribed drug regimens to maximize patient outcomes. The challenge remains to individualize treatments to account for variations in drug response among patients because of genetic, environmental, and lifestyle factors. Hence, research into combination therapy and pharmacological treatment individualization continues at the core of developing nephrology therapy. Ultimately, a balanced strategy combining new pharmacological approaches with traditional wellness philosophies could open the door to improved kidney disease management and patients' general well-being (Figure 5.11).

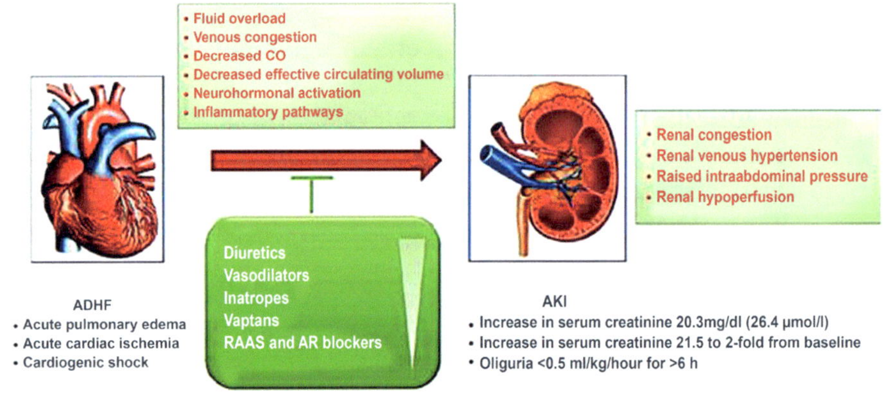

Figure 5.11. Pharmacological management of acute CRS (type 1). AKI = Acute kidney injury; AR = angiotensin receptor; CO = cardiac output.

Source: https://www.researchgate.net/profile/Bernard-Canaud/publication/265418457/figure/fig1/AS:295429020373001@1447447175424/Pathophysiology-and-pharmacological-management-of-acute-CRS-type-1-AKI-Acute-kidney.png.

5.4.2. Dialysis Options and Procedures

Dialysis is a critical treatment option for patients with end-stage renal disease (ESRD), with required renal replacement therapy when native kidney function is not feasible. Two modalities are generally available: hemodialysis (HD) and peritoneal dialysis (PD). Hemodialysis, typically performed in an outpatient setting, employs a machine that removes waste products from blood through an artificial membrane. This therapy involves creating a vascular access point, typically via an arteriovenous fistula or a central venous catheter, and can involve several sessions a week, lasting approximately 4 hours. Peritoneal dialysis, by contrast, utilizes the patient's own peritoneal membrane as a filter barrier, allowing continuous treatment by instilling dialysis fluid into the peritoneal cavity. Every modality has its advantages and limitations, requiring careful consideration of comorbidities, patient preferences, and lifestyle factors when developing a personalized treatment plan. The decision to start dialysis, as well as the choice between HD and PD, must also take into account individual patient circumstances and practice guidelines. It should be noted that the 2020 Kidney Disease: Improving Global Outcomes (KDIGO) guidelines provide an all-encompassing framework for evaluating candidates for kidney transplantation and, by extension, for dialysis initiation. The guidelines identify the need for integrated evaluation based on a patient's demographic and health status factors, including comorbid conditions such as diabetes, obesity, and cardiovascular disease. Besides, psychosocial considerations are involved in determining dialysis candidacy, where adherence to treatment protocols is essential to realizing the full benefits. Understanding these guiding principles is necessary for nephrology professionals to provide effective care for patients with ESRD, ensuring that treatment is tailored to individual patients' specific needs and circumstances. Most importantly, the relationship between dialysis procedures and transplantation candidates cannot be overstated. Patients undergoing dialysis are likely to experience changes in their overall health status that can impact their suitability for a transplant. As the KDIGO guidelines point out, immunologic considerations, a history of infection, and the patient's compliance must be assessed to develop an informed understanding of the patient's candidacy for kidney transplantation. Integration of dialysis management with transplant evaluation allows health care workers to not only prolong life via dialysis but also maximize quality of life and potentially further improve survival via successful renal transplantation. This multidimensional approach is a reminder of the importance of continuous education and adherence to constant clinical guidelines as they relate to dialysis options and interventions in nephrology management (Figure 5.12).

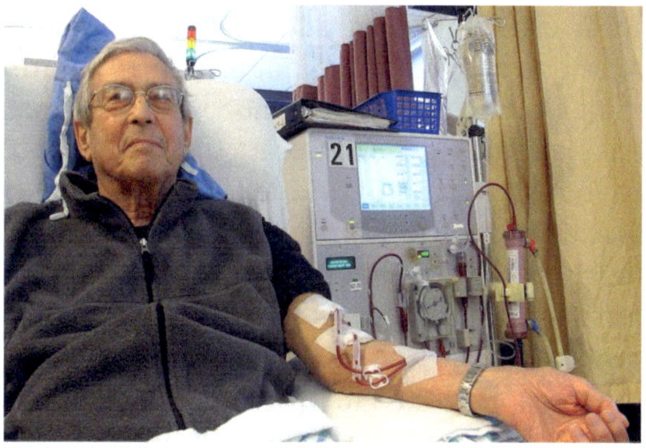

Figure 5.12. Patient receiving dialysis.

Source: https://upload.wikimedia.org/wikipedia/commons/thumb/c/c2/Patient_receiving_dialysis_03.jpg/1024px-Patient_receiving_dialysis_03.jpg.

5.4.3. Kidney Transplantation

Kidney transplantation is the process that marks a significant step forward in nephrology, providing an option for life salvage in end-stage renal disease (ESRD) patients. Not only does transplantation enhance the patient's quality of life, but it also prolongs survival compared with dialysis. The principle of this procedure lies in the replacement of a non-functioning or failing kidney with a functioning kidney from a living or cadaveric donor. Nephrologists should have a good understanding of immunology, as the risk of transplant rejection requires close observation and control through immunosuppressive treatment. Although a successful kidney transplant can lead to improved physiological function, ongoing problems such as graft rejection, infections, and complications in the long run justify extensive post-transplant care and regular follow-ups with the patients (Ali et al., 2023). Kidney transplant is increasingly becoming a necessity with rising cases of diabetes and hypertension—two of the leading causes of renal failure. Concerns such as donor shortages and rising numbers of transplantable patients pose significant challenges to the nephrology landscape. Nephrologists not only play a central role in addressing the medical issues of transplantation but also in advocating policies that could raise donor rates and make transplantation easier. Education on the benefits and complexities of kidney transplantation should also be prioritized in nephrology training programs. Despite such issues, the general success rate of kidney transplantation is also higher due to improved surgical techniques and post-transplant care. Institutions that specialize in blending research with clinical practice, such as those affiliated with the Harold Simmons Center for Kidney Disease Research and Epidemiology, contribute to optimal outcomes (Tantisattamo et al., 2020). Patient education and psychological support are equally important components of kidney transplantation. Ensuring that patients are provided with complete information regarding the risks and benefits of transplantation can reduce anxiety and enhance overall outcomes. Nephrologists must promote open communication with patients to reduce anxiety regarding post-operative care and lifestyle modifications needed for long-term success. The inherent kidney transplant challenges, such as the challenges of organ rejection and lifelong medication adherence, necessitate a collaborative intervention by patients, clinicians, and support systems. These strategies are crucial because they significantly influence patient satisfaction and treatment adherence. In future practice in nephrology, consideration must also be given to rectifying disparities in access to transplantation services, thereby advocating for an equitable system for all patients in need of this life-sustaining measure (Ali et al., 2023) (Figure 5.13).

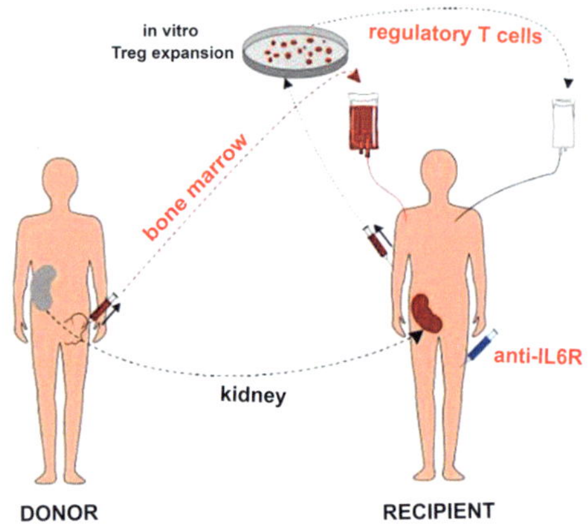

Figure 5.13. Living donor kidney transplant recipients are treated with in vitro expanded polyclonal recipient Tregs, donor BM cells and anti-IL6R mAb (tocilizumab).

Source: https://www.researchgate.net/publication/348810822/figure/fig1/AS:11431281187544096@1694277151782/of-the-study-concept-Living-donor-kidney-transplant-recipients-are-treated-with-in-vitro.tif.

Test Your Knowledge

1. What are the common treatment options for managing kidney diseases?
2. How do dialysis and medication help patients with kidney failure?

5.5. Role of Internal Medicine in Nephrology

Learning Outcome

1. Identify the integration of nephrology with other specialties
2. Describe the management of comorbid conditions
3. Define the patient-centered care in nephrology

The role of internal medicine in nephrology is focal, as internists are the first-line providers and specialists in the management of complex renal diseases. Nephrology is a broad and general area encompassing chronic kidney disease, acute kidney injury, and hypertension, all of which necessitate extensive diagnosis and treatment schemes. Internal medicine physicians possess comprehensive experience in systemic diseases with renal implications, such as diabetes mellitus and cardiovascular disease. This generalist mindset is required to develop individualized treatment plans that are not only directed toward kidney function but also toward their interconnectedness with other organ systems. Internists are also typically the point of initial detection and management, effectively connecting care across multiple specialties to achieve the best patient outcomes. Perhaps most importantly, a key aspect of internal medicine's contribution to nephrology is the ongoing monitoring and intervention required for the treatment of progressive kidney diseases. Chronic kidney disease patients must be monitored regularly to gauge the progression of their conditions, adjust therapeutic regimens, and treat comorbid conditions. Internists are in the best position to use evidence-based guidelines and to employ referral pathways for more sophisticated treatments, such as dialysis or transplantation, if necessary. Additionally, they play a role in educating the patients about lifestyle modifications, such as diet and physical exercise, that can significantly improve renal function. This holistic model, in addition to helping keep the kidneys functioning, enhances the patient's overall well-being, demonstrating the value of a holistic healthcare model. Additionally, the meeting of internal medicine and nephrology extends to the management and comprehension of industry pressures on healthcare. Recent studies demonstrate the disparity in payments from the industry to physicians, with some specialties receiving significantly higher economic incentives. For instance, male doctors and doctors with more practice experience are associated with higher payments, as research shows that industry payments are concentrated in select specialties, including nephrology (Blumenthal et al., 2019). Internalists who are aware of these forces can engage in informed debates on the ethical considerations surrounding industry relationships and how these can shape practices in the clinic. Such knowledge enhances patient-centered care, in which treatment decisions are made on the basis of clinical evidence rather than other determinants, thereby strengthening the integrity of nephrology practice in internal medicine (Silva et al., 2014).

5.5.1. Integration of Nephrology with Other Specialties

Integration of nephrology with other specialties in medicine is essential in maximizing patient outcomes, most particularly in the management of chronic kidney disease (CKD) and end-stage renal disease (ESRD). Nephrologists usually collaborate with primary care physicians, endocrinologists, cardiologists, and urologists to offer integrated care to individuals with complex medical conditions. For instance, CKD usually comes in conjunction with diabetes and hypertension, and necessitates an interdisciplinary team to ensure the optimization of glycemic control as well as blood pressure management. Interprofessional care is superior at ensuring care coordination and promoting a holistic understanding of each patient's complex medical condition, thereby preventing additional renal damage. Moreover, integrating nephrology with genetic counselors and transplant specialists would greatly enhance the care of patients at risk of inherited kidney disease or seeking kidney transplants, based on current genetic insights into nephrology (Canning, 2020). Furthermore, involvement in patient-focused models of care is facilitated by multidisciplinary teams that encompass nephrology, oncology, and palliative care. Interdisciplinary close contact advantages patient management for complications of cancer treatments or renal cancers. The collaboration offers a mechanism for oncologists to provide necessary cancer therapy and nephrologists to manage resulting kidney complications, achieving maximal survivorship and quality of life. For example, when patients like Shirley Roberson are faced with serious ailments, the integration of nephrology and oncology allows one to have a clear picture and control of how cancer treatment can impact kidney function (Broyles, 2019). Therefore, better communication and collaborative decision-making across specialized fields ensure the fulfillment of individual patient preferences, ultimately enabling an enabling healthcare environment to address the complexity of co-occurring health issues. Finally, integrating nephrology into community health programs is imperative for mitigating inequalities in access to and care, especially for rural and underprivileged populations. The delivery of integrated services encompassing prevention, early diagnosis, and long-term management has tremendous potential to minimize the severity of kidney disease before it worsens. Outreach programs, kidney health education, and routine screening can facilitate early intervention, reducing the need for high-level nephrology care. Through this, health systems can not only minimize hospitalization but also mortality among CKD or ESRD patients. Through collaboration between public health officials and community organizations, such actions can be initiated, facilitating equal access to nephrology care across various populations (Canning, 2020). This multifaceted integration actually strengthens the entire health care system, emphasizing the essential role nephrology plays as it crosses multiple specialties (Figure 5.14).

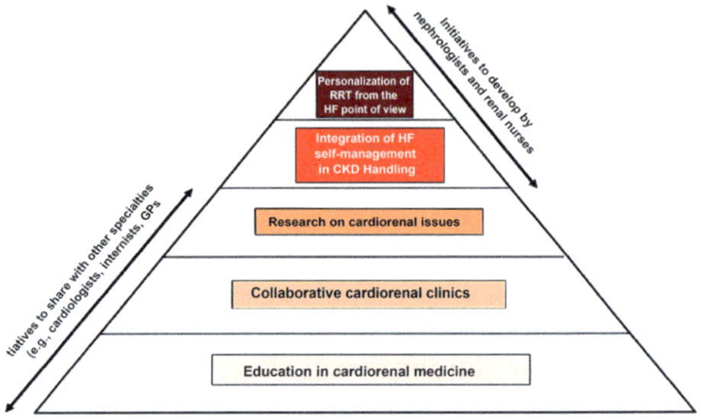

Figure 5.14. Initiatives to be promoted by nephrologists and renal nurses in order to make true cardiorenal medicine for patients with chronic kidney disease (CKD) and heart failure (HF) (GPs, general practitioners; RRT, renal replacement therapy).

Source: https://www.researchgate.net/publication/338283014/figure/fig5/AS:869821759643659@1584393076686/nitiatives-to-be-promoted-by-nephrologists-and-renal-nurses-in-order-to-make-true.png.

5.5.2. Management of Comorbid Conditions

Management of comorbid conditions is a central aspect of nephrology since chronic kidney disease (CKD) frequently coexists with other medical conditions, significantly complicating patient management. A high standard of management steps is essential to optimize patient outcomes and avoid additional kidney disease. Primary care doctors (PCPs) are at the heart of this process, often the first point of contact for patients with newly diagnosed CKD. However, current studies have determined that PCPs are faced with numerous barriers in providing optimal CKD care, including insufficient patient knowledge about the disease and trouble following through with guidelines. By breaking down such barriers and designing supportive strategies, for example, electronic alerts on medical charts and clear guidelines for CKD management, health systems can improve PCPs' capacities, ultimately enhancing the management of comorbid conditions in patients with kidney disease (Abdel-Kader et al., 2019). Furthermore, the relationship between acute kidney injury (AKI) and chronic kidney disease is pivotal in understanding comorbid conditions in nephrology. Evidence shows that patients having severe AKI usually require dialysis, and although some usually recover normal renal function, an extremely high risk of developing CKD later in life has been found in them. Evidence has shown that, besides increased age, diabetes, and vascular disease, the likelihood of developing CKD after a bout of AKI requiring dialysis is increased. This underscores the need to closely observe patients with such risk factors for kidney function compromise. Hence, individualized care plans that include the control of such comorbid conditions are pivotal in nephrology, as they can improve long-term outcomes for patients recovering from AKI or with established CKD (Geddes et al., 2017). In addition, effective communication and coordinated care among healthcare providers are required to manage nephrology comorbidities. Multidisciplinary management with nephrologists, PCPs, specialists, and allied healthcare professionals can significantly improve patient outcomes. Integration of all facets of a patient's health, ranging from cardiovascular to metabolic comorbidities and beyond, by bringing together the implications of pharmacotherapy on each of those conditions treated simultaneously, is provided through such collaboration. Better communication breaks down the barriers outlined by PCPs, establishing a healthcare environment where knowledge is exchanged and leading to better, tailored treatment plans. Ultimately, this model of care addresses the nuance of treating comorbid conditions in nephrology, offering a harmonizing strategy that prioritizes patient health and optimal disease control across the continuum of renal care (Abdel-Kader et al., 2019) (Figure 5.15).

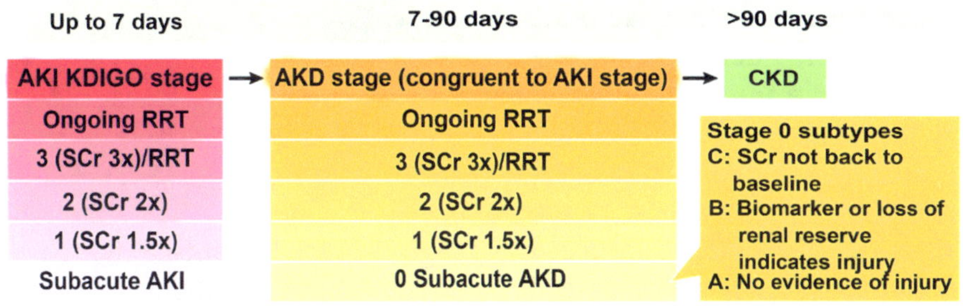

Figure 5.15. Interplay between acute kidney injury (AKI), acute kidney disease (AKD) and chronic kidney disease (CKD).

Source: https://www.researchgate.net/profile/Lakhmir-Chawla/publication/314088358/figure/fig1/AS:476442598350848@1490604175447/Interplay-between-acute-kidney-injury-AKI-acute-kidney-disease-AKD-and-chronic.png.

5.5.3. Patient-Centered Care in Nephrology

The patient-centered care concept in nephrology emphasizes the need to personalize treatment in accordance with a patient's needs, preferences, and values. In the management of chronic kidney disease (CKD), this paradigm is not only about managing the clinical aspects of the disease but also its psychological, social, and emotional aspects, which play a role in patients' well-being. Patient involvement in shared decision-making is a major element of this paradigm, aimed at improving communication between patients and medical professionals. It facilitates trust and greater adherence to treatment plans, empowering patients to be active participants in their health care. However, patient-centered care in nephrology is laden with challenges, particularly in primary care settings where primary care physicians (PCPs) are likely to face difficulty with CKD management and a lack of proper training in such a specialty area (Abdel-Kader et al., 2019). Barriers faced by PCPs can impede the optimal use of patient-centered strategies. Many PCPs report difficulty keeping up with shifting CKD guidelines, which subsequently affects their ability to provide care tailored to individual patients (Abdel-Kader et al., 2019). Other system barriers in healthcare, such as inflexible electronic medical records and time constraints on patient consultations, also affect the overall care for CKD patients. To overcome these challenges, the development of facilitating tools and resources that facilitate communication between providers and patients is required. By using electronic prompts and decision support systems, PCPs can simplify workflows and facilitate more meaningful interactions centered on patient needs. In the end, resolving these barriers might improve nephrology care quality, leading to enhanced patient outcomes and satisfaction. Also, new modes of communication, such as e-consultation, can significantly aid patient-centered care in nephrology. E-consultation enables PCPs to work effectively with nephrologists by providing a real-time advice space without face-to-face referrals. This not only reinforces continuity of care but also ensures better accessibility for patients who may find it challenging to attend specialist consultations. By using technology to drive communication, health care systems can guarantee patients receive timely interventions appropriate to their unique situations. Successful e-consultation adoption is possible, however, only by overcoming potential hurdles such as access to technology and provider training. By resolving these problems, nephrology can transition to a more cohesive, patient-oriented model that aligns health care practices with the needs of various populations with kidney disease (Figure 5.16).

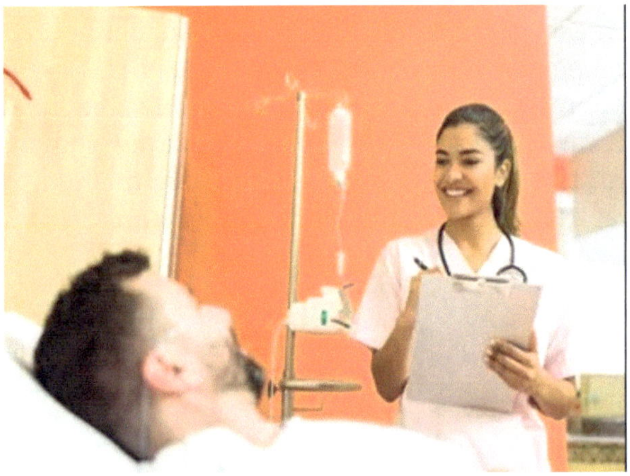

Figure 5.16. Patient-centric care in nephrology enhancing engagement and outcomes.

Source: https://www.apollodialysis.com/wp-content/uploads/2024/12/patient-centric-care-in-nephrology-enhancing-engagement-and-outcomes.webp.

Test Your Knowledge

1. How do internists contribute to the early detection of kidney diseases?
2. What role does internal medicine play in managing chronic kidney disease and its complications?

5.6. Current Research and Advances in Nephrology

Learning Outcome

1. Describe the innovations in kidney disease treatment
2. Define the genetic studies and their implications
3. Focus on future directions in nephrology research

Recent advances in nephrology underscore the importance of understanding kidney disease pathogenesis, which is applicable to diagnosis and treatment. Scientists increasingly recognize the multifactorial nature of diseases such as CKD and nephrolithiasis, which genetic, environmental, and lifestyle factors can induce. New research focuses on identifying biomarkers that could signal the early development of kidney disease and enable early interventions. This preventive strategy not only aims to slow disease progression but also enhances patient care by developing treatment programs tailored to individual risk profiles. Recent research also highlights the interconnectedness of renal function and global well-being, underscoring the need for nephrologists to consider the interplay between renal and more advanced medical conditions, including the recent findings on the relationship between kidney stones and metabolic diseases. Among the concerns in treating and preventing kidney stones, recent guidelines highlight a shift toward more balanced approaches. Traditional urinary crystallization testing and surgery are now complemented by new knowledge of idiopathic calcium nephrolithiasis. A recent review underscored functional collaborations among urologists and nephrologists to treat challenging cases of stone disease with possible manifestations of underlying systemic disease. Identifying patients who require preventive measures is now a necessity, as evidenced by recent research demonstrating the value of individualized dietary and drug management for recurrence prevention. The involvement of multidisciplinary teams in the treatment of kidney stone patients marks a new trend in nephrology, aimed at addressing gaps among specialties and facilitating integrative care (Kawachi et al., 2017). Moreover, emerging technologies are crucial to advancing nephrology research, particularly in imaging and genomics. Technologies such as high-resolution imaging modalities improve visualization of renal anatomy and enable early detection of congenital and acquired renal pathology. On the molecular side, next-generation sequencing is revolutionising the diagnosis of inherited renal disorders, enabling clinicians to deploy targeted treatment modalities. All these technological advances work in tandem with increased understanding of nephron physiology and pathology to provide effective therapeutic interventions. The translation of these advances to the clinic highlights an evolving paradigm in nephrology that prioritizes precision medicine, ultimately aiming to optimize patient management and improve quality of life in patients with kidney disease (Kawachi et al., 2017).

5.6.1. Innovations in Kidney Disease Treatment

Advances in kidney disease treatment have transformed the field of nephrology over the last few years. One of the significant developments has occurred in the field of early detection and management of chronic kidney disease (CKD). Improved screening methods and the use of advanced biomarkers enable clinicians to diagnose CKD earlier in the disease process, allowing intervention to slow disease progression. Specifically, interventions such as electronic decision-support systems in primary care are significant because they enable the identification of vulnerable populations. These systems can assist PCPs with alerts and decision support triggered by predefined clinical guidelines. In this way, PCPs are well positioned to address the complexities of kidney disease care, which often entail overcoming entrenched barriers in the healthcare system, promoting patient adherence, and keeping up with the evolving evidence base (Abdel-Kader et al., 2019). Telehealth technology use is another significant advancement in kidney disease treatment. Through remote monitoring and virtual consultation, nephrologists can enhance patient engagement and follow-up care, particularly among rural or underserved patients. Patient monitoring can be conducted regularly via telehealth, enabling real-time adjustments to treatment plans without requiring face-to-face visits, thereby reducing the burden on patients and healthcare systems. Also, telemedicine fosters a culture of collaboration among patients, their loved ones, and their providers, thereby increasing adherence to treatment. With accelerating technological innovations in healthcare, integrating telehealth into nephrology is an essential milestone towards more personalized, accessible care for patients with kidney disease (Crowther et al., 2009).

In addition, technological improvements in dialysis have revolutionized treatment modalities for end-stage renal disease (ESRD) to the point where patients now enjoy a greater quality of life and survival outcomes. Technologies such as home dialysis systems give patients greater independence in managing their treatment protocols, increasing flexibility and convenience. The development of more biocompatible dialysis membranes and the introduction of portable dialysis machines exemplify how technological advances can mitigate some of the physical and psychological burdens associated with traditional dialysis. Moreover, these innovations have significantly impacted the patient-provider relationship, fostering a more collaborative environment in which patients are active participants in their care journey. With nephrology's advancement as a discipline, the integration of these technological revolutions promises an impeccable future for kidney disease management and treatment (Crowther et al., 2009; Abdel-Kader et al., 2019).

5.6.2. Genetic Studies and Their Implications

Genetic studies have gained prominence in nephrology, particularly in understanding and managing kidney diseases. The study of genetic susceptibility helps identify individuals who may be at higher risk for illnesses such as end-stage renal disease (ESRD). The recognition that racial and ethnic minorities, especially African Americans, have a disproportionate number of cases of ESRD underscores the importance of the role genetic factors have in health disparities. The disparities are driven by social determinants of health, including access to health care and variations in treatment outcomes.

By interfacing genetic data with clinical practice, nephrologists can create more tailored treatment that addresses the patient's particular genetic make-up and, consequently, improve the general care outcome for patients who are prone to renal complications, as stipulated in the racial differences in the care of ESRD report (Boulware et al., 2017). Moreover, the genetic discovery is not limited to mere risk identification but also includes potential interventions that may suppress the development of renal disease. Genetic studies have yielded important insights into the pathophysiology of idiopathic calcium nephrolithiasis, a common cause of kidney stones.

By observing the genetic aetiology of stone formation, nephrologists can refine diagnostic criteria and modify prevention strategies. For instance, urologist-nephrologist coordination, informed by genetic data, will enhance the treatment of patients with recurrent kidney stones. In addition, a framework based on a systematic literature review validates the identification of secondary etiologies of calcium nephrolithiasis, as central to clinical practice.

These cooperative approaches not only improve patient care but also advance research into the genetic determinants of kidney stone disease (Bartoletti et al., 2016). Lastly, the evolving nature of genetic studies in nephrology necessitates ongoing research and interdisciplinarity to fully realize their potential. Investigating genetic differences and their contribution to renal disease can help elucidate mechanisms underlying new therapeutic strategies that could forestall disease progression or enhance patient tolerance. Future studies should focus on integrating genetic counseling and screening as central tenets of nephrologic practice, especially in high-risk populations with particular renal diseases. By recognizing the interplay among genetic, environmental, and lifestyle factors, nephrologists can facilitate whole-person management plans through education and individualized care. With advances in the discipline, the incorporation of genetic information will transform nephrology practice in internal medicine and, ultimately, improve patient outcomes and health equity for those with kidney disease.

5.6.3. Future Directions in Nephrology Research

The future of nephrology research is increasingly shaped by the integration of advanced technologies, particularly artificial intelligence (AI). While the field advances towards improved patient outcomes and therapy, the ability of AIs to process data and make predictions offers promising avenues for study. The application of AI in nephrology can enhance workflow accuracy and, consequently, earlier detection of kidney disease, an important factor due to the often asymptomatic course of its progression. Studies have found that AI applications in nephrology's neighboring specialties, including radiology, have already demonstrated effectiveness in enhancing workflows and supporting diagnosis, an indicator of the potential to do the same in nephrology. Through collaborations between nephrologists and AI developers, the field can leverage innovative solutions to address the complexities of kidney disease care and improve patient engagement in their treatment (Najjar, 2023). Furthermore, nephrology has to address systemic issues related to research grants and innovation within the field. Contrary to the long-established and dire state of end-stage kidney disease (ESKD), federal research funding is still lagging behind money invested in other areas, including cardiovascular and cancer research. This disparity underscores the need for a paradigm shift, prioritizing research endeavors that promote patient-centered care and innovative treatment modalities. Recent perspectives on the 2019 U.S. Presidential Executive Order on Advancing American Kidney Health observe industry pushback against moving away from the status quo, with dialysis being the default treatment for the majority as it stands. Transitioning to new technologies and expanding access to home-based therapy can change the ESKD care landscape, significantly increasing patient control and outcomes while simultaneously decreasing the cost to the healthcare system (Conway et al., 2022). Lastly, stringent interdisciplinary approaches are the solution to novel therapeutic prospects in nephrology. Biomedical engineers, nephrologists, and other healthcare professionals have to collaborate to develop novel treatment strategies. Initiatives like KidneyX demonstrate the potential of public-private partnerships to accelerate technological advances that address the unmet needs of patients with kidney disease. By aiming bioengineering solutions at self-care in renal failure, the field can address concerns about cost, access, and patient choice. If successful, these interventions can set in motion a revolutionary shift in the treatment of kidney disease, based on patient experiences and outcomes rather than entrenched, more rigid models of care. The future of nephrology research is therefore to be in a position to promote innovation while keeping very much in mind the real needs of patients and the overall health system, to ensure that the advances reach those who most benefit from kidney disease (Conway et al., 2022) (Figure 5.17).

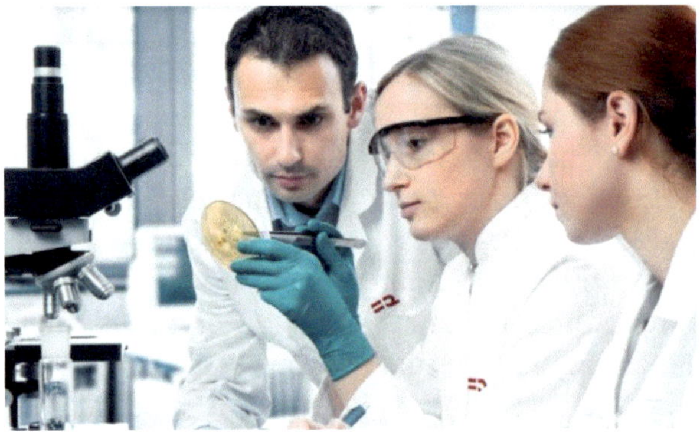

Figure 5.17. The future of nephrology research is focused on personalized medicine, advanced technologies, and novel therapies.

Source: https://images.zapnito.com/cdn-cgi/image/metadata=copyright,format=auto,quality=95,fit=scale-down/https://images.zapnito.com/users/196664/posters/1612550361-62-4506/d499b040-7ff3-4ffa-a9c6-90795e32ef51_large.jpeg.

Test Your Knowledge

1. What recent advances have improved the treatment of chronic kidney disease?
2. How is ongoing research shaping the future of nephrology care?

SUMMARY

The specialty of internal medicine in nephrology underscores the critical importance of a multidimensional approach to chronic kidney disease (CKD) and related disorders. Consistent with the conceptualization of barriers in primary care settings, including patient knowledge and healthcare system process constraints, healthcare professionals have to implement interventions that empower both patients and physicians. Identification of the challenges lies at the heart of developing effective management strategies to enhance the quality of care delivered to CKD patients. Further, implementing tools such as electronic reminders and abridged guidelines can alleviate the workload on primary care physicians, thereby improving patient outcomes (Abdel-Kader et al., 2019). In addition, the promising results of trials like the C-DIRECT trial suggest the potential effectiveness of nurse-led models to improve self-management and blood glucose control in people with complicating illnesses such as diabetes and end-stage renal disease. The research demonstrated improvements in quality of life, even though not all clinical indicators showed varying levels. These findings urge nephrology professionals to encourage innovative, evidence-based treatment for CKD involving behavioral health interventions alongside traditional medical care (e.g., Jakobson et al., 2019). As the prevalence of kidney disease continues to rise globally, the call for action among nephrology professionals is amplified. A transition to an integrated model of care will not only address the complexity of CKD but also enhance interdisciplinary collaboration among healthcare professionals. By a persistent commitment to learning and overcoming both provider and patient challenges, the nephrology community will be empowered to create meaningful changes in patient care. On the heels of learning from numerous studies, creating guidelines that ensure effective management pathways in the ever-changing setting of kidney health (Abdel-Kader et al., 2019; Jacobson et al., 2019) will be the key. Healthcare providers ought to gain insight into the intricacies of nephrology within the framework of internal medicine, as they deal with renal health. The highlights in this field are the imperative management of acute kidney injury (AKI) and chronic kidney disease (CKD). Providers must comprehend the multifactorial etiology of these conditions, from hemodynamic instability to toxic nephropathies. With an emphasis on the need for individually tailored intervention, healthcare professionals must be proficient in initiating renal replacement therapy where indicated. Effective patient treatment also includes vigilant monitoring of fluid and electrolyte status, underscoring the importance of a dynamic clinical approach. A practical understanding of these principles allows clinicians to enhance patient care in the more complex settings of nephrology, thereby elevating the quality of care in internal medicine (Bonilla et al., 2025). In addition to acute and chronic kidney disease, the integration of genetic testing into nephrology is one of the most significant advancements in internal medicine. Genetic evaluation has two primary clinical roles: diagnostic evaluation in symptomatic patients and predisposition evaluation in asymptomatic patients with a hereditary risk factor. This dual approach enables early diagnosis of genetic nephropathies and affects prevention and treatment strategies. Exome sequencing and other techniques have been crucial in identifying silent disorders and developing personalized management strategies in the past. Moreover, clinicians are required to navigate the subtleties of variant interpretation as the definition of genetic variants continues to evolve, creating both challenges and opportunities in the practice of nephrology. This is an expanding field that combines genetics and renal medicine, underscoring the growing significance of continuing education for healthcare professionals (Kiryluk et al., 2019). Moreover, the nephrology subspecialty of critical care plays a key role in the management of renal complications in intensive care. It not only addresses complex renal issues in critically ill patients but also encompasses a wide range of interventions, including extended renal replacement therapy. Knowing the distinct clinical scenarios associated with acute kidney injury in intensive care environments enables nephrologists to appropriately apply evidence-based practice. The combination of various multidisciplinary methods provides for streamlined therapy, allowing patients to benefit from integrated treatment approaches as required. As the field evolves, ongoing studies and training will be necessary to refine management techniques and maximize patient outcomes in critical care nephrology, ultimately highlighting the central role of nephrology within internal medicine (Bonilla et al., 2025).

KEY TERMS FROM THIS CHAPTER

- Kidney
- Glomerulonephritis
- Acute Kidney Injury (AKI)
- Hemodialysis
- Kidney Transplant
- Hematuria
- Hypertension
- Nephritic Syndrome
- Creatinine
- Nephron
- Chronic Kidney Disease (CKD)
- Dialysis
- Peritoneal Dialysis
- Proteinuria
- Electrolyte Imbalance
- Nephrotic Syndrome
- Uremia
- Blood Urea Nitrogen (BUN)

CRITICAL THINKING QUESTIONS

1. **Which of the following structures in the kidney is primarily responsible for the filtration of blood to form urine?**
   a. Glomerulus
   b. Proximal convoluted tubule
   c. Distal convoluted tubule
   d. Renal pelvis
2. **Which of the following is the most commonly used marker to estimate glomerular filtration rate (GFR) in clinical practice?**
   a. Blood urea nitrogen (BUN)
   b. Serum creatinine
   c. Urinary sodium concentration
   d. Urinary albumin
3. **Which of the following is the first-line treatment for a patient with stage 1 chronic kidney disease (CKD) due to hypertension?**
   a. Angiotensin-converting enzyme (ACE) inhibitors
   b. Diuretics
   c. Statins
   d. Beta-blockers
4. **What is the most common treatment modality for end-stage kidney disease (ESKD) when a kidney transplant is not an option?**
   a. Peritoneal dialysis
   b. Conservative management
   c. Hemodialysis
   d. Renal artery angioplasty
5. **In patients with acute kidney injury (AKI), which of the following is the primary role of internal medicine specialists?**
   a. Performing kidney transplantation
   b. Providing dialysis immediately after diagnosis
   c. Initiating long-term dialysis therapy
   d. Identifying and managing underlying causes of AKI

Short Answer Questions

1. What is the primary function of the nephron in the kidney?
2. Describe the process of glomerular filtration and its significance in kidney function.
3. What is the role of serum creatinine levels in assessing kidney function?
4. How is a urinalysis used in diagnosing kidney diseases?
5. What are the key differences between hemodialysis and peritoneal dialysis?
6. What pharmacological agents are commonly used to manage hypertension in patients with chronic kidney disease?
7. How do internists collaborate with nephrologists in managing patients with acute kidney injury (AKI)?
8. What are some promising areas of research in nephrology related to kidney transplantation?

Answers to Critical Thinking Questions

1. (a); 2. (b) ; 3. (a); 4. (c); 5. (d)

REFERENCES

1. Abassi, Z., Hamoud, S., Hassan, A., Khamaysi, I., Nativ, O., Heyman, S. N., Muhammad, R. S., Ilan, N., Singh, P., Hammond, E., Zaza, G., Lupo, A., Onisto, M., Bellin, G., Masola, V., Vlodavsky, I., & Gambaro, G. (2017). Involvement of heparanase in the pathogenesis of acute kidney injury: nephroprotective effect of PG545. *Oncotarget, 8*(21), 34191–34204. https://doi.org/10.18632/oncotarget.16573Abdel-Kader, K., Agrawal, V., Cavanaugh, K., Choi, M., et al. (2019). Primary care physicians' perceptions of barriers and facilitators to management of chronic kidney disease: A mixed methods study. https://core.ac.uk/download/323073389.pdf (accessed on 16th July 2025).

2. Aigner, F., Pratschke, J., Schumann, T., Stockmann, M., et al. (2020). Recent advances and the potential for clinical use of autofluorescence detection of extra-ophthalmic tissues. https://core.ac.uk/download/323257980.pdf (accessed on 16th July 2025).

3. Ajaimy, M., & Melamed, M. L. (2020). COVID-19 in patients with kidney disease. *Clinical Journal of the American Society of Nephrology, 15*, 1087–1089. https://doi.org/10.2215/cjn.09730620 (accessed on 16th July 2025).

4. Alexander, R., Alvarado, A., Lakshmanaperumal, N., McClain, J., et al. (2015). Stem cells and fluid flow drive cyst formation in an invertebrate excretory organ.

5. Ali, A., Al-Omar, D., Lami, F. H., & Bhandari, S. (2023). Perception and satisfaction of nephrology education and training in Iraq. *Journal of the Royal College of Physicians of Edinburgh, 53*, 13–18. https://www.semanticscholar.org/paper/196163f2f056895af3bb999d95be5ab6f2641116 (accessed on 16th July 2025).

6. Arici, M., Assaad-Khalil, S. H., Bertoluci, M., Choo, J., Lee, Y. J., Madero, M., Rosa Diez, G. J., et al. (2024). Results from a cross-specialty consensus on optimal management of patients with chronic kidney disease (CKD): From screening to complications. *BMJ Open, 14*. https://www.semanticscholar.org/paper/2302863625a03ce31a6ee5574134b2f77c006dcd (accessed on 16th July 2025).

7. Bajema, I. M., Bertsias, G. K., Boumpas, D. T., Gordon, C., et al. (2015). Lupus nephritis management guidelines compared. https://core.ac.uk/download/77009956.pdf (accessed on 16th July 2025).

8. Bamias, A., Cheung, M., Conference Participants, Danesh, F., et al. (2020). KDIGO Controversies Conference on onco-nephrology: Understanding kidney impairment and solid-organ malignancies, and managing kidney cancer. https://core.ac.uk/download/346619147.pdf (accessed on 16th July 2025).

9. Bartoletti, R., Buchholz, N., Buchholz, N. N. P. (Noor), Bushinsky, D., et al. (2016). Metabolic diagnosis and medical prevention of calcium nephrolithiasis and its systemic manifestations: A consensus statement. https://core.ac.uk/download/72001809.pdf (accessed on 16th July 2025).

10. Berney, M., Bühler, R., Chheang, C., Cominetti, F., Decker, F., Dévaud, M., Fidalgo, C., et al. (2025). [The year 2024 placed in perspective by hospital internists]. *Revue Médicale Suisse, 21*(903), 164–166. https://www.semanticscholar.org/paper/c3aca11db8e8882a13b44d3543f33bd651afe425 (accessed on 16th July 2025).

11. Blumenthal, D. M., Elashoff, D., Inoue, K., Tsugawa, Y., et al. (2019). Association between physician characteristics and payments from industry in 2015–2017: Observational study. https://core.ac.uk/download/323076301.pdf (accessed on 16th July 2025).
12. Böbel, I., & Martis, A. (2025). *Value Creation in Health Care: The Case of the Princesses Grace Hospital (CHPG) Monaco*. https://core.ac.uk/download/pdf/6586022.pdf (accessed on 16th July 2025).
13. Bonilla, M. A., Koyner, J. L., & Neyra, J. A. (2025). Acute kidney injury and critical care nephrology. *Advances in Kidney Disease and Health, 32*(1), 12–23. https://www.semanticscholar.org/paper/e51d4d0bfbb7f73cef903eec0ff4d1031b9e70af (accessed on 16th July 2025).
14. Borniche, D., Claus, S., Correa-Rotter, R., Crestani, R., et al. (2010). When the Earth trembles in the Americas: The experience of Haiti and Chile 2010. https://core.ac.uk/download/pdf/9417860.pdf (accessed on 16th July 2025).
15. Boulware, E. B., Kalantar-Zadeh, K., Kovesdy, C. P., Nicholas, S. B., et al. (2017). Hemodialysis disparities in African Americans: The deeply integrated concept of race in the social fabric of our society. https://core.ac.uk/download/231897279.pdf (accessed on 16th July 2025).
16. Braun, G. S., Horster, S., Ihrler, S., Schmid, H., et al. (2007). Cryoglobulinaemic vasculitis: Classification and clinical and therapeutic aspects. https://core.ac.uk/download/12175185.pdf (accessed on 16th July 2025).
17. Broyles, J. (2019). 175,000 blue chairs. *Journal of the American Geriatrics Society, 67*. https://www.semanticscholar.org/paper/a65453447efd5f82afcf0ee1c7fb1e3439ddb2c0 (accessed on 16th July 2025).
18. Canning, D. (2020). Re: Adolescent testicular microlithiasis: A case-based, multinational survey of clinical management practices. *The Journal of Urology*. https://www.semanticscholar.org/paper/5cd9475f644e842afd6f16a8bb7cb2af6c423ece (accessed on 16th July 2025).
19. Chadban, S. J., Ahn, C., Axelrod, D. A., Foster, B. J., Kasiske, B. L., Kher, V., Kumar, D., et al. (2020). KDIGO clinical practice guideline on the evaluation and management of candidates for kidney transplantation. *Transplantation, 104*, S11–S103. https://doi.org/10.1097/tp.0000000000003136 (accessed on 16th July 2025).
20. Chávez-Íñiguez, J. S., & Madero, M. (2022). Global perspectives in acute kidney injury: Mexico. *Kidney360, 3*, 737–739. https://doi.org/10.34067/kid.0006592021 (accessed on 16th July 2025).
21. Chawla, L. S., Bellomo, R., Bihorac, A., Goldstein, S. L., Siew, E. D., Bagshaw, S. M., Bittleman, D., et al. (2017). Acute kidney disease and renal recovery: Consensus report of the Acute Disease Quality Initiative (ADQI) 16 Workgroup. *Nature Reviews Nephrology, 13*, 241–257. https://doi.org/10.1038/nrneph.2017.2 (accessed on 16th July 2025).
22. Ciccariello, M., D'Angelo, A. R., Di Gaeta, A., Ferrigno, L., et al. (2018). Magnetic resonance imaging 3T and total fibrotic volume in autosomal dominant polycystic kidney disease. https://core.ac.uk/download/188827782.pdf (accessed on 16th July 2025).
23. Collins, C. A., Daugherty, A. L., Hreha, T. N., Hunstad, D. A., et al. (2020). TGFβ1 orchestrates renal fibrosis following *Escherichia coli* pyelonephritis. https://core.ac.uk/download/297573955.pdf (accessed on 16th July 2025).

24. Conway, P. T., Gedney, N., Roy, S., & Fissell, W. H. (2022). The Advancing American Kidney Health Initiative: The challenge of overcoming the status quo. *Journal of the American Society of Nephrology, 33*, 1797–1798. https://doi.org/10.1681/asn.2022040510 (accessed on 16th July 2025).

25. Crowther, S. M., Reynolds, L. A., & Tansey, E. M. (2009). *History of Dialysis in the UK: c.1950–1980*. https://core.ac.uk/download/30696171.pdf (accessed on 16th July 2025).

26. De Hert, S. (2020). Burnout in healthcare workers: Prevalence, impact and preventative strategies. *Local and Regional Anesthesia, 13*, 171–183. https://doi.org/10.2147/lra.s240564 (accessed on 16th July 2025).

27. Elliott, J., Jepson, R. E., Lawson, J. S., Syme, H., et al. (2015). Renal fibrosis in feline chronic kidney disease: Known mediators and mechanisms of injury. https://core.ac.uk/download/36777966.pdf (accessed on 16th July 2025).

28. Fink, E., Fischer, K. G., Henger, A., Huber, T. B., et al. (2002). Eluate derived by extracorporeal antibody-based immunoadsorption elevates the cytosolic Ca^{2+} concentration in podocytes via B-2 kinin receptors. https://core.ac.uk/download/16432528.pdf (accessed on 16th July 2025).

29. Garcia-Finana, M., Murray, P., Park, B. K., Poptani, H., et al. (2016). Imaging technologies for monitoring the safety, efficacy and mechanisms of action of cell-based regenerative medicine therapies in models of kidney disease. https://core.ac.uk/download/80777055.pdf (accessed on 16th July 2025).

30. Geddes, C. C., Mark, P. B., McQuarrie, E. P., Stoumpos, S., et al. (2017). Continued monitoring of acute kidney injury survivors might not be necessary in those regaining an estimated glomerular filtration rate > 60 mL/min at 1 year. https://core.ac.uk/download/74230017.pdf (accessed on 16th July 2025).

31. Guedes, M., Dias, P. T., Réa, R. R., Cálice-Silva, V., Lopes, M., Brandão, A. A., Bauer, A. C., et al. (2024). Patterns of kidney function and risk assessment in a nationwide laboratory database: The Brazilian CHECK-CKD study. *BMC Nephrology, 25*. https://www.semanticscholar.org/paper/5f1b9898a625f097efadbdab715f6fd2b174e8e5 (accessed on 16th July 2025).

32. Hernández Miramontes, J. A., Méndez Durán, A., & Hernández Villanueva, J. A. (2024). Tricarboxylic cycle intermediates in combination with calcium phosphate chelators and sodium bicarbonate increases eGFR in patients with stages 3b, 4 and 5 CKD: A retrospective observational study. *Revita Colombiana de Nephrology*. https://www.semanticscholar.org/paper/f6d6c11c6cbb1bc2dea49fa58fcd0238e270833b (accessed on 16th July 2025).

33. Jacobson, A. M., Zigmond, A. S., Lai, A. Y., Chua, C. G., Eigenmann, C. A., Goh, C. S. Y., Toobert, D. J., et al. (2019). The combined diabetes and renal control trial (C-DIRECT)–a feasibility randomized controlled trial to evaluate outcomes in multi-morbid patients with diabetes and on dialysis using a mixed methods approach. https://core.ac.uk/download/163076809.pdf (accessed on 16th July 2025).

34. Kawachi, I., Kivimaki, M., & Pulakka, A. (2017). Distance from home to the nearest tobacco outlet may not reflect the true accessibility: Reply. https://core.ac.uk/download/84363373.pdf (accessed on 16th July 2025).

35. Kirsztajn, G., Silva Júnior, G. S., Bezerra da Silva, A. Q., Abensur, H., Romão Junior, J. E., Bastos, M. G., Cálice-Silva, V., et al. (2024). Estimated glomerular filtration rate in clinical practice: Consensus positioning of the Brazilian Society of Nephrology (SBN) and Brazilian Society of

Clinical Pathology and Laboratory Medicine (SBPC/ML). *Jornal Brasileiro de Nefrologia, 46*. https://www.semanticscholar.org/paper/ed924aa7318ddfe4aba667d6a4d20d6912fb6d21 (accessed on 16th July 2025).

36. Kiryluk, K., Goldstein, D., Rowe, J., Gharavi, A., Wapner, R., & Chung, W. (2019). Precision medicine in internal medicine. *Annals of Internal Medicine, 170*, 635–642. https://www.semanticscholar.org/paper/c7199e8a5226f8d9d55777da0e15e91797bb459a (accessed on 16th July 2025).
37. Lameire, N. (2014). Wars, disasters and kidneys. https://core.ac.uk/download/55847404.pdf (accessed on 16th July 2025).
38. Lechien, J. R., Chiesa-Estomba, C. M., Hans, S., Barillari, M. R., Jouffe, L., & Saussez, S. (2020). Loss of smell and taste in 2013 European patients with mild to moderate COVID-19. *Annals of Internal Medicine, 173*, 672–675. https://doi.org/10.7326/m20-2428 (accessed on 16th July 2025).
39. Miao, J., Thongprayoon, C., Garcia Valencia, O. A., Craici, I. M., & Cheungpasitporn, W. (2024). Navigating nephrology's decline through a GPT-4 analysis of internal medicine specialties in the United States: Qualitative study. *JMIR Medical Education, 10*. https://www.semanticscholar.org/paper/ee9ee73b86f96fb5a2416a3b16b8eeffff05ef84 (accessed on 16th July 2025).
40. Najjar, R. (2023). Redefining radiology: A review of artificial intelligence integration in medical imaging. *Diagnostics, 13*, 2760. https://doi.org/10.3390/diagnostics13172760 (accessed on 16th July 2025).
41. Perkins, R. M., & Yuan, C. M. (2011). Renal replacement therapy in austere environments. https://core.ac.uk/download/pdf/8566584.pdf (accessed on 16th July 2025).
42. Rodby, R. A. (2022). Kidney biopsy should remain a required procedure for nephrology training programs: CON. *Kidney360, 3*, 1667–1669. https://doi.org/10.34067/kid.0007762021 (accessed on 16th July 2025).
43. Schalkwijk, C. G., van der Sande, F. M., Kooman, J. P., Kaysen, G. A., Usvyat, L. A., Dekker, M. J., Shiels, P. G., et al. (2017). Inflammation and premature aging in advanced chronic kidney disease. https://core.ac.uk/download/84591453.pdf (accessed on 16th July 2025).
44. Silva, P. A. B. da. (2014). Estágio em gestão de dados e estatística numa CRO. https://core.ac.uk/download/32243844.pdf (accessed on 16th July 2025).
45. Tantisattamo, E., & Kalantar-Zadeh, K. (2020). Novel therapeutic approaches in chronic kidney disease, uremia and kidney transplantation: Past, present and future. *Current Opinion in Nephrology & Hypertension*. https://www.semanticscholar.org/paper/b5fdc279afb09371c6f1154c2bb796c18cedd9b6 (accessed on 16th July 2025).
46. Wagner, E., Tufano, J., & Horner, K. (2011). Electronic consultations between primary and specialty care clinicians: Early insights. https://core.ac.uk/download/71358065.pdf (accessed on 16th July 2025).
47. Yates, M., Watts, R. A., Bajema, I. M., Cid, M. C., Crestani, B., Häuser, T., Hellmich, B., et al. (2016). EULAR/ERA-EDTA recommendations for the management of ANCA-associated vasculitis. *Annals of the Rheumatic Diseases, 75*, 1583–1594. https://doi.org/10.1136/annrheumdis-2016-209133 (accessed on 16th July 2025).

ENDOCRINOLOGY

6

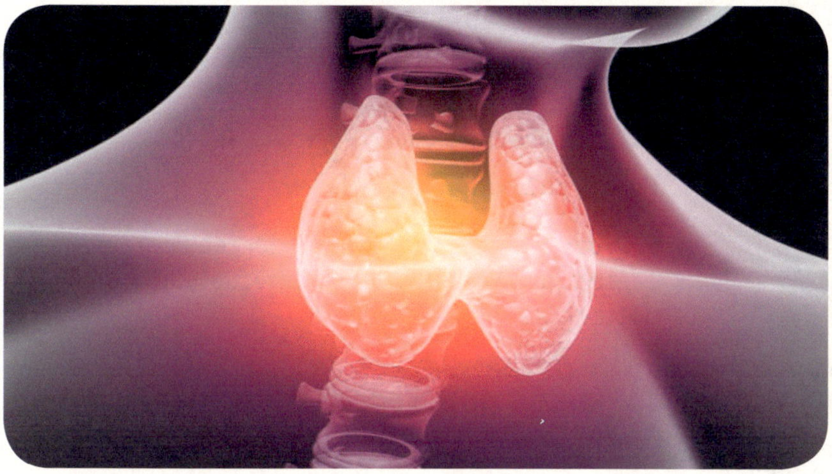

LEARNING OBJECTIVES

After studying this chapter, you will be able to:

1. Understand the fundamentals of endocrinology
2. Identify the common endocrine disorders
3. Define diagnostic approaches in endocrinology
4. Discuss treatment modalities in endocrinology
5. Describe the role of technology in endocrinology
6. Explain the challenges in endocrinology

Introduction

To comprehend the complexities of internal medicine, particularly endocrinology, it is first important to grasp the multidimensional nature of adult patient care. Internal medicine is a precursor to understanding various health disorders that occur episodically in patients throughout their lifetimes. It places emphasis on the prevention, diagnosis, and treatment of internal organ diseases, with the internist serving as the first-line doctor responsible for comprehensive care. The interfacial nature of internal medicine is reflected in the overlap of many subspecialties, which is crucial when patients present with overlapping conditions, such as diabetes or thyroid disease. This foundation provides a platform for internists not only to manage chronic illnesses but also to recognize patterns of comorbidities that will require expert interventions, thereby rendering the role of internal medicine particularly critical in endocrinology, where endocrine disorders have far-reaching health implications. Internal medicine sound practice includes recognizing that chronic illnesses require multidisciplinary care, particularly in endocrinology. For instance, adult patients with complex rare genetic syndromes (CRGS) usually require coordinated care, given the multifactorial etiology of their symptoms, quite a number of which may have endocrine implications. With the spotlight shed by recent developments on specialized clinics for the management of adults with CRGS, internists' efforts become increasingly important in ensuring syndrome-specific care, which tends to be in short supply as patients transition from pediatric to adult medical environments. Establishment of such multidisciplinary outpatient clinics is an initial step in which internists diagnose patients and provide the best possible management pathways based on each patient's needs, after a proper understanding of their conditions. By identifying such special health concerns, internists can formulate management options that escape risks of delayed diagnoses as well as excessive, invasive interventions, and therefore act in patients' best interest (Rosenberg et al., 2021). The effectiveness of integrated care programs in managing endocrine disorders also points towards the importance of internal medicine here. Studies have shown that multidisciplinary team educational interventions can help modulate patient outcomes, particularly in the management of chronic conditions such as diabetes.

By integrating multiple healthcare professionals, such as dietitians, pharmacists, and specialists, diabetes management can lead to better blood glucose control and improved overall health outcomes. This underscores the value of collective efforts in addressing endocrinological issues, as coordination among medical professionals leads to more comprehensive care plans. Because internists will usually be patients' first points of entry, familiarity with the interdependence of services and how to activate these resources is paramount. This integrative approach not only ensures that patients are healed of their specific ailments but also equips them to maintain their long-term health, leading to improved patient satisfaction and reduced healthcare costs (Kim et al., 2018) (Figure 6.1).

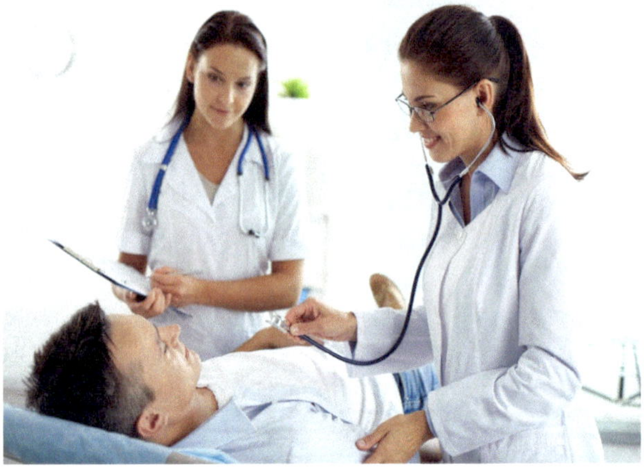

Figure 6.1. Internal medicine.

Source: https://www.onlinedegree.com/wp-content/uploads/2017/02/internalmedicine_doctor.jpg..

Definition and Scope of Internal Medicine

Internal medicine is a broad branch of medical practice that encompasses the diagnosis, management, and prevention of diseases in adults. Internists are physicians specializing in internal medicine who undergo extensive training to deliver care for complex patient health conditions. Unlike specialists, internists are trained to diagnose and manage multiple diseases in a patient to provide holistic care, taking into account comorbidities and patient-specific factors. The scope of internal medicine is broad, encompassing diverse areas such as cardiology, gastroenterology, and endocrinology, creating a large knowledge base that enables internists to appreciate the complexities of systemic illness and to coordinate care in an interdisciplinary approach across specialties, emphasizing the interdependence of these collaborations toward better patient outcomes. In endocrinology, internal medicine plays a vital role in the treatment of hormonal imbalances and associated disorders, such as diabetes, thyroid disease, and metabolic syndromes. Internists specializing in this subspecialty develop a clearer understanding of the intricacy of the endocrine system, resulting in more targeted and effective treatment modalities for patients. Endocrinology also relies heavily on broad-based internal medicine information, since treatment protocols need to be both effective and patient-centered and are developed from clinical data, lab results, and patient history. As such, internal medicine practitioners play a crucial role in integrating evidence-based practice into the treatment of endocrine illness, honing their skills to effectively navigate the subtleties of patients' presentations and the evolving literature. The revolution in internal medicine is also reflected by innovations in technology and telemedicine, both of which are now central to improving access to care, particularly for chronic conditions such as those encompassed in endocrinology. Improvements in telehealth enable internists to treat and monitor endocrine disease remotely, thereby improving patient engagement and compliance with treatment protocols. Moreover, current studies indicate that telemedicine delivery facilitates timely treatment and enhances patient satisfaction across several health systems.

In accordance with N/A (2010), it is essential to overcome difficulties surrounding telehealth adoption for the lasting continuity of the practices. Lastly, the intersection of internal medicine and endocrinology /demonstrates how comprehensive training and dynamic healthcare interventions are essential to providing outstanding medical care. The creation and quality assessment of registries such as the I-DSD and I-CAH are another instance of the role of research in furthering the study and treatment of endocrine disorders, as quoted by Ahmed et al. (2017).

Importance of Specialization in Internal Medicine

Specialization in internal medicine is a critical method of advancing the quality of patient care, particularly in the division of endocrinology. Because internal medicine encompasses such a broad range of medical conditions, the establishment of specialty branches allows it to analyze specific diseases and their complexities in greater depth. Endocrinologists, for example, deal with the intricate hormone systems and how they affect the body's functions. Specialization not only contributes to a deeper understanding of disease pathology but also gives physicians the ability to personalize treatment regimes that best address individual patient needs. Focus on internal medicine's specialty areas optimizes the allocation of healthcare resources, leading to improved patient outcomes and satisfaction. With advancing medical knowledge, it is becoming increasingly apparent that specialization in internal medicine is a key component in addressing today's healthcare challenges. Specialization in internal medicine is also promoted by physician productivity and patient outcomes dynamics. Research suggests that more competent doctors enter specialties with lower risk of moral hazard and stronger performance incentives, and that, in turn, quality of care improves in those specialties. Endocrinologists are a case in point when it comes to the benefits of specialization from this perspective. They have advanced training that enables them to diagnose and treat complex illnesses such as diabetes mellitus, thyroid disorders, and metabolic syndromes, providing patients with evidence-based, tailor-made treatment. This interconnection between specialization and the quality of care culminates in an environment where professionals can conduct extensive research and development within their fields, ultimately advancing medical science. Hence, the ongoing inconsistency in healthcare quality can be traced to the uncertainty surrounding physician specialization and its impact on the effective management of patients (Courty et al., 2025). The necessity of specialization in internal medicine, particularly in endocrinology, is also driven by evolving dynamics in healthcare and the imperative to keep up with emerging health concerns. The increasing prevalence of chronic diseases has compelled healthcare systems to focus on hiring specialized practitioners to adequately manage these vital conditions. As populations age and lifestyle-related disorders become prevalent, the role of endocrinologists becomes pivotal in appropriately managing such complex scenarios. Furthermore, institutions like Boston University Medical Center emphasize the imperative of creating adaptive health care responsive to societal needs, thereby also highlighting the necessity of advanced training to meet the challenges of contemporary times (Black et al., 1981). By fostering a culture of continuous education and professional development, specialization in internal medicine contributes to better patient care and positions the health system to effectively respond to the evolving medical landscape. Through specialization, internal medicine thus secures its vital role in promoting health and wellness across various patient populations (Figure 6.2).

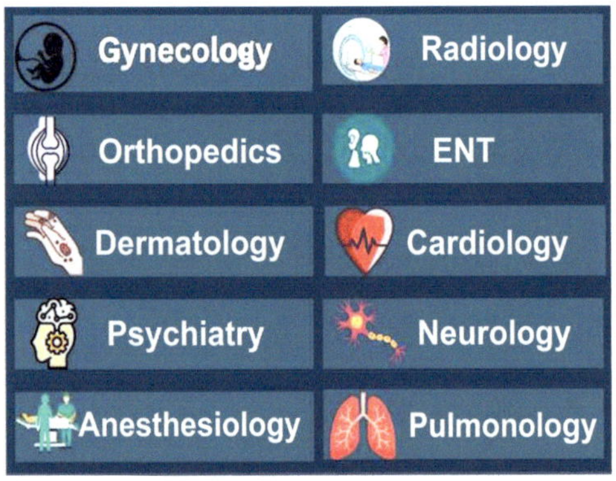

Figure 6.2. Importance of specialization in internal medicine.

Source: https://1852771943.rsc.cdn77.org/wp-content/uploads/2023/10/Specialization-in-Medicine.jpg..

Overview of the Role of Endocrinology Within Internal Medicine

Endocrinology occupies a central place in internal medicine, in part because of its focus on the endocrine system's far-reaching influence on a wide range of physiological processes. Physicians of internal medicine are most likely first to see patients with signs of hormonal imbalance, such as diabetes, thyroid disorders, and reproductive system ailments. These conditions also require a sound understanding of endocrinological concepts, along with the integration of thorough patient histories, physical examinations, and laboratory testing. Internists thus need to remain current with developments in endocrinology so they can effectively manage such intricate conditions and offer patients evidence-based treatment options that include lifestyle interventions alongside drug therapy. As advances continue to unfold in endocrinology, the combination of new diagnostic techniques and treatment strategies is transforming patient management in internal medicine. The most recent advances, like hormone replacement therapies (HRTs) and individualized medicine interventions, enable clinicians to personalize treatment approaches based on distinct genetic and physiological profiles. Such tailored approaches enhance therapy effectiveness while reducing the risk of side effects, further underscoring the necessity of a nuanced understanding of endocrinological principles. Additionally, with the aid of sophisticated diagnostic methods, internal medicine physicians can identify endocrine disorders more promptly, enabling quicker intervention and improved patient outcomes. This dynamic intersection of changing treatments and innovation within the specialty demonstrates that endocrinology not only remains relevant but is essential to internal medicine practice worldwide (Pandey, 2024). Also, the relationship between endocrinology and other subspecialties of internal medicine highlights the multidisciplinary approach needed to ensure optimal care. PCOS, obesity, and metabolic syndrome require a multidisciplinary approach that integrates endocrinologic expertise with consideration of other systemic factors. Internists deal with the complexity of such relationships while drawing on evidence from nutrition, genetics, and behavioral sciences to expand their practice domain. Moreover, an understanding of the implications of stress and environmental factors on endocrine function, as provided by classical approaches such as Unani medicine, can add substance to contemporary clinical practices. Internal medicine, by adopting a holistic approach, becomes better attuned to endocrine disorders, thereby improving patient health outcomes (Tasleem et al., 2025).

Test Your Knowledge

1. Describe the definition and significance of endocrinology
2. Discuss on major endocrine glands and their functions
3. Identify the hormonal regulation and feedback mechanisms

6.1. Fundamentals of Endocrinology

Learning Outcome

1. Understand hotel maintenance management and its impact
2. Perform preventive maintenance
3. Discuss about breakdown maintenance

The study of endocrinology encompasses an integrated view of the hormone regulatory systems that govern physiologic processes. Essentially, hormones are messengers, carried by blood to receiving tissues and organs, coordinating a variety of body processes from metabolism to growth and sexual health. The endocrine system's four major glands are the pituitary, thyroid, adrenal, and pancreas, each contributing to maintaining the body in homeostasis. Dysregulation of hormone secretion or function can cause a variety of health issues, including diabetes mellitus, thyroid disease, and adrenal insufficiency. A firm grasp of these fundamental ideas is essential to internal medicine clinicians since accurate diagnosis and therapy depend on an integration of this knowledge to manage endocrine disorders successfully, ultimately propelling better patient outcomes through targeted therapeutic interventions. Furthermore, developments in endocrinology have recognized the intricate relationship between endocrine function and overall health. Research breakthroughs indicate that stress, diet, and physical exercise can significantly influence endocrine function. Stress, for instance, has been shown to exacerbate diseases such as atopic dermatitis and metabolic syndrome, which demonstrates the interconnectedness of the body's systems. Each of these organizations enables internal medicine practitioners to design inclusive management plans that account for endocrine and environmental influences on health. The integration of lifestyle interventions with pharmacotherapy could lead to more efficient, patient-oriented therapy, as treating the underlying causes of endocrine disorders encourages holistic approaches. This convergence is most relevant in the management of chronic disease, where both treatment and lifestyle changes can complement each other to improve outcomes for the patient. Lastly, the integration of evidence-based guidelines into practice must be achieved to maximize care for patients with endocrine disease. Initiatives such as Choosing Wisely® are helpful frameworks that provide recommendations to reduce unnecessary tests and treatments and increase high-quality, evidence-based care. For example, best-practice guidelines underpinning the management of diseases such as venous thromboembolism and sickle cell disease emphasize the importance of responsible, necessity-driven actions in the provision of patient care. Internal medicine residents' instruction in applying such guidelines not only better equips them to understand endocrine disorders but also instills in them a responsibility to provide care that is efficient and cost-effective. Education on these basic principles equips prospective doctors with the competencies to manage complex clinical scenarios, ultimately paving the way for a patient-focused model of health care provision that delivers quality care par excellence (May et al., 2021; Ventura et al., 2024) (Figure 6.3).

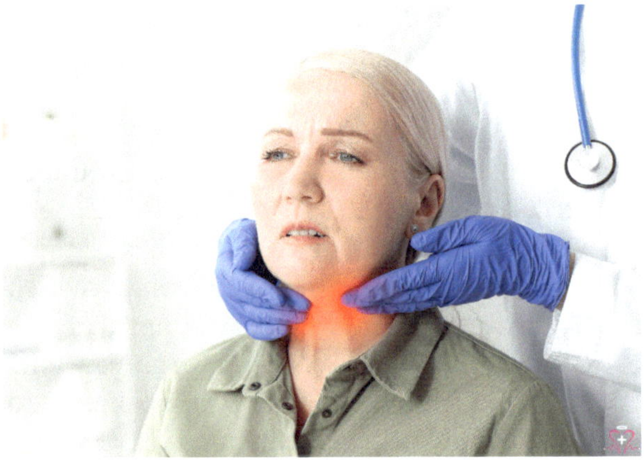

Figure 6.3. Fundamentals of endocrinology.

Source: https://allseniors.org/wp-content/uploads/2024/06/doctors-1-1536x1024.png.

6.1.1. Definition and Significance of Endocrinology

Endocrinology is a medical discipline that specifically investigates the endocrine system, which comprises glands that secrete and control hormones. The endocrine system plays a significant role in regulating various physiological functions, such as metabolism, growth, and reproduction. The significance of endocrinology extends beyond its specialty of diagnosing and treating endocrine illnesses, such as diabetes and thyroid disease, to encompass overall health. Because hormones exert broad control over the body, it is crucial to understand their functions and interactions to disentangle more complex biological processes. indicating. In the field of endocrinology, we see an echo of how hormonal imbalances can be pathogenetic for disease, underscoring the significance of this science within the general paradigm of internal medicine. In addition, the historical progress in endocrinology reflects its evolving significance within medical science. Early notions of health depended on the equilibrium of fluid states within the organism, as illustrated by Galen's humoral theory, yielding seminal concepts of homeostasis. Claude Bernard and Walter Cannon then elaborated on these concepts to better understand the stability of the internal environment. Over time, the association between endocrine function and the stress response has remained a crucial area of research. Hans Selye's general adaptation syndrome is a prime example of the body's physiological response to stress and its impact on endocrine control. Such knowledge has gone on to shape contemporary concepts regarding how physical and emotional stressors might influence hormonal health, illustrating the interdependent relationship between the endocrine system and various aspects of human health, and thereby enhancing the application of endocrinology in internal medicine. Notably, recent work emphasizes the intricate interplay among the endocrine system, the microbiota, and overall health, particularly through the microbiota-gut-brain axis. This new field of research examines how gut microbes communicate with the brain and the endocrine system, revealing the complexity of biological information systems within the body. Substances that influence microbiota composition, such as diet and stress, also have a potent impact on hormone function and metabolic health. Furthermore, conditions such as obesity and mental disorders have been linked to dysbiosis—a disruption in gut microbiota—highlighting the importance of hormonal and microbial interactions. With the advancement of research, understanding these associations may yield new therapeutic approaches, a crucial landmark in endocrinology's role in internal medicine. Through the exploration of such relationships, the role of endocrinology continues to expand and illuminate its underpinning importance to integrated health care (Cryan et al., 2019; McCarty, 2020).

6.1.2. Major Endocrine Glands and Their Functions

The endocrine system comprises a few large glands that regulate many physiological processes by secreting hormones. The pituitary gland, or the master gland, controls the other endocrine glands by secreting hormones that influence growth, metabolism, and reproduction. Its anterior lobe secretes hormones such as growth hormone (GH) and prolactin, which are involved in growth and lactation, while the posterior lobe secretes vasopressin (ADH) and oxytocin, which are involved in water retention and childbirth.

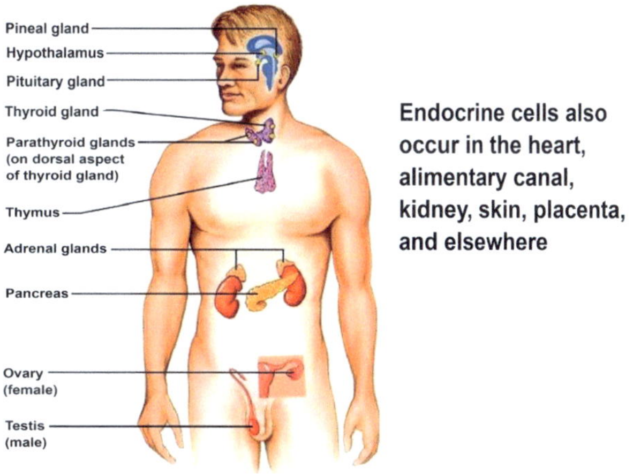

Figure 6.4. Major endocrine glands and their functions.

Source: https://overallscience.com/wp-content/uploads/2018/06/location-major-endocrine-glands-pineal-hypothalamus-pituitary-thyroid-shocking-celss-also-occur-heart-alimentary-canal-kidney-skin-placenta.jpg.

The adrenal glands also secrete hormones such as cortisol and adrenaline that are important in responses to stress, illustrating the coordination of endocrine functions in maintaining homeostasis and responding to environmental change. The thyroid gland is also an essential component of the endocrine system and plays a significant role in regulating metabolism by secreting thyroid hormones, such as thyroxine (T4) and triiodothyronine (T3). These are essential for regulating metabolic rate, energy balance, and overall growth and development. The thyroid also secretes calcitonin, which helps maintain calcium homeostasis by lowering blood calcium levels. Thyroid dysfunction, whether with hypo- or hyperthyroidism, can result in incredibly profound systemic effects, including fatigue, weight changes, and compromise of intellect, highlighting the demand for accurate metabolic control. Through such relations, the thyroid is a master regulator of energy balance in the human body. Equally essential are the pancreatic islets, which play a crucial role in glucose metabolism. The pancreas secretes insulin and glucagon, which exert an antagonistic effect to maintain blood glucose within a narrow range. Insulin encourages glucose entry into cells, while glucagon stimulates the release of glucose from the liver by breaking down glycogen. It is an essential balance to prevent metabolic illnesses such as diabetes mellitus, which may lead to severe morbidity if left untreated. Given the increasing prevalence of such disorders, knowledge of the pancreas's role in endocrine regulation is necessary. The relationships among these major glands account for the complexity of endocrine functions and the complex process of maintaining body homeostasis (Figure 6.4).

6.1.3. Hormonal Regulation and Feedback Mechanisms

The intricate relationship between feedback and hormonal control is a key element in endocrine homeostasis. Hormones, secreted by various glands, are chemical messengers that circulate through the bloodstream to influence target organs. Such a regulatory system is primarily regulated by two feedback mechanisms: negative and positive. Harmful feedback mechanisms function as a biological thermostat, where an increase in a particular hormone provokes a reaction that ultimately stops its production to restore equilibrium. To illustrate, elevated thyroid hormones inhibit hypothalamic and pituitary secretion, providing a classic example of negative feedback that helps regulate metabolic rate. This accurate orchestration is crucial for preventing disorders caused by excess or lack of hormones. In contrast, positive feedback mechanisms intensify physiological responses, with a tendency to have an ultimate, absolute outcome. A time-honored example is the role of oxytocin in delivery, where its release during contractions triggers further release, progressing towards birth. Though less frequent, these processes are equally crucial, as they allow for rapid biological modifications essential for specific stages of life or situations. The applications of these feedback loops are not limited to general health conditions; for example, dysfunction of negative feedback in metabolic pathways can lead to the progression of type 2 diabetes mellitus (T2DM) and other endocrine diseases. Knowing these feedback mechanisms helps us understand the pathophysiology underlying the conditions commonly seen in internal medicine. Additionally, recent studies have elucidated the complex roles of hormones beyond their classic regulatory functions. Exploring the adipose tissue function in hormonal pathways illustrates the complexity of the endocrine system. In particular, dysfunctional adipose tissue has been postulated to exacerbate metabolic diseases, such as T2DM and CVD, by secreting pro-inflammatory adipokines that disrupt healthy hormone signaling. The adipokines can alter glucose metabolism and insulin sensitivity, which illustrates the involvement of systemic inflammation in hormone regulation. Furthermore, gut microbiota metabolism may interact with such hormonal pathways, reflecting the actively developing field of research on the microbiota-gut-brain axis and its role in hormonal effects (Cryan et al., 2019). This growing understanding of hormonal systems highlights their importance not just in internal medicine but also in the development of potential therapeutic strategies for associated diseases.

Test Your Knowledge

1. What is the primary function of the endocrine system?
2. How do hormones regulate body processes?

6.2. Common Endocrine Disorders

Learning Outcome

1. Understand the diabetes mellitus: types and management
2. Describe the thyroid disorders: hypothyroidism and hyperthyroidism
3. Focus on adrenal disorders: cushing's syndrome and addison's disease

The endocrine system of man regulates many of the body's physiological functions, and its failure leads to a wide variety of diseases. Among these, diabetes mellitus is a prevalent endocrine disease characterized by chronic hyperglycemia resulting from insulin deficiency, impaired insulin action, or both. This disease comes primarily in two forms: Type 1 diabetes, an autoimmune destruction of insulin-secreting pancreatic beta cells, and Type 2 diabetes, typically associated with obesity and insulin resistance. Both are dangerous health conditions, with such complications as cardiovascular disease, nephropathy, and neuropathy. Current clinical practices revolve around general management strategies, including lifestyle therapy and drug therapy, which seek to achieve glycemic control and avoid related complications with this chronic illness. The rising incidence of diabetes globally gives its pathophysiology and treatment equal relevance within internal medicine, alongside endocrinology (Leidi et al., 2025). Thyroid illness is another prevalent category of endocrine system disturbances, including diseases like hypothyroidism and hyperthyroidism that significantly affect metabolic processes. Hypothyroidism, resulting from underproduction of thyroid hormones, produces symptoms like weakness, weight gain, and depression. In contrast, hyperthyroidism results from overproduction of the hormone, producing symptoms like weight loss, nervousness, and trembling. The conditions have the potential to create serious complications like cardiovascular disease and osteoporosis. Thyroid disorders are challenging to treat and can either involve hormone replacement in hypothyroidism or antithyroid drugs and radioiodine therapy in hyperthyroidism. Thyroid function test monitoring is a requirement for successful management, ensuring that treatment is tailored to the specific needs of individual patients. Given the high prevalence of thyroid disease, proper awareness and diagnosis are essential components of a successful internal medicine practice (Leidi et al., 2025). The second area of prime importance of endocrine disorders is abnormalities of the adrenal glands that manifest as diseases like Cushing's syndrome and Addison's disease.

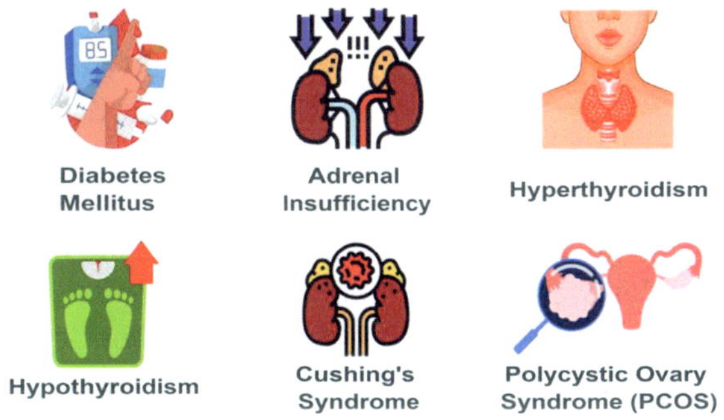

Figure 6.5. Common endocrine disorders.

Source: https://cdn.shopify.com/s/files/1/0789/3781/7379/files/25.png?v=1720715274.

Cushing's syndrome due to excess cortisol production usually has a presentation of features such as central obesity, hypertension, and glucose intolerance, with possible development of a variety of metabolic derangements. Addison's disease, which is characterized by underproduction of adrenal hormones, can have a presentation of lethargy, loss of weight, and hypotension. Understanding the basic pathophysiology of these disorders is vital for accurate diagnosis and management. Treatment would be surgical treatment in

Cushing's or hormone replacement therapy in Addison's disease. Also, recent evidence suggests a relationship between autoimmunity and adrenal disease, and the need for further exploration of the role of immune modulation in treatment strategies. As our understanding of these disorders advances, clinicians can better handle the intricacies involved in adrenal disorders, ultimately leading to better patient outcomes in the practice of internal medicine for endocrinology (Figure 6.5).

6.2.1. Diabetes Mellitus: Types and Management

Diabetes Mellitus is primarily categorized into three types: Type 1, Type 2, and diabetes in pregnancy. Type 1 diabetes is characterized by an autoimmune destruction of the beta cells in the pancreas that release insulin, thereby causing an absolute insulin deficiency. Type 1 diabetes is most commonly diagnosed in adolescents or children, but it may be diagnosed at any age. In contrast, Type 2 diabetes, the more prevalent form, is defined by insulin resistance and a relative insulin deficiency. It is frequently associated with obesity and lack of exercise. Gestational diabetes is encountered during pregnancy and is linked to various maternal and fetal complications, and it must be well-managed. The global emergence of diabetes has produced significant public health concerns, with nearly 100 million people projected to be diagnosed with the disorder. This emphasizes the importance of public awareness and education on its forms and impact on health (Ambrosiadou et al., 2000). Effective Diabetes Mellitus control is crucial in sustaining blood glucose control and preventing complications. Glycemic control assessment remains a high priority, with the majority of patients using home glucose monitoring systems and frequent consultations with healthcare providers to assess HbA1c levels. Several pharmacologic treatments, including insulin therapy in Type 1 diabetes and oral antihyperglycemic agents in Type 2 diabetes, exist. Lifestyle changes—dietary modifications and physical exercise—are also significant components of management, particularly of Type 2 diabetes. In addition to helping achieve optimal glycemic control, lifestyle changes can prevent complications, thereby enhancing the patient's quality of life. Furthermore, new technologies, including insulin pumps and continuous glucose monitors, have transformed the treatment of diabetes and have given patients additional strategies for managing their disease (Ambrosiadou et al., 2000). Lifestyle modification, particularly in at-risk populations, cannot be stressed too incredibly. Obese and overweight women, for example, are at extremely high risk for developing gestational diabetes mellitus (GDM), and accordingly, lifestyle prevention programs are highly relevant. Evidence shows that quality education and care have a significant impact on women's ability to control their health during pregnancy. Pregnant women have been shown to report the need for accurate information regarding their own risk of developing GDM, and this can motivate them towards adopting healthier lifestyles. However, perceived barriers like pregnancy-related fatigue and time constraints, especially on the mother's part, serve as barriers towards implementing these lifestyle modifications. Therefore, healthcare professionals must engage pregnant women in discussions of customized lifestyle changes based on their individual circumstances to prevent and manage gestational diabetes effectively.

6.2.2. Thyroid Disorders: Hypothyroidism and Hyperthyroidism

Thyroid illnesses, hypothyroidism, and hyperthyroidism are significant in influencing general health due to the role of thyroid hormones in controlling metabolism, growth, and development. Hypothyroidism, or a deficiency of thyroid hormone secretion, often causes a variety of symptoms such as tiredness, weight gain, depression, and cold intolerance. Diagnoses are usually made based on elevated thyroid-stimulating hormone (TSH) and decreased free thyroxine (T4). Ongoing treatment involves hormone replacement therapy with levothyroxine. Untreated, hypothyroidism can cause severe complications, including cardiovascular complications, myxedema coma, and impairment of mental processes, particularly in older patients whose clinical presentation may already be compromised by comorbid illnesses. Hyperthyroidism, in contrast, results from overproduction of thyroid hormone, with associated findings of weight loss, anxiety, tremors, and heat intolerance. Conditions such as Graves' disease or toxic adenomas are common etiologies of hyperthyroidism.

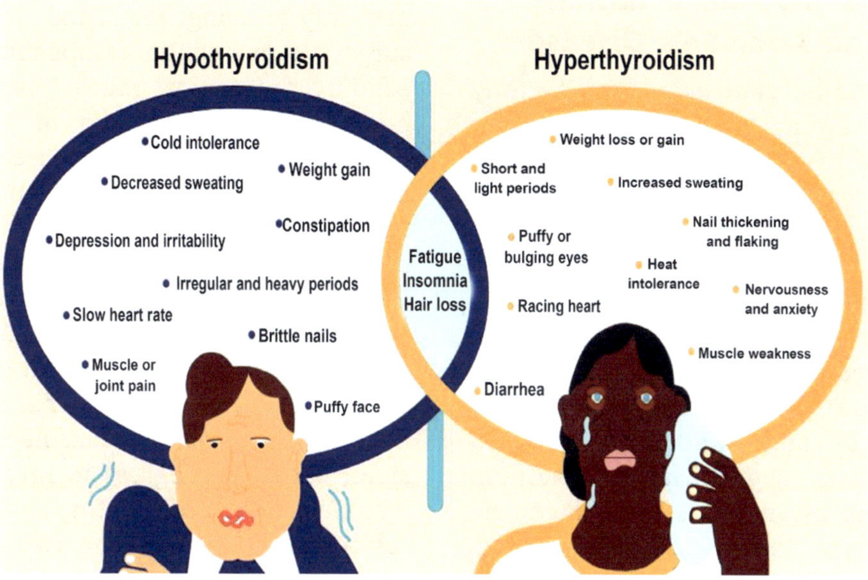

Figure 6.6. Thyroid Disorders: Hypothyroidism and Hyperthyroidism.

Source: https://www.verywellhealth.com/thmb/XBdgIUhlNw6AmO55fwqyP5joQ28=/1500x1000/filters:no_upscale():max_bytes(150000):strip_icc()/Hypothyroidism-hyperthyroidism-5180646_final-82b76c2edd074f59aa005f72ba2a3994.jpg.

Diagnosis typically involves clinical evaluation, with elevated free T4 and suppressed TSH. Treatment is successful with antithyroid medications, radioactive iodine ablation, or, in some situations, surgical resection of half of the thyroid gland. One of the important aspects of treating hyperthyroidism, particularly among older patients, is hormone level control to prevent osteoporosis and thyroid storm, both of which have a significant impact on the patients' quality of life and overall healthcare outcomes. Furthermore, the interrelation of thyroid diseases with other diseases accounts for their common implications. Notably, hyperthyroidism also has a bone component, with high thyroid hormone levels contributing to lower bone mineral density, particularly in postmenopausal women. They are at an increased risk of fragility fractures, added to by reduced bone density owing to the effect of excess thyroid hormones on remodeling processes. In contrast, hypothyroidism patients can also present with co-morbidities in the form of depression, a situation that is reinforced by the interplaying relationships between mental health and thyroid function. There is evidence that dysfunctional thyroid states in the form of subnormal T3 levels and disrupted TSH responses are common among depressed patients, affirming the need for integrated treatment protocols that find harmony between thyroid function and mental conditions (Azar et al., 2012). With further research, these relationships must be understood to create effective, multidisciplinary care for patients in endocrinology (Barbagallo et al., 2016) (Figure 6.6).

6.2.3. Adrenal Disorders: Cushing's Syndrome and Addison's Disease

Disorders of the adrenal gland significantly impact endocrine function, Cushing's syndrome and Addison's disease being graphic examples. Cushing's syndrome, defined by the long-term exposure to inappropriately elevated cortisol, can be caused either by endogenous origins, including adrenal adenomas, or exogenous glucocorticoid administration. On a clinical note, patients usually present with weight gain, hypertension, and glucose intolerance, accompanied by more specific signs and symptoms such as purple striae and plethora of the face. The diagnosis is often made by biochemical tests such as 24-hour urinary free cortisol or late-night salivary cortisol measurement. Effective management typically involves a multidisciplinary approach, including endocrinologists, surgeons, and primary care physicians, to tailor treatment programs aimed at restoring hormonal balance and preventing associated comorbidities in subjects with complex adrenal disease. Addison's disease, however, is defined as adrenal hormone deficiency, predominantly due to autoimmune adrenal cortical cell destruction. The disease results in severe clinical manifestations, including fatigue, weight loss, hyperpigmentation, and hypotension. Of significance is the fact that the diagnosis of Addison's relies almost entirely on hormone studies showing low serum cortisol and elevated adrenocorticotropic hormone (ACTH) levels. Those afflicted with the disease may frequently need lifelong hormone replacement with glucocorticoids and mineralocorticoids to provide sufficient physiological function. Since a crisis of the adrenals is a possibility, educating the patient about stress management and the necessity to change medication during illness or surgery is an essential component of treatment, echoing the critical mutual responsibility of healthcare professionals in the successful treatment of Addison's disease. The need for discovery and appropriate management of these adrenal disorders cannot be overstated since they have the potential for considerable morbidity. The interplay between Cushing's syndrome and Addison's disease underscores the dazzling complexity of adrenal physiology and the consequences of hormonal imbalance. For instance, chronic hypercortisolemia in Cushing's syndrome may progress to secondary adrenal insufficiency, demonstrating a cause-and-effect relationship between the two conditions. In addition, the growing awareness of autoimmune associations with adrenal insufficiency, as well as related complications such as metabolic syndrome and thromboembolic events, underscores the necessity for continued research and clinical suspicion. The managerial approaches outlined in contemporary literature target the imperative to personalize treatment protocols, synchronizing advances in diagnostic technology and therapeutic interventions to maximize patient outcomes within adrenal disorders (Nicola et al., 2022; Santos et al., 2025).

Test Your Knowledge

1. What are the most common disorders of the endocrine system?
2. How does hormonal imbalance affect normal body functions?

6.3. Diagnostic Approaches in Endocrinology

Learning Outcome

1. Understand the laboratory tests for hormone levels
2. Discuss the imaging techniques for endocrine evaluation
3. Define the clinical assessment and patient history

Endocrinology practice relies on practical diagnostic approaches to diagnose and manage the majority of hormonal disorders. Traditional methods have mainly concentrated on biochemical tests and imaging techniques in evaluating endocrine function. Blood hormone measurements, e.g., insulin, cortisol, and thyroid hormones, are standard equipment in the diagnostic workup. Radiologic tests such as MRI and ultrasound help visualize glandular anatomy to detect tumors or other pathology. Advances in individualized medicine methods further validate the efficacy of diagnosis, enabling tailored treatment programs for each patient's profile. The addition of genetic and epigenetic factors to diagnostic tests has also opened new horizons in understanding complex endocrine illnesses, highlighting the importance of developing methodologies in the field (Pandey, 2024). Artificial intelligence (AI) is increasingly becoming a key tool in endocrinology diagnostics. By working on large datasets, AI algorithms can identify patterns and correlations that are not visible to human practitioners, thereby enhancing diagnosis. A recent study found that physicians who used AI tools achieved improved diagnostic accuracy and therapeutic outcomes, particularly across various internal medicine specialties, including endocrinology (Mansoor et al., 2024). The ability of AI to interpret clinical data alongside genetic data or imaging reports is a significant step towards better diagnostics. Alongside this, however, comes the question of the algorithms' interpretability and transparency, which can affect trust among physicians and patient outcomes. As AI continues to evolve, its application in endocrinology must be met with hope and cautious optimism if best outcomes are to be achieved.

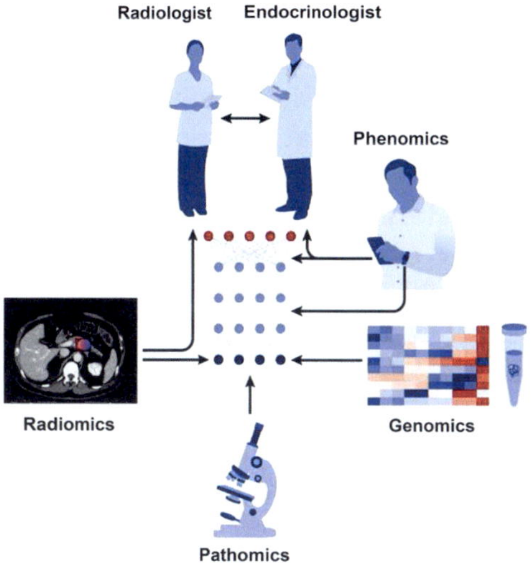

Figure 6.7. Diagnostic approaches in endocrinology.

Source: https://media.springernature.com/full/springer-static/image/art%3A10.1038%2Fs41574-021-00543-9/MediaObjects/41574_2021_543_Fig1_HTML.png.

Furthermore, the application of extensive biomarker panels in the diagnostic workup of endocrine diseases is more common. Such panels may help uncover hormone imbalances and metabolic dysfunctions, enabling a more accurate understanding of a patient's endocrine status. For instance, biomarker assessment of adrenal, calcium metabolic, or thyroid function can diagnose Addison's disease or hyperthyroidism with greater precision. Additionally, advances in point-of-care testing methods provide faster diagnoses to improve patient management in acute. However, the challenge lies in integrating these practices into clinical environments to ensure uniformity and consistency in results. As the endocrinology environment continues to evolve with advances in science, clinicians need to stay up to date with the latest diagnostic equipment to provide the best patient care possible (Pandey, 2024) (Figure 6.7).

6.3.1. Laboratory Tests for Hormone Levels

Laboratory testing of hormone levels is a pillar of endocrinology that enables the diagnosis and management of a wide range of endocrine disorders. Hormone imbalances may manifest as various clinical presentations, such as menstrual disorder, metabolic syndrome, or reproductive disorder, and thus necessitate precise and comprehensive testing. Laboratory measurements for hormone assays typically include quantification of substances such as follicle-stimulating hormone (FSH), luteinizing hormone (LH), estradiol, and sex hormone-binding globulin (SHBG). Integrate these hormone levels into forecasting models, as shown in investigations using machine learning platforms, to enhance early detection power, particularly for illnesses such as Polycystic Ovary Syndrome (PCOS). Such advances allow clinicians to identify at-risk patients in advance and initiate the appropriate therapeutic interventions to prevent downstream health consequences associated with hormonal dysregulation (Zad et al., 2024). In addition, advances in laboratory testing have shifted the focus from mere detection of aberrant hormone levels to a better understanding of the molecular mechanisms of endocrine disease. Current diagnostic methods require a multidisciplinary approach, in which the clinician must interpret complex hormonal patterns alongside genetic and clinical data. For instance, differentiating between Type I and Type II diabetes isn't merely a matter of measuring insulin and blood glucose levels but also of interpreting the genetic influences on these disorders. This integrated strategy emphasizes the need to select appropriate tests based on patient demographics and potential endocrine disorders, as outlined in landmark research on optimal testing practices (Grigorescu, 2010). Such considerations are crucial in reducing diagnostic delay and ensuring appropriate treatment planning.

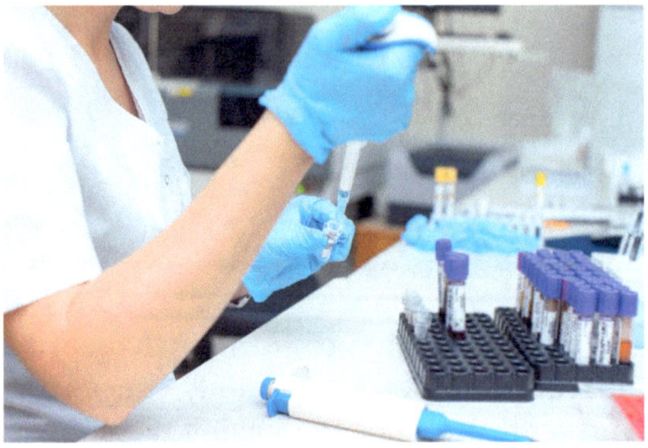

Figure 6.8. Laboratory tests for hormone levels.

Source: https://chapelhillhormonetherapy.com/wp-content/uploads/2022/07/AdobeStock_244908924.jpeg.

Also, developments in genetic testing and personalized medicine have revolutionized laboratory practice in the handling of hormone-related disease. Endocrinologists today must navigate a set of sophisticated tests designed to clarify the genetic origins of various endocrine disorders. For instance, congenital hypothyroidism and Multiple Endocrine Neoplasia tests not only enable accurate diagnosis of these conditions but also guide treatment that is specific to patient profiles. With the evolution of the specialty, the salient interest in educating clinicians regarding the various tests and their implications must be sustained. Without full awareness of laboratory assays and interpretation, clinicians are exposed to the risk of using ineffective treatment strategies. The present era of pharmacogenomics highlights the incorporation of expertise in genetic diagnostics to enable endocrinologists to maximize patient outcomes and embrace the challenges of modern hormonal therapies (Figure 6.8) (Grigorescu, 2010).

6.3.2. Imaging Techniques for Endocrine Evaluation

Endocrine disorder evaluation relies heavily on advanced imaging modalities, which have advanced significantly to enhance diagnostic yield. One of the most important areas of focus is thyroid gland evaluation, where ultrasonography is an essential modality for the primary thyroid nodule work-up. Ultrasound's strength lies in its real-time imaging and nodular feature evaluation. While there is wide interobserver variability in interpreting ultrasound results, numerous classification systems, including AACE/ACE/AME and ACR, have been established to improve assessment consistency. These not only grade the probability of malignancy but also guide the decision for FNA biopsy. More agreement among observers, especially after targeted training, has been reported, demonstrating that uniform protocols can greatly enhance diagnostic reliability in the evaluation of thyroid pathologies. In contrast to ultrasonography, however, other imaging tests have essential functions to fulfil in the full endocrine evaluation. MRI and CT are increasingly used in the evaluation of complex endocrine disorders, particularly adrenal disorders and pituitary adenomas. These modalities provide superior visualization of soft-tissue anatomy and are particularly useful for localizing disease processes spreading from the initial area of interest. For instance, MRI plays a crucial role in the identification of pituitary adenomas and in assessing their impact on surrounding anatomical structures. Further, newer imaging modalities can be combined in multichannel applications, capitalizing on each modality's strengths to enhance diagnosis. These techniques continue to evolve and hold the potential for even more accurate management plans tailored to each patient's pathology. Lastly, the role of functional imaging in endocrinology cannot be overemphasized, especially in differentiated thyroid cancer (DTC). The evolving pattern of imaging modality has transformed the follow-up and management of patients with DTC, focusing on dynamic assessment of recurrence risk. Current imaging modalities yield both structural change and metabolic activity data, allowing clinicians to tailor post-treatment surveillance optimally. As established in existing studies, modalities such as Positron Emission Tomography (PET) combined with CT play a central role in detecting metastatic disease that is not readily evident on conventional imaging. This combined modality not only helps with accurate staging but also impacts therapeutic intervention, highlighting the central relationship between imaging technology and clinical outcome in endocrine evaluation (Deandreis et al., 2016; Cantisani et al., 2017).

6.3.3. Clinical Assessment and Patient History

Clinical assessment of a patient's history in the practice of internal medicine for endocrinology is the secret of successful therapy and diagnosis. A thorough patient history not only reveals pertinent symptoms but also identifies risk factors and comorbidities that may influence endocrine disorders. Physicians must delve into a patient's medical history, including family history, lifestyle, and prior medical treatments. Such detailed questioning helps build a more informed clinical picture, which can guide subsequent testing and imaging schedules. For instance, awareness of a patient's diabetic history can direct the clinician's focus to the disease's complications and treatment, enabling targeted interventions that improve patient outcomes. In addition, adding structured tools and evaluation to the clinical assessment process deepens the patient history. Applying uniform risk assessment models, such as those that have been investigated in multidimensional studies of venous thromboembolism (VTE), may lead clinicians to categorize patients on their personal risk profiles. For example, the Shijitan Risk Assessment Model (SJT RAM) has been shown to have higher predictive power for VTE in inpatients of internal medicine than other models, thereby enabling personalized interventions for different patient populations (Chen et al., 2024). This is a result of the authority that detailed information about past health events and prevalent risk factors provides, driving individualized medicine in endocrinology. It ultimately favors clinicians by enabling them to make decisions about the management of endocrine disorders based on effective, efficient treatment measures. In addition, emerging modalities such as point-of-care ultrasound (PoCUS) enhance clinical assessment by providing real-time diagnostic information, with the potential to alter patient care dramatically. In a prospective study, it was found that multi-organ PoCUS performed within the first 24 hours of hospitalization yielded helpful diagnostic information in nearly 28% of patients, with significant therapeutic changes in over 19% of these patients (Casado-lópez et al., 2022). These findings highlight the importance of integrating advanced diagnosis techniques into routine clinical assessment, especially for conditions prevalent in endocrinology, such as thyroid disorders or adrenal illness. By leveraging the potential of such diagnostic techniques, healthcare professionals can refine knowledge of a patient's status, correspondingly modify treatment protocols in a timely manner, and thereby enhance patient outcomes within the scope of internal medicine (Figure 6.9).

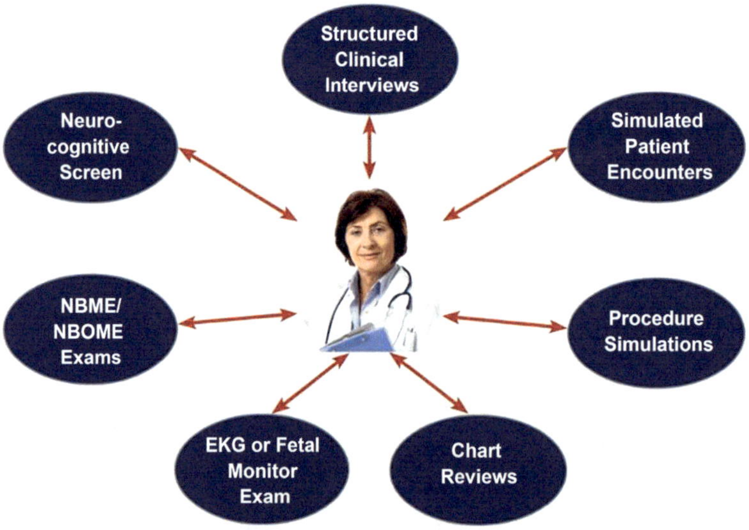

Figure 6.9. Clinical assessment and patient history.

Source: https://external-content.duckduckgo.com/iu/?u=http%3A%2F%2Fwww.cpepdoc.org%2Fwp-content%2Fuploads%2F2016%2F10%2FassessmentflowchartwithChartReviews-1030x713.png&f=1&nofb=1&ipt=81d4b9ebb61102d96a241a7014b5e0e14cd0a69425f0c0a5a6c2ca692255e2ee.

Test Your Knowledge

1. What laboratory tests are commonly used to diagnose endocrine disorders?
2. Why are hormone level assessments important in endocrinology?

6.4. Treatment Modalities in Endocrinology

Learning Outcome

1. Discuss on pharmacological interventions
2. Identify the lifestyle modifications and patient education
3. Describe the surgical options for endocrine disorders

The treatment modalities in endocrinology consist of a range of methods tailored to manage various hormonal disorders. One of the most prevalent is hormone replacement therapy (HRT), which is essential for individuals with deficiencies arising due to conditions such as hypothyroidism or hypogonadism. HRT aims to restore hormone levels to normal, along the way alleviating symptoms and reducing the risk of comorbidities that could be associated. Moreover, the integration of cutting-edge technologies, including artificial intelligence and machine learning, is revolutionizing the monitoring and modulation of treatment responses. These technologies make treatment more personalized, enhancing patient compliance and therapeutic success. Using evidence-based information, healthcare providers can better personalize HRT therapy to address individual patient needs, thereby improving quality of life and reducing healthcare costs (N/A, 2025). In addition to HRT, endocrine disorder treatment may involve pharmacotherapy in certain conditions. Medications such as metformin for diabetes and antihypertensive drugs for endocrine disorder-induced hypertension provide an example of the magnitude of pharmaceutical interventions available. These treatments are not solely symptomatic; they also aim to address underlying hormonal imbalances that drive the development of the disease. For instance, for the disease polycystic ovary syndrome (PCOS), lifestyle modifications coupled with pharmacological treatments like ovulation induction medications recognize interdisciplinary practices in endocrinology. Also, an interprofessional approach to healthcare involving endocrinologists, primary care providers, and other specialists is necessary to provide comprehensive care, optimizing all aspects of a patient's health (Rosenberg et al., 2021). Surgical interventions also play an important role in the management of certain endocrine disorders, particularly when pharmacotherapy is ineffective or inappropriate. Disease states such as hyperparathyroidism or thyroid cancers are likely to require surgical ablation or removal to avoid complications and achieve homeostasis. Surgery offers more effective disease control in disease-refractory conditions, underscoring the need for a diversified approach in endocrinology. Additionally, patients with complicated rare genetic syndromes (CRGS) might have specific challenges, since the routine treatment modalities can prove insufficient. Establishment of specialty outpatient clinics aims to provide multidisciplinary adult care with CRGS, and the focus is on syndrome-specific, targeted treatment to achieve the best patient outcomes and reduce misdiagnosis and unnecessary therapy (Rosenberg et al., 2021) (Figure 6.10).

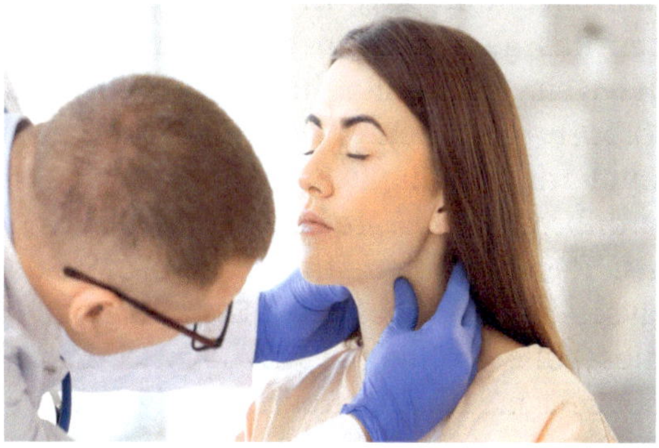

Figure 6.10. Treatment modalities in endocrinology.

Source: https://storage.googleapis.com/treatspace-prod-media/pracimg/u-1995/shutterstock_1757021699-1-1.jpeg.

6.4.1. Pharmacological Interventions

Pharmacotherapies are increasingly central to the management of endocrine disorders, significantly improving outcomes and quality of life for patients with these conditions. A prime example is the treatment of Type 2 diabetes, which now often involves a multidrug approach, using drugs from various classes. These include metformin, sulfonylureas, and newer agents such as GLP-1 receptor agonists and SGLT2 inhibitors, all of which work via distinct mechanisms of glucose metabolism. The use of continuous glucose monitoring (CGM) systems has proven to be an important adjuvant to pharmacotherapy, enabling real-time tracking of glycaemia variability and optimizing individual treatment plans. As presented, educational interventions among internal medicine residents have significantly increased their confidence in prescribing CGM, underscoring the growing need for an effective combination of pharmacological treatment and current technological innovations in diabetes management (Abbas et al., 2025). This union of drug and monitoring optimizes therapeutic efficiency and allows patients to act as protagonists in self-management programs. Pharmacologic therapy also plays a pivotal role in the management of other diseases such as non-alcoholic fatty liver disease (NAFLD), which has generated increasing interest due to its rising incidence linked to obesity and metabolic syndrome. Various therapeutic compounds, ranging from metabolic modifiers to antifibrotic drugs, are being studied in clinical trials. Recent systematic reviews and meta-analyses have emphasized the pathogenic role of metabolic profiling in NAFLD, with patterns of specific metabolites, particularly lipids and amino acids, associated with disease severity (Abbas et al., 2025). Even though the current pharmacologic treatment options are limited and generally not curative, they do represent a significant step towards the development of targeted treatments. Incorporation of metabolic signatures into treatment protocols can further individualize pharmacotherapy and optimize patient care in endocrinology. Last but not least, the establishment of pharmacological therapies in endocrinology has its challenges. The polygenic etiology of endocrine diseases necessitates a distinct awareness of individual patient histories to coordinate treatment accordingly. Existing research underscores the importance of standardized protocols to ensure the reproducibility of metabolic profiling for clinical use. Additionally, transitioning into daily practice remains problematic; barriers such as provider lack of awareness and variability in patient adherence to therapy can undermine the optimal achievement of outcomes. Educational interventions, such as the improved performance among internal medicine residents in using CGM, are needed to overcome these barriers and translate pharmacologic strategies across various clinical settings (Ponvilawan et al., 2025). Ultimately, ongoing research and education will determine the course of pharmacological management in endocrinology, enabling enhanced patient care and improved public health.

6.4.2. Lifestyle Modifications and Patient Education

Lifestyle modification is essential for the management of chronic endocrine diseases, including obesity and hormonal imbalance. Healthy dietary habits, physical activity, and weight control are not suggestions but interventions that can significantly enhance patient outcomes. Studies show that nutrition education can help patients make smart food choices, mitigating the effects of diseases such as Type 2 diabetes and metabolic syndrome. Furthermore, a supportive environment that encourages physical activity can help patients overcome exercise barriers, which are often the result of misinformation or social stigma about weight. Placing these changes in a broader health context is one way to create an upbeat message promoting long-term wellness habits that can enhance patients' treatment outcomes (Rubino et al., 2020). Patient education is an integral part of treating endocrine disorders because educated patients are more compliant with treatment and more willing to accept lifestyle changes. An effective education plan should be customized to the individual, taking into account their health issues, challenges, and goals. The use of visual aids, interactive classes, and regular consultation with healthcare providers may enhance learning and memorization. For chronic diseases like X-linked hypophosphatemia (XLH), in which misdiagnosis has a delaying effect, intensive educational strategies are all the more critical.

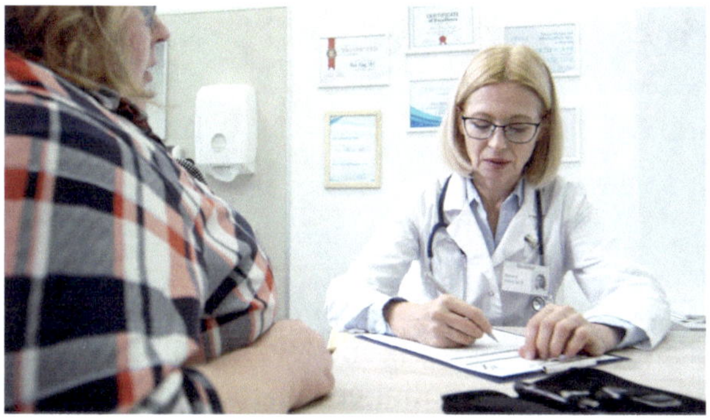

Figure 6.11. Lifestyle modifications and patient education.

Source: https://images.drlogy.com/assets/uploads/img/admin/blog/patient-counselling-lifestyle-modification.webp.

These interventions can underscore the complex nature of diseases and the importance of routine monitoring. Lastly, by providing patients with comprehensive information, healthcare providers can foster a sense of responsibility and autonomy, improve health outcomes, and reduce healthcare costs (Haffner et al., 2019). The integration of patient education and lifestyle change is not just desirable on an individual basis but can have broader public health effects. Through the alteration of societal perspectives and treatment of endocrine disorders, it is possible to deconstruct weight stigma and promote inclusivity. Healthcare professionals and policymakers must collaborate to establish programs that emphasize educating individuals about the impact of lifestyle choices and the societal constraints that surround them. Programs aimed at improving awareness of weight bias and its impact can help create a healthier environment for patients seeking to improve their health. Through promoting empathy and compassion within the healthcare system and among the population at large, these programs can ultimately lead towards a healthier population, establishing a culture in which lifestyle modification is embraced as an integral part of integrative patient care (Rubino et al., 2020) (Figure 6.11).

6.4.3. Surgical Options for Endocrine Disorders

Surgery is still a central method in the treatment of numerous endocrine diseases, especially when conservative management is inadequate. Hyperthyroidism, thyroid cancer, and adrenal tumors are some of the conditions that usually require surgical intervention. An example is thyroidectomy, where either part or all of the thyroid gland is removed in a patient presenting with malignancies or extensive hyperthyroidism. Surgical resection not only alleviates symptoms but also decreases the risk for cancer development, a significant consideration in the management of thyroid disease. Moreover, innovation in surgical techniques, including minimally invasive surgery, has decreased recovery time, minimized complications, and thus made surgery possible for a broader population of patients. Another area in which surgical therapy becomes essential is that of pancreatic endocrine tumors and insulinomas, with the ability to produce hyperinsulinemic hypoglycemia. These tumors have severe metabolic derangements, and treatment usually requires surgical resection. Despite the availability of medical management, the rarity of these conditions underscores the need for surgical treatment. The nuances of differentiating between a variety of hypoglycemic states demand a sensitive approach, and surgery provides both a therapeutic and diagnostic avenue for those who are having symptoms severely impairing the quality of their lives (Colao et al., 2016). The benefit of tumor excision is more than the risks of surgery in most cases if patients are otherwise healthy and can recover. Surgical intervention is not limited to resection only but may involve additional procedures, like adrenalectomy, which includes the removal of adrenal glands to manage Cushing's syndrome or pheochromocytoma. Such an operation can have a profound effect on endocrine function, and appropriate management in the postoperative period is crucial. Patients might require regular follow-up and supportive therapies to manage possible post-operative complications or hormonal imbalance that may ensue. Further, psychosocial support is beneficial after extensive surgical interventions, as hormonal level changes can impact mental health and wellness. Overall, surgery options are a significant, often life-altering part of endocrine disorder therapy in symptom relief as well as in effective correction of underlying pathological conditions. Individualized treatment with surgery and other interventions is, however, required for optimum benefit for the patient.

Test Your Knowledge

1. What are the common treatment options for managing endocrine disorders?
2. How does hormone replacement therapy help in endocrine diseases?

6.5. The Role of Technology in Endocrinology

Learning Outcome

1. Explain the advancements in diagnostic tools
2. Focus on telemedicine and remote patient monitoring
3. Define the emerging therapies and research in endocrinology

The application of technology to endocrinology has revolutionized the management and diagnosis of endocrine diseases. New imaging technologies, such as MRI and CT scans, enable endocrinologists to visualize tumors and assess hormonal imbalance with high precision. These technologies enable non-invasive testing, reducing the need for exploratory surgery significantly and enabling timely intervention. Moreover, laboratory technologies, including high-throughput screening and mass spectrometry, make it easy to test for hormones, enabling quick, accurate measurement of hormone levels. Not only does this technology enhance diagnostic skill, but it also enables more personalized treatment. By combining patient-specific data with new technologies, endocrinologists can now tailor therapeutic regimens to ensure the best possible outcomes for patients with endocrine disease. Moreover, telemedicine is an essential tool in endocrinology, particularly because it helps overcome the hurdle of patient accessibility. Through virtual consultations, endocrinologists can treat patients in remote locations, bypassing geographic limitations, and improve follow-up in chronic diseases, such as diabetes and thyroid disease. It facilitates patient activation and ongoing tracking, which are required for coping with complex endocrine illnesses. Secondly, the use of mobile health apps and wearable technologies provides real-time information regarding patient health parameters, enabling anticipatory adjustments to treatment regimens. With smooth coordination between patients and healthcare professionals, telemedicine represents a shift towards a more participative model of care that empowers patients while ensuring timely interventions, which are critical in managing their health.

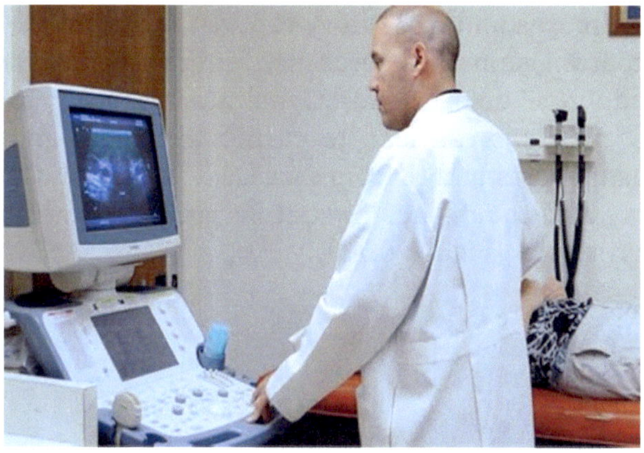

Figure 6.12. Role of technology in endocrinology.

Source: https://external-content.duckduckgo.com/iu/?u=https%3A%2F%2Ftse4.mm.bing.net%2Fth%2Fid%2FOIP.3J-xCJ8s7R4d_FBQVC98cwHaEn%3F pid%3DApi&f=1&ipt=85c58cf471215f9bfe6d525bddafc8fbfefb00910cdc0800 b9ea01fdc383f9cb.

Lastly, emerging technologies, such as machine learning and artificial intelligence (AI), will further transform endocrinology practice. These technologies enhance the precision of diagnosis by analyzing vast amounts of data to identify patterns that human clinicians may miss. For instance, AI algorithms can improve the accuracy of diagnosing insulin resistance and adrenal insufficiency. Moreover, AI platforms have tremendous potential for predicting patient response to various treatment regimens, enabling more effective, individualized therapeutic regimens. As endocrinology increasingly embraces such technologies, future research and investment will undoubtedly yield a greater understanding of endocrine disorders, ultimately improving patient outcomes. The potential for technological innovation in endocrinology underscores the need to integrate these tools into clinical practice, setting the stage for an era of personalized, data-driven medicine (Figure 6.12).

6.5.1. Advancements in Diagnostic Tools

The landscape of diagnostic tools in endocrinology has changed dramatically, with improvements that not only enhance precision but also the patient's experience. Among the technologies, imaging is exceptional. For instance, gamma cameras have come to play a pivotal role in nuclear medicine, giving information about the physiological action of endocrine glands. These gamma-ray detectors, which convert gamma rays into images, evolved from rudimentary designs to sophisticated machines with advanced imaging software and solid-state detectors. This evolution has yielded improved image quality and diagnostic accuracy, particularly in cardiology and endocrinology, where precise assessment of hormone-secreting glands is crucial. These advances underscore the importance of technology-based imaging modalities in the diagnosis of endocrine disorders, ultimately leading to more individualized and effective treatment protocols. Echocardiography, another invaluable diagnostic tool, is an example of the innovative approaches becoming increasingly popular in internal medicine for endocrinology. The cardiology manpower crisis is to be addressed through a pilot curriculum for physician assistants (PAs), according to the American College of Cardiology. This is expected to further PAs' skills in performing and interpreting echocardiograms, expanding healthcare practitioners' capability to diagnose cardiovascular conditions that may be entangled with endocrine issues, such as hypertension due to hormonal imbalance. Interactive blending of didactic online instruction and supervised clinical practice can lead to echocardiographic proficiency and, subsequently, enhanced patient care. By making such diagnostic equipment more accessible to more medical professionals, the healthcare system can better address heightened demand and provide timely, accurate evaluations for patients with complex endocrine illnesses. The integration of artificial intelligence (AI) into diagnostic platforms represents a paradigm shift in how endocrinology benefits from technology to improve patient outcomes. AI-powered algorithms are being developed to search massive volumes of medical data, enabling early detection and tailored treatment regimens. These technologies not only promise greater accuracy but also improve efficiency in interpreting complex diagnostic images and laboratory reports. For example, AI can significantly enhance the interpretation of data from gamma cameras and echocardiography, thereby streamlining the diagnostic process in endocrine disease. Additionally, AI's ability to recognize patterns that may not be visible even to clinicians can lead to earlier treatment and improved disease management for conditions such as diabetes and thyroid disease. With advances in technology, these diagnostic tools will increasingly find their place in routine practice, with a multidimensional approach to patient care in endocrinology (Figure 6.13).

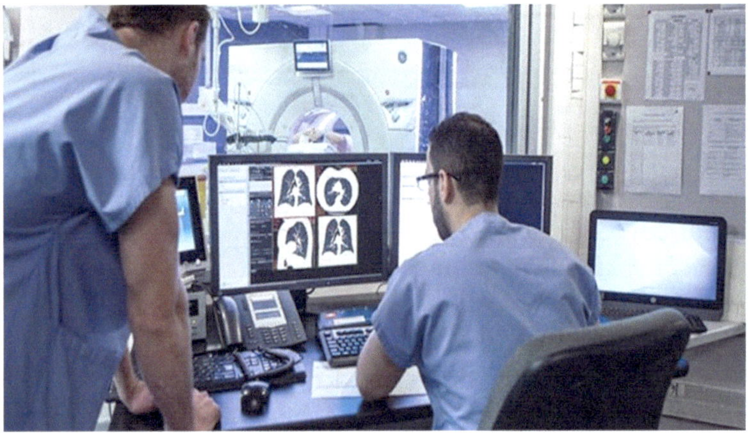

Figure 6.13. Advancements in diagnostic tools.

Source: https://www.healthcareoutlook.net/wp-content/uploads/2022/03/AI-based-Medical-Diagnostic-Tools-800x400.jpg.

6.5.2. Telemedicine and Remote Patient Monitoring

The integration of telemedicine and remote patient monitoring is a breakthrough in chronic disease treatment in internal medicine, particularly in endocrinology. In addition to enabling healthcare professionals to monitor patients' health parameters in real time and from remote locations, such technologies also enhance the effectiveness of clinical care. Telemonitoring, for instance, facilitates regular blood glucose monitoring in patients with diabetes. This continuous monitoring not only enables prompt intervention but also empowers patients to be engaged participants in their care pathways. In addition, the cost savings from telemedicine allow healthcare systems to focus resources on high-risk populations, ultimately providing timely care to patients and reducing unnecessary hospitalizations (van Steenkiste et al., 2025). Furthermore, the problems arising from improper compliance with the treatment underscore the need for robust monitoring systems. Medication non-adherence is a chronic obstacle to managing chronic illnesses and amplifies complications and healthcare costs (Garanin et al., 2025). Telemedicine offers solutions that enhance medication adherence through enhanced interaction between patients and healthcare providers. Telemonitoring devices are often equipped with reminders and educational content to help patients adhere to treatment plans. The coordination of tools, such as the COP-25 questionnaire, enables the effective measurement of patient compliance. The coordination not only streamlines data collection but also provides healthcare providers with valuable information about individual patients' behavior, thereby enabling more customized treatment approaches. Furthermore, telemedicine in endocrinology has a bright future, with ongoing advancements aimed at improving the effectiveness of care delivery. Enhancing telemonitoring programs involves an objective analysis of alert systems and the formulation of personalized algorithms that can detect potential health risks and provide preventive guidance. By analyzing alert information from telemonitoring schemes, healthcare practitioners can personalize their interventions and lower preventable alert levels, which may burden patients and healthcare providers. Finally, the establishment of an infrastructure for effective telemonitoring not only enhances patient health outcomes but also aligns with the evolving needs of the 21st-century healthcare landscape, serving as a step in the right direction for chronic disease management and patient activation (van Steenkiste et al., 2025).

6.5.3. Emerging Therapies and Research in Endocrinology

Endocrinology is undergoing a significant revolution due to new therapies and research. One of the most promising developments is the refinement of hormone replacement treatments (HRTs), particularly in disorders like diabetes and thyroid disorders. HRTs are now tailored to individual patient profiles based on genetic, environmental, and lifestyle determinants.

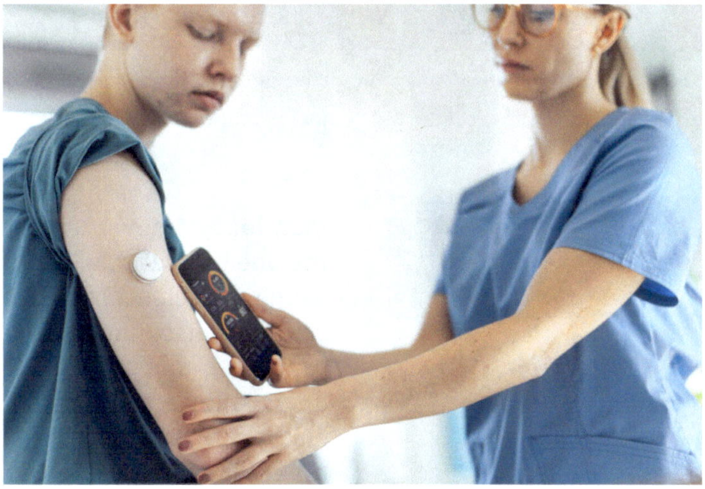

Figure 6.14. Emerging therapies and research in endocrinology.

Source: https://wp04-media.cdn.ihealthspot.com/wp-content/uploads/sites/464/2024/03/iStock-1796960382-1.jpeg.

This increases treatment efficacy and minimizes side effects, a primary concern in the treatment of endocrine disorders. Additionally, advances in drug delivery systems are making it possible to deliver therapies more selectively, thereby achieving improved therapeutic benefits with reduced risk of side effects, a valuable factor in the context of chronic endocrine disorders. Finally, the convergence of epigenetics and molecular genetics is revolutionizing diagnosis in endocrinology. Research is unearthing intricate interconnections between genetic mutations and hormonal diseases, enabling more precise diagnosis. For instance, the discovery of biomarkers has enabled early diagnosis and well-defined treatment regimens for diseases such as polycystic ovary syndrome (PCOS) and insulin resistance. This evolution towards precision medicine not only enhances diagnostic selectivity but also facilitates proactive treatment of endocrine disease, reducing the burden of complications from delayed diagnosis. Moreover, with ongoing research in these areas, the prospects for developing innovative therapeutic drugs that specifically target individual hormonal pathways are increasingly likely, with improved patient outcomes for those suffering from hormone-related diseases (Tereda, 2025). The quest for new treatments also extends to immunotherapy and its application in endocrinology, namely in the treatment of autoimmune illnesses such as Addison's disease and Graves' disease. New evidence suggests that modulating the immune response is a promising new area of treatment. Research is now investigating the use of biologics to dampen the underlying autoimmune process, promising better control of these chronic diseases. On top of that, new therapeutic technologies, such as CRISPR gene editing, are under investigation to repair the genetic defects underlying certain endocrine diseases, theoretically eradicating disease at the molecular level. Not only do these technologies highlight the utility of interdisciplinary research in endocrinology, but they also portend an era in which specialized treatments can dramatically improve quality of life in patients, combining efficacy and safety into treatment protocols (Tereda, 2025) (Figure 6.14).

Test Your Knowledge

1. How has technology improved the diagnosis and monitoring of endocrine disorders?
2. What role do digital tools play in the management of diabetes and other hormonal diseases?

6.6. Challenges in Endocrinology

Learning Outcome

1. Discuss the managing chronic endocrine diseases
2. Identify the addressing disparities in healthcare access
3. Understand the impact of obesity and lifestyle factors on endocrine health

Endocrinology is afflicted with numerous challenges, particularly in coping with the complexity and diversity of endocrine disease. Among the significant challenges is the lack of sound systems for systematically assessing the physician workforce in this subspecialty. As mentioned above, no national system akin to the one the National Science Foundation uses to gauge the scientific community exists. This gap creates a disconnected view of clinical research capability and personnel dynamics, watering down efforts to enhance clinical practice and endocrinology research. Without comprehensive, timely information to inform decision-making, the potential for endocrinologists to make a significant contribution towards clinical advancement is kept in check. Having a national workforce assessment system is crucial to improving buildings and to ensuring endocrinologists are provided with the optimal tools and information to address the evolving issues of this medical specialty (Bach et al., 2011). A second top challenge in endocrinology is the management of prevalent conditions, such as polycystic ovary syndrome (PCOS), affecting a high percentage of women. The complexity of PCOS, including its multifactorial aetiology, presents huge barriers to effective diagnosis and management. Owing to the integration of traditional diagnostic criteria, the absence of a definitive cure compels more difficulties in management. Weight reduction remains a pivotal intervention, but the variability of symptomatology of PCOS necessitates customized treatment plans addressing individual patient needs. This multidimensionality of the disorder underscores the challenge of designing integrative approaches that address not only weight regulation but also concomitant metabolic and reproductive disturbances. Finally, advancing PCOS and its treatment as a science remains a key challenge for endocrinologists seeking to optimize patient outcomes (Ghazeeri et al., 2021). This intersection of endocrinology and advancing research fields also makes the politics of challenges to practitioners more challenging. With each new finding about the genetic and environmental determinants of endocrine disorders, endocrinologists are confronted with the task of adapting their practice to utilize this knowledge in patient care. The rapid pace of scientific progress often outstrips practitioners' access to relevant information, creating gaps in understanding and use. Overcoming these challenges requires a concerted effort to expand educational materials and to sustain continuous professional development activities for endocrinologists. Besides, promoting coordination among clinical settings and research institutions can bring scientific discoveries into practice. Filling the knowledge gap by ensuring clinical practices align with the latest research will enable endocrinologists to manage the myriad problems characteristic of this dynamic field more effectively.

6.6.1. Managing Chronic Endocrine Diseases

Chronic endocrine disorders present significant clinical management challenges, necessitating an interdisciplinary approach integrating medical, nutritional, and psychological management. Careful management is crucial, as these disorders are likely to cause a range of complications that affect the quality of life and overall health of patients. Regular monitoring of hormone levels, titration of therapy, and patient education are the cornerstones of endocrine management. Diabetic patients, for example, need to have their glycemic control monitored continuously, and the dose of insulin or oral hypoglycemic medication titrated to individual needs. The individualized care not only avoids acute complications, e.g., diabetic ketoacidosis, but also avoids chronic sequelae such as neuropathy or cardiovascular disease, all of which emphasize the need for an active and individualized management plan in chronic endocrinology. The importance of nutrition in the treatment of chronic endocrine diseases cannot be overstated, particularly in conditions such as diabetes and thyroid disease. A combined meal plan that accounts for macronutrient intake and fiber can have a profound impact on disease progression and patient outcomes. In the case of diabetes, higher glycemic index foods, increased intake of complex carbohydrates, and greater soluble fiber intake play a beneficial role in glycemic control by slowing satiety, which decreases glucose absorption. The best dietary modification is also linked to beneficial results for patients' health and quality of life and reduced complications based on research in many settings, including acute pancreatitis, by maintaining intestinal barrier homeostasis and reducing the risk of infection. These nutritional nuances underscore the need for an individualized nutritional program, underscoring the relationship between diet, endocrine regulation, and overall health in the management of chronic endocrine disorders (Badiali et al., 2019). Psychosocial factors also play a significant role in the regulation of chronic endocrine disorders. Patients typically have various types of emotional and psychological challenges, including anxiety and depression, which may also play a significant role in affecting their adherence to treatment regimens. Institutions that support care models, including counseling and support groups, will help address such issues and enhance health behaviors. In addition, health providers must establish a collaborative relationship with patients through open communication of their disease and treatment modalities to achieve adherence. As management strategies are being fine-tuned, it is important to operate within the biopsychosocial model and to foster a global approach that integrates medical treatment with psychological and social care. This multifaceted approach will not only improve clinical outcomes but also allow patients to become active stakeholders in their health and chronic endocrine disease management (Dear et al., 2020) (Figure 6.15).

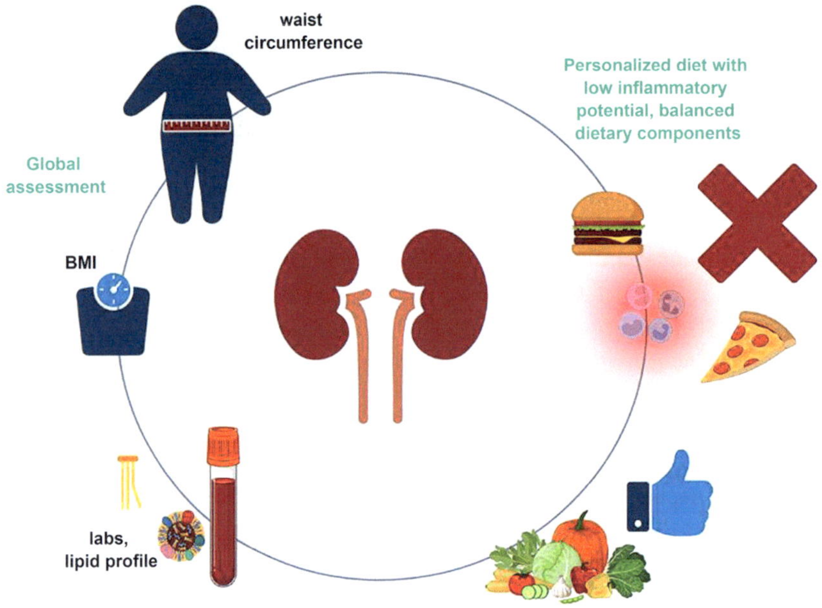

Figure 6.15. Managing chronic endocrine diseases.

Source: https://www.frontiersin.org/files/Articles/1212700/fnut-10-1212700-HTML-r1/image_m/fnut-10-1212700-g001.jpg.

6.6.2. Addressing Disparities in Healthcare Access

Overcoming disparities in healthcare access in internal medicine, specifically in the subspecialty of endocrinology, is essential to improving outcomes among diverse populations. Recent statistics indicate a disconcerting disparity: only 0.21% of editorial board members of top internal medicine journals come from low-income countries, while 89.8% come from high-income countries. This disparity is significant to note, given that this may represent broader issues in healthcare systems contributing to inequality, such as diminished access to relevant research and clinical practices for vulnerable groups. To enhance such inequities, enacting policies that increase the visibility and input of low- and middle-income country research and local voices is essential to enhance a more global approach towards healthcare with an indirect impact on endocrinology by enhancing equitable dissemination of clinical skills and knowledge to influence policy and practice worldwide (Singh et al., 2025). Additionally, systemic variation in postgraduate medical education, particularly in internal medicine, directly impacts access to and the quality of healthcare. In India, the extreme variation in the availability of residency programs, in terms of both numbers and quality, compared to resource-rich countries like the United States, severely restricts the scope of training for future internists and endocrinologists. Current evidence indicates that graduate medical education is heavily skewed, creating bottlenecks in the delivery of healthcare workers with the capacity to address complex medical issues, including endocrine diseases. The resulting shortage of trained internists exacerbates inherent healthcare inequalities, particularly among rural and underserved populations, where long-term illness tends to be underdiagnosed and undertreated. Encouraging equal training opportunities can improve the delivery and outcomes of healthcare, thereby meeting the urgent demand for endocrinology specialists (Nadella et al., 2025). Lastly, strategies need to be implemented comprehensively to close these gaps in healthcare access, especially in endocrinology. Strategies could include boosting research and medical education funding in low-resource settings, incentivizing collaborative partnerships between institutions of high-income countries and low-income countries, and fielding technology solutions such as telemedicine. Such solutions have the potential to enhance access to endocrinological expertise needed to manage diseases such as diabetes and thyroid disease. In addition, engaging in capacity-building through collective training programs can empower local healthcare workers with the capabilities and competencies needed to meet the specific healthcare needs of the populations. These multidimensional approaches will enhance access and contribute to a staggering reduction in health disparities, ultimately driving the practice of internal medicine forward through improved equality (Nadella et al., 2025; Singh et al., 2025).

6.6.3. The Impact of Obesity and Lifestyle Factors on Endocrine Health

Obesity is an essential player in endocrine health, particularly in metabolic diseases such as polycystic ovary syndrome (PCOS). PCOS is one of the most prevalent endocrine disorders in reproductive-aged women, and while its etiology remains multifactorial and complex, obesity has now been definitively related to PCOS. First-line treatment for the symptoms of PCOS, such as insulin resistance, hirsutism, and infertility is often administered in the form of weight loss. Therapy of obesity through dietary modification—e.g., reduction of saturated fats and control of carbohydrate intake—may improve insulin sensitivity, thereby reducing many of the associated endocrine symptoms. During therapy, a normal lifestyle that includes regular physical exercise is a determining factor, as it not only aids weight loss but also promotes better metabolic health, thereby playing a role in overall endocrine function (Ghazeeri et al., 2021). Lifestyle, for example, diet and physical activity, has a direct bearing on endocrine health, particularly in the context of obesity disorders that set the stage for diabetes mellitus. Evidence in a rural sub-Saharan African environment revealed a striking association between the prevalence of obesity and diabetes, pointing to the increasing public health issue of obesity among this population. In a subsequent period, the data indicated a substantial rise in abdominal obesity, demonstrating its specific link with metabolic syndrome and diabetes. The findings underscore the need to promote preventive lifestyle interventions targeting diet and physical exercise to combat the rising prevalence of obesity and its consequent endocrine disorders. By encouraging healthier living, it is possible to reverse the direct impact of obesity on endocrine conditions such as diabetes, thereby mitigating health outcomes for sufferers (Evaristo-Neto et al., 2016). The overlap among obesity, lifestyle, and endocrine function highlights the need for collaborative intervention and prevention. Treatment of obesity with comprehensive lifestyle modification can yield significant improvement in endocrine function, underscoring the importance of internal medicine to endocrinology. For patients with difficulties involving diseases such as PCOS or diabetes, an individualized treatment plan involving diet counseling, exercise therapy, and routine medical care can yield satisfactory results. This interdisciplinary strategy, along with addressing weight management, optimizes the hormonal milieu, favoring quality of life and reducing the risk of long-term sequelae of endocrine disorders. Therefore, physicians and other health-care providers must accord high priority to lifestyle interventions in clinical practice, bearing in mind their dramatic impact on endocrine health in obese patients and related metabolic disorders.

Test Your Knowledge

1. What challenges do clinicians face in diagnosing endocrine disorders early?
2. How does long-term management complicate the treatment of chronic endocrine diseases?

SUMMARY

The results of the study in internal medicine on endocrinology underscore the importance of effective communication and family involvement. With the development of healthcare systems, the use of technology such as video calls has become a key facilitator of closing the patient-healthcare provider gap and the patient-family gap. Patients have desired greater involvement with healthcare providers, especially during hospital admission. This need is particularly important in situations where in-person visits are not feasible, underscoring the need for additional communication channels to optimize family support and engagement in the care process. Family members have articulated that adequate advice and technical assistance are essential to ensuring that such interactions are optimized and effective, thereby enabling them to become positive contributors to patient outcomes (de Braekt et al., 2024). Furthermore, improvements in education and training among healthcare professionals, particularly in the context of chronic illnesses such as Type 2 Diabetes Mellitus (T2DM), have a significant impact on endocrinology practice in internal medicine. Effectively planned continuing medical education (CME) activities have amply demonstrated their effectiveness in improving clinicians' knowledge and self-efficacy in using insulin replacement therapy. Evaluation of these educational programs has indicated improved clinical practice among learners, suggesting the need for continuous learning to keep pace with evolving treatment strategies. This, in addition to reflecting enhanced patient care management, further increases overall patient satisfaction and outcomes, underscoring the two-way interdependence between provider education and patient care management (Turell et al., 2020). In summary, evidence from clinician education and family participation points to primary care pathways to enhance endocrinological care in internal medicine. The combination of technological innovation and educational campaigns sets the stage for patient-centered practice to thrive. Keeping families engaged and health professionals well-trained will be essential in bringing about future change in endocrinology practice. By recognizing the importance of these issues, the healthcare system can better address the complex needs of patients and families, resulting in better health outcomes and quality of care in internal medicine and endocrinology. By putting these issues at top priority, we are ensuring that we are on the way to a more integrated and holistic form of providing healthcare.

Endocrinology is one of the most important subspecialties of internal medicine, focusing on the diagnosis and management of hormonal disorders and their effects on the body as a whole. The distinguishing feature of this specialty lies in knowledge of endocrine signaling pathways and the effects of endocrine disease. Diabetes, thyroid disease, and adrenal disease are examples of the variety and complexity of endocrine illnesses that impact patient health. Practitioners should apply an integrative style to symptom assessment and laboratory reports, consistent with the multifactorial etiology of endocrine disorders. Hence, careful comprehension of the underlying mechanisms and the interdependencies among various hormonal axes is essential to manage and treat the conditions efficiently, as per existing research on hormonal regulation and patient outcomes (Thillai et al., 2020). In particular, endocrine disease management often requires frequent coordination of care across multiple specialties, underscoring the need for a multidisciplinary model. Cardiovascular disease, metabolic derangement, as well as even oncologic disorders, can often directly result quite significantly from hormone imbalance and therefore require large-scale evaluations beyond just the levels of hormones. New research underscores the need to employ modalities that integrate clinical evaluation with contemporary diagnostic methods, including imaging and genetic testing. This interdisciplinary paradigm supports a thorough understanding of disease onset and presentation, which, in turn, can increase the precision of therapeutic strategies for specific patients, as indicated in state-of-the-art research within the field (Kondadi et al., 2020). Furthermore, patient education and empowerment are essential factors in the management of endocrine disorders. The complexity of treatment protocols, for example, insulin therapy with injections for diabetes or hormone replacement for thyroid disease, necessitates that patients grasp their conditions and participate in their treatment plans. Inter-generational dialogue between healthcare professionals and patients can solidify treatment adherence and improve outcomes. Moreover, the evolving context of tailored medicine, driven by genetic and lifestyle factors, offers room for differentiated treatments that address personal risk profiles. This shift not only facilitates improved patient engagement but also reflects a broader valuation of endocrine well-being as part of overall wellness within internal medicine (Thillai et al., 2020).

KEY TERMS FROM THIS CHAPTER

- Hormones
- Pituitary Gland
- Thyroid Gland
- Adrenal Glands
- Insulin
- Diabetes Mellitus
- Hypothyroidism
- Growth Hormone
- Estrogen
- Endocrine Glands
- Hypothalamus
- Parathyroid Glands
- Pancreas
- Glucagon
- Hyperthyroidism
- Cortisol
- Testosterone
- Metabolism

CRITICAL THINKING QUESTIONS

1. **A 35-year-old woman presents with weight loss, palpitations, and heat intolerance. Her thyroid is diffusely enlarged. Which of the following is the most likely diagnosis?**
   a. Hashimoto's thyroiditis
   b. Subacute thyroiditis
   c. Graves' disease
   d. Toxic multinodular goiter
2. **Which of the following electrolyte abnormalities is most commonly associated with Addison's disease?**
   a. Hypernatremia and hypokalemia
   b. Hyponatremia and hyperkalemia
   c. Hypercalcemia and hypophosphatemia
   d. Hypomagnesemia and hypernatremia
3. **Which hormone is secreted in excess in acromegaly?**
   a. Insulin
   b. Prolactin
   c. Growth hormone
   d. Cortisol
4. **Which of the following is the first-line treatment for a patient with type 2 diabetes mellitus?**
   a. Insulin
   b. Sulfonylureas
   c. Metformin
   d. DPP-4 inhibitors
5. **A "moon face," central obesity, and purple striae are classic signs of which endocrine disorder?**
   a. Addison's disease
   b. Hyperthyroidism
   c. Cushing's syndrome
   d. Acromegaly

Short Answer Questions

1. What are the primary functions of the endocrine system in the human body?
2. Name three common endocrine disorders.
3. What diagnostic tools are commonly used to assess endocrine function?
4. How is hormone replacement therapy used in the treatment of endocrine disorders?
5. What role does imaging play in diagnosing endocrine gland abnormalities?
6. How has technology improved the management of endocrine conditions such as diabetes?
7. What are some key challenges faced in diagnosing and treating endocrine disorders?

Answers to Critical Thinking Questions

1. (c); 2. (b) ; 3. (c); 4. (c); 5. (c)

REFERENCES

1. Abbas, S. M., Hussain, Z., Asghar, N., Shabbir, M., Akhlaq, M. A., Mughal, H. M. F., Hussain, A., Asif, A. E., & Mzahri, E. U. H. (2025). Schematic assessment of metabolic signatures of non-alcoholic fatty liver disease by bridging endocrinology and internal medicine: a precision Therapy-Based Meta-Analysis. *Cureus, 17*(4), e83133. https://doi.org/10.7759/cureus.83133Adelantado, J. M., Andersen, L. L., Bertolotto, A., Bunn, F., et al. (2016). Beliefs, barriers and preferences of European overweight women to adopt a healthier lifestyle in pregnancy to minimize risk of developing gestational diabetes mellitus: An explorative study. https://core.ac.uk/download/42366567.pdf (accessed on 16th July 2025).
2. Ahmed, S. F., Bryce, J., Jiang, J., Kourime, A., et al. (2017). An assessment of the quality of the I-DSD and the I-CAH registries–international registries for rare conditions affecting sex development. https://core.ac.uk/download/80697838.pdf (accessed on 16th July 2025).
3. Ambrosiadou, B. V., Gogou, G., Goulis, D., Shankaramani, R., et al. (2000). Decision support methods in diabetic patient management by insulin administration neural network vs. induction methods for knowledge classification. https://core.ac.uk/download/1661424.pdf (accessed on 16th July 2025).
4. Aslam, J., Sohailuddin, M., Abbas, S. M., Shaikh, M. T. A., Saleem, S., Mubeen, A., Ahmad, B., et al. (2025). The schematic assessment of vitamin D deficiency in relation to autoimmune disorders and its implications in internal medicine. *Cureus, 17*. https://www.semanticscholar.org/paper/89908be9d781d65e0600ff982047b32b762e1eb6 (accessed on 16th July 2025).
5. Bach, M. A., Cappola, A. R., Desjardins, C., Ehrenberg, D., et al. (2011). Dissecting the workforce and workplace for clinical endocrinology, and the work of endocrinologists early in their careers. https://core.ac.uk/download/19958844.pdf (accessed on 16th July 2025).
6. Badiali, D., Bruno, G., Ribichini, E., Rossi, A., et al. (2019). Role of fiber in nutritional management of pancreatic diseases. https://core.ac.uk/download/231748461.pdf (accessed on 16th July 2025).
7. Barbagallo, M., & Dominguez Rodriguez, L. (2016). Fragility fractures in older persons with altered thyroid function. https://core.ac.uk/download/98111654.pdf (accessed on 16th July 2025).
8. Black, P. H. (1981). *Centre Scope*. https://open.bu.edu/bitstream/2144/21093/1/Centerscope1981v12n1_web.pdf (accessed on 16th July 2025).
9. Cantisani, V., Durante, C., Grani, G., Lamartina, L., et al. (2017). Interobserver agreement of various thyroid imaging reporting and data systems. https://core.ac.uk/download/141696499.pdf (accessed on 16th July 2025).
10. Capiau, S., Stove, C., & Velghe, S. (2016). Opening the toolbox of alternative sampling strategies in clinical routine: A key-role for (LC-)MS/MS. https://core.ac.uk/download/84043363.pdf (accessed on 16th July 2025).
11. Casado-López, I., Tung-Chen, Y., Torres-Arrese, M., Luordo-Tedesco, D., Mata-Martínez, A., Casas-Rojo, J., Montero-Hernández, E., et al. (2022). Usefulness of multi-organ point-of-care ultrasound as a complement to the decision-making process in internal medicine. *Journal of Clinical Medicine, 11*. https://www.semanticscholar.org/paper/433542ad22a8bb9fc54272ec24cde10f24ab8f51 (accessed on 16th July 2025).

12. Chait, A., & den Hartigh, L. J. (2020). Adipose tissue distribution, inflammation and its metabolic consequences, including diabetes and cardiovascular disease. *Frontiers in Cardiovascular Medicine, 7*. https://doi.org/10.3389/fcvm.2020.00022 (accessed on 16th July 2025).
13. Chen, X., Shi, H., Chang, J., Guo, W., Yang, Y., Wang, Y., & Pan, L. (2024). External validation of the risk assessment model of venous thromboembolism in multicenter internal medicine inpatients. *Clinical and Applied Thrombosis/Hemostasis, 30*. https://www.semanticscholar.org/paper/e7fea547296f8717646339048a5e998366393a8a (accessed on 16th July 2025).
14. Colao, A., Faggiano, A., Pia, A., Pizza, G., Davi', M. V., Guarnotta, V., et al. (2016). The treatment of hyperinsulinemia hypoglycemia in adults: An update. https://core.ac.uk/download/80166445.pdf (accessed on 16th July 2025).
15. Courty, P., & Marschke, G. (2025). On the sorting of physicians across medical occupations. https://core.ac.uk/download/pdf/7141445.pdf (accessed on 16th July 2025).
16. Cryan, J. F., O'Riordan, K. J., Cowan, C. S. M., Sandhu, K. V., Bastiaanssen, T. F. S., Boehme, M., Codagnone, M. G., et al. (2019). The microbiota-gut-brain axis. *Physiological Reviews, 99*, 1877–2013. https://doi.org/10.1152/physrev.00018.2018 (accessed on 16th July 2025).
17. Davis, S. R., Gompel, A., Lumsden, M. A., Pinkerton, J., et al. (2017). Managing menopausal symptoms and associated clinical issues in breast cancer survivors. https://core.ac.uk/download/96884955.pdf (accessed on 16th July 2025).
18. Deandreis, D., Durante, C., Filetti, S., Lamartina, L., et al. (2016). Endocrine tumors: Imaging in the follow-up of differentiated thyroid cancer: Current evidence and future perspectives for a risk-adapted approach. https://core.ac.uk/download/74318453.pdf (accessed on 16th July 2025).
19. Dear, J. D. (2020). Bacterial pneumonia in dogs and cats: An update. https://core.ac.uk/download/286361309.pdf (accessed on 16th July 2025).
20. Evaristo-Neto, A. D., Sumner, A. E., Ziraba, A. K., Melidonis, A. M., Sadiki, A., Baleke, A., Longo-Mbenza, B., et al. (2016). Obesity and diabetes mellitus association in rural community of Katana, South Kivu, in Eastern Democratic Republic of Congo: Bukavu Observ Cohort study results. https://core.ac.uk/download/74614012.pdf (accessed on 16th July 2025).
21. Garanin, A., & Trusov, Y. A. (2025). The program of remote compliance assessment based on the COP-25 questionnaire: A new telemedicine tool for remote assessment of treatment adherence. *Science and Innovations in Medicine*. https://www.semanticscholar.org/paper/37f449984f385f40010a98d231d00a2282dc5e3a (accessed on 16th July 2025).
22. Ghazeeri, G., Hmedeh, C., et al. (2021). Nutritional management in polycystic ovary syndrome: Challenges and opportunities. https://core.ac.uk/download/161103740.pdf (accessed on 16th July 2025).
23. Grigorescu, F. (2010). Genetic diagnosis of endocrine disorders. *Acta Endocrinological-Bucharest, 6*, 287–288. https://www.semanticscholar.org/paper/96759e343b71470d52a925c36d792a11b702fb90 (accessed on 16th July 2025).
24. Haffner, D., Emma, F., Eastwood, D. M., Biosse Duplan, M., Bacchetta, J., Schnabel, D., Wicart, P., et al. (2019). Clinical practice recommendations for the diagnosis and management of X-linked hypophosphatemia. *Nature Reviews Nephrology, 15*, 435–455. https://doi.org/10.1038/s41581-019-0152-5 (accessed on 16th July 2025).
25. In de Braekt, A., Coolen, C. M., Maaskant, J., de Man-van Ginkel, J. M., Eskes, A. M., & Jongerden,

I. (2024). Views of family members on using video calls during the hospital admission of a patient: A qualitative study. *Journal of Advanced Nursing*. https://www.semanticscholar.org/paper/aebeacb76798a0082121aa4f95651406eacdfede (accessed on 16th July 2025).

26. Khare, J., Kalra, S., & Jindal, S. (2023). Sociocrinology: Impact of social media on endocrine health–A review. *Indian Journal of Endocrinology and Metabolism, 27*, 480–485. https://www.semanticscholar.org/paper/c09e5d48d670ceb4ee91599fc2dde705dca6d771 (accessed on 16th July 2025).

27. Kim, J. H., Nam, Y., Kim, W. J., Lee, K. A., Baek, A., Park, J. N., Kim, J. M., et al. (2018). The effectiveness of multidisciplinary team-based education in the management of type 2 diabetes. *The Journal of Korean Diabetes, 19*, 119–133. https://www.semanticscholar.org/paper/787e89677a172d35b41bba7eb30c01e9e023c806 (accessed on 16th July 2025).

28. Kondadi, A. K., Anand, R., Hänsch, S., Urbach, J., Zobel, T., Wolf, D. M., Segawa, M., et al. (2020). Cristae undergo continuous cycles of membrane remodeling in a MICOS-dependent manner. *EMBO Reports, 21*. https://doi.org/10.15252/embr.201949776 (accessed on 16th July 2025).

29. Leidi, A., Porto, V., Mazza, T., Reinmann, M., Andreoli, G., Berner, A., Coen, M., et al. (2025). [Perspectives in internal medicine]. *Revue Médicale Suisse, 21*(903), 172–175. https://www.semanticscholar.org/paper/6bbd07b4f850cbece8cb3c54fa8ea7f936adcefc (accessed on 16th July 2025).

30. Mansoor, M. A., Ibrahim, A. F., & Kidd, N. (2024). The impact of artificial intelligence on internal medicine physicians: A survey of procedural and non-procedural specialties. *Cureus, 16*. https://www.semanticscholar.org/paper/dd8f6eff52fea5d1e88efa4a39b6632888d27a30 (accessed on 16th July 2025).

31. May, J. E., Paschal, R. D., Morris, J. L., & Willett, L. (2021). Choosing non-malignant hematologic care wisely: An educational pilot study for internal medicine residents. *Blood*. https://www.semanticscholar.org/paper/385e753f873888947c9fbed092e7eea7ec77b117 (accessed on 16th July 2025).

32. McCarty, R. (2020). *Evolution of the Stress Concept*. Oxford University Press eBooks. https://doi.org/10.1093/med-psych/9780190697266.003.0003 (accessed on 16th July 2025).

33. Mishra, A. (2024). Gamma cameras: Exploring the technology, applications, and future prospects. https://core.ac.uk/download/617006397.pdf (accessed on 16th July 2025).

34. Moon, S. (2017). Echocardiography curriculum development for physician assistants using entrustable professional activities. https://core.ac.uk/download/215924737.pdf (accessed on 16th July 2025).

35. N/A. (2010). *Staying Connected: A Progress Report: Reimbursement Under the Telemedicine Development Act of 1996*. https://core.ac.uk/download/71355210.pdf (accessed on 16th July 2025).

36. Nadella, N., & Edara, L. (2025). From primary care to super specialty: A comparison of workforce expansion and capacity building in internal medicine in India and the United States. *Cureus, 17*. https://www.semanticscholar.org/paper/70f65c9cdfeedec13ad5f51af0b1784c1c428fa6 (accessed on 16th July 2025).

37. Nicola, A., Carsote, M., Gheorghe, A., Petrova, E., Popescu, A., Staicu, A. N., Ţuculină, M., et al. (2022). Approach of heterogeneous spectrum involving 3beta-hydroxysteroid dehydrogenase

2 deficiency. *Diagnostics, 12*. https://www.semanticscholar.org/paper/8db5969dc71adc0aac2f75f4ee1ebb03c5369b13 (accessed on 16th July 2025).

38. Pandey, A. (2024). Advancements in endocrinology: Exploring novel therapies and diagnostic innovations. *Endocrinology and Disorders*. https://www.semanticscholar.org/paper/6ba69493122f605f17a8880b31bfe8e307c3da1e (accessed on 16th July 2025).

39. Ponvilawan, B., Mohammed, S., Wooldridge, D., Barthel, B., & Tselovalnikova, T. (2025). 1039-P: A quality improvement project to increase understanding and confidence in continuous glucose monitor utilization among internal medicine residents at a community-based primary care clinic. *Diabetes*. https://www.semanticscholar.org/paper/6b5c608761987bf618add1a136482e75d80a896b (accessed on 16th July 2025).

40. Rosenberg, A. G. W., Mochèl, K., Hähner, L. M., Ruules, L., Davidse, K., Bos-Roubos, A., van Dijk, S. A., et al. (2024). Endocrine and non-endocrine causes of fatigue in adults with Neurofibromatosis type 1. *Frontiers in Endocrinology, 14*. https://www.semanticscholar.org/paper/0d6b6452736b1e82f56e1a58fc3678b97223566a (accessed on 16th July 2025).

41. Rosenberg, A., Pater, M. R. A., Davidse, K., Kattentidt-Mouravieva, A., Kersseboom, R., Bos-Roubos, A., van Eeghen, A. M., et al. (2021). What every internist should know about rare genetic syndromes in order to prevent needless diagnostics, missed diagnoses and medical complications: Five-year experience of internal medicine for complex rare genetic syndromes. *Journal of the Endocrine Society, 5*, A513–A514. https://www.semanticscholar.org/paper/b2a905b3a4f7104c7ce635e168e7e4df5e8cb044 (accessed on 16th July 2025).

42. Rubino, F., Puhl, R. M., Cummings, D. E., Eckel, R. H., Ryan, D. H., Mechanick, J. I., Nadglowski, J., et al. (2020). Joint international consensus statement for ending stigma of obesity. *Nature Medicine, 26*, 485–497. https://doi.org/10.1038/s41591-020-0803-x (accessed on 16th July 2025).

43. Santos, M., Gago, L., Gama, C., Marques, B., Saldanha, T., Lourenço, M., Gonçalves, M., et al. (2025). Adrenal failure: When antiphospholipid syndrome leaves scars. *The Journal of Rheumatology*. https://www.semanticscholar.org/paper/54542cab0a49dc7203b4fc029eabb1f6d0729dbb (accessed on 16th July 2025).

44. Singh, J., Kumar, P., & Kumar, A. (2025). Global disparities and data transparency in editorial boards of prominent internal medicine journals including allied super specialities: A wake-up call. *Indian Journal of Medical Ethics*. https://www.semanticscholar.org/paper/6f10f5bdc5eee2cadc2d53a176b72e6dedfe58eb (accessed on 16th July 2025).

45. Tasleem, S. A., Pasha, S. O., Saffura, S., Begum, K., Khan, P. A., & Maheboob Mogle, A. B. (2025). Hairfall (*Intithar al Sha'r*) in Unani medicine: Exploring preventive and curative remedies–An overview. *International Journal of Innovative Science and Research Technology*. https://www.semanticscholar.org/paper/288baa88ba3d98b06e985ff952b11c03dc80ea4a (accessed on 16th July 2025).

46. Tereda, A. (2025). Advancements in pancreatic cancer management: From epidemiology to emerging therapies. *PriMera Scientific Medicine and Public Health*. https://www.semanticscholar.org/paper/28c7f532e239c693be4e1246ae0df403041b052f (accessed on 16th July 2025).

47. The role of artificial intelligence in early disease detection: Current applications and future prospects. (2025). *Global Journal of Emerging AI and Computing*. https://www.semanticscholar.org/paper/39ddbd51af5d7ad3b153a5277e03e8aca14fbbb2 (accessed on 16th July 2025).

48. Thillai, M., Atkins, C., Crawshaw, A., Hart, S. P., Ho, L. P., Kouranos, V., Patterson, K., et al. (2020). BTS clinical statement on pulmonary sarcoidosis. *Thorax, 76*, 4–20. https://doi.org/10.1136/thoraxjnl-2019-214348 (accessed on 16th July 2025).

49. Turell, W., Drexel, C., & Beaser, R. (2020). 669-P: Serial online education helps break down primary care practitioner barriers to insulin therapy for T2DM management. *Diabetes*. https://www.semanticscholar.org/paper/107f757a70d8bd3bf794e06a307f745044dd484f (accessed on 16th July 2025).

50. van Steenkiste, J., Lupgens, N., Kool, M., Dohmen, D., & Verberk-Jonkers, I. (2025). Alert reduction and telemonitoring process optimization for improving efficiency in remote patient monitoring programs: Framework development study. *JMIR Medical Informatics, 13*. https://www.semanticscholar.org/paper/05693e546dd801516c2679aef6e5cb9b6a1a5851 (accessed on 16th July 2025).

51. Ventura, N., & Soti, V. (2024). Integrating osteopathic principles for enhanced dermatological outcomes: A literature review. *Cureus, 16*. https://www.semanticscholar.org/paper/34ae2ae7727e4fff61d31af87f0a604196a3d7da (accessed on 16th July 2025).

52. Zad, Z., Jiang, V. S., Wolf, A. T., Wang, T., Cheng, J. J., Paschalidis, I., & Mahalingaiah, S. (2024). Predicting polycystic ovary syndrome with machine learning algorithms from electronic health records. *Frontiers in Endocrinology, 15*. https://www.semanticscholar.org/paper/27a313380b4e5e81cfeb11a5604710d3d0b0a4ec (accessed on 16th July 2025).

HEMATOLOGY

7

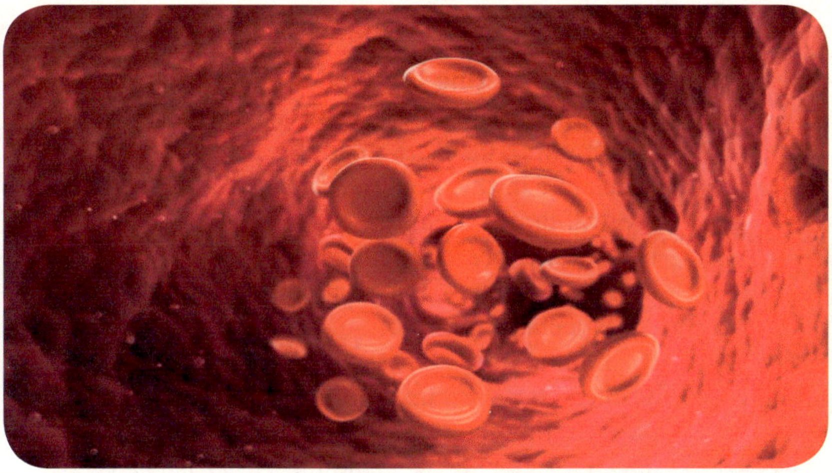

Introduction

Hematology-oncology (heme/onc) is an essential specialty in modern medicine, particularly given the rising prevalence of many malignancies, which significantly contribute to morbidity and mortality in the United States. Cancer is still the second most frequent cause of death, which emphasizes the necessity for effective education in this specialty among residents and medical students. Yet, while it is of extreme significance, there is a significant deficit in the didactic structures of formal education offered at medical schools, particularly during clinical rotations. Research shows that it is not unusual for medical students to feel uneasy about handling complex heme/onc dilemmas merely because actual clinical environments do not augment pre-clinical didactics. This lack of knowledge has a significant effect on their confidence in patient care, as was seen in revelations that students were less confident in knowing the treatment guidelines than in understanding the basics of cancer biology and diagnosis (Venugopal et al., 2024). Also, students' career-choice decisions by IM residents have a greater

LEARNING OBJECTIVES

After studying this chapter, you will be able to:

1. Understand the role of internal medicine in hematology
2. Explain the common hematological conditions
3. Discuss the diagnostic techniques in hematology
4. Focus on treatment modalities in hematology
5. Learn about challenges in hematological care
6. Evaluate the future directions in hematology

impact on the resultant hematology-oncology workforce. Growing evidence indicates that residency decisions can be affected by education exposure and immediate experience in the heme/onc specialty. In response to expanding needs for hematologist-oncologists, a static fellowship applicant volume implies a lack of alignment between interest and career choice.

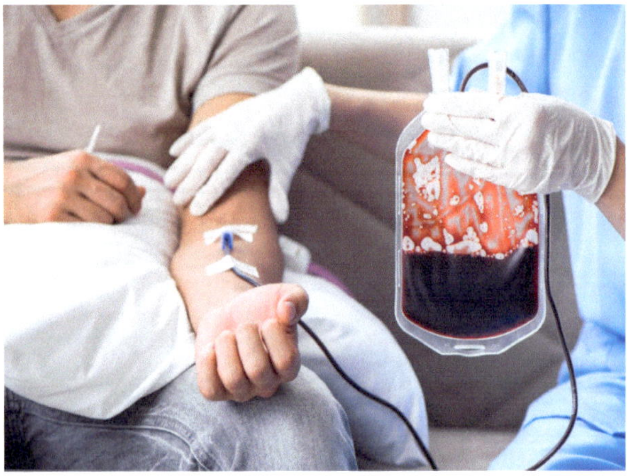

Figure 7.1. Internal medicine for hematology.

Source: https://www.news-medical.net/images/Article_Images/ImageForArticle_745_16624283204238538.jpg.

Results of surveys of IM residents offer complex motives and disincentives shaping their desire to pursue this specialty. Importantly, all recommend that increased exposure to heme/onc during their training would translate into increased interest, thereby helping mitigate the shortfall of doctors in this vital field of medicine (Parikh et al., 2024). In order to enhance the learning environment for future doctors practicing in this vital field of medicine, having organized and engaging curricula is most critical. As demonstrated by pilot programs to enhance heme/onc medical education, there exist focused lectures and laboratory learning experiences that can significantly improve knowledge levels as well as comfort levels among learners. These educational initiatives not only address gaps between theoretical foundations and clinical application but also aim to instill confidence among healthcare practitioners when dealing with patients with debilitating hematologic and oncologic conditions. With shifting horizons in medical education, it is all the more imperative to incorporate hematology-oncology training more comprehensively into the curriculum and thereby usher in a new generation of physicians better equipped to handle the intricacy of cancer care (Venugopal et al., 2024) (Figure 7.1).

Definition of Internal Medicine

Internal medicine is a field of medical practice that focuses on the prevention, diagnosis, and treatment of diseases in adults. Physicians who specialize in this field, referred to as internists, are trained to handle a wide range of medical issues and are particularly adept at treating patients with ongoing, complex conditions. This is a specialty based on a full understanding of the human body's systems and the interactions among the various organs. Through careful patient histories, physical examination, and advanced diagnostic techniques, internists strive to identify the etiology of diseases rather than merely their signs. The multidimensional nature of internal medicine enables comprehensive patient management, making it a crucial area of study in the health care setting, particularly in hematology, where intricate blood disorders require advanced knowledge (Linzer et al., 2022). One of the distinguishing characteristics of internal medicine is its focus on the patient as a whole rather than on individual symptoms. Such a holistic perspective is essential, especially in hematology, since diseases such as anemia and leukemia need a multifaceted approach to treatment. Internists collaborate with hematology experts to formulate treatment plans that succeed, monitoring the responses of patients to treatments closely and adapting interventions accordingly. Furthermore, internists play a central position in preventive medicine, emphasizing health education and lifestyle adjustments that are most critical in both hematologic and non-hematologic disorders. By engaging patients in their care, internists build an association that is vital for facilitating positive outcomes and long-term chronic disease management (Kiseleva et al., 2022). Besides, the evolving health care environment increasingly demands the application of technology and research. Internists must stay abreast of advancements in medical information, including new therapeutic techniques and diagnostic equipment introduced in hematology. As medical treatment becomes increasingly sophisticated, the demand for transparency and accountability in patient management increases. This is especially relevant when incorporating artificial intelligence and other high-tech technologies into clinical practice, where transparency can have a major influence on patient trust and quality of care. By accepting the ethical and pragmatic challenges that accompany our advances, internists consolidate their role not just as healers but as integral contributors to the ongoing evolution of healthcare systems, ultimately crafting improved lives for patients with diverse medical needs (Linzer et al., 2022).

Overview of Hematology

Hematology, as a fundamental subspecialty of internal medicine, is concerned with the study of blood and blood-forming organ diseases. Clinicians diagnose and manage a range of disorders from benign ailments, i.e., anemia, to malignant diseases like leukemia and lymphoma. An in-depth knowledge of hematology is necessary as pathologies of blood affect the whole body in terms of body systems. Also, blood ailments tend to present challenging diagnostic challenges that must be addressed through an integration of clinical findings, laboratory results, and patient history. Understanding the pathophysiology of hematologic disorders enables clinicians to develop an appropriate therapeutic approach and interventions, thereby improving patient outcomes. This reaffirms the importance of hematology training in internal medicine education, equipping medical practitioners with the necessary skills to address such challenges. Contemporary hematology practice emphasizes the need for early diagnosis and risk stratification in patients with blood disorders. For instance, the management of atherosclerotic cardiovascular disease (ASCVD) has progressively recognized Lipoprotein(a) (Lp(a)) as a risk factor in isolation. Unfortunately, there is widespread ignorance among internal medicine physicians about the need for Lp(a) testing, resulting in underutilization. Emerging evidence indicates that structured educational interventions, such as ASCVD risk assessment presentations, can enhance physicians' knowledge and comfort in applying Lp(a) tests. These initiatives have shown a significant increase in confidence and actual practice among residents and underscore the need for continuous education in hematology (Eidensohn et al., 2025). This necessity for successful training is indicative of the changing landscape of hematology, in which newer diagnostic and therapeutic developments require practitioners to stay up to date with the latest available information. Furthermore, the hematology curriculum must bridge gaps in medical education to improve the training of upcoming health professionals. Research has demonstrated that medical students lack confidence in managing complex hematologic and oncologic problems. Interactive lecture series programs have been found effective in enhancing students' knowledge and ease with hematology and oncology problems. For instance, targeted education sessions for disorders such as multiple myeloma and lymphoma resulted in statistically significant improvements in knowledge and self-assessed comfort levels among participants (Venugopal et al., 2024). This would mean that integrating comprehensive haematology education into clinical rotations not only promotes greater sensitivity to blood disorders but also spurs more competent and confident medical personnel to efficiently address public health challenges. As the field of hematology evolves, education systems must adapt to ensure that future physicians can manage these serious health conditions effectively.

Importance of Internal Medicine in Hematology

Internal medicine's contribution to hematology lies at the core, particularly in the management of complex hematologic diseases. Internal medicine specialists bring a holistic approach to such patients, who have multiple ailments caused by their hematologic disorders. This broad understanding enables targeted interventions that address not only specific hematological factors—such as anemia, coagulopathy, or blood malignancies—but also the broader range of medical comorbidities. As is evidenced by a study conducted in Iraq, among patients admitted to the internal medicine department, there was a high prevalence of red cell alloimmunization. Thus the necessity for experts who can handle this complexity is all the more present (Faisal et al., 2024). Understanding the interactions among different medical conditions and their hematologic manifestations is necessary to achieve optimal patient outcomes and prevent treatment complications. Training and education in hematology among internal medicine residents also highlights the importance of such overlap. Educational courses to enhance the knowledge and competence of internal medicine residents are significant, particularly in diagnosing and managing hematologic neoplasms effectively. A revised curriculum that applies a Reverse Morning Report approach demonstrates how formal learning environments can effectively close the knowledge gap between internal medicine residents when addressing hematological topics. The curriculum is case-based, focusing on specific hematologic diseases, where residents learn the nuances of diagnosis and management (Wallace et al., 2024). These educational frameworks not only enhance residents' capacity to manage challenging hematologic cases but also promote interdisciplinary collaboration between internal medicine and hematology specialists, thereby improving patient care and outcomes. Additionally, internal medicine and hematology are essential for the management of emergent hematologic complications that are likely to occur during treatment. For instance, patients undergoing chemotherapy for hematologic malignancies can develop life-threatening complications such as febrile neutropenia or tumor lysis syndrome. Internal medicine physicians typically take the lead in detecting and managing such emergencies due to their broad exposure to critical diseases and acute medical syndromes. The ability to detect and treat such complications in a timely manner can significantly improve patient survival and quality of life. Creating a solid collaboration between hematology and internal medicine not only facilitates whole-person care but also facilitates timely intervention that can avert unfavorable outcomes. Thus, this collaboration highlights the pivotal role of internal medicine specialists in efficiently handling hematology emergencies (Figure 7.2).

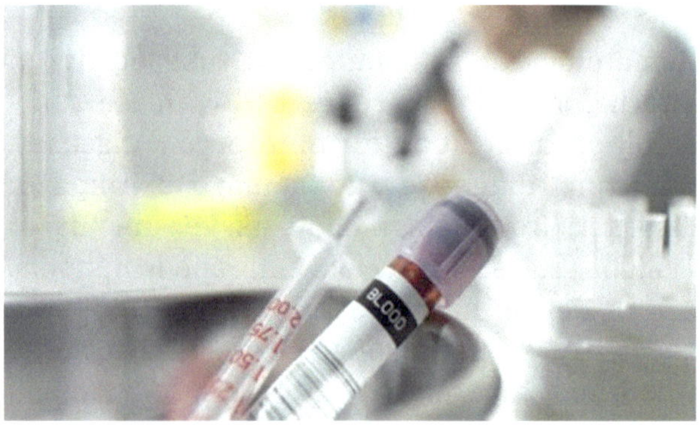

Figure 7.2. Importance of internal medicine in hematology.

Source: https://external-content.duckduckgo.com/iu/?u=https%3A%2F%2Ftse1.mm.bing.net%2Fth%2Fid%2FOIP.OuCM7VFKU4abi16mE4vJ1wHaEH%3Fpid%3DApi&f=1&ipt=4d974f9e63a755d7a67232872eeb23e7fa0dbc491a415b39bcc6d9e633901346.

7.1. Role of Internal Medicine in Hematology

Learning Outcome

1. Understand the diagnosis of hematological disorders
2. Define the management of chronic blood disorders
3. Describe the coordination of multidisciplinary care

Internal medicine lies at the heart of hematology, serving as a bridge between the general medical environment and the specialized interventions required for blood disorders. Internal medicine physicians are typically the first line of care a patient approaches when they present with a blood disorder, such as anemia, clotting disorders, or abnormal blood cell counts. This initial consultation is crucial for the appropriate diagnosis and early intervention. The high level of training internal medicine physicians receive enables them to consider a wide range of possible underlying conditions and, as a result, optimize patient results. The integration of internal medicine with hematology ensures that the patient benefits from an overall treatment approach for their condition, particularly when they have comorbidities that affect both blood health and overall disease resistance (Tavis et al., 2002, 2025). A central component of the hematology strategy under internal medicine is early detection and preventive medicine for hematologic diseases. Internal medicine doctors can identify risk factors, such as family history, lifestyle, and other illnesses, that predispose a patient to hematologic disease through thorough patient histories, physical examinations, and laboratory results. Early diagnosis and control of blood disorders such as chronic myelogenous leukemia or iron deficiency anemia can be highly aided by primary care settings through regular screening and lifestyle modification. Moreover, internal medicine physicians collaborate with hematologists to develop comprehensive treatment plans tailored to the specific needs of individual patients, further highlighting the importance of a multidisciplinary approach to caring for complex cases and achieving optimal patient outcomes in hematology (Tavis et al., 2002, 2025). Also, internal medicine's role in ongoing research and clinical trials is instrumental in broadening the practice of hematology. Internal medicine practitioners are often engaged in studies of innovative therapeutic approaches for blood diseases, guiding evidence-based practice that affects treatment protocols and patient care guidelines. The research is crucial to the development of new therapies and to improving patient outcomes in hematology, as the understanding of genetic and environmental factors affecting disease occurrence continues to evolve. In addition, as medicine advances toward precision medicine, the data derived from interactions between hematology and internal medicine will become central to the individualization of treatment models based on patient-specific profiles. Internal medicine, therefore, is an integral part of the ongoing evolution of hematological treatment and patient outcomes in this significant medical field (Tavis et al., 2002, 2025).

7.1.1. Diagnosis of Hematological Disorders

Hematology diagnosis of blood disorders is a complex, multi-faceted process that requires thorough knowledge of clinical assessment as well as laboratory examinations. CBC is typically the initial line of assessment and may detect abnormalities in red cells, white cells, and platelets. These are key indicators that guide physicians toward a potential diagnosis. For instance, low hemoglobin would suggest anemia, while an elevated white blood cell count would suggest leukemia or infection. Additional laboratory investigations, such as bone marrow biopsies, flow cytometry, and genetic studies, further enhance diagnostic precision, enabling personalized treatment plans. Such diagnostic investigation is incredibly critical since precise and early diagnosis of hematological disorders has a direct impact on the patient's outcome. The advent of molecular diagnostics has changed the diagnosis of hematological disorders. Innovation in genetic profiling, as in acute myeloid leukemia (AML), underscores the need to detect genetic mutations that cause disease. Recent research has yielded a comprehensive census of genes mutated in acute myeloid leukemia (AML). Our second challenge is to understand how this genetic diversity dictates the pathophysiology of AML and informs clinical practice. Awareness of these mutations not only aids diagnosis but also in prognostication as well as in therapeutic decisions.

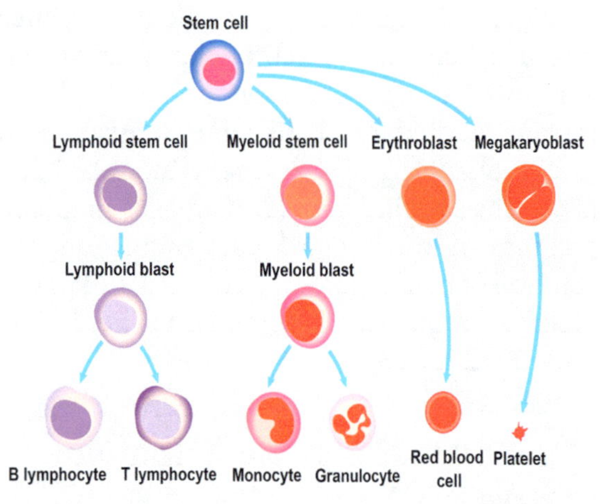

Figure 7.3. Diagnosis of hematological disorders.

Source: https://www.northerntrust.hscni.net//wp-content/uploads/2020/06/Diagram_showing_how_blood_cells_are_made_CRUK_125_svg.png.

Personalized medicine, with its focus on tailoring therapies for maximal effect based on a person's genetic profile, is the future of hematology diagnosis, enabling treatments that are both effective and specific to the individual's unique genetic environment. Secondly, the use of telemedicine in hematology has been an essential approach, especially brought to the forefront by the COVID-19 pandemic. When healthcare systems responded, remote consultation for hematological diagnosis became more widespread, creating opportunities for greater patient access to experts (Bashshur et al., 2020). A delivery model that reduced geographical limitations and enabled remote observation of chronic hematological diseases was implemented. Thus, telemedicine not only facilitates greater access to care but also allows earlier diagnosis of hematological diseases, triggering more timely interventions. Overall, the combination of traditional diagnostic methods with novel telehealth technologies presents an exciting roadmap for enhancing the precision and efficacy of hematological diagnosis, ultimately maximizing patient outcomes and experiences in internal medicine (Figure 7.3).

7.1.2. Management of Chronic Blood Disorders

The management of chronic blood disorders is a complex and multidisciplinary subspecialty of internal medicine, primarily hematology. Ailments such as CLL and other forms of anemia require specific therapeutic measures with attention to both symptomatic relief and disease progression. A 61-year-old female patient who experienced recurrent angioedema highlighted the significance of interprofessional communication in diagnosing and managing associated conditions, particularly when primary treatment like antihistamines and corticosteroids was unsuccessful. Additional workup diagnosed her lymphocytosis as CLL, to which Rituximab, a successful monoclonal antibody treatment, was administered. This case illustrates how precise diagnosis, along with a comprehensive management plan, can significantly reduce disease burden and improve the patient's quality of life, demonstrating the intricate interactions between chronic blood disorders and systemic complications (Kisakurek et al., 2021). Understanding the pathophysiology of chronic blood disorders is integral to proper management. For example, abnormalities in the normal production and regulation of blood components such as platelets and red blood cells can cause severe clinical issues. Chronic anemia, in most instances caused by nutritional inadequacies or chronic diseases, will necessitate a multidisciplinary approach that includes diet modification, supplementation, and, in some cases, transfusion. Alternatively, patients with diseases such as chronic myeloid leukemia can be treated with targeted drugs that block the activity of individual molecular pathways involved in disease formation. Regular checks of response to therapy and side effects remain crucial for optimizing treatment regimens for chronic blood disorders and achieving clinical outcomes aligned with patient-oriented goals (Motomura et al., 2018). The use of cutting-edge diagnostic tools and multidisciplinary care models makes the management of chronic blood disorders more effective. Modern hematology increasingly relies on devices such as flow cytometry and genetic analysis to inform management and monitor disease progression. Furthermore, multidisciplinary management involving hematologists, nutritionists, and other specialists is paramount for addressing the complex needs of patients with chronic blood conditions. Such a collaborative strategy not only improves clinical outcomes but is also conducive to increased patient education and involvement, facilitating informed decision-making on their treatment trajectory. As progress in medicine is made, the fusion of innovative therapy and holistic patient care will ultimately redefine the future of chronic blood disorder management, ultimately leading to better prognoses and increased quality of life for those with the disease (Kisakurek et al., 2021).

7.1.3. Coordination of Multidisciplinary Care

Effective multidisciplinary care coordination is a key to the management of complex hematological diseases. Hematology and internal medicine may include a range of specialists, from hematologists to nephrologists, nutritionists, and mental health professionals. Multidisciplinary care models enable effective patient management tailored to the complex needs of hematological patients. For instance, individuals with sickle cell disease may require coordination among various providers of health care to address physical, psychological, and social well-being. The multidisciplinary approach facilitates communication between specialties, fosters shared decision-making, and ultimately leads to improved health outcomes. The benefits of coordination of this kind are also more effectively realized in acute cases, where timely responses can contribute to patient prognosis and treatment outcomes, especially in high-burden systems like those experienced during the COVID-19 pandemic (N/A, 2020). Effective integration of evidence-based guideline use is also a major mechanism for leading multidisciplinary hematology care. As cited by the American Society of Hematology, these recommendations help prioritize interventions to prevent causation based on their relative clinical importance, ultimately to prevent the complications of conditions like sickle cell disease (DeBaun et al., 2020). By providing guidelines for routine screening and intervention for therapies, multidisciplinary teams are better placed to impose preventive treatment and intervention on time, accelerating the intervention of neurological morbidities and cognitive impairments that are endemic among patients who present with hematological disorders. This systematized strategy not only streamlines clinical procedures but also educates patients and their families through simplified channels of care and support, thereby enhancing the overall patient experience. Lastly, the challenges of managing multidisciplinary care must also be addressed, particularly where there are concerns regarding resource shortage and differentiated availability of care. The coordination of experts requires strong communication channels and organizational systems to function well, especially in health systems with high demand for services. During crises such as the COVID-19 pandemic, real-time information sharing and interprofessional collaboration became essential to address the immediate needs of hematology patients. Operations under these conditions provide valuable lessons in fostering resilience and flexibility in multidisciplinary teams. Future efforts should aim to develop innovative coordination strategies that keep patient-centered care at the center of hematology treatment, regardless of external pressures or systemic challenges (N/A, 2020).

Test Your Knowledge

1. How do internists assist in the early detection of hematological disorders?
2. What role does internal medicine play in managing anemia and bleeding disorders?

7.2. Common Hematological Conditions

Learning Outcome

1. Define the anemia: types and causes
2. Discuss the hemophilia: genetic considerations
3. Identify the leukemia: classification and treatment

Hematologic disorders include various diseases affecting blood cells and their production. Anemia, thrombocytopenia, and hemophilia are among the most common hematological disorders. Anemia due to red cell deficiency can result from various causes, including nutritional deficits, chronic disease, or bone marrow pathology. For instance, iron-deficiency anemia is prevalent and can be easily managed through dietary changes, supplementation, and addressing the root cause. In contrast, thrombocytopenia is characterized by reduced platelet counts, which can increase the risk of bleeding. It can be caused by conditions such as idiopathic thrombocytopenic purpura (ITP) or as a secondary issue of more intricate matters, including leukemia. Understanding the pathophysiologic processes involved in each of these conditions is important to permit effective treatment regimens and improved patient outcomes. The complicated interplay between hematologic complications and systemic diseases renders a holistic approach to diagnosis and treatment imperative. Chronic illness like diabetes or renal disease may have their treatment severely impacted by the occurrence of conditions such as anemia, and therefore require careful monitoring and adjustment in treatment by doctors. Hemophilia, a congenital defect in the coagulation system, is another example of how internal medicine requires a multidisciplinary approach. Hemophilia patients may suffer from spontaneous or excessive bleeding during surgery, and as such, healthcare professionals have to get specialists across disciplines to collaborate to provide adequate care. Collaboration with specialists in hematology and other disciplines can provide access to newer treatments and therapeutic interventions, thereby improving the patient's quality of life and addressing the multidisciplinary nature of these diseases. The development of new health complications, including infectious disease complications, has also advanced the study of hematological disorders. For example, recent studies have revealed the effects of SARS-CoV-2 on the hematopoietic system and uncovered such complications as thrombocytopenia and coagulopathy that contribute to unfavorable clinical outcomes. Venous thromboembolism and hemolytic anemia are now significant complications in COVID-19 patients that need close observation from healthcare providers. Furthermore, patients suffering from underlying hematological diseases are prone to exacerbation when they acquire such viral infections. The situation re-emphasises the central role internal medicine specialists play in managing common as well as emerging hematologic conditions, as they reprioritise therapies to provide well-balanced care amid escalating complexity and health risks. Understanding these interactions underpins coordinated, proactive healthcare interventions essential for optimal patient outcomes for internal medicine hematology (Kerna et al., 2024; Jogie, 2025) (Figure 7.4).

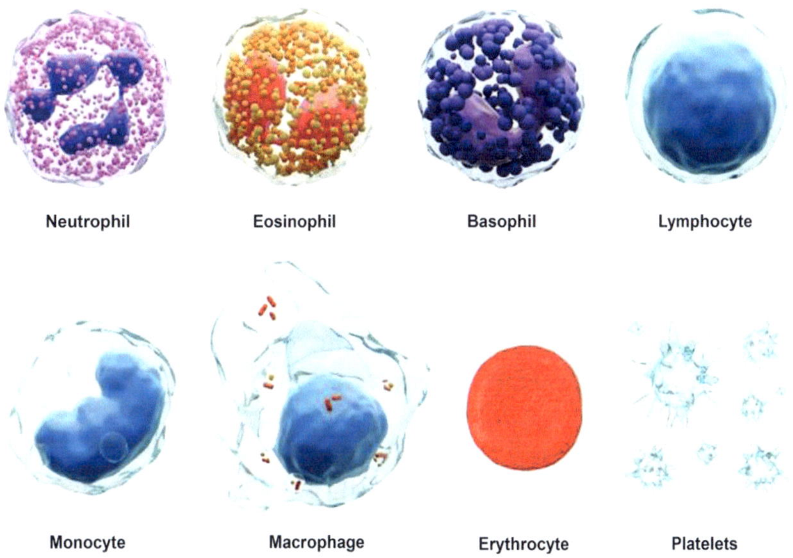

Figure 7.4. Common hematological conditions.

Source: https://www.news-medical.net/images/Article_Images/ImageForArticle_745_16624285963986525.jpg.

7.2.1. Anemia: Types and Causes

Anemia is a clinical syndrome characterized by a reduction in the number of red blood cells or in the hemoglobin content of red blood cells, leading to impaired oxygen delivery to tissues. This condition may be classified into many types based on etiology, each with its own pathophysiology. The most common of these are four: iron deficiency anemia, vitamin B12 deficiency anemia, aplastic anemia, and hemolytic anemia. Iron deficiency anemia occurs owing to inadequate intake or absorption of iron, while vitamin B12 deficiency anemia is often linked with poor dietary intake or malabsorption. Aplastic anemia arises from the failure of bone marrow, and hemolytic anemia arises from the premature destruction of red blood cells. Knowledge of both conditions is essential to proper diagnosis and treatment in internal medicine, particularly in hematology, because each has specific treatment approaches aimed at correcting its particular etiology. The causes of anemia are numerous and encompass nutritional deficiencies, chronic disease, genetic illness, and environmental toxins. Iron deficiency anemia is prevalent and can result from inadequate dietary intake, chronic blood loss, or increased physiological demands, such as during pregnancy. Vitamin B12 deficiency anemia can result from malabsorption disorders, such as pernicious anemia, in which intrinsic factor is lacking. Hemolytic anemia may be caused by an immune reaction to external agents, such as infections or drugs, or by intrinsic genetic factors, such as sickle cell disease. Also, chronic illnesses such as kidney disease may lead to anemia of chronic disease, a condition in which inflammation disrupts erythropoiesis. Anemia requires comprehensive analysis and awareness of its varied etiologies to develop an effective treatment plan that not only addresses symptoms but also the underlying etiology of the disorder. Awareness of the complexities of anemia and its varied manifestations is essential to improving patient outcomes in hematology. Determinants of these diseases can be complex and interrelated. For instance, genetic diseases like hereditary hemorrhagic telangiectasia (HHT) can have a significant impact on iron concentration depending on repetitive bleeding, which most often results in chronic anemia. Additionally, HHT patients can develop other medical conditions, such as arteriovenous malformations, which can lead to iron deficiency anemia due to increased blood loss. Identification of such associations underscores the importance of a multidisciplinary approach to managing anemia effectively. Individualizing treatment protocols based on accurate diagnoses, such as the use of transfusions for bleeding or supplementation for nutritional deficiency, is key to enhancing quality of life and overall patient outcomes in hematology practice (Jochen Rößler et al., 2021; Ajani et al., 2022).

7.2.2. Hemophilia: Genetic Considerations

The most significant characteristic of hemophilia is the lack of clotting factors, i.e., factor VIII in hemophilia A and factor IX in hemophilia B. These deficiencies are due to gene mutations, and their hereditary nature is central to the appropriate management and treatment. Genetic testing and counseling play a central role in identifying gene carriers of hemophilia, thereby helping families make reproductive choices. Because hemophilia is an X-linked recessive disorder, it would predominantly occur in males, while females can be carriers without being symptomatic. This genetic foundation underscores the need for early diagnosis and treatment, as improved gene therapy holds the promise of long-term outcomes. If one considers the genetic aspects of hemophilia, individuals and clinicians can better navigate the condition's complexities and optimize treatment options. New advances in gene therapy, such as the application of the CRISPR-Cas9 system, have introduced fresh hope for hemophilia treatment by gene-editing the underlying genetic flaws. Treatments using patients' own induced pluripotent stem cells (iPSCs) derived from peripheral blood mononuclear cells (PBMCs) may be a successful method of genetic correction, according to studies. By inserting human factor IX (hFIX) cDNA into specific genomic locations, consistent production of the required clotting factors can be ensured, and the lifetime dependence on replacement therapy can be eliminated. In addition, the safety profile of CRISPR-Cas9's low off-target activity enhances its prospects as a treatment for hereditary disorders such as hemophilia. This innovative approach not only emphasizes the role of genetic factors in therapy but also touches upon the future of personalized medicine in hematology, where therapies are tailored to individual genetic profiles and needs (Lyu et al., 2018). Unlike hereditary hemophilia, AHA presents a unique set of genetic factors and therapeutic challenges. This disease is brought about by the production of autoantibodies against endogenous factor VIII, initiating spontaneous and life-threatening bleeding complications. Curiously, AHA is more often found to develop in patients with underlying comorbidities, aggravating the course of therapy and increasing mortality rates. The interplay between genetic predispositions and environmental triggers underscores the pressing need for careful clinical evaluation. While treatment of AHA requires deep knowledge of immune mechanisms and hemostatic strategies, recommendations mandate that practitioners remain up to date on evidence-based practices for this disorder. It is therefore important to understand the genetic foundations of inherited and acquired hemophilia to improve patient outcomes in hematology (Kruse-Jarres et al., 2017).

7.2.3. Leukemia: Classification and Treatment

Leukemia, a heterogeneous group of hematologic malignancies, should be classified for prognostic and treatment-planning purposes. Thoroughly split into acute or chronic leukemia, leukemia also has subtypes based on lineage and morphology. Acute leukemias are those that occur rapidly and require immediate treatment, whereas chronic leukemias progress gradually. In this system, a distinction then occurs between myeloid and lymphoid lineages. For example, acute myeloid leukemia (AML) and acute lymphoblastic leukemia (ALL) are distinguished based on the type of immature cell line involved. Recent advances, particularly the International Consensus Classification of acute leukemias of indeterminate lineage (ALAL), have highlighted the detection of mixed-phenotype acute leukemias (MPAL), which exhibit characteristics of both lineages and complicate diagnosis and treatment (Weinberg et al., 2023). This dynamic classification accurately meets the need for differential diagnosis in leukemia as an internal medicine specialty with a hematology emphasis. Treatment of leukemia is multidisciplinary, employing chemotherapeutic agents, targeted therapy, and supportive therapy. For the acute leukemias, the urgency of treatment necessitates intensive chemotherapy protocols, often followed by stem cell transplantation to produce sustained remission. Therapeutic selection is also made in large measure by genetic mutations and chromosomal abnormalities that may dictate prognosis; thus, genetic profiling is increasingly a standard in treatment decision-making. In chronic leukemias, for instance, chronic myeloid leukemia (CML), newer molecular-targeted agents, like tyrosine kinase inhibitors (TKIs), have revolutionized management, from being able just to prolong life to potential functional remission. As researchers advance in linking treatment outcomes to genetic signatures, personalized medicine remains at the forefront of improving efficacy and reducing toxicity in the treatment of leukemia (Nie et al., 2021). Furthermore, the field of leukemia treatment continues to expand through new therapies and ongoing clinical trials. Immunotherapy, for example, using monoclonal antibodies and CAR T-cell therapy, has shown promise, especially in relapsed or refractory disease where traditional treatments are ineffective. These new techniques leverage the body's immune system to target and destroy cancer cells. Additionally, microbiome research is revealing the potential for leukemia treatment. For instance, understanding how gut microbiota, such as Roseburia intestinalis, plays a role in systemic inflammation provides new avenues to enhance treatment outcomes and overall patient health (Nie et al., 2021). As the discipline develops, it is important for healthcare workers in hematology and internal medicine to stay abreast of these advances to treat patients properly.

Test Your Knowledge

1. What are the most common hematological disorders encountered in clinical practice?
2. How do inherited blood disorders differ from acquired hematological conditions?

7.3. Diagnostic Techniques in Hematology

Learning Outcome

1. Define the complete blood count (CBC)
2. Describe the bone marrow biopsy (BMB)
3. Discuss on coagulation studies

Diagnostic approaches within the developing discipline of hematology have experienced significant changes, which are essential to efficient patient management within internal medicine. Hematologic system disorders, ranging from benign to malignant hematological neoplasms, necessitate timely and accurate diagnoses. Techniques such as complete blood counts (CBC), peripheral blood smears, and bone marrow biopsies form the foundation for assessing blood diseases. Recent Breakthroughs involve flow cytometry and molecular diagnosis, which enhance the accuracy in the characterization of leukemias and lymphomas. These technologies provide accurate information on cellular characteristics, enabling individualized treatment protocols. These diagnostic techniques have been incorporated into clinical practice to reflect their invaluable role in hematology, ensuring that clinicians can ensure patients with complex hematologic disease receive full treatment. Flow cytometry is an outstanding example of a modern diagnostic technique that has revolutionized the evaluation of hematologic neoplasias. Using this technique, multiple parameters within cells can be rapidly evaluated simultaneously, and critical information on cell surface antigens and intracellular components can be obtained. In the case of acute myeloid leukemia (AML) or non-Hodgkin lymphoma, the method of determining specific immunophenotypes is important in accurate classification and prognosis. Further, cytogenetic analyses, including fluorescence in situ hybridization (FISH) or karyotyping, are important for identifying chromosomal aberrations in specific malignancies. This information is significant in treatment decisions and therapeutic prognosis. Thus, the continuous refinement of these methods underscores the need for ongoing education of internal medicine practitioners to remain cognizant of the state of the art in hematology diagnostics.

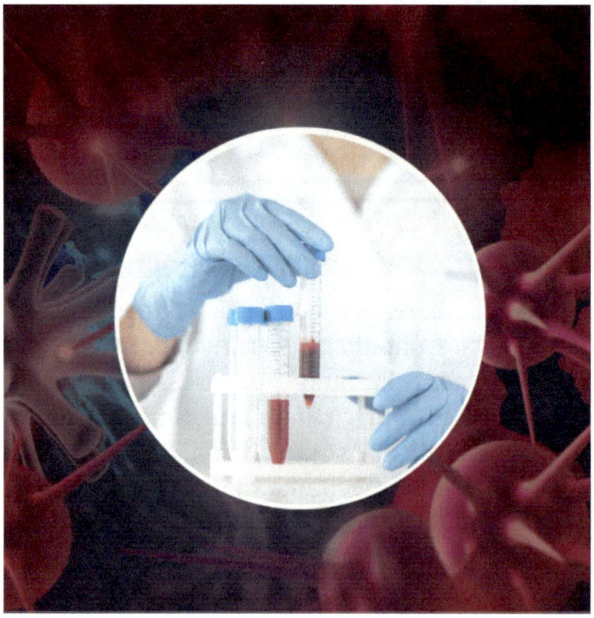

Figure 7.5. Diagnostic techniques in hematology.

Source: https://equineinstitute.org/cdn/shop/files/FundamentalsofEquineHematologyandLaboratoryTechniques_60d87e2d-13ae-4bfd-a2b0-dd00922352d2.png?v=1733568313&width=2048.

Furthermore, the correlation between traditional and new technologies emphasizes the role of the multidisciplinary approach in hematology. The clinicians must understand the role of integrating clinical data and the outcomes of laboratory investigations to arrive at an integrated diagnostic approach. For instance, diagnosis of complications like febrile neutropenia or tumor lysis syndrome cannot simply depend on the laboratory but also on a vigilant clinical acumen based on a patient's presentation. This is important for initiating early intervention, which eventually benefits patients. As suggested in recent educational curriculum plans for internal medicine residents, such as the Reverse Morning Report, emphasis on case-based education best facilitates an environment in which practitioners explore the finer points of hematologic diagnosis in real-time clinical settings (Wallace et al., 2024). Such programs underscore the imperative for designed educational models that enhance knowledge and use of diagnostic approaches in the discipline of hematology (Kucharz, 2023) (Figure 7.5).

7.3.1. Complete Blood Count (CBC)

The CBC is a critical diagnostic test in internal medicine, particularly in hematology. The test examines the components of blood, including red blood cells (RBCs), white blood cells (WBCs), and platelets, allowing medical professionals to assess a person's overall health and detect a range of medical conditions. Abnormalities in these values can mirror disorders such as anemia, infection, or hematologic malignancies. Therefore, the CBC is a valuable point of entry for further investigation in clinical practice. By employing advanced automated systems in CBC testing, such as the methods described in the Abbott Alinity h-series review, medical professionals can achieve greater precision and efficacy in determining hematological health, which is critical for developing treatment plans (Browning et al., 2024). Moreover, interpreting CBC results requires an understanding of one's biological variability. Recent studies have shown that values such as white blood cell count and platelet count can be highly personalized, suggesting that population-based reference ranges alone may not be sufficient for accurate diagnosis (Browning et al., 2024). These studies confirm the need for personalized medicine in hematology, as patients are likely to present with new hematological manifestations. By considering personal baseline values and using calculated reference change values (RCV), clinicians can enhance the sensitivity of their diagnostics, so that even the slightest pathologic changes are not overlooked. This is particularly necessary when standard reference ranges might obscure severe health abnormalities. In hematology, the CBC provides not only essential information about a person's general state of health but also informs treatment and monitoring. With advances in automation, such as those found in the Alinity h-series, the accuracy and speed of CBC testing have been greatly improved, enabling more rapid clinical assessments and interventions (Kwak et al., 2022). With more personalized reference intervals and improved analytical techniques, clinicians can make more informed choices regarding patient care. With the progress in hematology, the CBC remains a cornerstone of diagnostics, as an articulation of more overarching trends toward precision medicine and personalized care paradigms, eventually contributing to better patient outcomes in internal medicine (Figure 7.6).

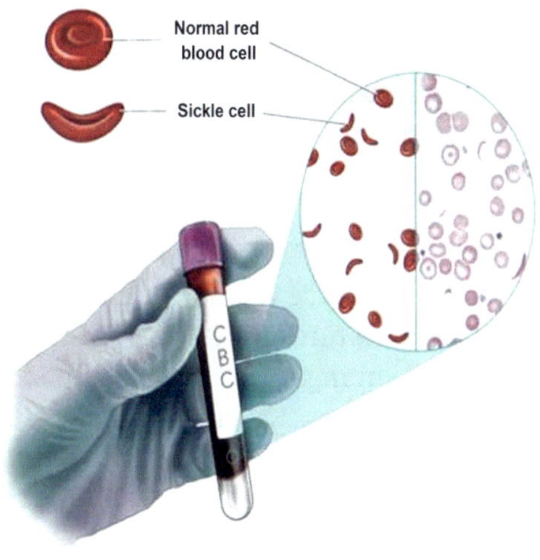

Figure 7.6. Complete blood count (CBC).

Source: https://stjude.scene7.com/is/image/stjude/sickle-cell-histology?wid=500.

7.3.2. Bone Marrow Biopsy (BMB)

BMB is a simple hematology test that can help diagnose many hematological diseases, including leukemias, lymphomas, and anemias. It is an invasive technique in which bone marrow tissue is aspirated for cytological, histological, and genetic examinations. It is significant because it can yield detailed information on hematopoiesis and the marrow microenvironment, which helps identify underlying pathologies. The process, however, demands that practitioners not only have technical skills but also understand the theoretical basis that enables them to formulate indications and contraindications. Constant training and competency testing for BMBs is required, as these directly influence the safety of patients and outcomes. Effective simulations and hands-on training programs have been best practices for enhancing medical trainees' competency in BMB procedures and achieving standardized care across facilities (Rosenstein, 2024). The challenges of skill acquisition in performing a BMB have led many hematology programs to adopt simulation-based training. For example, a structured simulation program used at the Gundersen Health System focuses on practice using cadaver models. The program not only enables fellows to become proficient in their technique but also assures their competence through a structured educational process. Throughout multiple phases of training, fellows participate in both observational and participatory roles. This multi-tier approach forms a learning culture within which knowledge sharing occurs naturally, triggering a culture of mentorship amongst learners. Furthermore, fellows have also shown significant increases in self-assessment scores following simulation training, suggesting its effectiveness in building confidence and competence in performing BMBs (Rosenstein, 2024). Moreover, continuous evaluation of procedural skills clinics demonstrates a perceivable effect on resident confidence and procedural expertise. A weekly procedural skills clinic implemented at the Odette Cancer Centre has led to significant improvements in residents' ability to perform BMBs and LPs. The clinic model combines didactic instruction with practical experience, allowing learners to receive immediate feedback. Such all-encompassing training fills knowledge gaps in procedural skills, safety measures, and post-procedure complications, specifically regarding local anesthetic use. Surveys indicate that residents appreciate these training sessions, as they give them the confidence to perform BMBs independently. This underscores the importance of including structured, faculty-directed training clinics in hematology residency programs to produce competent hematologists who are proficient in performing key procedures, such as BMBs.

7.3.3. Coagulation Studies

Coagulation tests are most important in internal medicine, particularly in hematology, because they provide significant information on the mechanisms of hemostasis during blood clotting and the maintenance of vascular integrity. Coagulation tests assess the function of the coagulation pathways, including the intrinsic, extrinsic, and common pathways. Conditions such as vitamin K deficiency and hemophilia highlight the importance of understanding these pathways, as they can lead to significant bleeding complications. Moreover, cross-talk between immune and coagulation systems, as seen in diseases such as paroxysmal nocturnal hemoglobinuria (PNH), demonstrates the interplay among these systems. As discussed by Dr. Panse in the context of PNH, advancements in the treatment of complement dysregulation highlight the relevance of coagulation studies not only in classical hematologic diseases but also in new therapeutic approaches in modern medicine (de Latour et al., 2023). Latest studies point out even more the relevance of coagulation studies in identifying systemic diseases, namely in the case of COVID-19. The pandemic has highlighted the capacity of viral infections to induce coagulopathies through mechanisms such as endothelial dysfunction and hyperactivation of the coagulation cascade. In a study assessing ischemia-modified albumin (IMA) in

COVID-19 patients, they demonstrated elevated levels, which were correlated with increased coagulation risk and highlighted the need to monitor coagulation factors in this population (Sağlam et al., 2023). These findings emphasize the importance of repeated coagulation testing in patients with COVID-19 complications, enabling clinicians to stratify risk and guide therapeutic interventions. Including coagulation testing in the overall clinical evaluation enables clinicians to maximize patient outcomes by early detection and treatment of potential coagulopathies. Last but not least, the interpretation of coagulation studies requires a nuanced understanding of both individual patient variables and the disease's pathophysiologic context. Clinicians must be able to correlate test findings with clinical presentation to choose appropriate therapeutic strategies. As new therapies evolve, particularly those targeting complement pathways, the relevance of coagulation studies grows, underscoring their role as part of an integrated approach to patient care. The development of new therapeutic drugs, including inhibitors of components of the complement cascade, exemplifies the interplay between coagulation research and novel therapeutic principles. These general appraisals provide hematologists with important information informing patient care, further underlining the pivotal role of coagulation tests in both traditional and modern internal medicine practice (de Latour et al., 2023).

Test Your Knowledge

1. What is the importance of a complete blood count (CBC) in diagnosing blood disorders?
2. Why is bone marrow examination used in hematological diagnosis?

7.4. Treatment Modalities in Hematology

Learning Outcome

1. Understand the pharmacological interventions
2. Define the blood transfusion therapy
3. Identify the stem cell transplantation

The field of hematology has evolved, with significant improvements in treatment modalities, providing options for a range of hematological conditions. Pharmacologic therapies, including chemotherapy, immunotherapy, and targeted therapy, are some of the most significant strategies. Chemotherapy remains a mainstay for cancers of hematology, such as leukemia and lymphoma, wherein drugs toxic to actively dividing cancer cells are employed to destroy them. New technologies in immunotherapy, including monoclonal antibodies and immune checkpoint inhibitors, have provided new mechanisms for using the patient's own immune system to target malignancies more effectively. These modalities have improved outcomes and radically changed the prognosis for patients with hematologic malignancies, leading to improved survival and better quality of life. In addition to pharmacotherapy, stem cell transplantation is a curative option for various hematologic malignancies. The treatment involves replacing tainted or damaged bone marrow with healthy stem cells, which can be harvested from the patient or a donor with a matching gene. The treatment combines high-dose chemotherapy or radiotherapy to destroy malignant cell populations with the administration of stem cells to enable hematopoietic engraftment, particularly in acute leukemia and certain myeloproliferative neoplasms. Stem cell transplantation can often provide lasting remission. However, the procedure requires stringent patient selection, as complications of graft-versus-host disease and the conditioning regimen require thorough pre-transplantation evaluation and supportive care. Cutting-edge therapies are being increasingly used in conjunction with traditional modalities to optimize hematology results.

For instance, the application of personalized medicine, in which therapy protocols are tailored to a patient's genetic or molecular characteristics of a disease, represents a significant shift in hematologic care. Doctors can use genomic data to identify specific mutations that respond to targeted treatments, thereby enhancing efficacy and preventing unnecessary side effects.

Furthermore, hematology-oncology educational curricula in internal medicine residency programs are necessary to equip future physicians with the knowledge and skills to apply these new treatment options appropriately. It is important to develop systematic hematology curricula in training programs, as outlined in recent studies, to bridge knowledge gaps and improve patient care outcomes in hematology (Parikh et al., 2024; Shilpakar et al., 2025) (Figure 7.7).

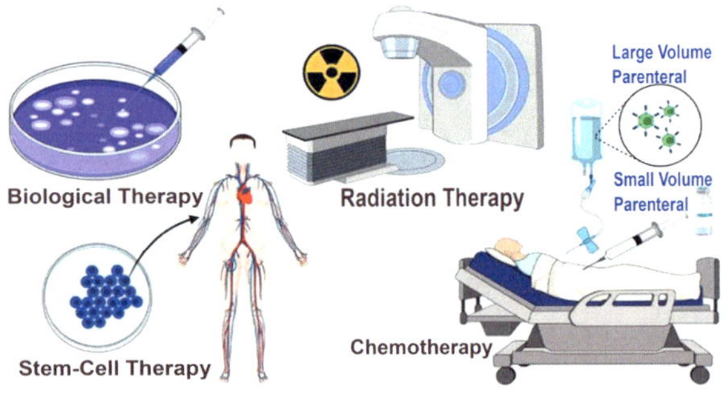

Figure 7.7. Treatment modalities in hematology.

Source: https://static.wixstatic.com/media/ff1dc2_80d254052c684920bb60d44c6ef0cb16~mv2.png/v1/fill/w_886,h_494,al_c,q_90,enc_auto/ff1dc2_80d254052c684920bb60d44c6ef0cb16~mv2.png.

7.4.1. Pharmacological Interventions

Pharmacological interventions in internal medicine and hematology form the core of the management of several hematological ailments. Drugs form the cornerstone of treatment for conditions such as anemia, thrombocytopenia, and hematologic malignancies, and it is crucial that healthcare providers better understand the actions of these therapies. Proper selection of successful pharmacotherapy is reliant on a thorough assessment of the patient's clinical presentation, disease pathology, and drug interaction. For instance, in the case of malignant hematology, pharmacologic interventions may consist of the employment of chemotherapy regimens that assault rapidly growing cancer cells while taking into account the patients' overall condition and comorbidities. All this sophisticated decision-making makes personalized pharmacologic interventions, which optimize the therapeutic effect while minimizing the toxicities, all the more pertinent. In addition, the internal medicine curriculum would require innovative training strategies to equip residents with the necessary skills in pharmacologic interventions. Clinical case discussion is an effective instructional method that enhances learning, as seen in the Reverse Morning Report model. This approach enables internal medicine residents to engage in retrospective evaluations of real patient cases, focusing on critical details such as pharmacotherapeutics, drug side effects, and emergent complications of their hematologic disorder. In this process, residents not only solidify their pharmacology concepts but also enhance clinical reasoning skills essential to patient care. Evidence from this curriculum indicates that residents reacted very favorably to these structured sessions, offering an example for other centers to emulate in improving their teaching content on hematology pharmacotherapy (Wallace et al., 2024). In addition, ongoing research aimed at clarifying resident outcomes related to pharmacologic instruction is important for the formulation of curricular approaches. For example, resident and hematology fellows' questionnaires can provide insight into perceptions of these skills and knowledge deficits in pharmacologic interventions. This feedback system plays an important role in continuous improvement and in adapting training strategies to keep pace with the evolving paradigm of hematology treatment, particularly with the advent of new therapies as a reality of everyday clinical practice. Analysis of residents' interest in hematology determinants can also reveal potential deterrents to participation, such as limited elective experience or exposure to procedures, and thereby guide institutions in creating evidence-based interventions to build a stronger pipeline of future hematologists (Parikh et al., 2024). Finally, by prioritizing pharmacologically sound internal medicine education, educators can maximize learners' proficiency in managing complex hematologic disorders, ultimately improving patient care outcomes.

7.4.2. Blood Transfusion Therapy

Blood transfusion therapy is a critical intervention in internal medicine, especially in hematology, where the management of various blood disorders is essential. Therapeutic use of packed red blood cells (pRBCs) is prevalent in clinical practice, wherein they are the cornerstone of therapy for complications such as acute anemia and hemorrhage. Decisions to start a transfusion depend on various factors, including patient hemoglobin levels, clinical stability, and guidelines set by blood banks. Guidelines, for instance, commonly recommend a hemoglobin level of < 7 g/dL to initiate transfusion in stable patients, reflecting the fine balance between therapeutic benefit and the complications of transfusion. Knowledge of such clinical decision-making is essential to optimizing patient outcomes and limiting unnecessary transfusion-related complications, such as transfusion reactions, and the consequent management complexity in hematologic practice. Also, the incidence of transfusion reactions is an important aspect of blood transfusion therapy that must be carefully managed. Existing studies have indicated that the incidence of acute transfusion reactions has been quite disparate, with a high rate of febrile nonhemolytic reactions and allergic reactions observed with the transfusion of pRBCs and plasma products. Specifically, the incidence of acute transfusion reaction was 8.9% with pRBCs in one comprehensive study involving over 850 dogs (Hall et al., 2024). Such information emphasizes the importance of strict adherence by healthcare professionals to standard protocols for blood product selection and transfusion, as prolonged storage of pRBCs has been linked to increased rates of adverse reactions. Such findings underscore the importance of strategic transfusion therapy tailored to the patient's risk profile, along with a complete appreciation of complications that may arise during treatment. Finally, a review of current transfusion practice is observed with major trends that affect the safety and effectiveness of blood transfusion therapy. A retrospective evaluation at an inner-city community Veterans Affairs hospital reported that a high proportion of multi-unit transfusion requests were inappropriate, with more than 63% failing to meet the clinical criteria for such treatment (Huynh et al., 2024). This finding suggests an evidence-based practice gap that may be linked to increased patient risk and resource waste. Establishing evidence-based guidelines, such as single-unit transfusion protocols, is crucial to enhancing the appropriateness of transfusion therapy and patient outcomes. As hospitals implement strategies to maximize the use of blood, ongoing education and adherence to transfusion practices will be crucial to preventing the risks of transfusion therapy while maximizing its therapeutic benefit across diverse patient populations.

7.4.3. Stem Cell Transplantation

Stem cell transplantation is an anchor therapeutic modality in hematology, particularly for hematologic malignancies such as acute myeloid leukemia (AML). In patients treated with intensive chemotherapy, hematopoietic cell reconstitution aims to restore normal blood cell production. The outcome of stem cell transplantation varies depending on factors such as the underlying disease, prior treatments, and the stem cell source, which can be peripheral blood, bone marrow, or umbilical cord blood. As noted, more recent studies have also implicated that the expression levels of immunological markers, i.e., CD200, may be significant in modulating therapeutic outcomes in AML patients and, therefore, highlight the intricate interplay between graft outcome and immunological characteristics (Hassan et al., 2023). Pre-transplant conditioning regimens also play a crucial role in determining the success of stem cell transplantation.

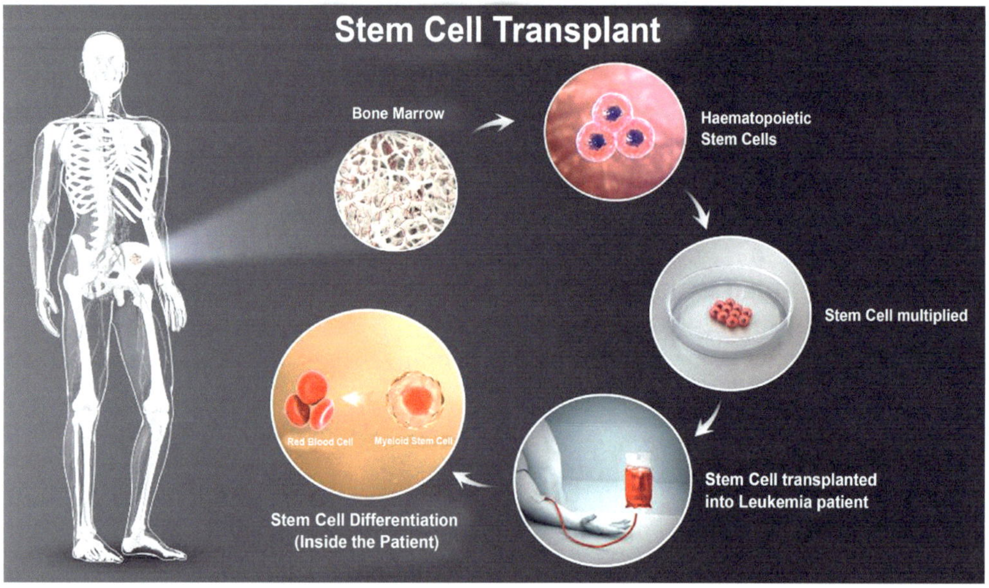

Figure 7.8. Stem cell transplantation.

Source: https://www.scientificanimations.com/wp-content/uploads/2015/10/StemCellTransplant-IOW47.jpg.

These regimens usually employ myeloablative therapies, which aim to destroy neoplastic cells while also immunosuppressing the host to reduce the risk of transplant rejection. However, the severity of myeloablative conditioning may also increase the treatment-related morbidity and mortality. Today's research focuses on optimizing such regimens by adding newer drugs that may enhance anti-tumor effects with minimal toxicity. For instance, the incorporation of directed therapies with conventional chemotherapy can potentially augment the success rate of stem cell transplantation, particularly in cases that have been resistant (McIlroy et al., 2020). Post-transplantation, immune system reconstitution, qualitative and quantitative, is very important to prevent infections as well as reduce relapse rates. Monitoring immune recovery using lymphocyte counts and functional assays could help us estimate how long the patient's recovery period will last. Along with this, understanding the roles of myeloid and lymphoid cell populations during this time can help clinicians plan effective supportive care and surveillance strategies. Recent advances in the characterization of immune checkpoints, such as CD200, have identified novel targets for therapeutic interventions capable of preventing hematological malignancy patient relapse following transplantation (Hassan et al., 2023). By illuminating the immune environment in which stem cell transplantation occurs, hematologists can move closer to improving the long-term prognosis of patients with such complex diseases (Figure 7.8).

Test Your Knowledge

1. What are the common treatment approaches for hematological disorders?
2. How do blood transfusions and medications help manage blood diseases?

7.5. Challenges in Hematological Care

Learning Outcome

1. Discuss the access to specialized care
2. Define the patient compliance and education
3. Describe the emerging resistance to treatments

Hematological practice faces various challenges that significantly impact patient outcomes and the effectiveness of treatment protocols. The most salient challenge is the complexity of diagnosing hematological illnesses, where presentations often feature double-hued symptoms that may be mistaken for other ailments. For instance, the patient may present with symptoms that overlap with those of both hematological malignancies and infectious diseases, complicating diagnosis. According to Conroy et al. (2025), it is critical to diagnose uncommon disorders, such as acute variegate porphyria, promptly and accurately, as misdiagnosis can delay therapy and lead to secondary consequences, such as multiorgan failure. It is a challenge that must be addressed through collaboration among several specialties, with joint input, to provide patients with appropriate care tailored to their unique presentations. In addition to diagnostic challenges, the management of hematological diseases is further complicated by patients' varying responses to treatment. The effectiveness and toxicity of therapy may be influenced by the patient's age, genetic traits, and underlying medical conditions. The advanced age of a patient, for example, may predispose him/her to treatment side effects, as was the case with a 77-year-old patient in Conroy et al. (2025). Additionally, healthcare professionals often face barriers, such as inadequate training and limited exposure to new therapies, particularly in resource-poor settings. These barriers may prevent healthcare professionals from effectively adopting evidence-based care, leading to compromised care and patient dissatisfaction. Besides, emotional and organizational support for hematology healthcare professionals is generally inadequate, potentially affecting their ability to deliver quality care. Research indicates that internal medicine staff frequently experience a deficiency of emotional support and insufficient organizational resources when handling complex cases, including those requiring palliative care. Insufficient specialized support systems may lead to greater burnout among medical professionals, affecting their motivation and the overall quality of patient interactions. Hence, addressing such systemic issues by prioritizing mentorship, enhancing organizational systems, and providing emotional support is essential to improving the landscape of hematological care. These shall not only enhance healthcare professionals' well-being but also pave the way for a setting that fosters better patient outcomes.

7.5.1. Access to Specialized Care

Availability of expert care remains a concern in hematology due to the uneven distribution of healthcare centers and professionals. The majority of community hospitals, which are usually the first source of care for patients with hematological syndromes, lack the infrastructure and manpower to manage and treat complex cases. This results in patients having a delay in receiving appropriate treatment, thereby worsening their conditions. It is crucial to fill this gap by building the capacity of general practice centers to manage hematological diseases. Measures such as specialized training programs for general practitioners and cooperative alliances between hematologists and community hospitals may enable appropriate initial treatment and help identify symptoms that require specialist care (Nakamura et al., 2025). Secondly, the lives of patients suffering from such diseases as sickle cell disease (SCD) demonstrate the vast need for accessible specialized services. Few health care practitioners, particularly those outside hematology, have emerged as SCD specialists, leaving a wide gap in the management of the chronic disease. Non-hematologist specialists of SCD (nhSCDe) have been able to develop new ways to enhance their knowledge through peer recognition and by fostering networks within the healthcare system. This bottom-up mechanism indicates the role of mentorship and community support in dismantling barriers to expertise development, thus improving patient outcomes. In addition, universalizing NHSCDe training can increase the number of trained professionals available to care for individuals with SCD and other hematologic diseases (Coyne et al., 2024). Addressing access to specialty care is not simply a matter of adding more experts, since it also needs to take into account how trainees become specialists and are deployed in the health system. Encouraging collaboration between hematologists and generalists in community practice can improve the standard of care. Continuous advances in hematology treatments and diagnostic equipment call for ensuring that community practice facilities have the appropriate equipment. Focusing on cooperative practice models and resource sharing can ensure the highest quality of care for patients with hematological conditions, enhancing their overall treatment experience. Innovative endeavors toward expanded access will ultimately contribute to better health outcomes and reduced care disparities among patients with hematological disorders (Nakamura et al., 2025).

7.5.2. Patient Compliance and Education

Patient compliance and education are crucial in hematology, particularly with the complexity of treatments and the high risk of non-compliance. Such patients with conditions such as venous thromboembolism (VTE) or immune thrombocytopenia (ITP) are likely to receive complex treatment regimens that require the complete understanding of their disease, medications, and necessary lifestyle adjustments. For instance, the American Society of Hematology (ASH) guidelines include cancer patients' prevention and treatment of VTE and emphasize not only medication therapy but also patient education to identify risks and maximize therapy. This is a crucial insight, given that non-adherence may lead to increased morbidity and mortality; hence, healthcare professionals should establish effective teaching programs that enhance patient involvement and ownership of their health outcomes (Lyman et al., 2021). Compliance is also extremely important in the management of ITP, as treatments differ dramatically between patients; hence, individualized treatment protocols are necessary. ASH guidelines prioritize shared decision-making in the treatment of ITP, recognizing that the patient's values and preferences should prevail. This introduces a greater appreciation of treatments available, along with their benefits and risks. By being involved in a discussion about their illness and treatment regimen, patients are helped by clinicians to build trust and adherence, since they are more compliant with a regimen they understand and feel responsible for. Education about the various management options, from corticosteroids to thrombopoietin receptor agonists, also helps address fears, ultimately leading to higher compliance rates (Neunert et al., 2019).

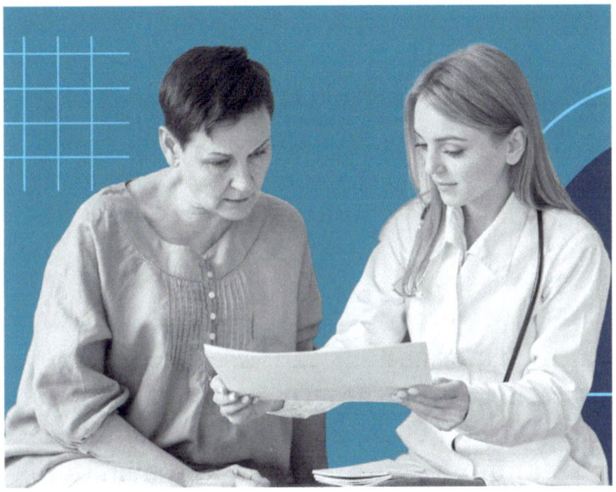

Figure 7.9. Patient compliance and education.

Source: https://creyos.com/hubfs/Patient%20 Compliance-1.png.

Furthermore, healthcare providers need to use multimodal education to address the various ways patients learn. The use of visual aids, computerized information, and support groups can supplement the patient's educational process, making it more accessible and comprehensible. Follow-up and compliance monitoring also facilitate ongoing conversations in which patients are comfortable bringing up issues they might have with their treatment interventions. By establishing a continuing education relationship, healthcare providers cannot only enhance compliance rates but also improve overall patient satisfaction and outcomes in hematology services. This emphasis on patient education and compliance is reinforced by the ASH guidelines, which encourage active, involved, and informed patients to co-manage their care effectively (Neunert et al., 2019; Lyman et al., 2021) (Figure 7.9).

7.5.3. Emerging Resistance to Treatments

The treatment landscape in hematology is under threat from the developing trend of resistance to existing therapies. As advances in treatment modalities and genetic manipulation remain promising for hematological disorders, it is becoming apparent that resistance mechanisms complicate patient care. Resistance can occur through several biological mechanisms, including genetic mutations that confer survival advantage in cancer cells and thereby render them less sensitive to targeted treatments. Such mutations have been thoroughly elucidated in various hematologic malignancies where conventional therapies in the form of chemotherapy and immunotherapy fail to yield favorable outcomes. With evolving treatment modalities, understanding resistance mechanisms is crucial to optimizing therapeutic strategies and improving patients' prognosis, rendering continuous research on this front obligatory (Naldini et al., 2022). Beyond genetic mutations, the tumor microenvironment's role in driving drug resistance cannot be overstated. The microenvironment provides a sanctuary for cancer cells to evade treatment. Mechanisms such as hypoxia, immune checkpoint signaling pathways, and metabolic reprogramming in the tumor microenvironment all contribute to selective pressure that drives resistant clones. This cross-talk illustrates the intricate dynamics between tumor cells and their microenvironment, which also has the potential to impact the response to treatment significantly. For instance, it has been shown that specific immune cells within the microenvironment can modulate the efficacy of CAR-T cell therapies, potentially leading to disease re-growth. As novel therapies, such as those involving genetically modified immune cells, evolve, learning and countering these environmental factors take precedence in overcoming resistance and maximizing therapeutic efficiency (Nie et al., 2021). The strategy for overcoming resistance requires a multidimensional approach by integrating new treatment modalities and individualized medicine. For instance, integrating comprehensive genomic profiling into the clinic enables clinicians to tailor interventions based on a patient's malignancy mutation profile. Additionally, modalities such as combination therapies, in which multiple agents converge on alternative pathways, may overcome neoplastic cell resistance. Furthermore, emerging technologies such as CRISPR and gene editing are imminent for direct targeting of genetic defects of resistance. With advances in the discipline of hematology, precision titration of the treatment regimen in line with specific tumor characteristics will enhance the responsiveness of therapy and limit the scope for the development of resistance, paving the way for longer-lasting patient outcomes in hematological malignancies (Naldini et al., 2022).

Test Your Knowledge

1. What challenges arise in the early diagnosis of hematological disorders?
2. How do treatment-related side effects complicate long-term hematological care?

7.6. Future Directions in Hematology

Learning Outcome

1. Describe the advances in genetic research
2. Define the innovations in treatment approaches
3. Identify the role of technology in patient monitoring

Hematology is leading the charge in innovation in the medical sciences, and future trends are guaranteed to transform patient treatment and therapy protocols revolutionarily. One of the most exciting innovations is the use of artificial intelligence (AI) in the practice of hematology. AI can enhance diagnosis and individualize treatment plans through advanced data analysis. Through systematic mapping of the existing literature, researchers are beginning to identify uses of AI that can aid personalized medicine, particularly in hematological disease. The model of AI education in medical education requires a robust re-evaluation so that future health professionals can take advantage of this technological progress with the requisite skills (Gordon et al., 2024). Thus, the interface of technology with traditional hematology practice will most likely result in improved patient outcomes and an improved clinical workflow. With continued research, the impact of cancer therapeutics, particularly in hematologic malignancies, becomes increasingly significant. Advances in treatment modalities such as immunotherapy and targeted therapy have, in fact, improved survival. However, these developments also hold complex challenges, such as cardiovascular toxicities, which are now a priority concern for hematology professionals. Current data indicate that underrepresented populations bear disproportionate burdens from these treatments. Addressing these disparities requires complex strategies to balance therapeutic effectiveness and the risk of adverse effects. Future directions in hematology will need to prioritize the development of consensus guidelines that integrate evidence-based practices to treat and counteract these divergent cardiotoxicities across diverse patient groups, reflecting a comprehensive approach to cancer care (Addison et al., 2023). In addition to planning for technological and therapeutic advances, future directions in hematology will also involve greater attention to patient-centered care. This includes creating a setting in which patient preferences and values take center stage in decision-making, particularly in the treatment of hematological disorders. While we recognize the multifaceted involvement with diverse patient populations, there is greater pressure to combine personalized strategies with treatment protocols based on unique genetic profiles and psychosocial factors. This shift towards individualized care can be achieved through the use of genomics and precision medicine, enabling clinicians to make informed choices that maximize treatment efficacy and minimize harm. Ultimately, the continued advancement of hematology will hinge on whether the field can embrace new approaches without forsaking compassionate and patient-centered practice.

7.6.1. Advances in Genetic Research

The field of genetic research has come a long way in relevance to internal medicine, particularly hematology. The discovery of the nature of gene mutations and their role in hematological malignancies has revealed the molecular basis of the disease. Genetic mutations that disrupt normal cellular function, for example, are now known to be pivotal in the etiology of most cancers of the blood, including leukemias and lymphomas. Through extensive genomic studies, healthcare workers can identify specific genetic markers that not only diagnose but also enable personalized therapeutic interventions. These interventions can enhance treatment efficacy and reduce side effects, paving the way for customized management of hematological diseases. This foundational shift towards precision medicine necessitates integrating genetic information into routine clinical practice, ultimately improving patient outcomes in the practice of internal medicine and hematology. In recent years, the application of high-complexity genetic testing techniques, such as next-generation sequencing (NGS), has revolutionized the diagnostic picture of hematology. NGS enables rapid screening of multiple genes simultaneously, exponentially increasing the efficiency and accuracy of genetic profiling in patients. Hematologists can now detect specific mutations relevant to prognostic stratification and predict therapy response. Innovations of this sort are particularly significant in conditions like acute myeloid leukemia (AML), where molecular characteristics can significantly influence treatment options and prognosis. Furthermore, such developments enable the identification of new therapeutic targets, which can be targeted with therapies based on this genetic information. Therefore, the application of genetic information in clinical decision-making transforms traditional hematological practices, underscoring the importance of continued research into the genetic basis of blood diseases. Its application to hematology is also highlighted by the potential for greater cost-effectiveness and improved patient management offered by advances in genetic research. Genetic information enables early intervention strategies and justifies the implementation of new therapies with potentially more successful rates. Furthermore, the application of artificial intelligence (AI) in genetic data analysis offers the promise of higher predictive value in genetic testing, enhanced patient care efficiency, and better resource use in clinical settings. For instance, machine learning models can analyze large datasets effectively and identify patterns, which are used to guide treatment approaches and improve patient stratification. Therefore, the integration of genetic research with AI technologies can facilitate better decision-making by hematologists when dealing with challenging cases. Lastly, ongoing research and its integration into practice are critical to advancing the field of internal medicine for hematology, with a solid groundwork for better patient outcomes in the future (Figure 7.10).

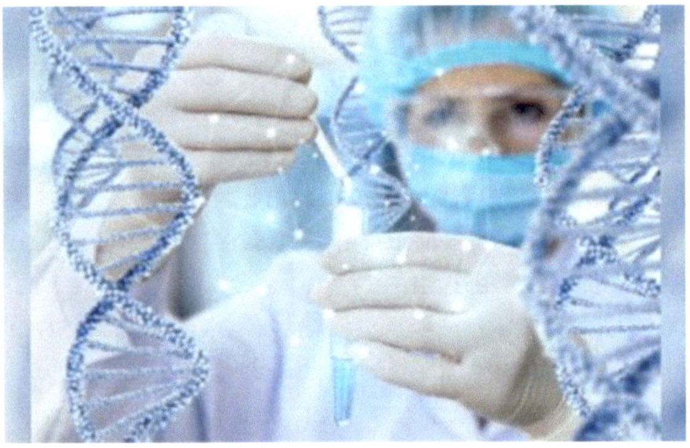

Figure 7.10. Advances in genetic research.

Source: https://external-content.duckduckgo.com/iu/?u=https%3A%2F%2Ftse4.mm.bing.net%2Fth%2Fid%2FOIP.ob1Ddv2pxa1apoARt4vjQQAAAA%3Fpid%3DApi&f=1&ipt=2e706274274343515ae2511e93c90563c330a70add076b766ed54b033556bfb1.

7.6.2. Innovations in Treatment Approaches

The discipline of hematology is undergoing a radical transformation, particularly with the advent of powerful tools such as AI and LLMs. The introduction of sophisticated AI solutions can aid clinical decision-making and enhance the efficiency of patient care. For example, AI platforms can assist clinicians with clinical documentation, speed up insurance pre-authorization procedures, and condense pertinent research evidence effectively. These solutions' deployment, however, should be closely monitored to prevent potential harm to patient care and data privacy. Regulatory systems must adjust to ensure that these technologies enhance the clinical practice of hematology without jeopardizing the medical and ethical standards of care expected for patients. As AI technology continues to improve, ongoing interaction among healthcare providers and regulatory bodies will be necessary to achieve maximum benefits and prevent adverse consequences (Meskó et al., 2023). In addition to technological advancements, advances in genetic treatments, particularly in hematology, are the most promising area of treatment development. Gene treatments for hematopoietic stem cells (HSCs) are a new avenue of therapy for many inherited blood diseases. These therapies aim to correct defects at their genetic origin and thereby promise cures rather than palliative relief. Treatments such as autologous HSC gene therapy employ patient-specific cells, providing significant therapeutic advantages, including reduced risks of graft-versus-host disease and increased compatibility. The European Hematology Associations updated Research Roadmap attaches greater significance to the need for research into genetically targeted therapies to effectively treat an increasing number of hematological diseases. As safety and efficacy profiles continue to develop in current trials, gene therapy will rapidly become a cornerstone of the treatment approach for numerous hematologic disorders (Naldini et al., 2022). Another milestone in the treatment approach has been the development of chimeric antigen receptor T-cell (CAR-T) therapies. This groundbreaking therapy harnesses the immune system to target specific cancers, including hematologic malignancies such as some types of leukemia and lymphoma. The engineered T-cells are designed to recognize and kill cancer cells more effectively, achieving impressive gains in patient prognosis, especially in patients who have survived the useful duration of conventional therapies. The potential of CAR-T therapy has once again generated interest in personalized medicine, underscoring the need for treatment tailored to the individual patient and disease biology. While studies are still ongoing, ensuring equitable access and cost-effectiveness of such groundbreaking therapies is a critical issue. The effectiveness of CAR-T treatments can revolutionize hematology treatment regimens; as such, it is important to integrate these advances into the wider clinical setting (Naldini et al., 2022).

7.6.3. Role of Technology in Patient Monitoring

The integration of technology into patient monitoring has revolutionized the practice of internal medicine, particularly in hematology. More advanced tools, such as remote monitoring devices and wearable technology, have become fundamental components in the treatment of hematological diseases. These developments enable continuous monitoring of patient vital signs, allowing clinicians to detect changes in health status in real time. In anemic or thrombocytopenic patients, early detection of alterations can lead to early intervention, thereby preventing complications. Such data collected from monitoring systems also contribute to a clearer picture of patient health, as technology and clinical observations are brought together, ultimately enhancing the quality of care offered in hematological practice. Artificial intelligence (AI) and machine learning also play crucial roles in enhancing hematology patient monitoring systems. The ability of AI to handle large amounts of clinical information enables the identification of patterns that would not have been possible, which, in drug-induced cytopenias, is especially important. Algorithmic processing can predict potential side effects and identify high-risk patients, enabling intervention steps to be initiated before it is too late. In studies, this has been shown to significantly enhance the risk assessment role, leading to better management plans and patient outcomes (Andrès et al., 2025). Besides, AI-driven tools can deliver tailored monitoring solutions that adapt to individual patient needs and ensure interventions are derived from their unique health profiles, which is particularly vital in the management of hematological disorders. Digital twins are among the innovative ways to monitor patients, demonstrating the meeting points of state-of-the-art technology and tailored medicine in hematology. By creating virtual patient replicas, health professionals can simulate health scenarios, test treatments, and predict disease progression without risking the patient. The technology is not only beneficial for understanding patient-specific conditions but also impacts clinical trials and therapy planning. As virtual twins advance, they demand a high level of balancing, fostering patient care and addressing ethical issues related to data confidentiality and consent (Vallée, 2024). The prospect of using digital twins in the management of hematological patients enhances predictive capability, leading to anticipatory healthcare interventions as well as raising important questions about the ethical considerations of using such technology in patient care.

Test Your Knowledge

1. What emerging therapies are shaping the future of hematological treatment?
2. How is personalized medicine influencing advancements in hematology?

SUMMARY

In summary, integrating new curricula for new-style education into the hematology arena is essential for producing competent healthcare professionals. The use of the Reverse Morning Report program, as described in the pertinent research, emphasizes its efficacy in enhancing internal medicine residents' knowledge of hematologic malignancies. This case-based approach not only facilitates understanding of diagnostic processes but also emphasizes practical management strategies. By involving current patients as learning resources, the curriculum demonstrates how experience-based education can bridge the gap between academic knowledge and clinical practice and prepare residents for the realities of practical hematology care. As such, education programs within internal medicine must emphasize active learning to ensure residents have the critical thinking skills to handle complex hematologic cases effectively (Wallace et al., 2024). Furthermore, the effectiveness of hematology instruction is not limited to resident training; it also plays a major role in the overall quality of patient care in internal medicine settings. A pilot study using a targeted lecture curriculum with medical students demonstrated the liberating potential of a sound foundation in hematology and oncology education. By broadening the knowledge and confidence of students, the program not only serves to meet short-term educational needs but also fosters a long-term commitment to continued education in hematology/oncology. This focus on continued professional development enhances the capacity of future internists and hematologists to provide comprehensive care, ultimately benefiting patients with hematologic disease. It is thus necessary to ensure that medical students learn the fundamentals well to facilitate the development of a workforce able to navigate the complexities of oncologic care (Venugopal et al., 2024). In summary, these advancements in the educational structures illustrate a broad commitment towards improving hematology-focused training in internal medicine. The obvious positive outcomes of the Reverse Morning Report and lecture-based, curriculum-rich curricula are worthy of consideration for broader adoption across all medical schools. With support for an environment that fosters innovative pedagogical methods, medical education can better prepare future healthcare professionals to manage the nuances of hematologic disease. Besides, the impact of such programs concerns not only student success at the individual level but also the enhanced quality of patient care, creating space for collaborative approaches to hematologic malignancy treatment. As healthcare continues to evolve, education in this field remains a top priority and sets the stage for future patient improvement (Venugopal et al., 2024; Wallace et al., 2024).

Hematology is a foundation of internal medicine and involves a wide range of disorders of coagulation and blood cells. Appropriate evaluation and management of conditions like hematologic malignancies, coagulopathies, and anemia are essential components of effective hematological practice. These conditions necessitate adequate knowledge of not only pathophysiology but also of treatment and diagnostic modalities. Sophisticated laboratory techniques, including flow cytometry and molecular diagnostics, are essential for advanced diagnosis of hematologic diseases, enabling practitioners to tailor treatment to patient needs. Moreover, the integration of new therapeutic techniques testifies to progress in this area, which calls on practitioners in hematological practice to continue their education and adaptation. The prevalence underscores the significance of recognizing such complexities and widespread morbidity figures reported for hematological diseases. Professional standards and quality assurance criteria shape the evolution of hematology within internal medicine. Quality assurance programs continued to ensure the reliability of the laboratory data, which form the basis of accurate diagnosis and effective treatment choices. Moreover, longstanding organizations, such as the American Society for Hematology, play a vital role in codifying practice standards, keeping hematologists current with the latest research and treatment standards. These guidelines not only improve clinical practice at the individual level but also public health at large by improving outcomes through the maximization of patient management across a variety of hematological disorders. Adherence to evidence-based practices not only guarantees the safety of patients but also guarantees the proper allocation of healthcare resources, which ultimately enhances the efficiency of hematological interventions in a clinical setting. The last decade has seen the regulatory frameworks adjust to address the sophistication of hematology and internal medicine. For instance, in the United States, the Clinical Laboratory Improvement Amendments (CLIA) establish a regulatory framework that ensures laboratory testing is of high quality and complies with stringent quality standards. While the emphasis remains primarily on human medicine, similar principles are beginning to find their way into veterinary laboratory diagnostics, promising a broader trend towards standardization and improvement. Such controls are intended to minimize diagnostic testing errors, which have very real consequences for patient care. But the dynamic state of hematological science also calls for practitioners to be sensitive to ongoing changes initiated by technological progress, such as the development of targeted therapies and genetic assays. A general knowledge of the current state of affairs and potential future directions in hematology is required of healthcare professionals committed to delivering high-quality care in this demanding discipline.

KEY TERMS FROM THIS CHAPTER

- Activated partial thromboplastin time (aPTT)
- Anemia
- Bone marrow biopsy
- Coagulation cascade
- Complete blood count (CBC)
- Erythropoiesis
- Folic acid deficiency
- Hemophilia
- Iron deficiency
- Leukemia
- Lymphoma
- Multiple myeloma
- Peripheral smear
- Prothrombin time (PT)
- Reticulocyte count
- Sickle cell disease
- Thalassemia
- Thrombocytopenia

CRITICAL THINKING QUESTIONS

1. **Which of the following is the most common cause of microcytic hypochromic anemia worldwide?**
   a. Vitamin B12 deficiency
   b. Iron deficiency
   c. Aplastic anemia
   d. Chronic kidney disease
2. **Which laboratory finding is most consistent with hemolytic anemia?**
   a. Low lactate dehydrogenase (LDH)
   b. Decreased reticulocyte count
   c. Elevated indirect bilirubin
   d. Decreased unconjugated bilirubin
3. **The presence of Reed-Sternberg cells in a lymph node biopsy is diagnostic of:**
   a. Chronic lymphocytic leukemia
   b. Multiple myeloma
   c. Hodgkin lymphoma
   d. Non-Hodgkin lymphoma
4. **Which coagulation abnormality is most commonly seen in disseminated intravascular coagulation (DIC)?**
   a. Elevated platelet count
   b. Shortened prothrombin time (PT)
   c. Decreased fibrinogen levels
   d. Normal D-dimer
5. **Which of the following is a key feature of vitamin B12 deficiency that differentiates it from folate deficiency?**
   a. Microcytosis
   b. Iron overload
   c. Neurological symptoms (e.g., paresthesias)
   d. Rapid onset anemia

Short Answer Questions

1. What are the common causes of microcytic anemia, and how are they differentiated?
2. How is iron deficiency anemia diagnosed and managed in adults?
3. Describe the clinical features and lab findings in vitamin B12 deficiency.
4. What is the difference between intrinsic and extrinsic hemolytic anemia?
5. What are the diagnostic criteria for acute leukemia?
6. What is the role of the bone marrow biopsy in the diagnosis of hematologic disorders?
7. List the key differences between Hodgkin and non-Hodgkin lymphoma.
8. What are the indications for blood transfusion in chronic anemia?

Answers to Critical Thinking Questions

1. (b); 2. (c) ; 3. (c) ; 4. (c) ; 5. (c)

REFERENCES

1. Group, D. O. N. C. U. V. C. O. P. W., & Group, D. O. N. C. U. V. C. O. P. W. (2020). Disaster Response to the COVID-19 Pandemic for Patients with Kidney Disease in New York City. *Journal of the American Society of Nephrology, 31*(7), 1371–1379. https://doi.org/10.1681/asn.2020040520Addison, D., Branch, M., Baik, A. H., Fradley, M. G., Okwuosa, T. M., Reding, K. W., Simpson, K. E., et al. (2023). Equity in cardio-oncology care and research: A scientific statement from the American Heart Association. *Circulation, 148*, 297–308. https://doi.org/10.1161/cir.0000000000001158 (accessed on 16th July 2025).
2. Ajani, J. A., D'Amico, T. A., Bentrem, D. J., Chao, J., Cooke, D. T., Corvera, C. U., Das, P., et al. (2022). Gastric cancer, version 2.2022, NCCN Clinical Practice Guidelines in Oncology. *Journal of the National Comprehensive Cancer Network, 20*, 167–192. https://doi.org/10.6004/jnccn.2022.0008 (accessed on 16th July 2025).
3. Andrès, E., El Hassani Hajjam, A., Maloisel, F., Alonso-Ortiz, M. B., Méndez-Bailón, M., Lavigne, T., Jannot, X., et al. (2025). Artificial intelligence (AI) and drug-induced and idiosyncratic cytopenia: The role of AI in prevention, prediction, and patient participation. *Hematology Reports, 17*. https://www.semanticscholar.org/paper/62188717c487d0a5154868d2101df526da91913c (accessed on 16th July 2025).
4. Arnold, J. E., Camus, M. S., Freeman, K. P., Giori, L., Hooijberg, E. H., Jeffery, U., Korchia, J., et al. (2019). *ASVCP* Guidelines: Principles of quality assurance and standards for veterinary clinical pathology (version 3.0). *Veterinary Clinical Pathology, 48*, 542–618. https://doi.org/10.1111/vcp.12810 (accessed on 16th July 2025).
5. Bashshur, R. L., Doarn, C. R., Frenk, J., Kvedar, J. C., & Woolliscroft, J. O. (2020). Telemedicine and the COVID-19 pandemic, lessons for the future. *Telemedicine Journal and e-Health, 26*, 571–573. https://doi.org/10.1089/tmj.2020.29040.rb (accessed on 16th July 2025).
6. Browning, G. R., Kjelgaard-Hansen, M., Howard, L. L., Keener, L., LaFarga, M., & Perrin, K. L. (2024). Biological variation of hematology parameters and clinical application in African elephants (*Loxodonta africana*). *Journal of Zoo and Wildlife Medicine, 55*, 173–181. https://www.semanticscholar.org/paper/357911e53ec0801bc2ad58745f8f8951e463548e (accessed on 16th July 2025).
7. Conroy, P. B., Davel, S., Malherbe, J., Carrivick, S. J., & Briggs, E. N. (2025). Diagnostic and therapeutic challenges in an acute variegate porphyric crisis complicated by anuric renal failure and multiorgan dysfunction: A case report. *The American Journal of Case Reports, 26*. https://www.semanticscholar.org/paper/8d41710e35e48d3606135a45bf55e35a6a78ceaa (accessed on 16th July 2025).
8. Coyne, F. W., Terrell, D. R., Lang, V., Jenkins, A. M., King, A. A., & Smith, W. R. (2024). "It was bootstrap all the way": Exploring the barriers and facilitators to the development of non-hematology sickle cell disease experts in the United States. *Blood*. https://www.semanticscholar.org/paper/5db6509b2048976527509af352bd67d7c4a3f27d (accessed on 16th July 2025).
9. DeBaun, M. R., Jordan, L. C., King, A. A., Schatz, J., Vichinsky, E., Fox, C. K., McKinstry, R. C., et al. (2020). American Society of Hematology 2020 guidelines for sickle cell disease: Prevention, diagnosis, and treatment of cerebrovascular disease in children and adults. *Blood Advances, 4*, 1554–1588. https://doi.org/10.1182/bloodadvances.2019001142 (accessed on 16th July 2025).

10. Eidensohn, Y., & O'Rourke, P. (2025). Implementation and assessment of a lipoprotein(a) curriculum for internal medicine residents: A longitudinal study. *Cureus, 17*. https://www.semanticscholar.org/paper/706f16d27ffd4e7189d3ea37fc6d9cc8bbcd2380 (accessed on 16th July 2025).

11. Esteva, A., Chou, K., Yeung, S., Naik, N., Madani, A., Mottaghi, A., Liu, Y., et al. (2021). Deep learning-enabled medical computer vision. *npj Digital Medicine, 4*. https://doi.org/10.1038/s41746-020-00376-2 (accessed on 16th July 2025).

12. Faisal, I. B., Abbas, M. S., Thabit, Z. A., Aljebouri, D. M., & Almusawi, Y. A. (2024). The prevalence of erythrocyte alloimmunization in clinical practice: A hospital-based study. *Iraqi Journal of Hematology*. https://www.semanticscholar.org/paper/23317b5f2e51817b3ba0ab9ff47e8952a803e602 (accessed on 16th July 2025).

13. Gordon, M., Daniel, M., Ajiboye, A., Uraiby, H., Xu, N. Y., Bartlett, R., Hanson, J. L., et al. (2024). A scoping review of artificial intelligence in medical education: BEME Guide No. 84. *Medical Teacher, 46*, 446–470. https://doi.org/10.1080/0142159x.2024.2314198 (accessed on 16th July 2025).

14. Hall, G. B. F., Birkbeck, R., Brainard, B., Camacho, F., Davidow, E. B., LeVine, D., Mackin, A. J., et al. (2024). A prospective multicenter observational study assessing incidence and risk factors for acute blood transfusion reactions in dogs. *Journal of Veterinary Internal Medicine, 38*, 2495–2506. https://www.semanticscholar.org/paper/d0479422b90859014017a4a8d990c98449ae8541 (accessed on 16th July 2025).

15. Hassan, N., Nabih, N., Ibrahim, T., & Abdelfatah, R. G. (2023). Correlation between CD200 expression on leukemic stem cells and response to treatment in de-novo adult acute myeloid leukemia patients. *Ain Shams Medical Journal*. https://www.semanticscholar.org/paper/b26fe7cb90b6c49b81dbd05e145a0fd9065debe6 (accessed on 16th July 2025).

16. Huynh, N., Dayal, S., Sama, S., Eljabali, A., Mahmood, O., Meyer, W., Liman, A., et al. (2024). Inpatient blood transfusion usage at a community Veterans Affairs teaching hospital. *Blood*. https://www.semanticscholar.org/paper/07da10e702042be66f908f6ec21e2f5de884570a (accessed on 16th July 2025).

17. Jogie, J. A. (2025). A comprehensive review of occupational medicine in the paint industry: Roles of family medicine and internal medicine. *Cureus, 17*. https://www.semanticscholar.org/paper/f0e4687134fe4fba5dd7b7919870aed828701b1d (accessed on 16th July 2025).

18. Kerna, N. A., Flores, J. V., Pruitt, K. D., Carsrud, N. V., Ngwu, D. C., Rodriguez, D., Holets, H. M., et al. (2024). Hematological conditions associated with COVID-19: Pathophysiology, clinical manifestations, and therapeutic approaches. *European Journal of Medical and Health Research*. https://www.semanticscholar.org/paper/8e585d6a858ef00e74e4af1d00928c3a41bf9edd (accessed on 16th July 2025).

19. Kisakurek, Z., Sönmez, S. C., Osmanbaşoğlu, E., Öztürk, E., & Öztürk, A. (2021). Larynx angioedema as a signal in chronic lymphocytic leukemia: A case-based guide for acquired angioedema in the setting of lymphoproliferative disorders. *Asthma Allergy Immunology*. https://www.semanticscholar.org/paper/5605f949d2cd551e3f43082c47062a119d5fbc58 (accessed on 16th July 2025).

20. Kiseleva, A., Kotzinos, D., & De Hert, P. (2022). Transparency of AI in healthcare as a multilayered system of accountabilities: Between legal requirements and technical limitations.

Frontiers in Artificial Intelligence, 5. https://doi.org/10.3389/frai.2022.879603 (accessed on 16th July 2025).

21. Kruse-Jarres, R., Kempton, C. L., Baudo, F., Collins, P. W., Knoebl, P., Leissinger, C., Tiede, A., et al. (2017). Acquired hemophilia A: Updated review of evidence and treatment guidance. *American Journal of Hematology, 92*, 695–705. https://doi.org/10.1002/ajh.24777 (accessed on 16th July 2025).
22. Kucharz, E. (2023). A journal as a mirror of continued progress in internal medicine. A century of *Polish Archives of Internal Medicine. Polish Archives of Internal Medicine, 133*(4). https://www.semanticscholar.org/paper/52da3d30d410a344ced7cc007dcaffa5356a5d6e (accessed on 16th July 2025).
23. Kwak, M. S., Jeong, I. H., Cho, S. S., Woo, K., & Han, J. Y. (2022). Performance evaluation of the Abbott Alinity hs blood slide maker/stainer. *Annals of Laboratory Medicine, 42*, 482–484. https://www.semanticscholar.org/paper/c6f8bc6eb7616c592c35fbbb5355b55880ebb810 (accessed on 16th July 2025).
24. Lifshits, I., Agbaria, H., Zoabi Sawaed, A., Neuberger, A., & Darawshi, S. (2025). The approach of internal medicine healthcare personnel to palliative care. *Annals of Palliative Medicine, 14*(2), 128–135. https://www.semanticscholar.org/paper/b451acf1a9a1abc3a9f98321d92b397a34f102fa (accessed on 16th July 2025).
25. Linzer, M., Jin, J., Shah, P., Stillman, M., Brown, R., Poplau, S., Nankivil, N., et al. (2022). Trends in clinician burnout with associated mitigating and aggravating factors during the COVID-19 pandemic. *JAMA Health Forum, 3*, e224163–e224163. https://doi.org/10.1001/jamahealthforum.2022.4163 (accessed on 16th July 2025).
26. Lyman, G. H., Carrier, M., Ay, C., Di Nisio, M., Hicks, L. K., Khorana, A. A., Leavitt, A. D., et al. (2021). American Society of Hematology 2021 guidelines for management of venous thromboembolism: Prevention and treatment in patients with cancer. *Blood Advances, 5*, 927–974. https://doi.org/10.1182/bloodadvances.2020003442 (accessed on 16th July 2025).
27. Lyu, C., Shen, J., Wang, R., Gu, H., Zhang, J., Xue, F., Liu, X. F., et al. (2018). Targeted genome engineering in human induced pluripotent stem cells from patients with hemophilia B using the CRISPR-Cas9 system. *Stem Cell Research & Therapy, 9.* https://doi.org/10.1186/s13287-018-0839-8 (accessed on 16th July 2025).
28. McIlroy, G., Nikolousis, E., Abou-Zeid, N., Shankara, P., Kishore, B., Kaparou, M., Lovell, R., et al. (2020). Mixed T-cell chimerism at 3 months followed by donor lymphocyte infusion is independently associated with favorable outcomes in alemtuzumab-based reduced-intensity allogeneic hematopoietic stem cell transplantation. *Leukemia & Lymphoma, 61*, 202–205. https://www.semanticscholar.org/paper/5e320da8e521c568181be287d5bb8f878548f80b (accessed on 16th July 2025).
29. Meskó, B., & Topol, E. J. (2023). The imperative for regulatory oversight of large language models (or generative AI) in healthcare. *npj Digital Medicine, 6.* https://doi.org/10.1038/s41746-023-00873-0 (accessed on 16th July 2025).
30. Motomura, D. I. N., & Cameron, P. (2018). A curious case of hypercalcemia. *Canadian Journal of General Internal Medicine, 13.* https://www.semanticscholar.org/paper/efd1397fabee0e890a3a7d7d4eb28a4b43e75b72 (accessed on 16th July 2025).

31. Nakamura, S., Maeda, Y., Hori, T., & Oura, M. (2025). Hematology in community medical care. *The Journal of Medical Investigation: JMI, 72*(1.2), 21–25. https://www.semanticscholar.org/paper/0f7271b78222ebc86a047bd743a25c427ac76122 (accessed on 16th July 2025).

32. Naldini, L., Cicalese, M. P., Bernardo, M. E., Gentner, B., Gabaldo, M., Ferrari, G., & Aiuti, A. (2022). The EHA research roadmap: Hematopoietic stem cell gene therapy. *Hemisphere, 6*, e671. https://doi.org/10.1097/hs9.0000000000000671 (accessed on 16th July 2025).

33. Neunert, C., Terrell, D. R., Arnold, D. M., Buchanan, G. R., Cines, D. B., Cooper, N., Cuker, A., et al. (2019). American Society of Hematology 2019 guidelines for immune thrombocytopenia. *Blood Advances, 3*, 3829–3866. https://doi.org/10.1182/bloodadvances.2019000966 (accessed on 16th July 2025).

34. Nie, K., Ma, K., Luo, W., Shen, Z., Yang, Z., Xiao, M., Tong, T., et al. (2021). *Roseburia intestinalis*: A beneficial gut organism from the discoveries in genus and species. *Frontiers in Cellular and Infection Microbiology, 11*. https://doi.org/10.3389/fcimb.2021.757718 (accessed on 16th July 2025).

35. Papaemmanuil, E., Gerstung, M., Bullinger, L., Gaidzik, V. I., Paschka, P., Roberts, N. D., Potter, N., et al. (2016). Genomic classification and prognosis in acute myeloid leukemia. *New England Journal of Medicine, 374*, 2209–2221. https://doi.org/10.1056/nejmoa1516192 (accessed on 16th July 2025).

36. Parikh, E. N., Sharma, P., Steinberg, A., & Reddy, R. P. (2024). A survey-based analysis of factors influencing interest in hematology-oncology in internal medicine residents: A pilot study at an academic center. *Blood*. https://www.semanticscholar.org/paper/0bdeccd2556dc60e83ede8e22ea67a67eb4aa114 (accessed on 16th July 2025).

37. Peffault de Latour, R., & Risitano, A. (2023). Complement inhibition in medicine: Hematology and beyond; complement inhibition in hematology: PNH and beyond. *American Journal of Hematology, 98*. https://www.semanticscholar.org/paper/d3ba785a6fe44078a35223b1f6ff5d8903d71c0f (accessed on 16th July 2025).

38. Rosenstein, L. J. (2024). Practice makes perfect: Using simulation to build and assess competency in bone marrow biopsy for heme/onc fellows. *Journal of Clinical Oncology*. https://www.semanticscholar.org/paper/c57255061474e1117d17a3739a3d07046bcf1037 (accessed on 16th July 2025).

39. Rößler, J., Baumgärtner, I., & Kremer Hovinga, J. A. (2021). EHA endorsement of the Second International Guidelines for the diagnosis and management of hereditary hemorrhagic telangiectasia. *HemaSphere, 5*, e647–e647. https://doi.org/10.1097/hs9.0000000000000647 (accessed on 16th July 2025).

40. Sağlam, E., Şener, G., Bayrak, T., Bayrak, A. T., & Gorgulu, N. (2023). Analysis of ischemia-modified albumin (IMA) and coagulation parameters in patients with SARS-CoV-2 pneumonia. *Journal of Clinical Medicine, 12*. https://www.semanticscholar.org/paper/6ae1f0f7118d4d0f4c812029e674be9f6854cabd (accessed on 16th July 2025).

41. Shilpakar, R., Acharya, B., Neupane, P. C., Paudel, B., Acharya, S. C., Paudel, B., et al. (2025). Hematology-oncology education in postgraduate internal medicine programs in Nepal: Current status and the pressing need for improvement. *Journal of Clinical Oncology*. https://www.semanticscholar.org/paper/df596a8839dbc3985a986c5557edafd0bb3eda3a (accessed on 16th July 2025).

42. Tavis, L. A. (2002). *Novartis and the United Nations Global Compact Initiative.* https://www.wdi.umich.edu/files/Publications/WorkingPapers/wp526.pdf (accessed on 16th July 2025).

43. Tavis, L. A. (2025). *Novartis and the United Nations Global Compact Initiative.* https://core.ac.uk/download/pdf/7051026.pdf (accessed on 16th July 2025).

44. Teichman, J. (2024). Development and evaluation of a procedural skills clinic for teaching residents bone marrow biopsies and lumbar punctures on adult hematology patients. *Blood.* https://www.semanticscholar.org/paper/603eb690b2e29f06944c6920ebc56e187ca529bd (accessed on 16th July 2025).

45. Vallée, A. (2024). Envisioning the future of personalized medicine: Role and realities of digital twins. *Journal of Medical Internet Research, 26.* https://www.semanticscholar.org/paper/d03637d052fb73e10f83213798cd29ef27c25415 (accessed on 16th July 2025).

46. Venugopal, N., Louis, P., McInnis, C., Ssentongo, P., & Akhtar, N. (2024). Pilot: Hematology/oncology curriculum for the internal medicine and hematology/oncology sub-internships. *Blood.* https://www.semanticscholar.org/paper/eb4acaff455135512e414d2e8d918ff2c516cbaf (accessed on 16th July 2025).

47. Wallace, D. S., Maguire, C., Moore, J., Passero, F., Mariano, J., Casulo, C., & O'Connor, A. B. (2024). Reverse morning report: A case-based, fellow-lead, curriculum for internal medicine residents rotating on the inpatient malignant hematology service. *Blood.* https://www.semanticscholar.org/paper/9c04844b445a2e04c0e3b91480f5507543f7afd8 (accessed on 16th July 2025).

48. Weinberg, O. K., Arber, D. A., Döhner, H., Mullighan, C. G., Orgel, E., Porwit, A., Stone, R. M., et al. (2023). The International Consensus Classification of acute leukemias of ambiguous lineage. *Blood.* https://doi.org/10.1182/blood.2022019493 (accessed on 16th July 2025).

49. Yi, Z., Arvola, R. M., Myers, S., Dilsavor, C. N., Abu Alhasan, R., Carter, B. N., Patton, R. D., et al. (2022). Mammalian UPF3A and UPF3B can activate nonsense-mediated mRNA decay independently of their exon junction complex binding. *The EMBO Journal, 41.* https://doi.org/10.15252/embj.2021109202 (accessed on 16th July 2025).

INFECTIOUS DISEASES

8

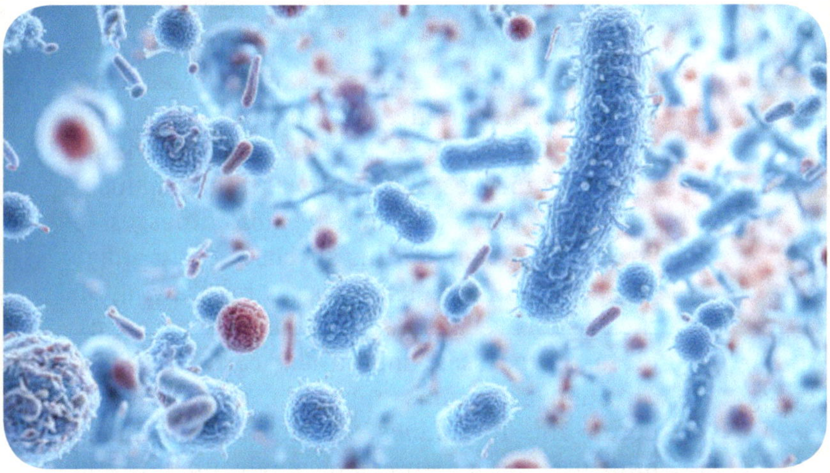

LEARNING OBJECTIVES

After studying this chapter, you will be able to:

1. Define historical context of Infectious Diseases
2. Identify the common infectious diseases
3. Understand the diagnostic techniques of infectious diseases
4. Explain the treatment modalities of infectious disease
5. Discus the challenges in of infectious diseases management

Introduction

The field of Infectious Diseases in Internal Medicine has a significant role in shaping healthcare delivery and patient outcomes against increasingly changing microbial threats. With changes in the world, infectious diseases are not only left in the history books but remain leading causes of sickness and mortality worldwide. The complexity of human-pathogen interactions, particularly in today's more urbanized and globalized setting, underscores the importance of knowledge of infectious agents and the intricacies of the human immune response. These need to be well understood by clinicians and public health experts so that effective strategies can be formulated to address infections, thereby avoiding overburdening the healthcare system. With greater focus on emerging diseases, including antibiotic resistance and the functions of microbial communities in humans, internal medicine specialists are at the forefront of solving today's infectious disease challenges. The dynamic process between human beings and microbes, and the concept conveyed by the microbiota notion, further indicate the relevance of Internal Medicine to Infectious Diseases. In the gastrointestinal tract, trillions of microbes play a role in our health by breaking down food, modulating the immune system, and regulating our metabolism. Dysbiosis, or an imbalance in this microbiota, however, can cause various diseases, such as inflammatory bowel conditions, and increase susceptibility to infections.

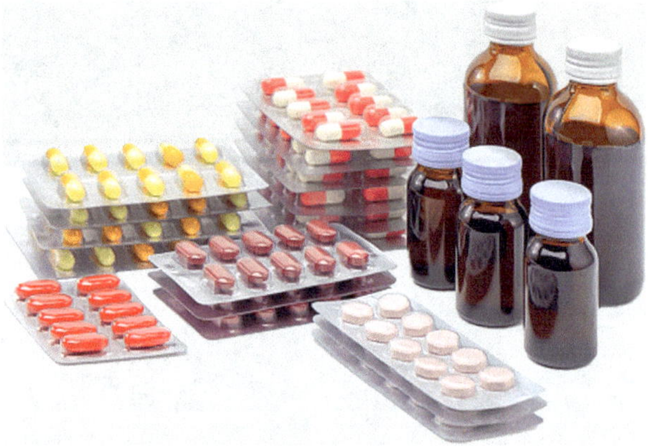

Figure 8.1. Internal medicine for infectious diseases.

Source: https://spshospitals.com/wp-content/uploads/2022/10/Internal-Medicine.png.

Recent research investigated these correlations and highlighted the need for a better understanding of the role of the microbiota in disease mechanisms. These new findings in grasping the sophistication of human-microbe interactions are essential in guiding clinical practice and therapeutic management, highlighting the necessity of an integrated approach in managing infectious diseases. Also, the social and economic impact of diseases necessitates a holistic response that integrates clinical practice and public health interventions. The association of over-the-counter (OTC) medicine sales and patient visits to urgent care clinics illustrates the social processes of accessing and utilizing healthcare. Research has shown that OTC sales can strongly forecast patient volume across different seasons, indicating the public's use of self-medication and its implications for managing healthcare resources. These trends need to be identified by internal medicine professionals who work at the intersection of patient treatment and broader healthcare trends. More generally, the complexity of infectious diseases requires an agile, multifaceted strategy, making Internal Medicine for Infectious Diseases a crucial area of study in contemporary medicine (Figure 8.1).

Definition of Internal Medicine

Internal medicine is the basis of adult medicine, encompassing numerous subspecialties, such as infectious diseases. Internal medicine primarily focuses on the prevention, diagnosis, and management of non-surgical illnesses in adults. Physicians in this specialty can manage common and complex illnesses by drawing on their extensive knowledge of the body's systems, disease processes, and patient care strategies. Through a systems approach, internists are better able to balance the interactions among multiple factors—lifestyle, environment, and genetics—that may affect a patient's well-being. This is particularly crucial for infectious diseases, where knowledge of pathophysiology and epidemiology plays a key role in managing and treating them effectively, thereby underscoring the role of internal medicine in modern healthcare (Escota et al., 2020). In the field of infectious diseases, internal medicine clinicians are taught to address the threats posed by pathogens such as fungi, viruses, bacteria, and parasites. They perform a thorough patient evaluation, including infection history, symptomatology, and clinical manifestations, to guide diagnosis and treatment. The task of an internist in the healthcare profession is not merely treatment; it also entails preventive care initiatives to contain the spread of infectious diseases. Preventive care interventions are more essential given the current globalized threat of emerging infectious diseases. This knowledge, once acquired, is not only used in the management of existing conditions but is also essential for establishing public health programs that aim to prevent infectious disease outbreaks, thereby underscoring the multidimensional role of internists in infectious disease control (Anderson et al., 2018). Infectious disease control also needs to be approached from a multidisciplinary aspect, as well as adherence to best practices in medicine. Internal medicine is the vehicle that promotes this team effort through interdisciplinary cooperation and the sharing of resources between physicians. By embracing a multidisciplinary approach to comprehensive care, internists are better positioned to address the complex nature of infectious diseases, which often require input from microbiologists, epidemiologists, and public health experts. Diversity of input ensures a more effective fight against infectious disease threats, resulting in better patient outcomes. Hence, the concept of internal medicine extends into a paradigm for education and response to the evolving dynamics of infectious disease, underscoring the crucial role of internists in combating such health threats (Anderson et al., 2018; Escota et al., 2020).

Overview of Infectious Diseases

Infectious diseases constitute a significant component of the global health profile and continue to pose challenges to public health systems worldwide. These diseases, caused by pathogens such as bacteria, viruses, fungi, and parasites, are transmitted from individuals or animals and may cause severe health challenges. The relationships between environmental determinants, social determinants, and human actions make infection epidemiology more complex. One example worth mentioning is the emergence of zoonotic diseases, which occur in animals but can be transmitted to humans, underscoring the need for a One Health approach that integrates human, animal, and environmental health to address infectious diseases effectively (Anderson et al., 2018). To understand these diseases, one needs a multi-perspective approach that considers the causative biological mechanisms, patterns of transmission, and determinants of outbreaks. The global infectious disease burden is not only evident in morbidity and mortality but also in its substantial economic costs. Research indicates that the cost of managing outbreaks tends to exceed initial healthcare costs, underscoring the need for proactive actions and public health interventions. This can be particularly evident during influenza seasons, when non-pharmaceutical interventions and off-the-shelf sales of over-the-counter (OTC) drugs can have substantial implications for healthcare utilization patterns. An analysis of the relationship between patient volume in urgent care clinics and sales of over-the-counter medications illustrates how consumer behavior can reflect and shape public health trends (Kaufmann et al., 2013). Healthcare providers and policymakers, in their quest to control infectious diseases, should understand these interactions to have effective control and prevention efforts. Control of infectious diseases requires coordination across multiple sectors, indicating the need to adopt multidisciplinary approaches. Projects like the Southern African Centre for Infectious Disease Surveillance (SACIDS) mirror this integrated approach, inviting convergence among various actors to achieve better health outcomes. Evaluation of such initiatives identifies strengths in systematic coordination and infrastructure sharing, as well as problems such as resource distribution and limitations in data sharing, which are critical to successful implementation (Anderson et al., 2018). These reviews highlight the importance of reactive, adaptability and responsiveness to emerging threats, and remind us that combating infectious diseases is not limited to clinical treatment alone. A combination of education, research, and community mobilization is critical to preventing the spread of these diseases and enhancing global health security (Figure 8.2).

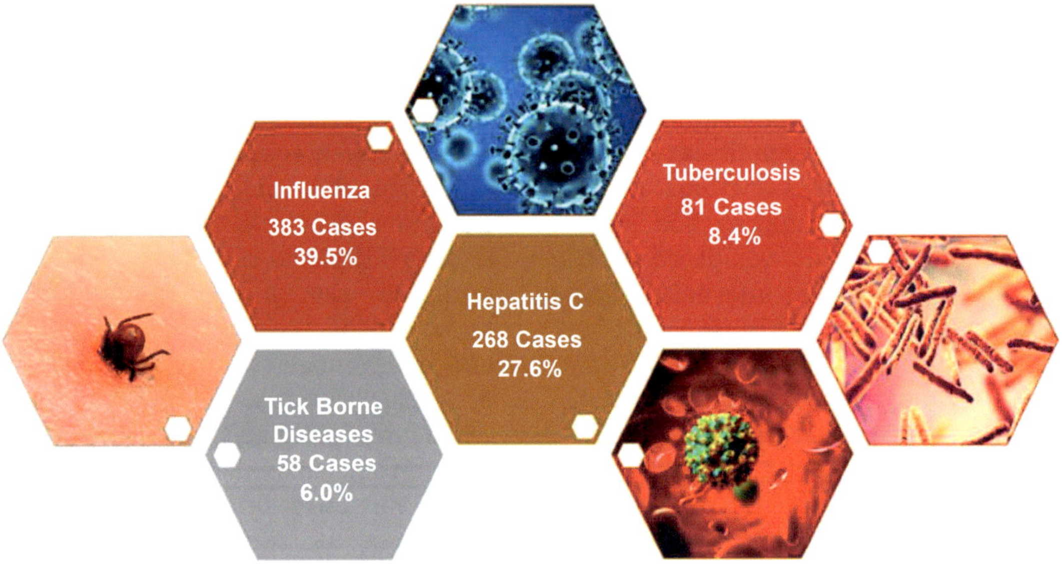

Figure 8.2. Overview of infectious diseases.

Source: https://webster-ma.gov/ImageRepository/Document?documentId=13544.

Importance of Internal Medicine in Treating Infectious Diseases

Internal medicine is the cornerstone of the treatment of infectious diseases and serves as the pillar of the healthcare system for the treatment of complex cases. Internists undergo extensive training in the diagnosis and management of diverse infections, with essential knowledge for appropriate management. Their skill is not just the mere treatment course; it is the ability to incorporate patient histories, symptoms, and laboratory tests to design overall treatment plans. For instance, the very lack of consistency in following antimicrobial guidelines emphasizes the importance of internists handling these complexities effectively. In a research study, compliance was much better with lower respiratory tract infections than with sepsis and urinary tract infections, indicating the need for sound clinical judgment (Alvarez et al., 2005). The internists' capacity to integrate multiple pieces of information prepares them to prevent the risks of inappropriate antimicrobial prescribing and, consequently, to promote the advancement of public health. The management of infectious diseases by internal medicine physicians is of vital importance, particularly in the era of rising antibiotic resistance and emerging pathogens. Internists are proficient at assessing the suitability of initial therapy and the pivotal transition to culture-directed treatment. Nevertheless, the majority of practitioners lean more towards defensive prescribing at the cost of long-term resistance consequences compared to short-term patient outcomes (Alvarez et al., 2005). This is a testament to the balancing act that internists have to perform between patient safety and public health concerns. Furthermore, given the ever-evolving nature of infectious diseases, the internal medicine community must remain vigilant to detect trends in disease recurrence and drug resistance. For instance, metronidazole monotherapy has been shown to significantly influence recurrence rates in Clostridium difficile infection, particularly among high-risk ribotype patients. The above indicates the utmost importance of internal medicine's function in reforming treatment strategies to decrease recurrence and optimize patient outcomes. Moreover, internists' interprofessional collaborations greatly enhance infectious disease management. Internal medicine physicians have an optimal position, by collaborating with infectious disease specialists, pharmacists, and public health professionals, as gatekeepers for the provision of full-care services. The interdisciplinary model is more important than ever in addressing the multifaceted challenge posed by infectious diseases, such as that of Clostridium difficile infection. The study found stark differences in predictors of recurrence between patient groups, underscoring the imperative for tailored therapeutic approaches that consider individual risk profiles. As specialists in internal medicine, internists are ideally suited to offer these collaborations, ensuring that treatment guidelines are not only evidence-based but also attuned to patients' needs. With infectious diseases able to travel so quickly across borders, the role of internal medicine in this collaborative environment is more critical than ever.

8.1. Historical Context

Learning Outcome

1. Define the evolution of infectious disease treatment
2. Discuss on internal medicine
3. Understand the milestones in infectious disease research

The historical background of internal medicine, particularly in infectious diseases, illustrates how previous epidemics and advances in medicine have shaped practice today. For instance, the late 20th-century emergence of HIV/AIDS brought a fresh epidemic spotlight to infectious diseases that triggered revolutionary changes in treatment paradigms. Early studies, including the EMERALD trial, established combination therapies, particularly those involving antiretrovirals such as Darunavir/cobicistat/emtricitabine/tenofovir alafenamide (D/C/F/TAF) (Ajana et al., 2019), as effective. These developments highlight the importance of a historical context in understanding the development of treatment methods informed by past epidemics and current research. Additionally, knowledge of the social response to such conditions can help explain existing stigmas and policy decisions that impact patient care today. The historical effects of infectious diseases are not limited to clinical outcomes; they significantly shape public health policies and community reactions. For example, Prof. Stillwaggon's chapter touches on diseases prevalent in sub-Saharan Africa and shows that differences in HIV incidence among populations cannot be explained solely by differences in behavior, but instead reflect greater socioeconomic and health disparities (Sawers et al., 2018). This emphasizes the intricate association between historical context, disease prevalence, and the evolution of medical concepts in internal medicine for infectious diseases. An appreciation of this rich, multifaceted history can inform modern treatment and prevention interventions, particularly for diseases disproportionately affecting disenfranchised populations. Furthermore, the historical background of infectious diseases underlines the paramount value of multidisciplinary collaboration in internal medicine. The synergistic interaction between infectious disease physicians, epidemiologists, and public health activists has assisted in contending with the challenges posed by such diseases as HIV/AIDS. The results of the EMERALD trials can be seen as reflecting lessons learned from previous outbreaks and treatment failures, underscoring the efficacy and safety of new treatments (Ajana et al., 2019). In addition, recognizing the social factors' contribution to disease transmission and control can inform more effective, culturally sensitive healthcare interventions. Thus, historical understanding not only adds to our experience of infectious disease but also provides invaluable blueprints for the setting up of lasting remedies in internal medicine.

8.1.1. Evolution of Infectious Disease Treatment

The history of the treatment of infectious diseases has been principally shaped by advances in biomedical science and technology. Conventionally, procedures such as bloodletting and the use of herbal medicine have formed the bulk of medical practice. But with the discovery of antibiotics in the middle of the 20th century came a vital turning point, essentially transforming previously fatal infections into curable conditions.

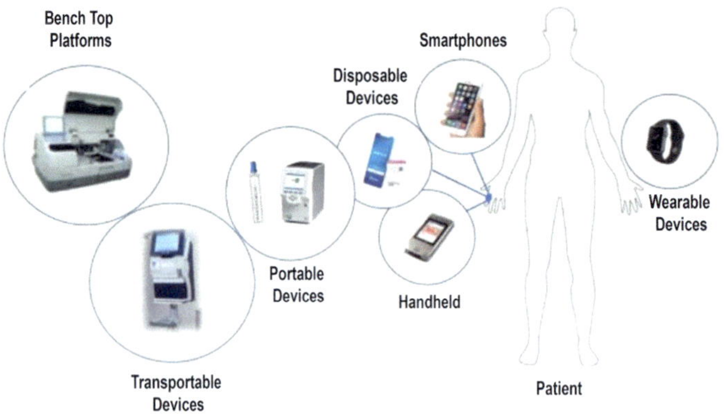

Figure 8.3. Evolution of infectious disease treatment.

Source: https://incacare.live/wp-content/uploads/2022/04/Capture2-1024x568.png.

After the discovery of penicillin, physicians saw death rates from bacterial infections dwindle, and this ushered in a revolution in disease management. Furthermore, as our understanding of microbial resistance grew, the focus of infectious disease treatment evolved from merely eradicating pathogens to implementing strategies that prevent resistance, demonstrating a significant progression in medical methodologies and philosophies in the field of internal medicine for infectious diseases. In the contemporary landscape of infectious disease management, innovative treatments such as clinical metagenomic next-generation sequencing (mNGS) represent the next frontier in bacterial diagnostics. This is a sophisticated technique that allows for the thorough analysis of the host and microbial genetic material isolated from patients to quickly and effectively detect the pathogens. Such technological advancements have the potential to promote antimicrobial resistance research and the role of the human microbiome in disease and health. By integrating mNGS applications into clinical laboratories, physicians are more likely to tailor treatments to each patient's needs and thereby improve therapeutic outcomes. However, there is a challenge in bringing these new technologies together, necessitating the development of robust frameworks to best leverage their application in clinical settings and to ensure they effectively guide infectious disease treatment strategies (Chiu et al., 2019). Moreover, the importance of cooperation in managing infectious diseases cannot be overstated, particularly across global networks dedicated to disease surveillance and response. The Rockefeller Foundation evaluation of the Disease Surveillance Networks (DSN) Initiative highlights the challenges of trans-boundary, multi-sectoral collaboration in addressing the efficacy of disease surveillance. The evidence shows that more coordinated, collaborative networks can strengthen the identification, tracking, and response to infectious threats across borders. This multi-faceted approach to infectious diseases not only affirms the conviction that health is everyone's responsibility worldwide but also validates existing treatment practices by addressing the systemic aspect of treating infectious diseases. As such, collaborative platforms continue to evolve; they will play an increasingly significant role in defining public health policy and strategy, and ultimately, translating into better patient outcomes within internal medicine for infectious diseases (Kimball et al., 2011) (Figure 8.3).

8.1.2. Key Figures in Internal Medicine

Within the field of internal medicine, and more specifically in the specialty of infectious diseases, certain critical actors have made important contributions to our knowledge and care for clinical conditions. Dr. Paul Farmer is one of them, known for his work with Partners In Health, where he has led the way in providing healthcare in poor resource environments. Farmers' application of public health concepts to clinical practice stands out in particular, most notably in infectious diseases that disproportionately affect socially vulnerable groups. His call to tackle the social determinants of health emphasizes the value of a systems-based approach in internal medicine, calling for policies that cross customary clinical boundaries. The intricacy of disease control for infectious diseases often involves interdisciplinary collaboration, as noted in the Rockefeller Foundation's evaluation of the Disease Surveillance Networks program, which calls for strong, multi-sectoral partnerships to enhance disease surveillance and response (Kimball et al., 2011). Another prominent figure in internal medicine is Dr. Anthony Fauci, whose research during the HIV/AIDS epidemic and the more recent COVID-19 pandemic has guided public health interventions globally. His research on infectious disease pathogenesis and treatment has guided significant advances in clinical practice to the discovery of life-saving treatments that have rescued millions of lives. Fauci's tenure at the National Institute of Allergy and Infectious Diseases illustrates how central individuals can lead research efforts and tackle urgent public health problems. His focus on the significance of scientific communication during public health emergencies serves as a reminder of the role of internal medicine professionals beyond the clinic. The success of projects reliant on improved disease surveillance and response, such as in the Rockefeller Foundation's report, is consonant with Fauci's call for ongoing research and collaboration in infectious disease control (Kimball et al., 2011). Moreover, Dr. Ellenberg's work in epidemiology and prevention of infectious diseases has revolutionized knowledge of disease spread and intervention effectiveness. By the use of advanced statistical methods, she has illuminated infectious disease dynamics that can be applied to evidence-based clinical interventions. Her work has also highlighted the need for surveillance systems to monitor infectious disease trends, as explained in the Disease Surveillance Networks assessment. The ability to detect and respond to outbreaks in a timely way is crucial to mitigating the effects of infectious disease. The integration of empirical research and clinical practice, as embodied by figures like Dr. Ellenberg, is essential in internal medicine, especially in managing complex problems posed by infectious diseases (Kimball et al., 2011).

8.1.3. Milestones in Infectious Disease Research

Infectious disease research has been guided by milestones that have shaped public health policies and clinical practices. One such milestone is the discovery of antibiotics in the 20th century, which revolutionized the management of bacterial infections. Penicillin, discovered by Alexander Fleming in 1928, ushered in a new era of medicine in which what had been previously incurable infections became curable, significantly reducing mortality. This discovery was not only a scientific breakthrough but also the value of collaborative research efforts. With Kohrt (2025) hypothesizing that science, technology, and marketplace collaboration at the intersection have driven innovation in infectious disease control, illustrating how collaborative efforts can yield significant impacts on public health. In addition to advances in pharmacology, innovations in behavioral interventions have significantly impacted infectious disease control. Interventions targeting hygiene behaviors, such as handwashing, have proven highly effective in preventing the spread of contagious diseases. The Southeast Asia programs are a good case in point, specifically the Vietnam program, whose intervention was not only aimed at changing behavior but also at learning about local practices and customs to effect lasting change. This approach shows a growing recognition that the prevention of infectious diseases is as much a social issue as a health issue, involving community engagement and specific interventions. As N/A (2011) describes, tapping the resources of the private sector alongside public health systems can expand the reach and impact of such schemes, demonstrating an integrated effort in the battle against infectious diseases. Last but not least, the application of vaccination programs is a breakthrough in the success of infectious disease research. Vaccines have been invaluable in the prevention of contagious diseases like measles, polio, and hepatitis, and have saved millions of lives worldwide. Previous efforts, such as the global smallpox eradication campaign, have set precedents for the success of coordinated global vaccine implementation initiatives. These milestones are an actual reflection of the importance of international cooperation, as evidenced in Kohrt (2025), where multidisciplinary works propel ahead the disciplines of science and public health. Ultimately, future improvement in the field of infectious diseases hinges on such cooperation, pointing to the unity required to address future challenges in this ever-changing arena (Figure 8.4).

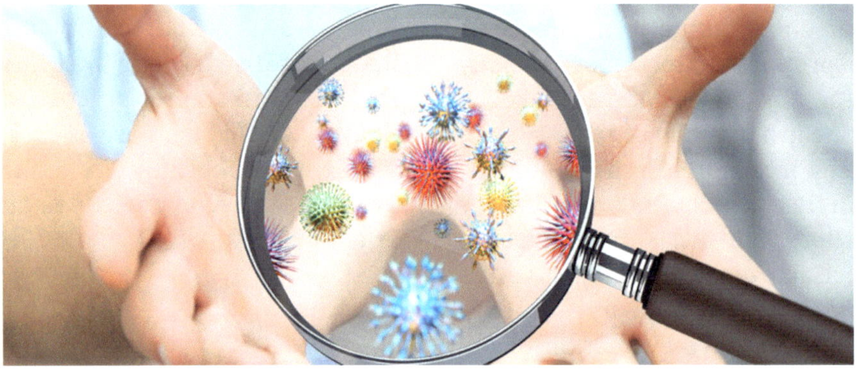

Figure 8.4. Milestones in infectious disease research.

Source: https://www.urmc.rochester.edu/MediaLibraries/URMCMedia/vaccine-research-unit/images/idrc-slider2.jpg.

Test Your Knowledge

1. How has the development of antibiotics transformed the treatment of infectious diseases?
2. What role has vaccination played in controlling infectious diseases over time?

8.2. Common Infectious Diseases

Learning Outcome

1. Define the bacterial infections
2. Describe the viral infections
3. Discuss on fungal infections

Treatment for common infectious diseases in internal medicine has evolved. There have been developments in diagnostic techniques, such as clinical metagenomic next-generation sequencing (mNGS), that have brought sophisticated methods for detecting pathogens. This integrative analysis allows clinicians to make diagnoses more accurately and, hence, individualize drug regimens to the microbial agents. This change is not just critical for fighting prevalent infections such as pneumonia, influenza, and urinary tract infections, but also for controlling emerging infections in complex patient populations. The integration of mNGS into practice represents a paradigm shift, providing important insights into infectious diseases, particularly when standard culturing methods are unsuccessful. These innovations contribute significantly to better patient outcomes and shorter duration of illness, demonstrating the immense capability of internal medicine in limiting infectious diseases (Chiu et al., 2019). Further, the intersection of public health and infectious diseases cannot be overstated, especially where vulnerable populations are concerned. All the studies that are currently being conducted, particularly in the Veterans Affairs (VA) system, are focusing on delivering quality healthcare services to those individuals afflicted with war-related ailments and associated infections. This group is most susceptible to various types of infectious diseases, including respiratory and sexually transmitted infections. A push to increase the provision of treatment and the delivery of healthcare is a positive for immediate medical needs, as well as long-term welfare and health for veterans. Healthcare professionals, aware of veterans' specific health problems, can ensure that they have dedicated programs in place that are attuned to the multifaceted nature of disease and recovery, ultimately seeking a holistic approach to care in internal medicine (N/A, 2014). The efforts of internal medicine specialists play a key role in the ongoing battle to reduce the prevalence and impact of common infectious diseases. Through constant learning, research, and practice, such specialists are spearheading the fight against not only current infections but also emerging new threats resulting from public health challenges. For instance, antibiotic resistance and the recrudescence of vaccine-preventable diseases call for preemptive prevention and treatment measures. Internal medicine practitioners can help create a resilient health infrastructure in the face of infectious disease pressures by leveraging advances in diagnostics and prevention. As the health landscape continually changes, so too must the methods used by internal medicine to be responsive to a diverse and evolving population, reaffirming, in turn, its fundamental position in public health (Chiu et al., 2019).

8.2.1. Bacterial Infections

Bacterial infections are a leading issue in internal medicine, particularly because they can cause a variety of clinical syndromes, ranging from harmless to life-threatening. The multifactorial etiology of these infections arises from the diversity of mechanisms of pathogenicity various bacterial species possess, coupled with the variability of the host immune response. For instance, Gram-positive bacterial infections, such as Streptococcus and Staphylococcus, can cause pneumonia and septicemia, while Gram-negative bacteria, such as Escherichia coli and Klebsiella, are generally responsible for urinary tract and hospital infections. The emergence of multidrug-resistant organisms complicates diagnosis and treatment and demands extensive knowledge of microbial behavior and host interaction to treat such an infection effectively. Recent advancements in diagnostic testing, including the emergence of clinical metagenomic next-generation sequencing (mNGS), have transformed the landscape of bacterial infection control. The technology opens the door to the simultaneous detection of a wide variety of pathogens, thereby improving the accuracy of diagnosis compared to traditional culture techniques. mNGS not only facilitates the identification of microbial pathogens but also provides details on antimicrobial resistance and the host's immune response. While integration of mNGS into standard practice is beneficial, there are challenges in its widespread use and standardization.

Overcoming these challenges can potentially optimize patient care and enhance public health returns from infectious disease, particularly because healthcare networks are struggling to keep pace with evolving bacterial threats (Chiu et al., 2019). The urgent issue of antibiotic resistance underscores the added intricacy of treating bacterial infections. Over the past several decades, the pace of antibiotic development has decreased considerably, leaving existing antibiotics increasingly ineffective against resistant bacteria. The pharmaceutical industry's abdication from antibiotic development, driven by the natural difficulty of finding new agents and the low returns of pursuing such projects, exacerbates the crisis (Coukell et al., 2016). As a result, healthcare providers are routinely confronted with stubborn infections that demand new treatment modalities, such as combination therapy or the use of last-resort antibiotics. The mutually reinforcing dynamic between antibiotic use and resistance underscores the importance of careful prescribing practices, ongoing monitoring of resistance patterns, and increased research into antibiotic development to safeguard the public from the rising tide of bacterial infections.

8.2.2. Viral Infections

The increasing number of viral infections highlights the seminal issues in internal medicine, particularly in infectious diseases. Influenza, HIV, and SARS-CoV-2 are examples of viruses that are highly contagious on a mass scale with severe morbidity and mortality. The effects of these infections extend past the immediate viral insult; secondary infection can complicate clinical courses. For example, bacterial pneumonia is persistent as a secondary complication following viral infection. It suggests that intrinsic pathogenic processes, such as viral infections, can establish a pattern for further pathogenic development and growth, necessitating an integrated management plan that includes not only antiviral medication but also prophylactic measures to control secondary complications (Dear et al., 2020). Consequently, it is essential for clinicians who see patients in an internal medicine clinic to grasp the relationship between viral and bacterial pathogens. Viral infections are often well-documented to trigger a series of immunological responses that can lead to an array of complications. For instance, critically ill patients with COVID-19 have been documented to progress to invasive pulmonary aspergillosis (IPA), a complication that is typically encountered by compromised immune systems. Notably, in patients where IPA initially occurs without pre-existing risk factors, the complexity of the interaction between viral infections and opportunistic pathogens is illustrated (Eller et al., 2021). These interactions have the potential to exacerbate the clinical presentation, thereby complicating diagnosis and treatment protocols. Thus, treatment of viral infections includes screening for potential opportunistic infections that may occur due to the immunocompromised state induced by the virus. As physicians work to address such intricacies, the need for coordinated care approaches grows, mandating even greater caution in patient treatment and observation. The advancement of antiviral drug treatments has transformed the therapeutic approach to viral infections, yet problems remain to be overcome. Development of resistance, particularly to chronic viral disorders like HIV, is the biggest deterrent to efficacious treatment. Besides, the emergence of new virus strains, as seen with influenza and SARS-CoV-2, calls for ongoing research and adjustments to treatment protocols. Targeted public health interventions based on vaccination are necessary to provide a preventive paradigm against viral infections with morbidity. However, as also observed with the current ongoing mutation of these pathogens, vaccination alone is not sufficient. Deep-thinking strategies that include public health policy, patient education, and tailored therapeutic interventions must be employed to effectively combat the pervasive threat of viral infections in the practice of internal medicine for infectious diseases (Figure 8.5).

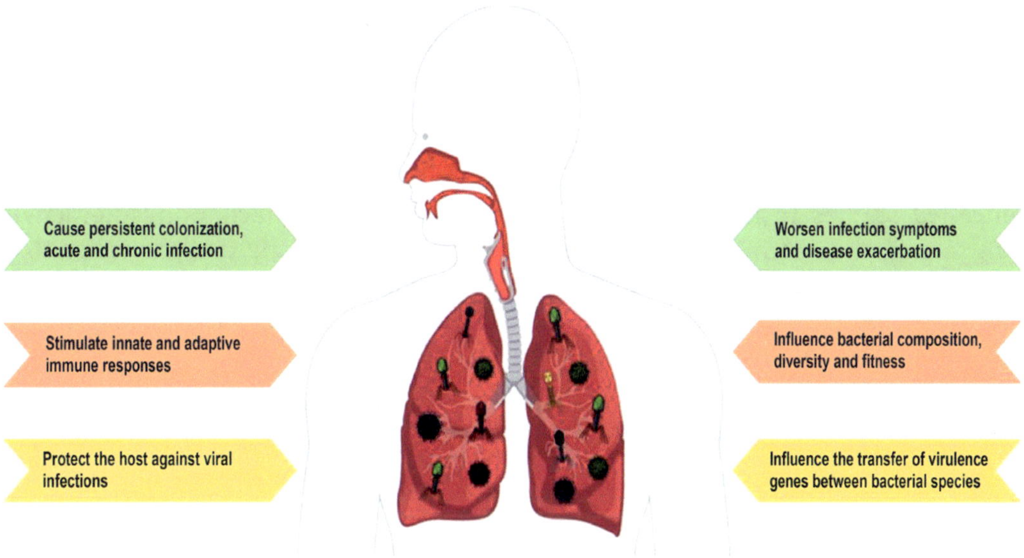

Figure 8.5. Viral infections.

Source: https://www.frontiersin.org/files/Articles/885341/fimmu-13-885341-HTML/image_m/fimmu-13-885341-g001.jpg.

8.2.3. Fungal Infections

Fungal infection is an emerging problem in the practice of internal medicine, particularly with morbidity and mortality from these conditions still on the rise. Fungal infections, which are caused by a spectrum of fungal pathogens ranging from benign yeasts to more pathogenic moulds, are predominantly prevalent in immunocompromised individuals, such as those with HIV/AIDS, cancer, or organ transplant recipients. Timely treatment and diagnosis are essential in managing these infections, which often can mimic bacterial or viral infections. Recent methods, such as clinical metagenomic next-generation sequencing (mNGS), have proven effective in this regard. mNGS facilitates the simultaneous, holistic examination of microbial pathogens, enhancing diagnostic accuracy and supporting appropriate therapeutic decisions, thereby maximizing patient outcomes in complex fungal infections (Chiu et al., 2019). The flexibility and variability of fungi pose formidable challenges to prevention and treatment maneuvers. Fungi are unique in that they possess specialized cellular structures and mechanisms that enable them to become resistant to conventional antifungal treatments. This is further compounded by the widespread use of antifungal drugs in the clinic and agriculture, heightening concerns for antimicrobial stewardship. Management of fungal infections requires not only specific therapy but also a proper understanding of the immune system of the hosts and comorbidities. In such situations, a multidisciplinary approach is necessary, bringing together expertise from across medicine to address the multidimensionality of fungal infections. Research workers continue to advocate for tightly controlled studies to further elucidate the mechanisms of the interactions between fungal pathogens and host defence, especially in vulnerable groups (Eijck et al., 2003). In addition to improved diagnostic and therapeutic strategies, public health interventions are also crucial in combating the epidemic of fungal disease. Health awareness programs and education can equip clinicians and patients to identify the signs and symptoms of such infections early, ultimately leading to better health outcomes. Surveillance programs are targeted to identify new fungal pathogens, especially those associated with agriculture and environmental advances. Increasing recognition that certain animal husbandry practices apply to zoonotic disease transmission of fungi has underscored the need for an increasingly integrative infectious disease control strategy. Evidence shows that organic farming practices, although commonly perceived as safer, can, in turn, create emerging problems, such as exposure to zoonotic fungal pathogens (Eijck et al., 2003). Hence, facilitating interactivity among scientists, clinicians, and public health officials is essential to the evolution of effective measures to address the threat of fungal infection in humans.

Test Your Knowledge

1. What are the most common infectious diseases affecting humans worldwide?
2. How are infectious diseases transmitted from person to person?

8.3. Diagnostic Techniques

Learning Outcome

1. Understand the laboratory testing in internal medicine infectious diseases
2. Define the imaging studies in internal medicine infectious diseases
3. Discuss the clinical evaluation in internal medicine infectious diseases

The diagnosis of internal medicine infectious diseases is changing, driven largely by the need for rapid, accurate detection of pathogens. Traditional diagnostics rely on microbiological culture and serological investigations, which, though effective, are time-consuming and can hamper the treatment of infectious diseases. To illustrate, tuberculosis is a significant global health problem, with its traditional diagnosis taking weeks to yield results. The lack of access to rapid point-of-care tests is also a significant contributing factor towards delays in diagnosis and treatment, thereby allowing continued transmission in populations (Harari et al., 2012). This underscores the need for advanced diagnostic technologies, including the development of new biomarker tests, to accelerate the identification of active infections and resistance patterns. The improvement in diagnostic techniques is therefore crucial to enhancing patient outcomes and control of disease transmission. Invasive fungal infections (IFDs) are another area where diagnostic innovation plays a significant role. Traditional IFD definitions and classification have mainly been described in reference to discrete patient populations, such as cancer patients and transplant patients. However, with the introduction of new diagnostic techniques, it became necessary to redefine the above systems. Recent efforts to reclassify IFDs have incorporated imaging and laboratory diagnostic information to aid in detecting infection in an increasing number of patients (Akan et al., 2019). This change is particularly necessary because it allows clinicians to detect IFDs, ultimately leading to more effective treatments more specifically.

Such a revision can address the diverse presentations of fungal infections in both immunocompetent and immunocompromised patients, underscoring the multidimensional nature of these diseases, even in current medicine. In addition, integrating technological frontiers such as molecular diagnostics can revolutionize the field. Polymerase chain reaction (PCR) and next-generation sequencing are among the tools enabling rapid pathogen identification and genetic material detection, providing invaluable insights into potential drug resistance and co-infection. These technologies facilitate individualized treatment regimens tailored to each patient's profile. Further, the ability to rapidly identify pathogens can significantly reduce hospitalizations and improve prognostic outcomes in the treatment of infectious diseases. However, despite the promising advances of these approaches, availability, cost, and the need for trained professionals to interpret complex results remain constraints. The continuous interest in optimizing and utilizing these diagnostic techniques is essential to advance the quality of care in internal medicine for infectious diseases (Figure 8.6).

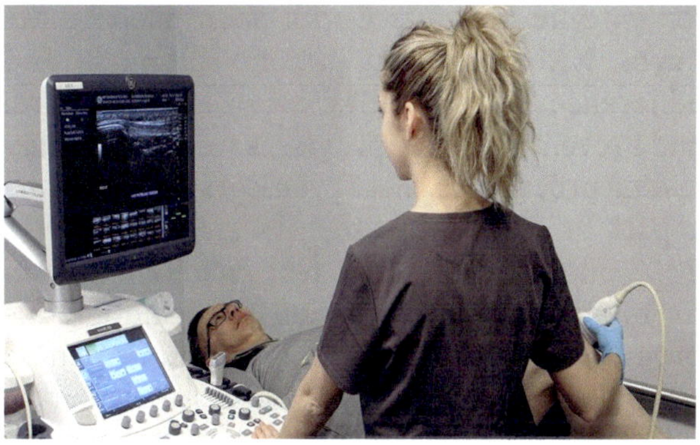

Figure 8.6. Diagnostic techniques in internal medicine.

Source: https://www.recomind.net/wp-content/uploads/2023/05/diagnostic-imaging-systems-875x528.jpg.

8.3.1. Laboratory Testing

Laboratory testing is a pillar of accurate diagnosis and effective treatment in internal medicine for infectious diseases. Without precise diagnostic tests, the management of infectious diseases can be complicated by misdiagnosis. The implementation of robust laboratory testing protocols enables the identification of causative agents of infections, leading to targeted therapies. However, it is crucial to remember that no diagnostic test is infallible; hence, understanding a test's sensitivity and specificity is vital. Particularly in diverse populations, the prevalence of a disease plays a massive role in test result interpretation, which is crucial in disease control efforts. As science advances, adherence to these principles in laboratory testing will enhance the efficacy of clinical decision-making and outcomes in infectious diseases. Progress in the laboratory over the last few years has altered our approach to evaluating infectious diseases, holding out the promise of new screening devices and therapies. The move away from invasive diagnosis, such as liver biopsy for the assessment of hepatitis C, has streamlined the diagnostic process. New evidence suggests that all-oral therapy for chronic hepatitis C will soon become the norm, with increased patient tolerance and adherence. As new Centers for Disease Control and Prevention (CDC) programs work to simplify testing procedures, these processes must become a part of regular practice. Notably, the CDC's 2012 one-time-only HCV test recommendation for individuals born between 1945 and 1965 is proof of the shift towards increased screening measures that can greatly improve detection rates. This evolution in laboratory testing is part of an overall commitment to optimizing patient care through informed, timely intervention. In the setting of infectious disease, communication between laboratory staff and primary care physicians is essential to optimal healthcare delivery. Open communication of laboratory test results is essential to facilitate timely decision-making and a thorough understanding of a patient's health state. By employing evidence-based practice when interpreting laboratory results, health care practitioners can make logical decisions about treatment modalities and disease management. Continuous consideration of laboratory evidence helps healthcare practitioners ensure they use tests that, in addition to informing treatment, also account for the broader implications of diagnostic testing for population health. On this point, prudent observation of laboratory findings can influence management strategies. In response, this affects how the co-infection and enduring pathogen complications are managed. Thus, there is a need for harmonious collaboration between clinical practice and laboratory investigation to combat infectious diseases and enhance patient well-being.

8.3.2. Imaging Studies

Imaging studies play an integral role within the practice of internal medicine and in the diagnosis and treatment of infectious diseases. These procedures, such as X-rays, computed tomography (CT), and magnetic resonance imaging (MRI), allow physicians to visualize pathological changes in organs and tissues without the need for extensive surgery. To illustrate, in pneumonia, imaging procedures assist in assessing the extent and presence of pulmonary involvement, specifically in classifying viral versus bacterial etiologies. It is essential, given the vast diversity of etiologic causes of pneumonia, that antimicrobial treatment be directed by accurate determination of the causative pathogen. Enhanced diagnostic accuracy from imaging studies significantly improves patient outcomes by providing unambiguous direction for personalized treatment protocols based on the specific infectious process identified (Dear et al., 2020). Besides, imaging tests are not limited to the evaluation of invasive fungal diseases (IFDs); they are also pertinent in immunocompromised hosts. As IFDs are varied and therefore conclusive diagnosis can be based on imaging studies that can yield lesions characteristic of fungal infection, they find frequent use for this purpose. The revised categorizations of proven, probable, and possible IFDs in the latest release highlight the importance of reliable imaging correlates for diagnosing IFDs. Clinicians ought to utilize high-end imaging modalities along with laboratory work to effectively treat and manage patients with symptoms consistent with IFDs. This synergy ensures definitions of fungal infection apply across a broad range of patient populations, consistent with the broad epidemiological trend of these diseases (Akan et al., 2019). In general, imaging tests are a key tool in the infectious disease expert's armamentarium and can identify not only pathogens but also host tissue responses to them. The integration of imaging findings with clinical and laboratory data enables a more accurate representation of infectious processes, enabling early and effective management. With technological advances, new imaging applications for infectious diseases will emerge, leading to further risk stratification and optimized disease management. Ultimately, appropriately using imaging enhances patient care and guides practitioners in making informed decisions with far-reaching effects on the management of infectious disease (Akan et al., 2019; Dear et al., 2020).

8.3.3. Clinical Evaluation

Clinical evaluation of infectious diseases is key to accurate diagnosis and effective treatment. Clinical evaluation comprises taking an appropriate patient history, performing a physical examination, and using appropriate diagnostic investigations. Critical leads, such as fever pattern, recent travel history, and exposure to sick contacts, tend to guide physicians toward limiting the potential pathogens. Additionally, with the advent of advanced diagnostic technologies, there is a need for traditional methods to more precisely identify the pathogen.

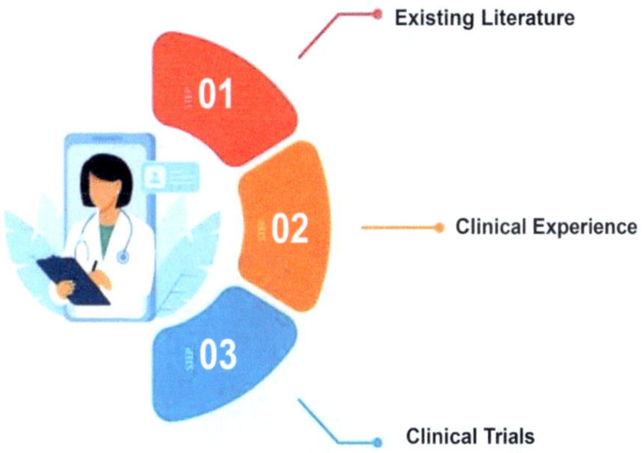

Figure 8.7. Clinical evaluation in the realm of infectious diseases.

Source: https://pubrica.com/academy/wp-content/uploads/2021/11/aca4.jpg.

For instance, molecular diagnostics can detect specific DNA or RNA sequences, enabling rapid detection of the etiologic infectious agent. All these advances are required to guide treatment regimens, particularly when early intervention can completely alter a patient's outcome, underscoring the central role of clinical assessment in the management of infectious diseases. Clinical assessment in internal medicine must also consider patients' predisposing conditions to infection. Diabetes, drug-induced immunosuppression, and congenital abnormalities are chronic diseases that complicate the clinical presentation of infections. Accurate symptom interpretation for such patients requires immense skill and analytic intelligence. In addition, incorporating infection prevention into the assessment process is important to reduce disease transmission, especially in the health care setting. Awareness of how underlying medical conditions affect infectious processes enables more comprehensive treatment. For example, bacterial pneumonia in patients with compromised respiratory systems requires a tailored clinical evaluation that focuses on both short- and long-term care protocols to support respiratory function and effectively treat the infection (Dear et al., 2020). Infectious disease specialists' specialty is now well recognized in enhancing hospital clinical evaluation processes. Evidence indicates that hospitals with in-house infectious disease experts have better antibiotic stewardship, by extension more prudent antibiotic use, and improved patient outcomes. Coupled with the primary care doctors, these experts share useful information on difficult cases and guide therapeutic decisions. This multidisciplinary approach has the potential to optimize clinical evaluation across various patient populations, especially those with complex comorbidities or infections. Moreover, practical clinical evaluation is also inextricably entwined with comprehensive education programs aimed at internal medicine and healthcare professionals, as well as patients, to ensure knowledge about proper procedures and practices. Specialist knowledge integration is also necessary to address the rapid evolution of infectious diseases and to promote efficient control practices within the internal medicine platform (Alexander et al., 2020) (Figure 8.7).

Test Your Knowledge

1. What laboratory tests are commonly used to diagnose infectious diseases?
2. Why is early and accurate diagnosis important in managing infections?

8.4. Treatment Modalities

Learning Outcome

1. Describe the antibiotic therapy
2. Discuss on antiviral medications
3. Define the supportive care

Treatment modalities applied in infectious diseases are fundamental blocks in the development of patient management. Empirical therapy is sometimes the initial response, especially in community-acquired infections where prompt intervention is necessary. Bacterial pneumonia treatment is a classic case of such a strategy, which often relies on broad-spectrum antibiotics until more targeted therapies can be determined. Successful management depends on the determination of underlying causes such as viral infection or foreign body aspiration, since these conditions have a strong potential to affect the treatment plan. In addition, risk factors of weakened immune systems or existing respiratory diseases require customized therapeutic protocols. Thus, the choice of treatment agents must be closely linked with causative organisms and individual patient circumstances, attesting to the complexity of infectious disease intervention in internal medicine (Dear et al., 2020). Prompt diagnosis and accurate pathogen identification are important for optimizing treatment regimens and improving patient outcomes. Advances in diagnostic technology, such as with the Accelerate Pheno™ system, demonstrate the application of novel technologies to accelerate both pathogen detection and antimicrobial susceptibility testing. For comparison, AXDX reduces such processes by quite a significant amount, reporting results in as few as 3.7 hours for identification and up to 9.0 hours for susceptibility testing. Such rapid turnaround enables clinicians to act quickly and accurately, optimizing antibiotic regimens based on susceptibilities. The value of AXDX is considerable; it can enable earlier treatment initiation in approximately 25% of patients and sharply reduce delays in proper therapy adjustment. Consequently, integrating sophisticated diagnostics into clinical practice maximizes antimicrobial stewardship, promoting objective-directed therapy and reducing unnecessary antibiotic use (Blevins et al., 2019). Therapeutic modalities are also not confined to pharmacotherapy, and supportive measures are strengthened to augment recovery in the patient. Adjunctive treatments, such as oxygen therapy for respiratory infections, are crucial for patient comfort and improved outcomes. Patient education on compliance with prescribed regimens and the importance of follow-up can also profoundly influence treatment effectiveness. Part and parcel of an integrated process is acting upon environment and lifestyle factors that place the person at risk of infection or impede their ability to recover. Lastly, efficient infectious disease management boils down to a multidisciplinary strategy that oscillates between high-tech medical modalities and holistic, patient-focused modes of treatment, and is required for optimizing outcomes. Such multimodal interventions must be compatible with current paradigms of internal medicine, ensuring that all aspects of a patient's health are considered in the intervention (Dear et al., 2020).

8.4.1. Antibiotic Therapy

Antibiotic treatment forms an integral part of infection management, and hence every effort should be made to adhere strictly to guidelines to prevent the dangers of antimicrobial resistance. Even as the clear advantage of antibiotic therapy is unequivocal, several studies report that physicians drift in adhering to recommended practices. For instance, an investigation in a prospective observational study revealed that guideline compliance varied significantly across infection types, with substantially higher concordance in lower respiratory tract infections (79%) compared to sepsis (53%) and urinary tract infections (40%) (Alvarez et al., 2005). These discrepancies suggest that factors such as underlying disease and physician behavior strongly influence prescribing patterns, which could undermine treatment efficacy while fostering conditions in which resistance can develop. One of the most significant challenges in antibiotic treatment is the management of Clostridium difficile infection (CDI), particularly recurrent disease after treatment. Research has identified factors associated with increased recurrence in patients infected with specific ribotypes of CDI. For instance, metronidazole monotherapy was recognized as a risk factor for recurrence in patients infected with the more virulent 027+ strain in a cohort that was examined (Aceti et al., 2018). The study findings showed that patients who underwent this treatment had a much higher recurrence rate, raising questions about the efficacy of metronidazole in these cases.

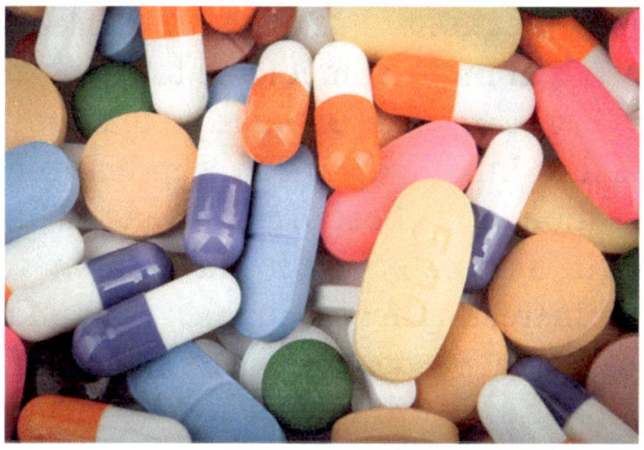

Figure 8.8. Antibiotic therapy.

Source: https://www.infectiousdiseaseadvisor.com/wp-content/uploads/sites/16/2019/03/antibiotics_G_639979482.jpg.

This points to the necessity for clinicians to personalize antibiotic treatment based on infection type and patient characteristics, ensuring therapy not only cures the acute infection but also prevents complications, such as recurrence. Secondly, the transition from broad-spectrum to narrow-spectrum antibiotic use is a key adaptation in the management of infectious diseases. Restricting the antimicrobial spectrum offers targeted treatment with minimal collateral damage to the microbiome, thereby avoiding resistance. However, the practice's deployment is less than optimal, as research indicates resistance among clinicians to adjusting initial broad-spectrum therapy based on culture results (Alvarez et al., 2005). Effective antibiotic stewardship requires an integrated approach combining ongoing education on appropriate prescribing practices with rigorous diagnostic testing to inform therapy selection. Ultimately, adherence to evidence-based practice guidelines in clinical practice is essential for maximizing antibiotic therapy while making certain that patient care is balanced with the long-term sustainability of antimicrobial drugs (Figure 8.8).

8.4.2. Antiviral Medications

The role of antiviral drugs in the treatment of infectious diseases, particularly viral pathogen-induced infections, has become increasingly significant in internal medicine today. Antiviral drugs are targeted explicitly against viral processes, inhibiting virus replication and propagation in the host organism. As examples, acyclovir and oseltamivir have been found effective in treating herpes simplex virus infection and influenza, respectively. Their mechanisms of action range from preventing viral DNA synthesis to restricting viral neuraminidase activity. Given the ever-changing nature of viral infections, such as the emergence of new strains and resistance patterns, the specific selection and application of antiviral drugs are imperative for improving patient outcomes and limiting morbidity associated with viral infections. Lastly, the integration of antiviral treatment and co-infections defines the complexity in treating patients with complex infectious diseases. For instance, HCV and HIV-co-infected individuals present a unique challenge, as HCV infection has been linked to progressive chronic kidney disease among HIV-positive individuals, with a resulting increase in the risk of adverse health outcomes. Evidence has shown that chronic HCV infection will exacerbate renal dysfunction among infected individuals, which necessitates vigilant monitoring and management of both viral infections (Bickel et al., 2012). Therefore, antiviral treatment not only aims to clear the infection but also requires a subtle understanding of the broader clinical impact an infection will have on a patient's overall health trajectory. Screening and early treatment with antiviral therapy should not be overestimated, particularly in high-risk individuals. The Centers for Disease Control and Prevention (CDC) recommends screening for HCV regularly among individuals born in the years 1945-1965, since it was in this population that the highest incidence of chronic infection has been found (Thompson et al., 2015). Screening in primary care remains inadequate, and the majority of individuals remain unaware of their infection status. Incorporating effective screening protocols within primary care models is fundamental for enhancing detection rates and enabling early intervention with antiviral therapy, ultimately leading to improved long-term health outcomes. Identifying screening gaps and actively treating antiviral diseases enable internal medicine to adapt and help prevent infectious disease.

8.4.3. Supportive Care

Supportive care in the context of internal medicine for infectious diseases involves a core element of patient care: symptom palliation and supportive measures. Patients with contagious diseases generally have a multitude of uncomfortable symptoms, including pain, weakness, and emotional distress. This necessitates multidisciplinary care management, not just to eliminate the infectious pathogen but also to alleviate the disease's pain and discomfort. Effective supportive care can enhance the patients' quality of life, achieve tolerance of complex treatment, and ultimately result in improved clinical outcomes. These holistic health strategies are called for, given the kaleidoscopic impact infectious diseases can have on patients across various aspects of their lives, be it physical, psychological, or social. Particularly with severe infections with resulting complications such as febrile neutropenia, the necessity for supportive care is particularly highlighted. In a deeper observational study, patients with lymphoma and solid tumors were seen to have a high cost of inpatient services due to infection complications like febrile neutropenia. Outcomes showed that the total mean hospital cost was US$4,193 per episode, with additional out-of-pocket expenses imposed on patients and their families (Bosly et al., 2014). This emphasizes the need for efficient supportive care methods that are not only effective in treating acute medical conditions but also budget-friendly. Developing targeted interventions that optimize costs without compromising adequate supportive care improves patient satisfaction and health outcomes, underscoring the intricacy and significance of such care in the infectious disease model. The incorporation of supportive care interventions during the treatment of infectious diseases also involves providing sensitive psychosocial care and rehabilitation. Patients suffering from severe infection commonly suffer from depression and anxiety regarding the course of the disease and treatment therapy. Counseling and effective communication can help curb these psychological problems, thereby increasing treatment compliance and reducing recovery time. Furthermore, recognizing the merit of family involvement in supportive care can facilitate the formation of an emotional support system for the patient. For cat patients with vestibular disorders, in particular, the need for effective supportive care that blends symptom management and emotional support becomes clear (LeCouteur et al., 1999). Incorporation not only addresses immediate clinical needs but also creates a therapeutic climate conducive to healing and well-being. These steps reinforce the general purpose of supportive care: to maximize health gains while maintaining patients' dignity and comfort in the morbidity of infectious disease (Figure 8.9).

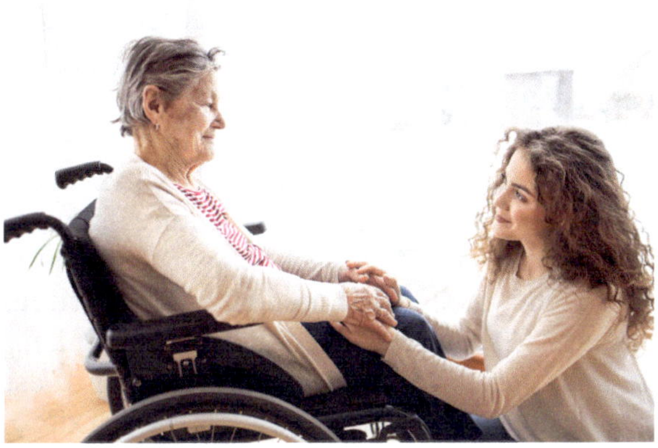

Figure 8.9. Supportive care.

Source: https://uploads-ssl.webflow.com/6202c570c269134c5f8e14d7/621417fa6ca4f681fb652bec_supportivecare-hero.jpg.

Test Your Knowledge

1. What are the common treatment options used for infectious diseases?
2. How do antibiotics and antiviral drugs help control infections?

8.5. Challenges in Management

Learning Outcome

1. Describe the antibiotic resistance
2. Identify the emerging infectious diseases
3. Discuss on socioeconomic factors

The treatment of infectious diseases is increasingly complex, reflecting broader problems in healthcare. One of the biggest challenges is the dynamic nature of pathogens; e.g., invasive candidiasis (IC) caused by Candida species has shifted from drug-susceptible organisms to a rise in non-albicans species driven by increasing rates of drug resistance. As healthcare environments adapt to such trends, they must then contend with the implications on therapy and prevention. Resistant organisms such as *C. auris* complicate management regimens, necessitating heightened vigilance and innovative approaches in clinical practice. This setting underscores the need for continuous education among physicians on up-to-date epidemiological data and optimal management practices, thereby creating a persistent demand for internal medicine resources and infectious disease training. In addition to the biological challenges introduced by infectious agents, problems in management within healthcare settings have the capacity to impact the efficacy of intervention and treatment procedures severely. The multidisciplinary nature of healthcare teams renders them victims to communication issues that can adversely affect patient outcomes. Effective management is not solely dependent on clinical expertise but also on effective leadership and interprofessional working among professionals. According to recent fellowship program director forums, topics such as assessment and feedback, performance management, and fellow well-being are critical areas that require focus to optimize the learning environment and overall competency in internal medicine for infectious diseases (Escota et al., 2020). By recognizing the need for continuous improvement in these areas, a more responsive and adaptive workforce will be fostered, able to meet the ever-growing, complex nature of infectious diseases. External factors cannot be overlooked in the context of management issues in infectious diseases. Financial constraints, policy changes, and alterations in healthcare expenditure can limit resources for research, training, and clinical practice. This setting creates an additional barrier for experts trying to implement evidence-based practice while maintaining their current pace in their line of work. Moreover, management of emergent infections typically requires a coordinated approach by more than a single stakeholder, from governmental institutions to hospital management and the population as a whole. Given the problems posed by resistant infections and the need for novel antifungals, multidisciplinary cooperation is necessary. Comprehensive management strategies that incorporate multidimensional perspectives can foster preparedness and adaptability, ultimately improving patient care processes in the otherwise chaotic environment of internal medicine for infectious diseases (Bays et al., 2024).

8.5.1. Antibiotic Resistance

Antibiotic resistance is a leading and growing threat to infectious diseases, endangering the effectiveness of medical interventions and treatments. As resistant strains become increasingly common, doctors are compelled to battle infections once thought easily curable. The World Health Organization has classified antibiotic resistance as a public health emergency, calling upon health systems to prioritize the development and implementation of strong antimicrobial stewardship (AMS) programs. These programs aim to guide appropriate antibiotic use, thereby constraining the selective pressure that favors resistance. In fact, a systems-level analysis of existing AMS efforts shows that although integration between healthcare sectors is underway, it is necessary for a global impact. This requires implementing One Health approaches to antibiotic use not only in human medicine but also in veterinary medicine and the environment, ultimately contributing to the broader antimicrobial resistance crisis (Ahmad et al., 2019). The arrival of new diagnostics is poised to revolutionize the therapy of antibiotic resistance. Clinical metagenomic next-generation sequencing (mNGS), for instance, provides an expansive survey of microbial genomic material from patient specimens, enabling accurate and rapid identification of pathogens and resistance patterns. As technology moves from a research tool to a routine part of the clinical laboratory, healthcare providers now have a powerful tool with which to individualize antibiotic therapy based on resistance patterns. Breaking away from empirical treatment toward a more targeted approach, mNGS can transform patient care and help counter the dangers of antibiotic misuse. Moreover, as mNGS technology continues to expand, its potential impact on public health can be immense, particularly in identifying emerging resistance patterns in advance and guiding public health interventions against infectious pathogens (Chiu et al., 2019). The interlinked problems of antibiotic resistance and continuous evolution of healthcare innovation necessitate a multifaceted intervention. With evolving mechanisms of resistance, constant research and surveillance are essential in informing effective interventions and policies implemented. Resistance strategies need to transcend traditional silos and increase collaboration among healthcare providers, researchers, and policy-makers. Importantly, evaluating the impact of combined multisectoral AMS interventions can yield lessons on effective interventions that could be replicated in individual healthcare contexts. Future research, particularly with robust research designs, will be critical to disentangle the complexities of antibiotic resistance in diverse health systems. By fostering a culture of collaboration and innovation, the medical community can effectively address the pressing issue of antibiotic resistance while ensuring the efficacy of treatment for future generations.

8.5.2. Emerging Infectious Diseases

The increased incidence of emerging infectious diseases is a complex problem that underscores the challenges of addressing global health. As the interfaces between human, animal, and environmental health become more interlinked, the likelihood of disease jumping across species lines increases exponentially. Initiatives like the Southern African Centre for Infectious Disease Surveillance (SACIDS) underscore the importance of the One Health approach in addressing such infectious threats. By coordinating efforts across sectors, SACIDS demonstrates how collaboration could enhance disease surveillance and response capabilities amid challenges such as inadequate infrastructure and uneven resources. The assessment of the programs identifies the importance of balancing contributions and ensuring equitable cooperation among member countries to achieve the highest level of coordinated action against emerging infectious threats. Such an integrated response not only sensitizes against health threats but also fosters a sense of community commitment to counter infectious threats with multifaceted strategies (Anderson et al., 2018). Further underscoring the need for a trans-boundary collaboration model, the Rockefeller Foundation's evaluation of Disease Surveillance Networks (DSN) programs highlights the benefits of cross-disciplinary exchange in responding to emerging infectious diseases. The foundations report concluded that strong networks can lead to improved disease surveillance and more effective responses, which are crucial for mitigating the impact of infectious diseases that lack geographical boundaries. This is important for internal medicine specialists and public health practitioners to recognize, as it shows that infectious disease outbreaks can have large-scale ramifications. Thus, the practice of internal medicine must embrace interdependent systems as core components of disease management, so that responses are not just guided by clinical evidence but also by evidence informed by multiple disciplines, in a bid to enhance health security and resilience in the face of emerging health challenges (Kimball et al., 2011). Keeping these considerations in mind, it becomes clear that a strategic focus on emerging infectious diseases requires coordination of clinical expertise and systemic collaboration. The magnitude of the burden these diseases pose, whether the potential for sudden spread or resulting morbidity, compels medical professionals to engage in overall surveillance and preventive action. Using the One Health philosophy, practitioners can apply their approach with modifications to how biological, social, and environmental factors combine to cause infectious diseases. The pursuit of innovative solutions enabled by practical training, as well as networking opportunities, is central to initiating effective responses that can match the dynamism of health threats. Since the epidemiologic profile of infectious diseases is changing, flexibility in the practice of internal medicine will be the essence of adequate preparedness and response and, ultimately, public health protection (Anderson et al., 2018) (Figure 8.10).

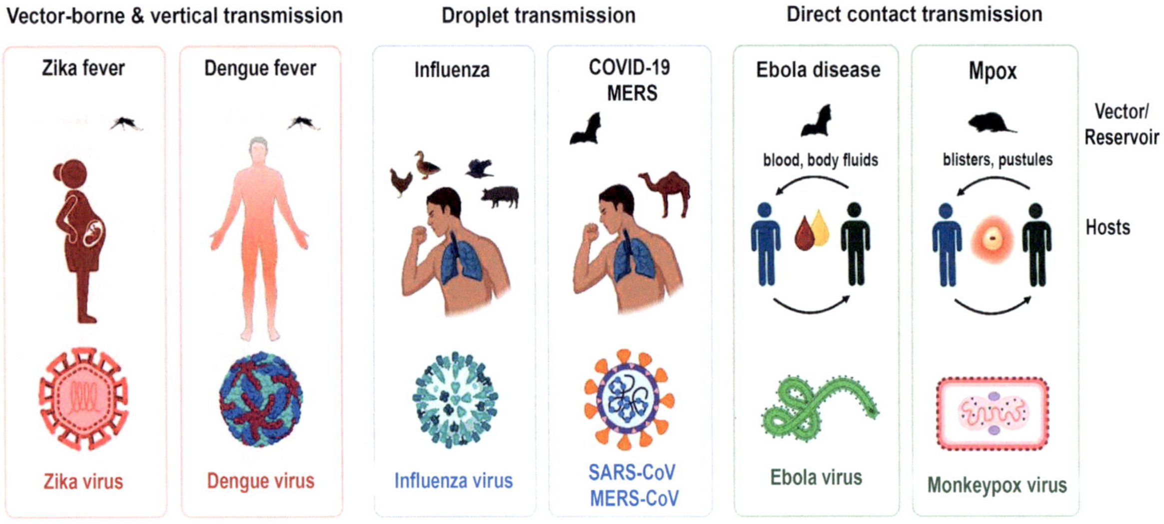

Figure 8.10. Emerging infectious diseases.

Source: https://pub.mdpi-res.com/microorganisms/microorganisms-11-02618/article_deploy/html/images/microorganisms-11-02618-g001.png?1698128705.

8.5.3. Socioeconomic Factors

Socioeconomic factors play a significant role in understanding the complexities of infectious diseases in internal medicine. Low socioeconomic communities are often subjected to inadequate access to healthcare services, low health literacy, and unfavorable living conditions that expose them to increased vulnerability to infectious pathogens. For instance, the increased incidence of chronic stress induced by financial hardships can lead to weak immunity and, therefore, increased susceptibility to infections. Furthermore, the interplay between socioeconomic status and access to preventive care also manifests, with lower-income groups facing barriers that may keep them from receiving timely vaccinations and screenings, thereby leading to elevated outcomes during infectious disease outbreaks. The influence of the above factors necessitates immediate review of how socioeconomic inequalities perpetuate mechanisms of health inequity, particularly as diseases such as influenza and tuberculosis disproportionately affect vulnerable populations. This association between childhood adversity and health outcomes further indicates the long-term influence of socioeconomic status on infectious diseases. Research indicates that childhood experiences of adversity, including socioeconomic disadvantage and illness, are linked with increased chances of developing adult chronic disease and demonstrate the direct link between early life circumstances and adult trajectories of health. Ferraro et al. (2018) highlight parental behavior and early-life socioeconomic status influencing adult vulnerabilities to cancer, indicating convergence in infectious disease susceptibility based on similar childhood adversities. Thus, a person who experienced adversity in early life may have neuroendocrine dysfunction, as indicated by aberrant cortisol circadian rhythms, which can impair the immune system's ability to combat infections. The evidence shows the need to adopt a multidimensional approach to mitigating health inequities, with particular emphasis on early-life interventions to reduce infectious disease burden among populations under socioeconomic disadvantage. Redressal of socioeconomic determinants of health is necessary for successful control of infectious diseases in internal medicine. A medical resource fair access policy, health education programs to enhance health literacy, and community intervention programs for high-risk groups are key components of a comprehensive strategy. For example, increased access to immunization programs in poor communities could significantly reduce the prevalence of infectious diseases. Furthermore, the inclusion of socioeconomic assessments in clinical practice can make healthcare professionals understand the unique problems that their patients need to endure, allowing them to come up with interventions that consider the social aspects of health. Collectively, these measures can break the cycle of ill health and destitution, paving the way for a healthier population capable of confronting the challenges posed by infectious diseases and further entrenching the role of socioeconomic determinants in public health outcomes overall.

Test Your Knowledge

1. Why is antibiotic resistance a major challenge in treating infectious diseases?
2. How does misuse of antibiotics contribute to the development of resistance?

8.6. Role of Preventive Medicine

Learning Outcome

1. Understand the vaccination strategies
2. Focus on public health initiatives
3. Identify the patient education

Preventive medicine plays a significant role in managing and containing infectious diseases, particularly in the internal medicine setting. By anticipating disease before they occur, preventive medicine aims to reduce the incidence and prevalence of infections that could have significant public health implications. The anticipatory strategy involves a range of interventions, from mass vaccination campaigns to health education programs, that not only inform individuals about risks but also empower them to make informed health choices. For example, vaccination has turned out to be one of the most effective preventive measures, substantially reducing diseases such as measles, influenza, and, more recently, COVID-19. This requirement is further elucidated when viewed in light of the growing problem of antibiotic resistance, which underscores the need for novel approaches based on prevention, not treatment. Furthermore, preventive medicine is not only about vaccines and pharmacologic therapy; it also emphasizes lifestyle modification and environmental prevention. With behaviors promoting healthier lifestyles, such as better diet, increased physical activity, and stress reduction, the likelihood of contracting infectious disease can be significantly diminished. Not only do these interventions improve health status, but they also reduce the healthcare burden caused by preventable diseases. Additionally, research in areas such as organic livestock production indicates that understanding the interdependence between animal husbandry practices and public health is required to prevent zoonotic diseases, which could otherwise be triggered by poor animal population management (Eijck et al., 2003). By incorporating multidisciplinary inputs, preventive medicine broadens understanding of disease prevention, thereby fostering a healthier population. Lastly, the economic aspects of preventive medicine are increasingly recognized as important in the context of infectious diseases. As demonstrated by the management of Porcine Reproductive and Respiratory Syndrome (PRRS), strategically used as preventive measures, it can bring significant financial gains to livestock farmers (Alarcon et al., 2018). By facilitating the adoption of low-cost intervention strategies, preventive medicine can promote productivity and limit the economic costs of disease epidemics. The economic rationale emphasizes the importance of public and private investment in preventive health programs that support personal wellness and the viability of the healthcare system. Hence, prevention strategies in everyday practice in internal medicine offer a possible way to combat infectious diseases, thereby serving as the cornerstone for maximizing global health (Figure 8.11).

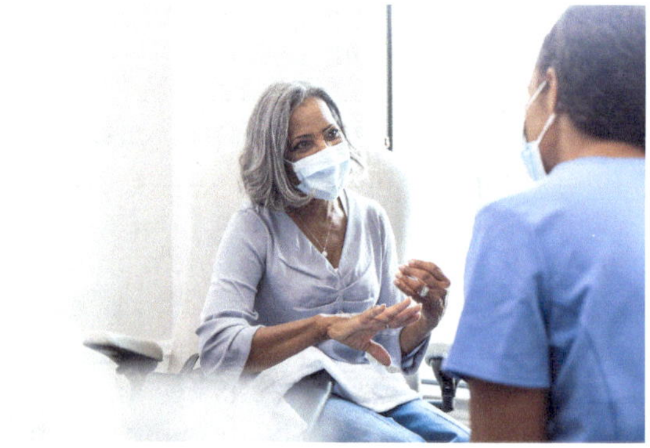

Figure 8.11. Role of preventive medicine.

Source: https://insights.ibx.com/wp-content/uploads/2021/01/woman-talking-nurse.jpg.

8.6.1. Vaccination Strategies

Implementation of effective vaccination strategies is core in internal medicine for infectious diseases. Vaccination not only safeguards individual patients but also enables herd immunity, ultimately decreasing the overall disease burden in populations. As indicated in a research study, adequate vaccination protection is an economical control measure in animal husbandry and could be applied in human health. Adequate introduction checks and vaccination measures significantly reduce the infection rate among livestock, demonstrating their comparable importance in human medicine. This strategic plan can maximize investment in healthcare resources to realize economic sustainability and enhanced health outcomes. Understanding the behavior of vaccination strategies enables the use of evidence-based decisions to strengthen public health programs and reduce the prevalence of infectious diseases. Furthermore, the emergence and spread of zoonotic diseases require sophisticated vaccination strategies tailored to specific epidemiological contexts. In regions particularly at risk for such diseases, such as Indonesia, collaborative efforts among health institutions and scientists are instrumental. Senior-level conferences between institutions such as the Pasteur Institute and local universities are used to identify cooperative avenues for managing infectious threats, such as rabies and zoonoses. The collaborative framework facilitates training healthcare personnel in vaccine administration and information sharing. As implied in rabies vaccination planning, complete solutions are required to address research gaps and develop robust vaccination strategies that can adapt to dynamic epidemiologic environments. Making such approaches effective is essential to controlling disease and improving public health. Finally, valuing the economic worth of vaccination campaigns illustrates their value above and beyond health outcomes. A conceptual framework that accounts for livestock disease shows that the best vaccination strategies minimize total disease costs, including both direct production losses and control costs. The framework can also be applied in human infectious disease interventions. By identifying the most efficient vaccination strategies, health systems can better allocate limited resources, thereby supporting productivity alongside health outcomes. Thus, vaccination strategies should not only focus on their medical impact but also on their economic impact. Bringing these perspectives together provides the whole landscape of vaccination as a key component of internal medicine for infectious diseases, both emphasizing individual protection as well as public health programs in general.

8.6.2. Public Health Initiatives

Public health interventions play a pivotal role in stemming the complex dynamics of infectious diseases. These initiatives, often supported by philanthropic organizations and government programs, aim to improve global disease surveillance and response mechanisms. For instance, the Rockefeller Foundation Disease Surveillance Networks (DSN) Initiative evaluates the effectiveness of collaborative networks in improving disease monitoring. Summative evaluation revealed that trans-boundary, multi-sectoral partnership leads to significant enhancements in the efficiency of disease surveillance (Kimball et al., 2011). These networks not only facilitate early detection of outbreaks but also enhance prevention of infectious disease transmission, underlining the necessity of integrated public health strategies in a connected world. Furthermore, having AMS programs in place is a quintessential example of how public health intervention can tackle infectious diseases programmatically by upgrading healthcare practice. Whereas several AMS strategies are traditionally limited to individual healthcare organizations, a One Health policy change has become unavoidable. Multisectoral AMS programs promote collaboration across, for instance, the human health and animal husbandry sectors to comprehensively address antimicrobial resistance (AMR) (Ahmad et al., 2019). Preliminary evaluations indicate that such multisectoral tactics can effectively limit rates of antimicrobial prescribing and ensuing healthcare infections. This extension of the AMS mandate reflects the imperative of harmonized public health interventions that leverage cross-sectoral resources to tackle the complexity of infectious diseases. Lastly, the potential for future public health programs against contagious diseases relies on continued monitoring and adaptive learning. The impact measurement of such programs is essential for establishing best practices and areas for improvement. The insights from rigorous research and program evaluations, such as the DSN and connected AMS, can inform policy and enhance funding decisions. By demonstrating successful collaborations and adaptability, such evaluations not only contribute to the understanding of the body of public health knowledge but also build a more effective counter-response system for infectious diseases (Kimball et al., 2011; Ahmad et al., 2019). Enhancing these efforts with evidence-based programs will be important in preparing healthcare systems better to address impending infectious threats (Figure 8.12).

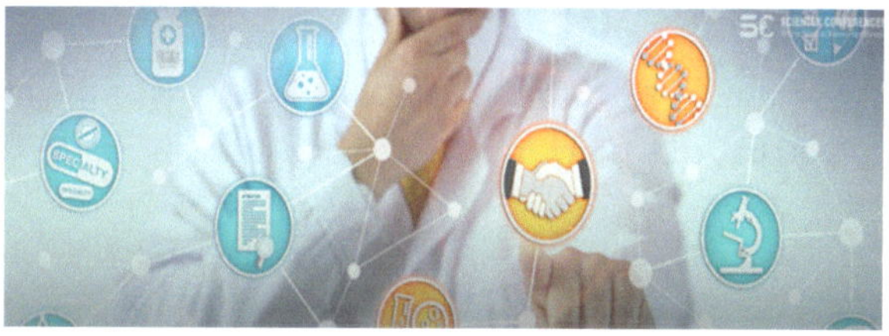

Figure 8.12. Public health initiatives.

Source: https://www.primarycare.scientexconference.com/cfiles/sessions/Global_Public_Health_Initiatives.jpg.

8.6.3. Patient Education

Effective patient education is a high priority in internal medicine, particularly in infectious diseases. Educating patients with substantial details about their illness, therapy, and preventive measures can have a significant impact on patient outcomes. Education facilitates active collaboration between patients and physicians, enabling individuals to take an active role in their own care and comply with recommended therapy. Also, educated patients are more likely to participate in shared decision-making, thereby enabling individualized treatment planning based on their needs. For infectious diseases, where timely intervention can significantly alter the disease course, educating patients to enable them is not only advantageous but also imperative. Furthermore, the integration of patient education into care pathways is essential for antibiotic stewardship and fighting the emerging threat of antibiotic resistance. Hospitals with in-house infectious disease specialists use fewer overall inpatient antibacterials, suggesting the merit of better-educated prescribing practices and drug-taking compliance (Alexander et al., 2020). By educating patients about appropriate antibiotic use and risks associated with abuse, healthcare professionals can prevent unjustified prescriptions, thereby ensuring proper drug handling. In addition, educating patients about their treatment plans helps inculcate responsibility and encourages questions about their care, further ingraining the culture of antibiotic stewardship in clinical practice. Finally, fulfilling patients' educational needs also entails the moral obligation of healthcare professionals to provide culturally sensitive care. This requires understanding patients' diverse backgrounds, literacy levels, and health perceptions, ensuring that educational materials are accessible and relevant to all demographics. Strategies such as using visual aids, simplifying complex medical concepts, and employing teach-back methods can enhance comprehension among diverse patient populations. Thus, effective patient education should not be founded on a one-size-fits-all approach but instead need to be adapted to the individualized obstacles patients face, aligned with the overall goal of increased health literacy and engagement in the field of internal medicine for infectious diseases (Escota et al., 2020).

Test Your Knowledge

1. How does preventive medicine help reduce the incidence of diseases?
2. What role do vaccination and health education play in preventive medicine?

SUMMARY

In discussing the internal medicine of infectious diseases, it is essential to mention that effective disease surveillance systems must be emphasized. As illustrated by the Rockefeller Foundation's review of the Disease Surveillance Networks (DSN) Initiative, good disease surveillance is a key element of public health programs. The initiative proved that trans-boundary and multi-sectoral alliances significantly raise the ability to monitor and respond to infectious diseases. This collaborative approach not only provides a comprehensive view of disease dynamics but also optimizes resource use in outbreak management. Participation in such networks may lead to improved patient and public health outcomes, which are most significant in the shifting picture of infectious diseases identified by internal medicine (Kimball et al., 2011). Furthermore, the implications of findings from various studies underscore the necessity of continuous research and evaluation in the field of infectious diseases. There are aspects of the shortage, based on the current literature, regarding the health impacts of organic and conventional farming methods that can directly affect public health through zoonotic diseases. For instance, the higher prevalence of certain zoonotic diseases associated with organic livestock production challenges the health claims made for organic commodities. It is imperative that a scientific study into the incidence of such infections and their management be undertaken to safeguard animal and human health (Eijck et al., 2003). Internal medicine practitioners must advocate for research to fill these gaps so that scientific data inform public health policy and clinical practice. Weaving together the considerations here, it is clear that where infectious diseases and internal medicine overlap, interdisciplinary approaches are the norm. Multidisciplinary collaboration between researchers, healthcare workers, and policymakers must exist to combat infectious disease threats. This synergy can lead to better disease prevention, more effective treatment strategies, and stronger public health measures. The dynamic nature of infectious diseases thus calls for adaptive, informed strategies in the practice of internal medicine, where continuous learning and evidence-based practice are cornerstones in striving for a healthier world. The integration of far-reaching surveillance, ongoing investigations, and interdisciplinarity is not only desirable but also imperative in the face of threats posed by infectious diseases (Eijck et al., 2003; Kimball et al., 2011).

In internal medicine, understanding the complexities of infectious diseases is central to providing the best patient care and achieving therapeutic success. Salient issues highlighting the need for accurate diagnosis and successful intervention provide the cornerstones for proceeding in clinical practice in this field. To illustrate, the determination of the etiologic causes of infectious enteritis in ruminants underscores the broad spectrum of viral, bacterial, and parasitic disease agents that clinicians must consider. The challenge is not only to identify these as potential agents, but also to understand the implications that they have on herd health and zoonotic risk. Therefore, diagnostic methods from fecal, blood, and tissue examinations become vital, as they provide information necessary for specific therapy and the treatment of dehydration and electrolyte imbalance caused by diarrhea, ultimately leading to improved patient care and control measures in the infected herd (Chigerwe et al., 2018). Educational factor regarding fellows working in the field is another significant factor within the scope of infectious diseases. Addressing the needs of struggling learners in infectious diseases fellowship programs is increasingly viewed as an imperative problem that calls for systematic intervention. By focusing on the issues of pertinence to contemporary program director dilemmas, such as performance management and remediation of fellows with knowledge deficits, education programs can enhance the education experience and efficacy of future clinicians. This proactive stance toward fellow development not only addresses immediate concerns but also reinforces the importance of mental well-being and career progression within the demanding specialty. The integration of feedback mechanisms, teaching skills, and time management strategies into the training regimen underscores an evolving framework that can improve learning outcomes and ultimately enhance patient care (Escota et al., 2020). Finally, the overall synthesis of knowledge from both clinical and teaching practices delineates an integrated vision of the infectious disease situation within internal medicine. Emphasis on collaborative strategies between healthcare practitioners and instructors enables a phased approach to addressing the complexities of infectious disease management. By developing a culture of continuous learning and adaptation, professionals can stay current with novel pathogens and treatment modalities, ensuring patient care remains at peak levels. In addition, integrating research and clinical practice guidelines helps shape the future direction of infectious disease care, fosters curiosity, and ensures evidence-based practice. Thus, the successful navigation of problems encountered in direct patient care and in educational systems can be a determining factor in shaping outcomes in the practice of infectious disease internal medicine.

KEY TERMS FROM THIS CHAPTER

- Pathogen
- Virus
- Parasite
- Contagion
- Antibiotic
- Antifungal
- Immunity
- Outbreak
- Pandemic
- Bacteria
- Fungi
- Infection
- Incubation Period
- Antiviral
- Vaccine
- Transmission
- Epidemic
- Zoonosis

CRITICAL THINKING QUESTIONS

1. **Which of the following is the most appropriate initial antibiotic for community-acquired pneumonia in a previously healthy adult with no comorbidities?**
   a. Vancomycin
   b. Azithromycin
   c. Ciprofloxacin
   d. Isoniazid
2. **A 30-year-old man presents with fever, night sweats, weight loss, and a persistent cough with blood-tinged sputum. Which disease is most likely?**
   a. Influenza
   b. Pneumocystis pneumonia
   c. Tuberculosis
   d. Bronchitis
3. **Which laboratory test is most specific for the diagnosis of HIV infection?**
   a. ELISA
   b. Western Blot
   c. CD4 Count
   d. Complete Blood Count (CBC)
4. **Which of the following infections is not typically caused by a virus?**
   a. Hepatitis C
   b. Influenza
   c. Tetanus
   d. Dengue
5. **What is the first-line treatment for Clostridioides difficile (C. difficile) infection in adults?**
   a. Metronidazole
   b. Vancomycin (oral)
   c. Ciprofloxacin
   d. Amoxicillin

Short Answer Questions

1. How has the historical context shaped our understanding and management of infectious diseases?
2. What are some of the most common infectious diseases globally, and how are they transmitted?
3. What diagnostic techniques are commonly used to identify infectious diseases?
4. What are the primary treatment modalities available for managing infectious diseases?
5. What are the significant challenges faced in the management and control of infectious diseases?
6. How have advancements in science and technology impacted the diagnosis and treatment of infectious diseases?

Answers to Critical Thinking Questions

1. (b); 2. (c) ; 3. (b); 4. (c); 5. (b)

REFERENCES

1. Green, L. (2010). Epidemiological information in sheep health management. *Small Ruminant Research*, *92*(1–3), 57–66. https://doi.org/10.1016/j.smallrumres.2010.04.006Aceti, A., Andreoni, M., Antonelli, G., Carfagna, P., et al. (2018). Risk factors for recurrence in patients with *Clostridium difficile* infection due to 027 and non-027 ribotypes. https://core.ac.uk/download/160466362.pdf (accessed on 16th July 2025).
2. Afdhal, N. H., Castera, L., Church, D. R., Dee, S., et al. (2013). The new paradigm of hepatitis C therapy: Integration of oral therapies into best practices. https://core.ac.uk/download/323065592.pdf (accessed on 16th July 2025).
3. Ahmad, R., Holmes, A., McLeod, M., Micallef, C., et al. (2019). A whole-health-economy approach to antimicrobial stewardship: Analysis of current models and future direction. https://core.ac.uk/download/323306206.pdf (accessed on 16th July 2025).
4. Ajana, F., Arribas, J. R., Bailey, J., Benson, C., et al. (2019). Week 96 efficacy and safety results of the phase 3, randomized EMERALD trial to evaluate switching from boosted-protease inhibitors plus emtricitabine/tenofovir disoproxil fumarate regimens to the once daily, single-tablet regimen of darunavir/cobicistat/emtricitabine/tenofovir alafenamide (D/C/F/TAF) in treatment-experienced, virologically-suppressed adults living with HIV-1. https://core.ac.uk/download/237011755.pdf (accessed on 16th July 2025).
5. Akan, H., Alexander, B. D., Andes, D., Azoulay, E., et al. (2019). Revision and update of the consensus definitions of invasive fungal disease from the European Organization for Research and Treatment of Cancer and the Mycoses Study Group Education and Research Consortium. https://core.ac.uk/download/287649722.pdf (accessed on 16th July 2025).
6. Alarcon, P., Alexopoulos, C., Amirpour Haredasht, S., Arruda, A. G., Nathues, H., Cano, J. P., Corzo, C. A., et al. (2018). Modelling the economic efficiency of using different strategies to control *Porcine Reproductive & Respiratory Syndrome* at herd level. https://core.ac.uk/download/153498728.pdf (accessed on 16th July 2025).
7. Alexander, B., Beck, B. F., Goetz, M. B., Goto, M., et al. (2020). Antibiotic stewardship implementation and antibiotic use at hospitals with and without on-site infectious disease specialists. https://core.ac.uk/download/323075232.pdf (accessed on 16th July 2025).
8. Alvarez, A., McCaig, D. J., Bearden, D. T., Ibrahim, E. H., Brown, E. M., European Antimicrobial Resistance Surveillance System, Haaijer-Ruskamp, F. M., et al. (2005). Limited effect of patient and disease characteristics on compliance with hospital antimicrobial guidelines. https://core.ac.uk/download/pdf/12919553.pdf (accessed on 16th July 2025).
9. Anderson, J., Aragrande, M., Argyris, Y., Chomel, B., Coker, R., Epstein, J., Gibbs, E., et al. (2018). A One Health evaluation of the Southern African Centre for Infectious Disease Surveillance. https://core.ac.uk/download/159106431.pdf (accessed on 16th July 2025).
10. Andrada, A., Dumitru, C., Sergiu, I., Micu, M., Manea, D., Elena, M. M., Marilena, S., et al. (2020). Microbiota: The missing link in the etiology of inflammatory bowel disease. https://core.ac.uk/download/304672907.pdf (accessed on 16th July 2025).
11. Bays, D. J., Chiller, T., Hoenigl, M., Jenkins, E. N., Lyman, M., Ostrosky-Zeichner, L., Pappas, P. G., et al. (2024). Epidemiology of invasive candidiasis. https://core.ac.uk/download/629270417.pdf (accessed on 16th July 2025).

12. Bergstrom, S., Gylfe, A., Henderson, B., Shamaei-Tousi, A., et al. (2009). Pathogen burden and cortisol profiles over the day. https://core.ac.uk/download/1778226.pdf (accessed on 16th July 2025).
13. Bickel, M., ESPRIT Study Group, Grint, D., INSIGHT SMART Study Group, et al. (2012). Hepatitis B and C co-infection are independent predictors of progressive kidney disease in HIV-positive, antiretroviral-treated adults. https://core.ac.uk/download/14525548.pdf (accessed on 16th July 2025).
14. Blevins, S., Bocian, B., Davis, T. E., Desai, M., et al. (2019). Susceptibility Provision Enhances Effective De-escalation (SPEED): Utilizing rapid phenotypic susceptibility testing in Gram-negative bloodstream infections and its potential clinical impact. https://core.ac.uk/download/188008375.pdf (accessed on 16th July 2025).
15. Bosly, A., Chan, A., Ihbe-Heffinger, A., Freifeld, A. G., Chan, A., Dulisse, B., O'Brien, C., et al. (2014). Costs associated with febrile neutropenia in solid tumor and lymphoma patients – an observational study in Singapore. https://core.ac.uk/download/287622414.pdf (accessed on 16th July 2025).
16. Bourhy, H., Gaidet, N., & Molia, S. (2012). *Mission to Indonesia to Participate to the 1st Indonesia-France Seminar in Medicine & Public Health and Investigate Potential Collaborations on Animal Health: 2nd–9th of November 2012*. http://agritrop.cirad.fr/567354/1/document_567354.pdf (accessed on 16th July 2025).
17. Chi, J., Keefe, G. P., Vanleeuwen, J. A., Weersink, A., et al. (2025). *The Economics of Controlling Infectious Diseases on Dairy Farms*. https://core.ac.uk/download/pdf/6995443.pdf (accessed on 16th July 2025).
18. Chigerwe, M., & Heller, M. C. (2018). Diagnosis and treatment of infectious enteritis in adult ruminants. https://core.ac.uk/download/323071914.pdf (accessed on 16th July 2025).
19. Chiu, C. Y., & Miller, S. A. (2019). Clinical metagenomics. https://core.ac.uk/download/323062552.pdf (accessed on 16th July 2025).
20. Coukell, A., Shore, C., Jungman, E., Talkington, K., Kothari, P., & Urahn, S. K. (2016). *A Scientific Roadmap for Antibiotic Discovery: A Sustained and Robust Pipeline of New Antibacterial Drugs and Therapies Is Critical to Preserve Public Health*. https://core.ac.uk/download/75785719.pdf (accessed on 16th July 2025).
21. Dear, J. D. (2020). Bacterial pneumonia in dogs and cats: An update. https://core.ac.uk/download/286361309.pdf (accessed on 16th July 2025).
22. Eijck, I., Groot, M., Kasteel, D., Kijlstra, A., et al. (2003). Analysis of black holes in our knowledge concerning animal health in the organic food production chain. https://core.ac.uk/download/10919416.pdf (accessed on 16th July 2025).
23. Eller, P., Hoenigl, M., Prattes, J., Reisinger, A. C., et al. (2021). Invasive pulmonary aspergillosis complicating COVID-19 in the ICU – A case report. https://core.ac.uk/download/323311046.pdf (accessed on 16th July 2025).
24. Escota, G., Melia, M. T., et al. (2020). The struggling infectious diseases fellow: Remediation challenges and opportunities. https://core.ac.uk/download/322802240.pdf (accessed on 16th July 2025).

25. Ferraro, K. F., Kemp, B. R., Morton, P. M., Mustillo, S., et al. (2018). Early origins of adult cancer risk among men and women: Influence of childhood misfortune? https://core.ac.uk/download/305123339.pdf (accessed on 16th July 2025).

26. Harari, A., Zumla, A., Armand, B., Axelsson-Robertson, R., Banada, P., Marais, B., Betsou, F., et al. (2012). Tuberculosis diagnostics and biomarkers: Needs, challenges, recent advances, and opportunities. https://core.ac.uk/download/9839032.pdf (accessed on 16th July 2025).

27. Kaufmann, A. F., Miller, B., Salisbury, C., Holleman, D. R., Tsui, F. C., Batal, H., Ginsberg, J., et al. (2013). Association of over-the-counter pharmaceutical sales with influenza-like illnesses to patient volume in an urgent care setting. https://core.ac.uk/download/12214723.pdf (accessed on 16th July 2025).

28. Kimball, A. M., Gugerty, M. K., Abernethy, N., & Curran, S. (2011). *Disease Surveillance Networks Initiative Global: Final Evaluation*. https://core.ac.uk/download/86445037.pdf (accessed on 16th July 2025).

29. Kohrt, C. F. (2025). *From Ideas to Innovations: Moving Technology Toward the Marketplace Through Universities and National Labs*. https://core.ac.uk/download/pdf/6755227.pdf (accessed on 16th July 2025).

30. LeCouteur, R. A., & Vernau, K. M. (1999). Feline vestibular disorders. Part II: Diagnostic approach and differential diagnosis. https://core.ac.uk/download/323068734.pdf (accessed on 16th July 2025).

31. N/A. (2011). *Handwashing with Soap–Two Paths to National-Scale Programs: Lessons from the Field: Vietnam and Indonesia*. https://core.ac.uk/download/75783149.pdf (accessed on 16th July 2025).

32. N/A. (2014). *Research Advances: January 2014*. https://core.ac.uk/download/75777581.pdf (accessed on 16th July 2025).

33. Sawers, L., & Stillwaggon, E. (2018). Understanding HIV/AIDS in the African context. https://cupola.gettysburg.edu/cgi/viewcontent.cgi?article=1030&context=econfac (accessed on 16th July 2025).

34. Thompson, J. A. (2015). *Practices of Nurse Practitioners in Screening for Hepatitis C*. https://core.ac.uk/download/162577448.pdf (accessed on 16th July 2025).

RHEUMATOLOGY

9

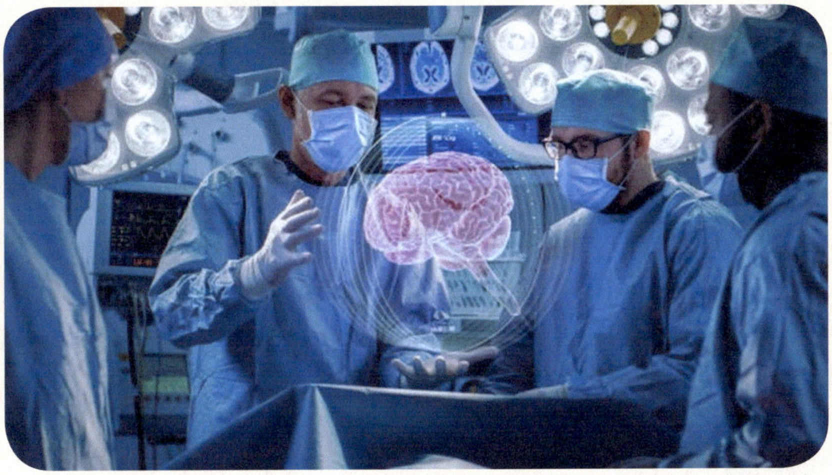

Introduction

Internal Medicine is the bedrock on which rheumatology stands, providing a general approach to the diagnosis and management of complex musculoskeletal illnesses. Rheumatology is an Internal Medicine subspecialty that addresses a wide variety of conditions characterized by inflammation and pain in the musculoskeletal system and surrounding tissues. A sound understanding of systemic illnesses such as rheumatoid arthritis, lupus, and scleroderma is essential for physicians who must manage them. Internists not only acquire expertise in pharmacologic interventions but also in non-pharmacologic management, such as lifestyle modification and self-management strategies, which are needed to enhance patients' quality of life. As the prevalence of rheumatic disorders is always on the rise globally, particularly in geriatric populations, Internal Medicine's contribution in providing holistic care becomes of the greatest concern. Exploration of psychological and behavioral dimensions of rheumatic disorders becomes highly important for effective patient management. Chronic pain, common in conditions like

LEARNING OBJECTIVES

After studying this chapter, you will be able to:

1. Describe the common rheumatological conditions
2. Describe the diagnostic approaches in rheumatology
3. Know the treatment modalities in rheumatology
4. Understand the role of the rheumatologist
5. Understand the challenges in rheumatology
6. Describe the advances in rheumatology

hemophilia and scleroderma, impacts the quality of life of patients considerably, necessitating holistic pain management approaches based on individual patient needs. For instance, research underscores that understanding psychological factors can improve patient outcomes, as seen in the association between pain acceptance and better mental quality of life. With the use of self-management interventions that heighten patients' awareness regarding their conditions and enable effective coping strategies, the adverse effects of chronic pain can be minimized. These interventions may include educating the patient about the distinction between acute and chronic pain, thereby enhancing comprehension and adaptation to their chronic conditions, which is a paramount factor in improving overall well-being (Acharya et al., 2014).

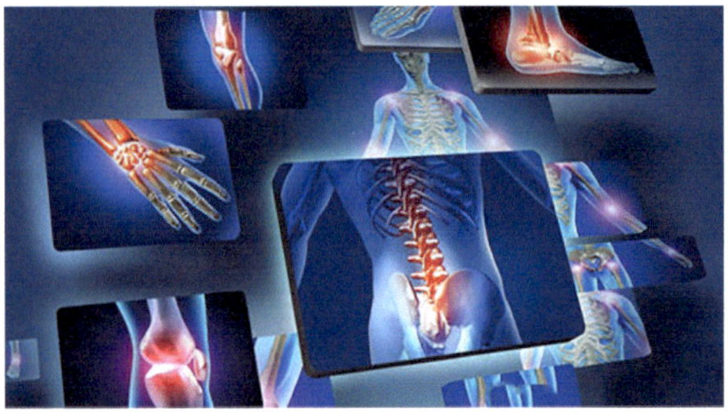

Figure 9.1. Internal medicine for rheumatology.

Source: https://admin.nmcth.edu/upload/images/departments/2024/05/08/1715171796Lightspring_Shutterstock_GenericJoints_500x270.jpg.

Fatigue has also been a prevalent characteristic in rheumatic disorder patients, particularly in systemic sclerosis (SSc) disease. Longitudinal studies have shown that fatigue severity correlates with various clinical, demographic, and psychosocial predictors, making the identification of these predictors during the early phases of the disease process essential for clinicians' assessment. Baseline patient evaluation can capture key variables, such as the severity of joint disease or coping ability, which are directly correlated with long-term fatigue levels. Their identification allows health practitioners to institute individualized treatment regimens that address the patient's physical symptoms and psychological distress. By targeting modifiable risk factors, such as the use of optimal coping mechanisms, healthcare professionals can substantially enhance the longitudinal quality of life of patients with chronic fatigue associated with rheumatic diseases (Assassi et al., 2011) (Figure 9.1).

Definition of Internal Medicine

Internal medicine is a fundamental pillar within the broader framework of medical specialties, with a primary focus on the prevention, diagnosis, and management of disease in adults. As a specialty, it is committed to a detailed understanding of the body's internal workings, enabling internists to effectively manage complex medical issues that often involve the interplay of several organ systems. The comprehensive treatment approach followed by internists is particularly valuable in rheumatology, where diseases like systemic lupus erythematosus (SLE) present complex symptom profiles. By integrating knowledge across various fields of medicine, internal medicine professionals are best positioned to address the intricate interplay of symptoms and treatment approaches in cases of rheumatology. This broad framework of internal medicine increases the ability of healthcare providers to provide patient-centered care and individualized therapeutic interventions based on the unique needs and circumstances of each. Within the scope of rheumatology, the contribution of internal medicine is enhanced through the application of advanced diagnostic methods that enable the proper identification of different rheumatic conditions. For instance, biomarker utilization, such as cell-bound complement activation products (CB-CAPs), allows clinicians to detect active complement activation in SLE-suspicious patients, providing information not normally detected by standard laboratory tests. The evidence from the recent past indicates a high rate of presumptive SLE patients presenting with raised levels of CB-CAP, which renders them a diagnostic agent relative to regular complement protein levels (Alexander et al., 2020). Also, understanding the evolution of diseases like SLE needs knowledge of internists who can properly appreciate such biomarker results in the context of the clinical syndromes. Thus, the multifaceted knowledge base of internal medicine proves most efficacious in dealing with rheumatologic diseases, underscoring the necessity of a strong foundation in internal medicine as the basis for sound clinical practice. Moreover, the use of validated testing instruments also prepares internists to treat individuals with autoimmune disease. The Fatigue Severity Scale (FSS) and the Pittsburgh Sleep Quality Index (PSQI) are tools that enable a comprehensive analysis of symptoms, a crucial element in the treatment of the multi-factorial condition SLE. Research has demonstrated that Maltese translations of these measurement tools are both reliable and valid, reflecting worldwide efforts to standardize patient treatment among multicultural groups (Borg et al., 2017). Using such tools, internists are not only able to monitor disease progression but also to prescribe interventions that address patients' physical and psychological health. This multidimensional model is one example of how the principles of internal medicine extend beyond mere disease control to create a holistic, patient-centered model of care that is essential to rheumatology (Figure 9.2).

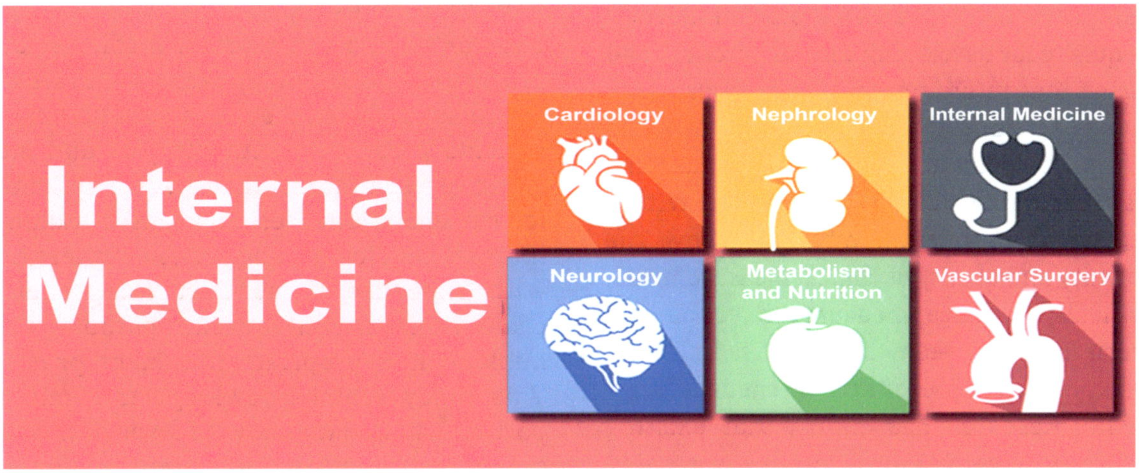

Figure 9.2. Internal medicine.

Source: https://wacpcoam.org/wp-content/uploads/2019/10/internal-Medicine.gif.

Overview of Rheumatology

Rheumatology, a significant subspecialty of internal medicine, is engaged with the analysis and treatment of musculoskeletal disorders and systemic autoimmune conditions. The variety of diseases managed in this specialty spans from rheumatoid arthritis and lupus to osteoarthritis and many other inflammatory and degenerative diseases. Rheumatologists play a key role in assessing not only the physical complications of these diseases but also their considerable impact on patients' quality of life, which justifies the use of a multidisciplinary treatment strategy. This need for whole-person care influences the generation of clinical practice guidelines and the application of research evidence to everyday clinical practice as well. As rheumatologic diseases become increasingly common globally, especially among older adults, the need for effective management practices tailored to individual patients' needs is growing. One of the most significant aspects of rheumatology is clinical research, which opens the door to new therapies and improved patient outcomes. Despite that possibility, there have been setbacks in the field, such as an enigmatic workforce and limited research activity among junior career rheumatologists. Current studies indicate a disturbing trend: few newly trained rheumatologists are minimally engaged in research or struggle to conduct clinical trials (Desjardins et al., 2009). Understanding the profile of early-career scientists and encouraging research activity are essential to improving the rheumatology workforce.

Therefore, efforts are underway to stimulate investigative activity among practitioners, a prerequisite for developing clinical practices and ensuring that future progress in rheumatology is driven by solid evidence. Additionally, the growing interest in standardized outcome measures signals a paradigm shift within the rheumatology community to improve the uniformity and quality of clinical measurements. Specifically, balance measures have been a concern in recent years due to their link with mobility and fall prevention in rheumatology patients. Research has shown that existing standing balance measures lack an integrated framework, thus hampering meaningful use within clinical practice (Shumway-Cook et al., 2015). The development of a core outcome set (COS) to measure balance in adults aims to bridge this gap and facilitate standardization that can affect research and patient management. With rheumatologists gaining prominence for the use of standardized evaluation in their clinics, the scope for comprehensive evaluation and individualized interventions improves, possibly for improved management of rheumatologic disorders (Figure 9.3).

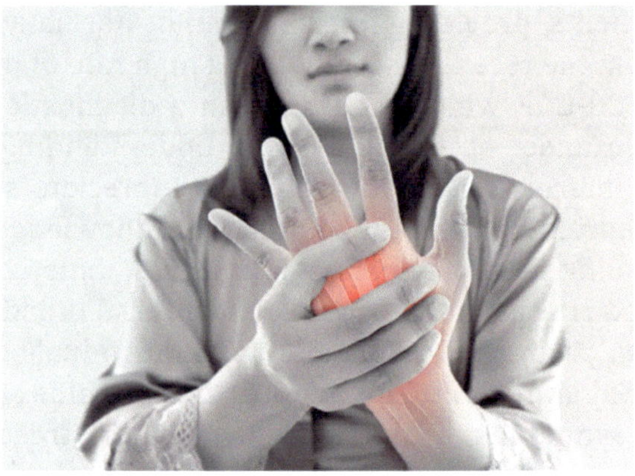

Figure 9.3. Rheumatology.

Source: https://www.felixhospital.com/sites/default/files/2024-07/rheumatology.jpg.

Importance of Internal Medicine in Rheumatology

The contribution of internal medicine to the practice of rheumatology cannot be overstated. Internists are often the first point of contact for patients presenting with complex and multi-organ presentations that have implications for rheumatic diseases. Substantial training in internal medicine equips such professionals with expertise to conduct comprehensive evaluations, identify occult pathology, and implement appropriate treatment protocols. This fundamental knowledge is significant, particularly in patients with fever of unknown origin (FUO) and inflammation of unknown origin (IUO). A study demonstrated the utility of Positron Emission Tomography-Computed Tomography (PET/CT) in accounting for such cases, reporting that a significant number of patients were definitively diagnosed through meticulous internal medicine investigations (Umut Yılmaz Koreli et al., 2025). Thus, the role of internal medicine is central in guiding early detection and management strategies in rheumatology. External to diagnosis, internal medicine's association with rheumatology also encompasses the management and care of patients with chronic rheumatic conditions.

Internists implement a multidisciplinary approach, collaborating with specialists to develop comprehensive treatment regimens tailored to patients' specific needs. For example, emphasizing comorbidities and complications specific to rheumatic conditions is integrated care that further improves patient outcomes. In regions with public health challenges, such as Sierra Leone, internal medicine becomes absolutely indispensable. Consideration of combating infectious diseases like malaria, tuberculosis, and HIV/AIDS indicates the intersection point of internal medicine and rheumatology, necessitating a robust healthcare system with the capability to address numerous health concerns simultaneously (Sankoh et al., 2024).

In enhancing coordination among healthcare professionals, internal medicine reinforces the overall care of rheumatologic patients. In addition to clinical practice, internal medicine in rheumatology also encompasses research and education. Internal medicine specialists are at the forefront in investigating disease mechanisms, efficacy of therapy, and outcomes for rheumatic illnesses, which are fundamental to advancing medical science. Their work in clinical trials and epidemiologic research is central to understanding the complex nature of diseases such as rheumatoid arthritis and lupus, thereby enabling the development of new therapeutic approaches.

Moreover, educating patients about their illnesses enhances self-management and treatment adherence. Hence, internal medicine not only provides needed diagnostic and therapeutic care but also serves as a foundation for continued research and improvement in rheumatology. The integration of these sciences is crucial for building a comprehensive picture of complex diseases and enhancing the overall quality of patient care for patients with rheumatic disorders.

9.1. Common Rheumatological Conditions

Learning Outcome

1. Describe the rheumatoid arthritis
2. Discuss the systemic lupus erythematosus (SLE)
3. Identify the osteoarthritis (OA)

Rheumatological disorders comprise a variety of disorders primarily affecting the joints and connective tissue, manifesting with chronic pain, inflammation, and functional impairment. Among the most frequent are rheumatoid arthritis and osteoarthritis. Rheumatoid arthritis, an autoimmune disease, causes generalized inflammation and joint destruction, most often generating severe disability if left untreated. Osteoarthritis, on the other hand, entails cartilage loss within the joint and ensuing bone changes, typically associated with aging and mechanical factors. Their etiology, clinical characteristics, and contribution to patient management practices require a complete review to understand these diseases. Proper diagnosis and treatment at an early stage are necessary to avoid the physical and psychological impact these conditions inflict on patients, and to improve their overall quality of life. Aside from joint-specific diseases, common rheumatological conditions include tendinopathies, for which a significant number of musculoskeletal consultations are attributed. Tendinopathy arises from repetitive stress or overuse and results in degenerative changes and tendon inflammation. In particular, heat shock proteins (HSPs) are recognized as mediators of tendon pathology and are demonstrated to be central to tissue responses to injury and inflammatory regulation. Exploring the HSPs provides insight into the molecular mechanisms underlying tendinopathies and offers potential therapeutic directions. The researchers are increasingly recognizing the importance of these molecular determinants, which may prove helpful in creating targeted therapies for tendinopathy and other chronic diseases of connective tissue patients. Integrating this information into rheumatological practice underlines the complexity of managing diseases in this area. Effective self-management strategies are valuable for patients with rheumatological disorders to become independent and maintain their quality of life. Despite evidence supporting the effectiveness of self-management assistance in significantly enhancing patient outcomes, findings indicate that large proportions of patients have limited access to organized programs.

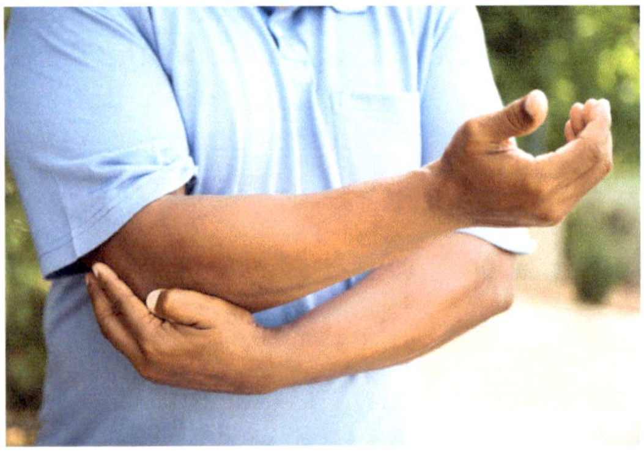

Figure 9.4. Common conditions in rheumatology.

Source: https://hoagmedicalgroup.com/wp-content/uploads/Common-Conditions-in-Rheumatology.jpg.

In inflammatory arthritis patients, studies ascertained that while the majority indicated they had the knowledge, skills, and confidence to manage their condition, not many reported receiving formal self-management education. Healthcare professionals recognize the significance of self-management support but struggle to initiate these interventions into routine care. This inconsistency underscores the need for greater communication and more equitable resource distribution in the clinical setting to increase patient engagement and empower patients to be active partners in their healthcare journey. Balanced integration of self-management concepts can reduce symptom severity and optimize the overall effectiveness of treatment regimens, thereby enhancing patient satisfaction and outcomes (Figure 9.4).

9.1.1. Rheumatoid Arthritis

The multifaceted nature of rheumatoid arthritis (RA) requires a strong understanding of its management in internal medicine. RA is an autoimmune condition that entails chronic inflammation of mostly the joints, causing pain, swelling, and ultimately joint destruction. The complexity of RA is compounded by the necessity for long-term therapy that all too often includes glucocorticoids, DMARDs, and biologics. Recent work has emphasized the significant role that low-dose glucocorticoids can play in perpetuating RA for many years, dispelling long-held concerns about the resultant risks. The American College of Rheumatology has additionally updated guidelines to prevent glucocorticoid-induced osteoporosis, emphasizing the assessment of fracture risk in these patients. These updates are essential for internal medicine physicians who encounter RA as part of their routine practice and must balance treatment effectiveness with side effects (Jalali et al., 2024). RA management is not just a pharmacologic intervention; it includes a comprehensive strategy with patient education and support for lifestyle modification. Because of the systemic and chronic nature of the disease, patients end up having comorbidities such as cardiovascular disease, osteoporotic fractures, and mental illnesses. Therefore, it is essential that healthcare professionals engage in shared decision-making with their patients to foster an environment where patients are enabled to participate actively in their care plan. Active participation from both the patient and the professional can also enhance compliance with the drug regimen and lifestyle adjustments, ultimately leading to improved quality of life. In addition, knowledge of the psychological effects of RA is essential because anxiety and depression can be factors that add to disease severity and treatment response. Internal medicine professionals should be able to identify such challenges and incorporate measures addressing the physical and emotional management of RA (Jalali et al., 2024). Research plays a central role in developing understanding and treating RA. The answer to the question of how standardization of core outcome sets for clinical trials is applied has become a critical method of ensuring that clinically important and pertinent outcomes are measured comparably. Standardization of outcomes is essential not only for comparing how different interventions work but also for informing RA management policy and clinical guidelines.

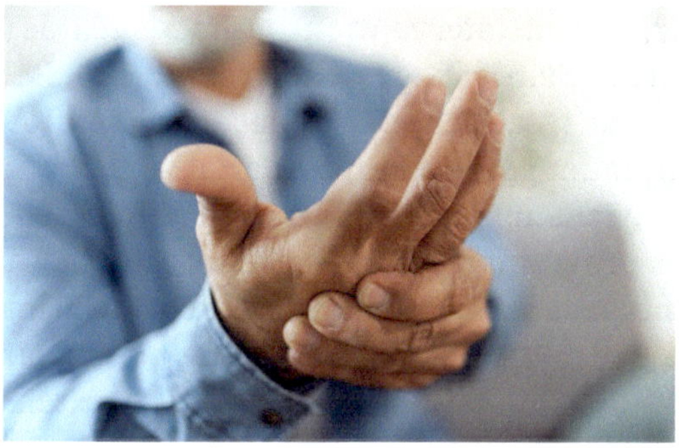

Figure 9.5. Rheumatoid arthritis.

Source: https://jnj-content-lab2.brightspotcdn.com/dims4/default/fa64da9/2147483647/strip/true/crop/1920x1080+0+0/resize/1440x810!/quality/90/?url=https%3A%2F%2Fjnj-production-jnj.s3.us-east-1.amazonaws.com%2Fbrightspot%2F18%2Fc0%2F5567046e4ac1a4b2a92a3635dfd7%2Fwhat-is-a-rheumatic-disease-1024.png.

Through a common framework, clinicians and researchers can address previously understudied aspects of patient care, improving treatments to more closely match the needs of patients with RA. Repeated updating of these core outcome sets will be needed as increasing evidence becomes available, so that the frameworks remain useful and practical. With advances in rheumatology, a collaborative strategy with patients, health practitioners, and researchers will be critical to maximizing outcomes in RA and other rheumatologic conditions (Figure 9.5).

9.1.2. Systemic Lupus Erythematosus (SLE)

SLE is a challenging condition in internal medicine because it is multifaceted and the clinical manifestations can be variable. It is an autoimmune disease characterized by the formation of autoantibodies against a broad range of self-antigens, leading to inflammation and damage across multiple organ systems. The illness is commonly characterized by nonspecific symptoms, such as fatigue, arthralgias, and rashes, which can make early diagnosis challenging. A comprehensive understanding of SLE's pathophysiology, including its genetic basis, can improve clinical management practices. For example, recent studies have demonstrated significant correlations between gene polymorphisms, such as ZNF76 and SCUBE3, and increased susceptibility to SLE, thereby emphasizing the application of genetic testing to inform targeted treatment in the future (Assar et al., 2024). Clinical heterogeneity of SLE is noted among children, where juvenile-onset SLE poses unusual diagnostic and treatment challenges. This patient population tends to have a higher incidence of specific manifestations, including arthritis and hematologic involvement. In a recent retrospective review, researchers found that musculoskeletal complaints were frequently the presenting symptoms of juvenile SLE, with a high correlation between hemolytic anemia and arthritis. The onset of age in such cases typically occurs before 16 years and necessitates a management approach tailored to the developing physiological status of the juvenile (Hannech et al., 2021). Engagement of holistic, multidisciplinary therapy by experts such as rheumatologists, pediatricians, and others is paramount to achieving the best therapeutic benefits for this underprivileged population. A sound management system for SLE must not only address the acute presentation but also aim to modify the disease in the long term. Pharmacotherapy, often with antimalarials such as hydroxychloroquine and corticosteroids, is an essential aspect of symptom control and flare prevention. However, the treatment must be individualized based on the patient's specific symptoms, comorbid medical conditions, and potential adverse effects. Better insight into doctors' understanding of disease expression will lead to earlier diagnosis and treatment, thereby improving prognosis. Moreover, more research into the genetic component of SLE and its etiology which is multifactorial, will be important in developing novel strategies for treatment and prevention based on patient profiles (Assar et al., 2024). With new information emerging from genetic research and clinical trials, the future of SLE treatment in internal medicine will differ significantly (Figure 9.6).

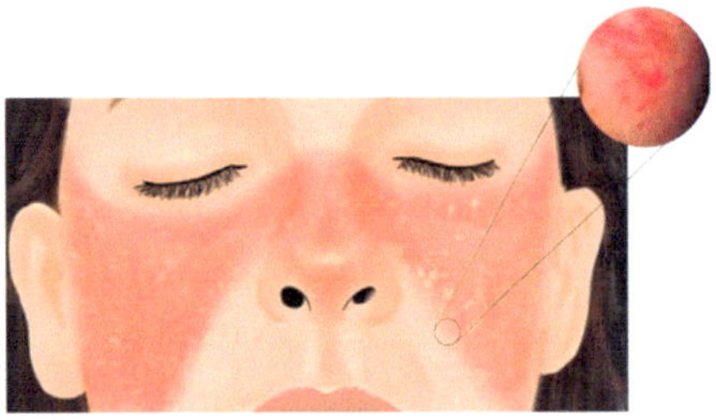

Figure 9.6. Systemic lupus erythematosus (SLE).

Source: https://aarc.sg/wp-content/uploads/2023/10/shutterstock_2180493141.jpg.

9.1.3. Osteoarthritis (OA)

OA is the most common form of arthritis, involving cartilage deterioration and underlying bone deterioration, and associated with pain and functional impairment. It primarily affects weight-bearing joints such as the knees, hips, and spine, which are very significant in causing problems with regular activities. The increased prevalence of OA, especially among geriatric populations, necessitates understanding proper management plans in the context of internal medicine. Health care professionals, particularly rheumatologists, play a critical role in addressing the multifaceted needs of OA patients, including not only pharmacotherapy but also lifestyle modifications that can maximize quality of life. With the complexity of OA, one must ensure a holistic perspective with both physical and psychosocial considerations, ensuring well-balanced care to those afflicted with this degenerative condition. Evidence-based practices have become key components of osteoarthritis treatment, particularly in primary care. Studies have indicated that programs with a structured intervention outline, such as the Arthritis Self-Management Programs (ASMPs), can make treatment more effective by improving pain management and increasing physical activity among patients. However, implementing such programs requires careful consideration of the peculiar challenges inherent in primary care settings. The PraxArt study, for instance, seeks to explore the influence of GPs' extensive medical education on the management of OA patients. By training GPs in OA management knowledge and tools, the program aims to enhance patient quality of life through greater treatment compliance and patient education, demonstrating that systematic training can improve healthcare outcomes in individuals with OA (Gensichen et al., 2005). Also, the development and validation of patient self-management skill assessment measures have become increasingly utilized in osteoarthritis research. The Effective Consumer Scale (EC-17) is a useful instrument for quantifying patients' capacity to take responsibility for their healthcare, thereby enabling personalized treatment. Its analysis of psychometric qualities demonstrates its applicability and potential for the patient's participation in his/her care process. Interestingly, high levels of person reliability and adequate test-retest reliability ensure that the scale is useful for gauging change over time, enabling healthcare practitioners to monitor and respond to the shifting needs of their OA patients. By Outcomes targeting both patient empowerment and clinical outcomes, incorporating such tools into daily practice can significantly enhance the quality of care in the rheumatology sector, leading to more effective health management for patients with osteoarthritis (Harmsen et al., 2012) (Figure 9.7).

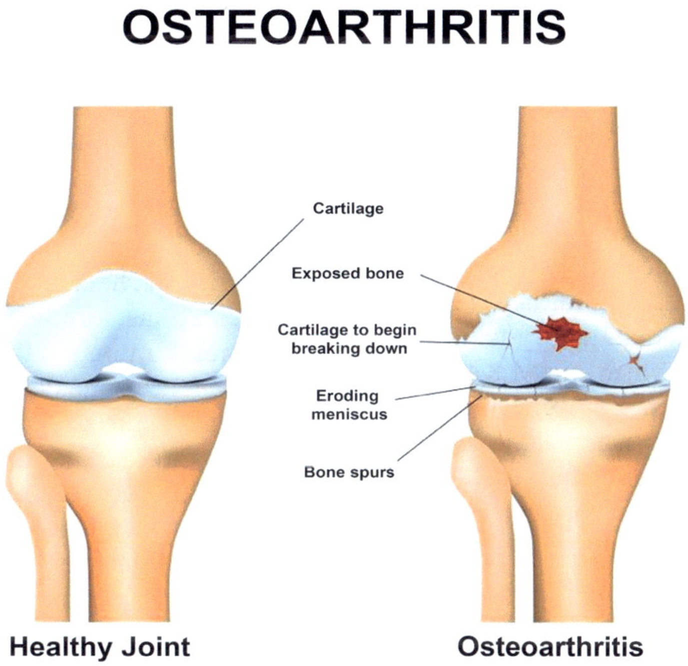

Figure 9.7. Osteoarthritis (OA).

Source: https://ocmc.in/wp-content/uploads/2024/04/osteo.png.

Test Your Knowledge

1. What are the most common rheumatological disorders affecting joints and connective tissues?
2. How do inflammatory rheumatological diseases differ from degenerative joint conditions?

9.2. Diagnostic Approaches in Rheumatology

Learning Outcome

1. Explain the clinical evaluation and history taking
2. Describe the laboratory tests and biomarkers
3. Explain the imaging techniques in diagnosis

The inherent complexity of diagnosing rheumatological conditions necessitates that the diagnosis be approached on many fronts, owing largely to the protean characteristics of diseases such as systemic lupus erythematosus and rheumatoid arthritis. The initial evaluation often consists of a detailed history-taking and physical examination, which may reveal joint effusions, tenderness, and systemic findings. These, however, may be nonspecific, and the next step would most likely require laboratory tests. Blood tests for inflammatory markers, autoantibodies, and a complete blood count provide valuable information. Imaging techniques such as X-rays and magnetic resonance imaging (MRI) are increasingly used to assess joint integrity and soft-tissue involvement, supplementing clinicians' capacity to establish an overall diagnosis. Clinical correlation with lab and imaging information is crucial to achieving an accurate diagnosis, underscoring the collaboration required in rheumatological assessment in internal medicine. Apart from conventional diagnostic methods, the use of advanced imaging techniques has significantly increased the precision of diagnosing rheumatological disorders. Imaging techniques such as MRI and ultrasound can detect subtle changes in joint structure, often before overt clinical manifestations. Ultrasound, on the other hand, has proven to be an invaluable tool for detecting erosions and synovitis, enabling timely intervention to alter the disease's trajectory. Equipment such as nailfold videocapillaroscopy has also been found to be beyond replacement in assessing systemic sclerosis (SSc), as capillary morphology can predict microvascular complications years before the onset of systemic symptoms. By categorizing these vascular abnormalities, physicians can tailor therapies more aptly, and thus the importance of a practical and systematic diagnostic process in rheumatology to ensure timely treatment and improved patient outcomes, as outlined in SSc literature (Cutolo et al., 2016). Recognition of the inner ear's involvement in systemic autoimmune diseases has introduced a new twist to the rheumatological diagnostic paradigm, as sensorineural hearing loss can represent an underlying systemic process. The interfusion of rheumatological and audiological manifestations implies the need for greater awareness among clinicians. Inconsistency of presentation means that there is room for misdiagnosis, thereby making early intervention difficult. Once audiovestibular symptoms like hearing fluctuations and intermittent tinnitus emerge in association with unmistakable autoimmune markers, corticosteroid therapy has also been successful in restoring auditory function. This highlights that audiological tests should be made a part of the routine examination of patients suspected to have rheumatological conditions because definitive diagnosis can significantly enhance the efficacy of treatment as per evidence obtained from case reports on immune-mediated inner ear disease (Adelchi et al., 2018).

9.2.1. Clinical Evaluation and History Taking

History and clinical assessment are the backbone of diagnosing and managing rheumatological disorders. It begins with taking an appropriate patient history, not just the chief complaint, but also past medical history, family history, and psychosocial problems. This approach assists the clinician in identifying patterns that would indicate associated rheumatological diseases, e.g., systemic lupus erythematosus (SLE), which is characteristically multi-systemic in its presentation and variability. Accurate history-taking ensures key symptoms are thoroughly documented, thereby facilitating the formulation of differential diagnoses. SLE, for instance, can affect renal function and thus necessitate specific queries regarding urinary symptoms, which will guide further investigative procedures, such as a biopsy. By pairing a thorough understanding of the patient's history and symptoms, clinicians can optimize diagnostic accuracy and outcomes for rheumatology patients. Significantly, clinical evaluation extends beyond history-taking to include an exhaustive physical examination, which is used to corroborate the patient's reported symptoms and to obtain data on disease activity. Systematic assessment of musculoskeletal findings, such as joint tenderness and swelling, is imperative in the setting of inflammatory arthritis. Furthermore, laboratory results supplement clinical information, with various biomarkers providing useful insights into disease activity and organ involvement in conditions like SLE. For instance, evidence indicates that urinary biomarkers, such as tissue factor pathway inhibitor (TFPI), have great potential in the assessment of lupus nephritis (LN) in SLE patients. By correlating clinical presentation with laboratory findings, rheumatologists can accurately measure disease activity and adapt management plans appropriately, demonstrating that well-organized assessments are paramount in rheumatological practice. Alongside physical and clinical evaluations, effective communication during history-taking helps establish a therapeutic relationship between the doctor and patient, making them more likely to disclose important details about their symptoms and concerns. The subtle coaction between history-taking and active listening helps clinicians establish trust, a determinant of effective management of common chronic diseases in rheumatology. Sharpening questions about systemic symptoms, e.g., fatigue or rash, may uncover instrumental diagnostic information typical of diseases such as SLE, in which interleukin 9 (IL-9) has been implicated. As clinical assessment language evolves, evidence-based practice and patient storytelling will remain crucial. A reflective, empathetic history-taking model not only enriches the clinical interview but also equips practitioners with the data needed for comprehensive management in rheumatology.

9.2.2. Laboratory Tests and Biomarkers

Laboratory tests and biomarkers are the hub of rheumatological practice, particularly in the diagnosis and treatment of SLE. The detection of individual biomarkers will allow for early diagnosis and improved disease stratification in patients. For instance, evidence indicates that cell-bound complement activation products (CB-CAPs) are excellent markers of complement activation in clinically suspected SLE patients. The frequency of positive CB-CAPs in likely SLE patients is considerably higher than that of routine serum complement levels; therefore, the markers are likely to enhance diagnostic accuracy. Notably, a multianalyte assay panel (MAP)—which includes CB-CAPs—was a predictor of patients who later fulfilled the classification criteria for SLE and, consequently, is a helpful instrument for rheumatologists in clinical practice (Alexander et al., 2020). Beyond complement proteins, cytokines have emerged as crucial biomarkers of disease activity in SLE. A recent article highlights the relationship between serum interleukin-2 (IL-2) levels and disease activity. Higher IL-2 levels also correlated strongly with the SLE disease activity index, suggesting that this cytokine is an ideal marker of disease severity. The ability to discriminate between active and inactive disease states using laboratory parameters, such as IL-2 levels, allows the clinician to better individualize treatment. Hence, these findings lend credence to the integration of such biomarkers into routine patient evaluation, therefore enabling more personalized treatment in SLE care and, consequently, other rheumatic disorders (Sedighi et al., 2014). More importantly, the pairing of laboratory analysis with biomarkers transcends their utility in diagnosis; it also guides disease prediction and therapy monitoring. The ability to measure biomarkers longitudinally enables clinicians to assess the efficacy of therapeutic regimens and make corresponding refinements. For example, in subjects with high CB-CAP or IL-2 levels, continuing assessment may facilitate expected flares or response to therapy. This adaptive approach not only maximizes therapeutic modalities but also engages patients in their care, with enhanced compliance with treatment regimens. Ultimately, with advances in scientific investigation, the increasing understanding and application of laboratory workup and biomarkers will be critical for rationalizing treatment protocols in rheumatology practice, leading to improved patient care and outcomes (Figure 9.8).

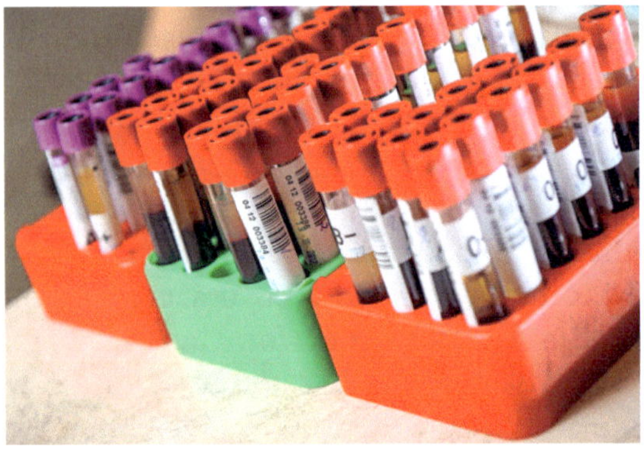

Figure 9.8. Blood tests used to diagnose rheumatoid arthritis.

Source: https://privatelondonrheumatologist.com/wp-content/uploads/2022/09/blood-tests.jpg.

9.2.3. Imaging Techniques in Diagnosis

Diagnostic imaging modalities play a significant role in the practice of rheumatology, particularly for conditions such as Takayasu arteritis, which can present with a broad spectrum of symptoms involving diverse bodily systems. Accurate imaging is particularly crucial for assessing vascular involvement and for follow-up of disease activity. Techniques such as ultrasound, magnetic resonance imaging (MRI), and computed tomography (CT) have gained prominence for their ability to demonstrate inflammatory changes in arterial walls and surrounding tissue. These modalities not only facilitate clinicians in reaching a final diagnosis but also allow prognostication. Current investigations highlight that, in the selection and interpretation of these imaging modalities, protocols should be standardized across the various presentations of Takayasu arteritis. An integrated approach leverages the clinician's ability to use imaging, ultimately improving patient outcomes in this multidimensional disease environment (N/A, 2025). At the same time, advanced digital imaging technologies have radically altered the practice of rheumatology diagnosis. Incorporating artificial intelligence (AI) into the interpretation of imaging, particularly algorithms that analyze chest X-rays and other imaging studies, has demonstrated great promise. For instance, HealthScan AI applies deep learning to analyze medical images for illnesses such as COVID-19 and pneumonia, providing timely, accurate diagnoses. In addition to streamlining the diagnostic process, the technology also provides patients with real-time information about their medical condition. By leveraging image analysis capabilities, rheumatologists can supplement traditional assessment methods with greater diagnostic accuracy and improved clinical decision-making. This imaging revolution points to the potential of AI to revolutionize everyday practice in rheumatology and other specialties (st Prudhvi et al., 2024). Further, imaging practices extend beyond diagnosis; they also involve ongoing monitoring and assessment of treatment efficacy. For patients with rheumatological conditions, regular imaging evaluation is essential to track disease activity and response to therapy. Using modalities such as ultrasonography and MRI, clinicians can identify subtle changes in joint inflammation, erosion, or trauma, which can inform treatment modifications. Visualization of these nuances promotes a more individualized therapeutic process, enabling clinicians to render evidence-based judgments that reflect the patient's changing clinical presentation. Moreover, the creation of imaging guidelines and consensus statements by expert panels points to the strength of their systematic use. Such sequential approaches not only benefit clinical practice but also elevate the general level of care in rheumatology (N/A, 2025).

Test Your Knowledge

1. What laboratory tests are commonly used to diagnose rheumatological diseases?
2. Why is imaging important in the evaluation of rheumatic conditions?

9.3. Treatment Modalities in Rheumatology

Learning Outcome

1. Understand the pharmacological treatments
2. Define the non-pharmacological interventions
3. Describe the emerging therapies and research

The landscape of treatment modalities in rheumatology is constantly shifting, with a merger of the traditional and innovative approaches. Conventional therapies, including non-steroidal anti-inflammatory drugs (NSAIDs) and glucocorticoids, have long been the cornerstone for the management of symptoms of diseases like osteoarthritis and rheumatoid arthritis. These provide symptomatic relief by modulating pain and inflammation. These have been substituted by newer, more specific therapies directed at altering the disease pathology of autoimmune diseases. Introduction of biologic agents, including tumor necrosis factor (TNF) inhibitors and interleukin inhibitors, represents a paradigm shift in treatment strategies, with precision medicine opportunities that can be further enhanced to significantly impact patient outcomes. As rheumatology continues to mature in embracing multidisciplinary care, the integration of new treatments underscores the rich potential for improved patient management in this complex discipline. With changing treatment modalities, stem cell therapy has risen to the forefront of rheumatology, driven by its regenerative capabilities. Stem cells, particularly mesenchymal stem cells, can differentiate into a variety of tissue types and possess a characteristic with far-reaching implications in the repair of injured soft tissues of rheumatic diseases. These cells contribute to healing through cell-matrix interaction and paracrine secretion of soluble factors that modulate the microenvironment. Early clinical trials have demonstrated the effectiveness of stem cell therapies in musculoskeletal diseases, providing an essential addition to existing treatment models. The rapid development of this sector, however, calls for prudent regulation and ethical considerations. While the stem cell therapy hype within rheumatology is valid, the need for strict scientific evidence and compliance with regulation is critical to therapeutic efficacy and safety as these treatments advance (Grange et al., 2011). Molecular imaging technology is yet another revolutionary field within rheumatology, enabling unprecedented insight into disease mechanisms and treatment response. By using non-invasive imaging agents that specifically target biological locations, clinicians can visualize and quantify cellular function in real time. This technology has the potential to enhance diagnosis, prognosis, and the monitoring of treatment protocols, particularly in inflammatory diseases such as rheumatoid arthritis. The advent of these advanced imaging modalities enables assessment of cellular targets and therapeutic effects at the molecular level. Furthermore, the new field of molecular imaging should enable the identification of new therapeutic agents and ultimately broaden the array of available treatments for rheumatologists. As this technology continues to advance, its integration into standard practice will redefine how rheumatic illnesses are diagnosed and managed (Funk et al., 2017).

9.3.1. Pharmacological Treatments

Pharmacological treatment is significant in managing many rheumatological illnesses, which are typically defined by multifaceted symptoms, e.g., chronic pain. Medications such as the non-steroidal anti-inflammatory drugs (NSAIDs) are utilized frequently to control pain and inflammation in conditions such as rheumatoid arthritis and systemic lupus erythematosus. The treatment needs to be tailored to individual patients, particularly taking into account the chronicity of pain in conditions such as systemic sclerosis and systemic lupus erythematosus, where it is commonly one of the initial presenting symptoms. Adequate pain control is essential, both to enhance the patient's quality of life and to avoid doctors finding themselves in unsafe over-treatment scenarios for patients with co-morbid syndromes, like fibromyalgia, commonly presented with connective tissue disorders (Atzeni et al., 2015). NSAIDs are used, along with corticosteroids, to alleviate inflammation in rheumatological disorders. These powerful anti-inflammatory medications can provide rapid relief of acute symptoms and are especially useful to control worsening exacerbations. Corticosteroids have also been shown to improve outcomes in conditions such as systemic lupus erythematosus, where treatment can lead to significant improvements in functional status and quality of life. Long-term use of these medications does demand close monitoring for the possibility of side effects, such as osteoporosis and susceptibility to infections. Thus, a comprehensive treatment plan may largely be based on an integrated approach involving pharmacological treatment, lifestyle modification, and supportive therapy to achieve optimal outcomes in patients with various rheumatological conditions. Advancements in immunosuppressive have expanded the pharmacological armamentarium for the management of autoimmune rheumatological diseases.

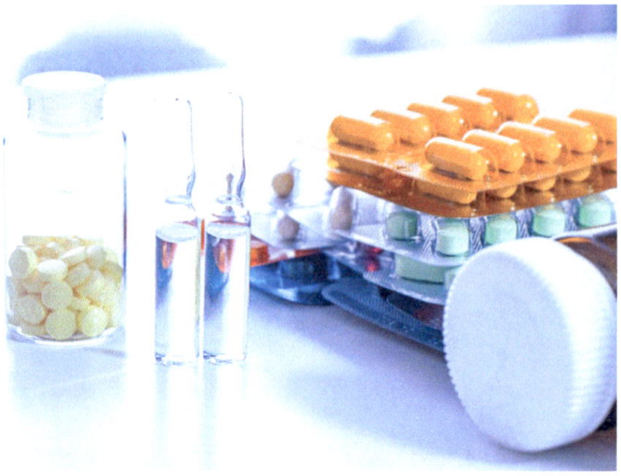

Figure 9.9. Pharmacological treatments for rheumatoid arthritis.

Source: https://images.ctfassets.net/yixw23k2v6vo/3vLi500FpODHC2JXKj2d5J/27e505102f4da25ddb1d9bb2cfc67c50/GettyImages-1252761829-3000x2000.jpg.

Agents such as methotrexate and biologics, including tumor necrosis factor inhibitors, have dramatically changed treatment patterns, making targeted therapy accessible for disease control. These therapies have been effective in reducing disease activity and improving long-term organ and joint function. In addition, in cases of hearing loss due to an autoimmune reaction, treatment with corticosteroids has responded favorably, often leading to significant improvement in auditory function (Adelchi et al., 2018). The availability of these advanced treatments in routine clinical practice emphasizes the importance of personalized therapy in rheumatology, reflecting the need for precise diagnosis and tailored treatment strategies to manage both systemic and focal manifestations efficiently (Figure 9.9).

9.3.2. Non-Pharmacological Interventions

Non-pharmacological management is a significant part of the internal medicine role in rheumatology, particularly for chronic diseases such as osteoarthritis and rheumatoid arthritis. Non-pharmacological interventions encompass physical therapy, exercise regimens, and multidisciplinary management that promote functional capacity and enhance quality of life. Systematic exercise programs, particularly progressive resistance training, have been found to be effective for reducing joint pain and promoting mobility. These types of interventions not only rehabilitate the physical results of such illnesses but also have psychological benefits since patients feel less anxiety and more confidence in managing their symptoms. Evidence supports that multi-disciplinary care systems with more than one health professional further increase these benefits, leading to improved symptom control and patient satisfaction (Adams et al., 2020). Moreover, the education and self-management roles cannot be overemphasized. Healthcare practitioners can empower patients by informing them about their disease and the behavioral changes needed. Cognitive behavior therapy and pain acceptance strategies have been adapted for patients with rheumatology, and these have played a significant role in effective pain management. It should be noted that psychological factors associated with chronic aches and pains must be addressed alongside physical treatments. Studies highlight a favorable correlation between effective pain control and improved physical and mental health, underscoring the need for an integrated model of care among rheumatologists (Acharya et al., 2014). These self-management strategies not only equip patients with coping mechanisms but also help them grasp the complexities of their treatment pathway. In addition, multidisciplinary teams are essential in the delivery of non-pharmacologic treatments. Different experts, such as physical therapists, occupational therapists, and dietitians, collaborate to prepare individualized care plans tailored to each patient's specific needs. Multidisciplinary teamwork has been promising in preventing complications of chronic rheumatologic conditions. For instance, specialist fracture liaison services provide comprehensive assessments and targeted interventions that have proven effective in reducing refracture rates in high-risk individuals. These approaches place great emphasis on the importance of interprofessional collaboration in healthcare and demonstrate how non-pharmacological care can be combined with traditional medical treatment to achieve better patient outcomes. As advancements in rheumatology continue, the incorporation of these different interventions into routine care will be ever more critical for enhancing the quality of life for patients (Adams et al., 2020) (Figure 9.10).

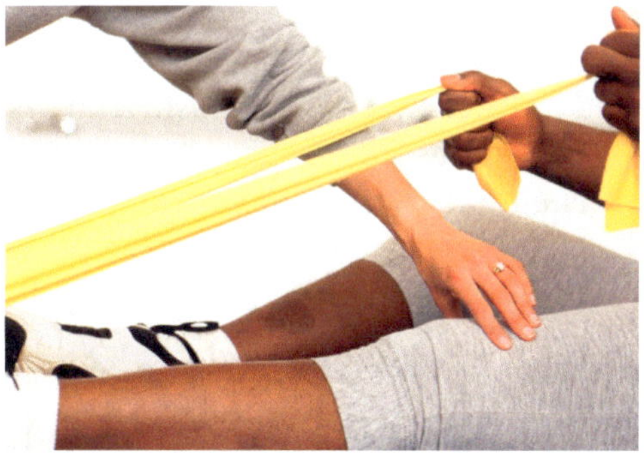

Figure 9.10. The role of physical therapy in rheumatoid arthritis management.

Source: https://centerforspecialtycare.com/wp-content/uploads/2024/01/Rheumatology-2-1000x675.png.

9.3.3. Emerging Therapies and Research

The latest advancements in rheumatology have underscored the importance of emerging therapies and ongoing research efforts to improve patient outcomes. For instance, improvements in the identification of myositis-specific antibodies have been instrumental in diagnosing dermatomyositis, a multifactorial inflammatory myopathy characterized by specific cutaneous manifestations. Identification of such antibodies allows clinicians to predict patient prognosis and tailor treatment protocols accordingly more reliably. A case report reported a 22-year-old male who had multifocal erythematous plaques and was diagnosed later with biopsy-proven dermatomyositis and was found to be seropositive for nuclear matrix protein 2 antibody (NXP-2). His treatment strategy changed from systemic corticosteroids to more targeted therapy like intravenous immune globulin therapy, which resulted in an excellent clinical response. This case demonstrates the significant role that personalized therapy and new therapeutic strategies play in the comprehensive treatment of rheumatologic disease (Cartron et al., 2020). Owing to the ongoing development of rheumatology, incorporating research-driven approaches is imperative to advancing innovative therapies. The clinical studies environment in rheumatology is evolving, as reflected in research on musculoskeletal disease and in the professional engagement of early-career rheumatologists. A recent study was designed to quantify the level of investigative activity among such practitioners, using both demographic and normative data, which are imperative for understanding their impact on clinical practice. The findings indicate an urgent need to enhance early-career rheumatologists' participation in research activities with the potential to be game-changing. Individuals focusing on research participation drivers, such as the availability of funding and the impact of research-oriented institutions, would shift their focus to discovering new therapies and fine-tuning existing treatment regimens (Desjardins et al., 2009). Moreover, ongoing research into targeted biologic therapies indicates the promising future of personalized rheumatology. Agents such as Janus kinase inhibitors and interleukin inhibitors are increasingly being used for their unique potential to modify immune function, thereby reducing disease activity with fewer side effects than traditional therapies. Emerging evidence suggests these drugs not only address patient symptoms but also potentially alter disease course, offering long-term solutions for managing the disease. Along with stringent assessment of therapy efficacy and safety, the adoption of advanced research techniques into clinical practice will play a crucial role in shaping rheumatology's future. Through an innovative, inquiry-based culture, rheumatologists can work toward better health outcomes by reshaping the face of care for people with autoimmune and inflammatory diseases (Desjardins et al., 2009; Cartron et al., 2020).

Test Your Knowledge

1. What are the common treatment options for rheumatological disorders?
2. How do disease-modifying antirheumatic drugs (DMARDs) help manage inflammatory arthritis?

9.4. Role of the Rheumatologist

Learning Outcome

1. Understand the patient management and care coordination
2. Identify the interdisciplinary collaboration
3. Focus on patient education and support

The rheumatologist plays a critical role in the diagnosis and management of inflammatory and autoimmune diseases, the most well-known being those involving arthritis. Rheumatologists use advanced diagnostic tools, including clinical evaluation and imaging, to accurately diagnose conditions such as rheumatoid arthritis, psoriatic arthritis, and systemic lupus erythematosus. Their education enables them to exclude these diseases from similar diseases, ensuring patients receive proper and timely treatment. Also, they monitor disease and treatment response using a thorough patient assessment. This focus on chronic conditions like rheumatoid arthritis, which affects over 400,000 Australians, underscores the utility of specialized disease management programs that can be provided by rheumatologists, potentially substantially improving patients' quality of life (N/A). In addition to diagnosis, rheumatologists play a key role in developing personalized treatment regimens that may include pharmacologic therapy and lifestyle modifications. They are educated about traditional disease-modifying antirheumatic drugs (DMARDs) as well as newer biologic agents, which have changed the direction of rheumatological management. Balancing the efficacy of treatments against potential side effects carefully, rheumatologists educate patients on compliance with treatment regimens while encouraging active self-management, emphasizing the importance of lifestyle aspects such as diet and exercise in the management of chronic disease. The development of national databases, such as the Australian Rheumatology Association Database (ARAD), also facilitates their ability to monitor treatment outcomes and maximize therapeutic interventions at the population health level (N/A). Rheumatologists also engage in continuous professional development to stay abreast of evolving treatment trends and evidence, fostering a culture of evidence-based practice. This lifelong learning ethos is reflected in initiatives such as the European Rheumatology Curriculum Framework, which aims to harmonize training across member states. By adhering to a structured training system, rheumatologists can ensure that skills are aligned, promoting high-quality care to patients throughout Europe. With medical care organizations striving for improved patient outcomes, these professionals are not only responsible for providing individual-level care but also contributing to a more macro-level dialogue of healthcare policy aligned with trending and pressing issues in rheumatologic care (Figure 9.11).

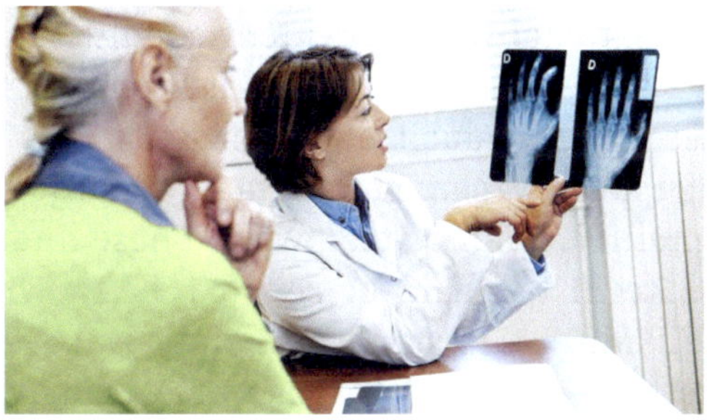

Figure 9.11. Role of the rheumatologist.

Source: https://i0.wp.com/post.medicalnewstoday.com/wp-content/uploads/sites/3/2021/11/rheumatologist_diagnose_GettyImages697568781_Header-1-1024x575.jpg?w=1155&h=1528.

9.4.1. Patient Management and Care Coordination

Effective patient care coordination and management are key determinants of the treatment of rheumatological illnesses, which are often multifaceted and difficult to manage. In rheumatology, where diseases such as rheumatoid arthritis and systemic lupus erythematosus require a multidisciplinary approach to management, the coordination of the efforts of various healthcare providers can have a dramatic effect on the outcomes of patients. Successful care coordination ensures that all team members—nurses, physicians, physical therapists, and social workers—are not only aware of the diagnostic and therapeutic strategy used but also cohesive in objectives to enhance patient adherence to treatment regimens. With open lines of communication and the power of shared decision-making, care coordination promotes patient satisfaction and enables holistic management strategies tailored to every individual's specific needs. Transition of adolescents and young adults with chronic rheumatological diseases into adult care settings presents particular issues that highlight the importance of an ordered approach to patient care. Systematic review in young patients with persistent conditions like Type 1 diabetes showed that transitional success hinges on individualized planning of care and vital support systems such as family engagement and multidisciplinary teamwork. These findings resonate in the field of rheumatology, where establishing a formal transition team—and processes—can lead to smoother transitions and better health outcomes in young adults. The application of transition coordinators, as brought to light in the review, calls for the empowering of both the healthcare practitioners and the patients to navigate the nuances of adulthood when ill with chronic diseases and hence prevent the risk of an acceleration of the health status over such formative years (Bagnall et al., 2013). The exploration of the research and workforce environment among early-career rheumatologists carries significant implications for coordinating patient care and management. Studies indicate that few early-career professionals engage in research, which ultimately informs clinical practice and patient care protocols. Insufficient data on research activities compromise the growth of knowledge about the development of evidence-based practice in rheumatology. The profession can bridge knowledge and innovation gaps that directly affect patient outcomes by advocating for efficient research and funding. As established in the research, developing a research-conducive environment also enhances the coordination of care and allows rheumatologists to implement new treatment models, ultimately improving the quality of patient care (Desjardins et al., 2009).

9.4.2. Interdisciplinary Collaboration

The nature of rheumatologic diseases necessitates an interdisciplinary model of patient care involving several medical specialties. Interdisciplinary collaboration enables the convergence of diverse knowledge to ensure a comprehensive treatment and assessment plan tailored to the unique needs of patients. Through collaboration, health workers such as rheumatologists, general practitioners, physiotherapists, and nutritionists can share ideas and develop well-integrated interventions that combine supportive and medical treatments. This model of collaboration not only enhances the quality of care but also addresses multifactorial problems commonly faced by patients with chronic rheumatic diseases, thereby improving patient outcomes. Notably, as the healthcare system continues to develop in response to rapidly changing patient requirements, promotion of collaborative settings can essentially bridge gaps in care provision commonly faced which may detract from efficient management of such complex conditions. In the field of rheumatology, team members' coordination and communication are of utmost significance. Effective multidisciplinary practice relies on the free flow of communication that enables a shared understanding of each discipline's strengths and its role. Interdisciplinary team meetings as a working forum for the sharing of patient progress and challenges, supplemented by the results of several specialties, can maximize clinical decision-making. Moreover, training across the professions directly impacting patient care can foster respect and trust among peers, thereby strengthening collaboration. Incorporating formalized training in team and interdisciplinary care into medical education curricula can prepare future healthcare practitioners to function efficiently in collaborative settings and maintain long-term effectiveness in managing complex rheumatic diseases. Furthermore, the increasing focus on patient-centered care naturally follows from interdisciplinary collaboration, which emphasizes the individualization of therapy needs. Including patients within the decision-making process not only ensures better treatment protocol compliance but also invites patients to become active participants in their own health care. Care models founded on these principles are more likely to be collaborative, featuring shared decision-making in which providers talk with patients to chart their values and preferences and thus have better health care experiences. The model has been shown to reduce barriers across specialties and improve outcomes more broadly, as evidenced by research conducted at various healthcare sites. By considering the patient's experience and perspective from a multidisciplinary perspective, healthcare providers can create more adaptive and responsive treatment options for the changing nature of rheumatologic diseases (Bagnall et al., 2013; Lehtsaar et al., 2017).

9.4.3. Patient Education and Support

Patient support and education during the rheumatology process are the determining factors in improving patient outcomes and treatment compliance. Effective patient-provider communication enables individuals to understand their conditions, treatments, and the need for lifestyle modifications. In rheumatology, chronic illnesses like lupus and rheumatoid arthritis require long-term management, making education a very important aspect. Educating patients through structured programs can reduce anxiety, enable them to be more actively involved in their care, and improve their quality of life. This approach is particularly crucial due to the complexity of conditions in rheumatic disease, where thorough knowledge of complex treatment regimens and symptom-control methods is critical for establishing a framework for symbiotic patient-caregiver interaction that ensures adherence and beneficial health outcomes. Moreover, the inclusion of support systems together with patient education enhances the effectiveness of treatment in rheumatology. Support can take many forms, including peer support groups, mental health services, and family members' participation in educational processes. Research has established that patients in support groups exhibit lower stress levels and greater patient satisfaction with care (Mendes et al., 2024). By providing opportunities for social interaction among patients with everyday issues, healthcare providers enable the sharing of valuable information and coping strategies. This social learning population not only promotes resilience but also key educational elements, such as self-management skills and recognition of early symptom exacerbation, which are essential for prompt intervention in rheumatic disorder management. Support systems are, therefore, a vital element for supplementing education programs and are a significant contributor to overall patient participation. Finally, the inclusion of technology in patient education and support represents a paradigm shift in the field of rheumatology. Telemedicine sites, mobile phone applications, and online educational materials enable patients to receive information at their convenience and interact with healthcare professionals without being bound by geography. The innovation enhances communication and equips patients with the tools needed to self-manage their conditions at a distance, thereby promoting treatment adherence (Song et al., 2024). Interventions using technology can also support specially developed learning material that caters to the specific needs of an individual patient, encouraging a process of personalized care. By embracing these innovations, healthcare providers can create an active patient-centered model of care that is well placed to meet the specific challenges of rheumatic diseases, with improved all-around health outcomes and sustained patient empowerment in their care.

Test Your Knowledge

1. How do rheumatologists contribute to the diagnosis of complex joint and connective tissue disorders?
2. What role do rheumatologists play in managing chronic rheumatological conditions?

9.5. Challenges in Rheumatology

Learning Outcome

1. Understand the diagnostic challenges in rheumatology
2. Define the treatment adherence issues in rheumatology
3. Discuss on access to care and health disparities in rheumatology

There are significant challenges in rheumatology, particularly in the management of systemic sclerosis (SSc), in which gastrointestinal tract (GIT) involvement is a frequent finding. This is a significant cause of disabling symptoms, which have a substantial impact on patients' quality of life. Despite the common manifestations of GIT disease, there are limited disease-modifying treatments for SSc, with treatment primarily symptomatic. This issue is further complicated by the complexity and heterogeneity of the clinical presentations with GIT involvement, which may be dissociated from skin disease. Symptoms are often nonspecific and can overlap across different anatomical sites, making precise diagnosis and timely intervention difficult. Moreover, some percentage of SSc patients develop serious GIT complications with increased mortality, highlighting the urgent need to understand its pathogenesis better and create effective therapeutic strategies (Abraham et al., 2017). Trends in research in rheumatology further complicate the clinical picture. The remit of clinical research in this specialty is often unclear, leading to significant gaps in our knowledge of disease mechanisms and effective therapies. Interestingly, the workforce currently engaged in rheumatology research remains largely unassessed, creating uncertainty about the sustainability of clinical developments in the field. Recent evidence indicates that early-career rheumatologists face specific challenges in becoming active in research, including inadequate support and resources. This, in turn, discourages research and the pursuit of new treatments, ultimately hindering progress in the field. Significantly increasing the size and sophistication of clinical trials in rheumatology is central to bridging these gaps and improving patient outcomes and treatment (Desjardins et al., 2010). In addition, application of new treatment regimens remains a challenge because disease mechanisms in rheumatology are elusive. For example, while advances have been made in understanding gastrointestinal dysmotility in SSc, the complex interactions between autoantibodies and their pathogenic roles remain to be translated into clear-cut treatments. Today, treatment strategies remain symptomatic relief and may not precisely rectify underlying mechanisms contributing to the disease. This limitation underscores the importance of sustained research aimed at developing targeted therapies that could alter disease course rather than merely relieve symptoms. By developing an interactive interface among clinicians and researchers, the field can move towards more effective interventions, ultimately improving the quality of treatment for patients with rheumatologic disorders (Abraham et al., 2017) (Figure 9.12).

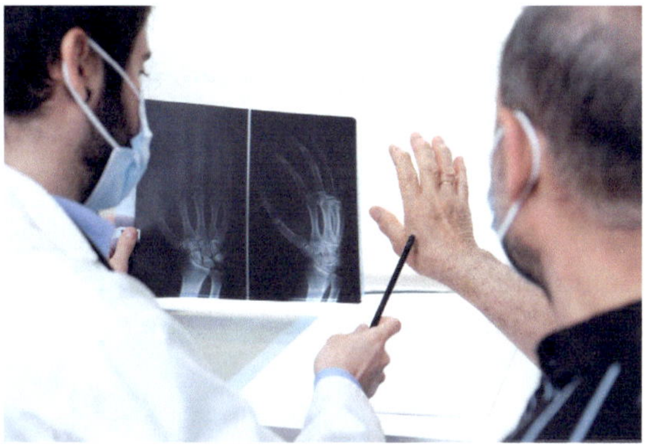

Figure 9.12. Challenges facing rheumatology.

Source: https://www.medicalindependent.ie/wp-content/uploads/2021/09/iStock-1315142723.jpg.

9.5.1. Diagnostic Challenges

The diagnostic challenge in rheumatological disease in internal medicine often stems from the overlapping manifestations and symptoms of several autoimmune conditions. Such diagnostic ambiguity is particularly significant in systemic sclerosis (SSc), with certain clinical manifestations, such as nailfold microangiopathy, potentially present years before characteristic symptoms. Nailfold videocapillaroscopy has also been a valuable tool in determining vascular damage associated with SSc. This technique allows clinicians to see peripheral capillary morphology, which can be highly informative in terms of the development of disease and treatment options. The ability to sort and score abnormality enables earlier detection of SSc, enabling timely intervention that can save patients in significant ways. Hence, despite the diagnostic challenges of SSc, the need to enhance the accuracy of diagnosis and patient care through advances in imaging modalities is imperative (Cutolo et al., 2016). Diagnostic challenges also arise in the detection of immune-mediated inner ear diseases associated with systemic autoimmune diseases. These illnesses can have indeterminate audiovestibular features, like sensorineural hearing loss, and are therefore more challenging to diagnose. The course is sudden, progressive, or fluctuating and can result in a misdiagnosis of primary inner ear disorders, such as Menière's disease. Patients can also exhibit a variety of associated symptoms, such as tinnitus and vestibular symptoms, further complicating the differential diagnosis. Knowledge of the mutual relationship between systemic autoimmune disorders and involvement of the inner ear is essential for proper diagnosis and management. The sensitivity of these diseases to corticosteroid treatment underscores the need for early identification and treatment, but the heterogeneity of clinical presentation and the lack of specific diagnostic methods pose significant obstacles (Adelchi et al., 2018). The convergence of clinical presentation and investigative methods gives evidence of the requirement for a multidisciplinary approach to rheumatological conditions. Since rheumatology involves a wide range of conditions with syndromic overlap, clinicians must rely on a series of clinical evaluations, high-resolution imaging modalities, and laboratory examinations to arrive at a definite diagnosis. This multidisciplinary approach not only enhances diagnostic accuracy but also ensures that treatments are individualized to the unique needs of patients. Furthermore, the use of novel diagnostic technologies will be paramount in mitigating the current burdens in rheumatology. By promoting collaboration among specialists, medical practitioners ensure that patients receive comprehensive care, which is crucial for managing the multifaceted nature of autoimmune disorders and their manifestations across various body systems. With ongoing research and clinical advancements, the future of rheumatological diagnosis appears promising, albeit not simple.

9.5.2. Treatment Adherence Issues

Compliance with treatment in patients with rheumatologic diseases, particularly rheumatoid arthritis (RA), is a significant challenge in treating such conditions. Compliance with DMARDs is crucial in optimizing treatment benefit and avoiding further disease progression. Nevertheless, multiple factors influence the level of adherence to the patient's drug regimen. Psychological barriers such as depression and anxiety, as well as ignorance about the advantages of medication, may result in non-compliance. Moreover, complexity in treatment regimens may leave patients uncertain, which in turn may lead to variation in medication use. Such multifaceted barriers must be overcome to improve patient outcomes and the efficacy of treatment strategies in rheumatology. The Compliance Questionnaire for Rheumatology (CQR), explicitly designed to measure treatment compliance among rheumatic patients, has enabled the examination of treatment compliance patterns. One limitation of the original CQR is its length, which may reduce patients' interest and response rates. To overcome this limitation, researchers have developed a shortened form of the instrument, the CQR5, which has been tested and validated. This five-point assessment effectively identifies patients who will adhere to their medication regimens, thereby allowing clinicians to earmark those at risk of non-adherence. The use of the CQR5 is more than mere identification; it adds value by providing insights into the factors driving compliance. Thus, the use of such specific measures in clinical practice can significantly enhance the management of compliance-related issues (Astorri et al., 2019; Done et al., 2013). Adherence determinants extend beyond patient-level characteristics to include social and environmental contexts. For instance, work status has been cited as a predictor of greater adherence, since working individuals may have a greater sense of responsibility to take better care of their health. Additionally, the treatment regimen, particularly the use of biologic DMARDs, has been shown to be associated with improved adherence outcomes. These findings suggest that medical practitioners should consider their patients' general life circumstances when addressing treatment compliance. Multidisciplinary approaches combining education, psychosocial interventions, and community resources can enhance compliance rates and eventually yield better clinical results. An integrative approach combining objective measurement and subjective patient report can serve as a basis for good internal medicine practice in rheumatology.

9.5.3. Access to Care and Health Disparities

The access and health disparities are stark in the backdrop of rheumatological disease, most importantly systemic lupus erythematosus (SLE). Research has revealed that SLE disproportionately affects people of color and the socioeconomically disadvantaged, which illustrates a central intersection of economic status, race, and health care access. For instance, in one retention in care study, 51% of Black SLE patients resided in the most deprived neighborhoods while only 5% of Whites did. This statistic illustrates how aspects of the neighborhood environment can determine health care involvement and, in the process, patient outcomes. Without targeted efforts to raise levels of engagement in care among these at-risk populations, such outcome differences in SLE will persist and even exacerbate, underscoring the necessity of immediate intervention to address health disparities in access and outcomes (Ahmad et al., 2020). Compounding these concerns is the failure to give sufficient attention to clinical research in rheumatology practice. Early-career rheumatologists' workforce and working conditions point to enormous research opportunities that are prevented from contributing to knowledge development and successful interventions. A lack of longitudinal studies of clinical research activity limits understanding of the specific needs and experiences of patients in rheumatology. Clearly, a more particular knowledge of the terrain of rheumatology research is required, strengthening the case for intervention to enhance the number and quality of clinical trials. In bridging these gaps, the field will be better able to respond to the complex realities of marginalized patients, and specifically those with rheumatologic disease, to maximize access to care and patient outcomes (Desjardins et al., 2010). Secondly, disparities in access to and treatment in rheumatology challenge the institutional machinery that sustains health care inequity. Insurance status, the geographical location of the care sites, and transportation availability are among the factors that affect patients' ability to maintain ongoing medical attention. Black patients and low socioeconomic communities are often subjected to various barriers that keep them away from access to specialists and services that are required. Hence, the pervasive occurrence of uncontrolled symptoms among such groups underscores the need for policies that promote greater access to rheumatological care. Such groups that mobilize for better health infrastructure and facilities can play a role in creating system-wide changes that lead to equal access to care in rheumatology and to an overall decrease in health disparities (Ahmad et al., 2020).

Test Your Knowledge

1. What challenges exist in the early diagnosis of rheumatological diseases?
2. How do treatment side effects complicate long-term management of rheumatic conditions?

9.6. Advances in Rheumatology

Learning Outcome

1. Discuss on innovations in treatment approaches in rheumatology
2. Define the research and clinical trials in rheumatology
3. Describe the future directions in rheumatology

Recent advances in rheumatology have brought about significant changes in research and clinical practice, particularly among early-career rheumatologists. The study of the current state of clinical inquiry reveals a compelling need to understand the number of new rheumatologists engaged in research. Findings indicate a critical gap in using investigative endeavors to refine treatment approaches and enhance patient outcomes. Research into how involved younger rheumatologists are has revealed that there is a need for an aggressive platform to promote and facilitate research activity. In addition to bolstering the practice clinically, it also encourages innovation. Such findings emphasize the importance of establishing a research-conducive climate and chart a course for further interventions aimed at stimulating clinical practice so that both current and emerging challenges in rheumatology are met effectively (Desjardins et al., 2009). Besides, psychological and behavioral factors in the management of chronic disease in rheumatology are becoming increasingly prominent. Particularly, the relationship between quality of life and joint pain is an essential concern in most rheumatic patients. Research concerning managing chronic pain indicates that interventions aimed at patients' psychological response to pain can enhance overall well-being. It is stated that patient self-management interventions can lead to a considerable reduction in pain intensity, thereby enhancing physical quality of life. For instance, improved pain acceptance and recognition of the difference between acute and chronic pain are essential variables that can empower patients. Patient-tailored self-management interventions can substantially improve how individuals manage their pain, promoting greater adherence to care and better psychological health outcomes. These results not only benefit patients with rheumatic diseases but also provide vital information that can shape care strategies across a wide range of chronic conditions (Acharya et al., 2014).

With the development of rheumatology as a science, there is a call for interdisciplinary collaboration for resolving the complexities involved in management and treatment. Advances in technology, including telemedicine and eHealth equipment, facilitate increased patient monitoring and care for patients with rheumatic conditions. The equipment allows the patient and healthcare team to communicate better, which leads to individualized and more effective care modalities.

Additionally, integrating behavioral science education into rheumatologists' medical school training can equip them with the skills to address the psychological aspects of chronic pain management and patient interaction. The juxtaposition of clinical research, psychological assessment, and technology marks a qualitative leap, promising to significantly improve patient outcomes. Consistent efforts must be made to sustain this momentum so that the potential of modern rheumatology is fully realized in clinical practice (Acharya et al., 2014; Desjardins et al., 2009) (Figure 9.13).

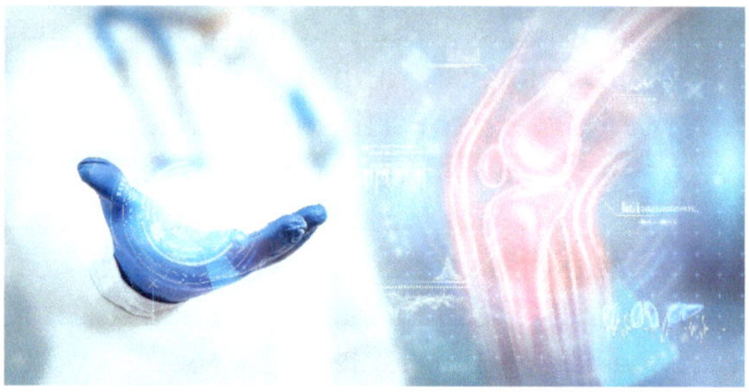

Figure 9.13. Advances in rheumatology.

Source: https://cpd.partners.org/sites/default/files/course/2023-04/Rheumatologist_shutterstock%20image.jpg.

9.6.1. Innovations in Treatment Approaches

The frontiers of rheumatology are increasingly being reshaped by treatment innovations, highlighting the promise of integrating laboratory discoveries with clinical application. With translational science in ascendance, it serves as the bridge between turning scientific discovery into practical treatments for rheumatologic patients. It is not merely a luxury of changing direction, but rather a matter of bridging so-called "translational gaps" and translating laboratory results into actual clinical application. By critically examining the paradigms surrounding translational research, particularly in rheumatology, stakeholders can more effectively identify the drivers and hindrances in this complex dynamic. This appreciation may enhance the effectiveness of treatment practices and ensure that the benefits of biomedical advances are transferred to those requiring novel care (Boenink et al., 2015). In examining the developments in treatment methods, the focus on personalized or targeted medicine has emerged as a cornerstone of innovation in rheumatology. Individualizing treatments to address the specific patient profile, including genetic, environmental, and lifestyle factors, enables improved management of chronic conditions such as lupus and rheumatoid arthritis. Research has shown that incorporating biomarkers and advanced diagnostic technologies into treatment approaches is highly promising for improving therapeutic outcomes. This shift towards personalization not only optimizes drug efficacy but also diminishes the likelihood of side effects, thereby increasing patient compliance with treatment regimens. Furthermore, by focusing on individual needs, rheumatologists can develop a more comprehensive system that enables patients to take a more active role in controlling their own health, ultimately leading to a higher quality of life (Desjardins et al., 2009). As the field of rheumatology advances, it is more essential than ever to invest in research methods that further advance clinical research. Early-career rheumatologists play a crucial role in this calculus because they must be proactive in investigative work to develop treatment modalities. Knowledge of the scope of clinical research and its bases by demographics among these practitioners can inform factors that allow or disallow innovation at practice. Studies aimed at developing a robust pipeline of research-oriented centers are key to providing both funding and mentorship opportunities for future clinicians. Such investment in holistic support not only prepares the next generation of rheumatologists but also improves the clinical practice of rheumatology through ongoing discovery and the translation of interventions to meet aligned patient needs (Desjardins et al., 2009).

9.6.2. Research and Clinical Trials

Clinical trials and research play a key role in advancing rheumatology within internal medicine, particularly by transforming approaches to treating musculoskeletal diseases. Rigorous protocols and the undertaking of clinical trials guarantee the efficacy and safety of new treatments, which is a priority given the complexity of rheumatic diseases. Also, applying research to practice not only enhances patient outcomes but also informs guidelines that establish standards of care. With each research endeavor carried out by rheumatologists, an expanding body of knowledge is created that facilitates evidence-based medicine and underlies the imperatives for ongoing inquiry in this specialty. Although research plays an important role in advancing rheumatology, the current situation reveals stark differences in the work conducted by investigators, especially among early-career rheumatologists. A majority of studies indicate that the scale of research involvement is not commensurate with the requirements of the rheumatic disorder-affected population of patients, something that requires serious notice. The determinants of this disparity, including institutional sponsorship and access to resources, are helpful in analyzing the problems facing early-career rheumatologists when it comes to conducting pertinent research. Overcoming such issues would enhance research activities, ultimately benefiting rheumatology as a whole and the quality of patient care. Analysis of the demographic setting and professional life of early-career rheumatologists is essential in understanding their involvement in clinical research. Current evidence shows that individual and institutional determinants influence engagement in investigative work, as does the importance of mentorship and access to resources. Early exposure to research can instill a more research-oriented mindset and reinforce interest in the discipline. Therefore, promoting programs that sponsor and reward research among rheumatologists would not only fill the gaps currently existing in clinical trials but also foster an environment of discovery and innovation in rheumatology, as outlined in more recent publications that document the necessity of remedial measures in the discipline as an imperative of immediacy (Desjardins et al., 2009, 2010).

9.6.3. Future Directions in Rheumatology

The promising field of rheumatology is on the cusp of great advancements, with a focus on incorporating personalized medicine principles. As science continues to advance, the relevance of individually tailored treatments based on patient profiles is more evident. Genetic, environmental, and immunological factors all play a role in variations in disease course and treatment response. For instance, data from genome-wide association studies (GWAS) could enhance understanding of RA susceptibility, enabling more effective personalized treatment approaches targeting underlying mechanisms. Moreover, employing cutting-edge technologies such as artificial intelligence and machine learning could enable the identification of patient-specific biomarkers, thereby easing the prediction of disease trajectory and therapeutic outcome. These innovations have the potential to enhance therapeutic efficacy while diminishing adverse effects, and they are likely to transform patient management in rheumatology. This tailored approach represents a new era of precision medicine that will potentially improve patients' quality of life. The integration of telemedicine and digital health technologies is also a notable future trend for rheumatology. Equipment such as mobile health apps and remote monitoring devices allows clinicians to monitor patient progress and treatment compliance more efficiently than ever. Not only do these technologies enable timely interventions, but they also empower patients by making their health information accessible, thereby promoting active engagement in self-management. Evidence shows that telemedicine can bridge the care gap faced by patients in rural areas and underserved communities, enabling uniform access to care. Again, evidence from studies implementing telemedicine in routine practice shows that patient outcomes, such as medication management and maintenance of disease control, can be significantly enhanced. By adopting these new solutions, rheumatology can enhance the overall quality of patient care while addressing longstanding healthcare inequalities in this field. Another very critical future path for rheumatology is a multidisciplinary management strategy, required by the intricate nature of rheumatic conditions. The cross-over between rheumatology and other clinical medicine disciplines—such as immunology, orthopedics, and physical therapy—nurtures an integrated approach to patient management. It is not only advantageous to clinical outcomes but also to comorbidities that are frequent in association with rheumatic disease, such as cardiovascular comorbidities and metabolic syndrome. Finally, ongoing education and interprofessional practice among health clinicians are essential to ensure that all clinicians are aware of the latest evidence-based guidelines and treatment protocols. Enhanced cross-disciplinary communication can result in the unification of a model of care that fosters patient-focused treatment addressing all aspects of health. As rheumatology evolves, the standard approach will enhance patients' quality of life, aligning with the universal goal of integrated care in internal medicine for rheumatology (Bashinskaya et al., 2016; Talele et al., 2024).

Test Your Knowledge

1. What recent advancements have improved the treatment of rheumatological diseases?
2. How have biologic therapies transformed the management of inflammatory arthritis?

SUMMARY

In attempting to summarize the complex relationship between internal medicine and rheumatology, it is evident that an extensive understanding of rheumatic disorders is crucial to ensuring effective patient care. The diseases have complex symptoms that need multidisciplinary management. Internal medicine specialists must stay up to date with the latest science and optimal rheumatology practice to effectively manage these conditions. This integration of practice not only enhances the doctor's ability to treat and diagnose but also improves patient outcomes by offering organized care. Adopting this integrated view eliminates the boundaries that normally segregate specialties, enabling a more robust healthcare system that is better suited to patients with rheumatic diseases. The evaluation of approaches in rheumatology is intended to highlight the need for research and data analysis to guide practice. Utilization of large electronic datasets, as seen in existing research, allows for greater understanding of disease prevalence and the effectiveness of treatments. Such datasets help illustrate where the healthcare system may collapse, providing the details needed to guide improvements in patient management. For instance, concordance analysis of health records attests to the importance of accurate data recording, which can drive the initiative to maximize the quality of information derived from various sources. Such research is pivotal in identifying discrepancies between treatment approaches and outcomes and can equip clinicians with authentic data that directly impacts their clinical decisions (Beral et al., 2013). Lastly, the nature of the workforce and workplace dynamics in rheumatology reveal a compelling need to further invest in research and education in the specialty. With new knowledge still emerging, albeit slowly, regarding the complexity of rheumatic disease, the professional community must ensure that it advocates for adequate training and resources to enable practitioners to stay abreast of evidence-based practice. It is crucial to understand the scope of clinical research and the challenges faced by rheumatology professionals to promote effective treatments and patient care. By addressing the knowledge gaps created by recent studies, such as deficiencies in the current research climate, stakeholders can better prepare rheumatologists to address the evolving needs of their patients. This initiative not only improves the practice of rheumatology but ultimately improves the quality of care delivered to patients afflicted with these chronic conditions (Desjardins et al., 2010).

In internal medicine and rheumatology, a critical component is the assessment of health-related quality of life (HRQoL) in patients with chronic illnesses such as rheumatoid arthritis (RA). The inclusion of HRQoL assessment in clinical practice has been proposed as a means to enhance patient care by improving psychosocial problem detection and evidence-based decision-making. However, studies show that although clinicians prefer the kind of information provided by such assessments, the effects on clinical outcomes are minimal. Studies have shown that the consistent feedback from HRQoL instruments does not directly alter the identification of mental disorders or improve overall psychosocial functioning in nonpsychiatric environments. Consequently, despite putatively helpful uses for such instruments, their application is called into question based on unspecified benefits and expenses (Gilbody et al., 2002). In addition, the understanding of musculoskeletal trauma, in particular in the case of rheumatoid arthritis, has been enhanced through the application of advanced technologies such as cadaver models. In a study exploring the application of such a technique, it was demonstrated that cadaver models could effectively simulate patterns of tendon damage typical of RA. In the survey analyzing tendon integrity, experts used ultrasonography (US) to assess surgically induced trauma in cadaver specimens. The findings had great concordance with US imaging and the actual tendinous lesions, thereby validating this imaging modality's effectiveness. In addition, intra- and interobserver reliability were extremely high, underscoring the robustness of US as a tool for tracking tendon injury in RA. Such advances in imaging modalities are significant milestones towards the efficient treatment of rheumatological conditions (Iagnocco et al., 2016). Lastly, ongoing innovation in assessment techniques and diagnostic tools remains key to enhanced care for rheumatology. The integration of high-quality HRQoL evaluation with advanced imaging technologies, such as ultrasonography, can offer improved insight into patient experience and treatment outcomes. The potential enhancement of clinical decision-making via these tools cannot be overstated, even amid debates over their usability and efficiency. By utilizing evidence-based methods, clinical practitioners can enhance not only the physical but also the psychosocial components of treatment, ultimately improving overall quality of life for patients with chronic rheumatological disease. Such ongoing evaluation of efficacy for these approaches will be critical for guiding future clinical treatments in rheumatology (Gilbody et al., 2002; Iagnocco et al., 2016).

KEY TERMS FROM THIS CHAPTER

- Rheumatoid Arthritis
- Systemic Lupus Erythematosus (SLE)
- Gout
- Vasculitis
- Synovitis
- Biologic Therapy
- Antinuclear Antibodies (ANA)
- C-Reactive Protein (CRP)
- Osteoarthritis
- Ankylosing Spondylitis
- Fibromyalgia
- Autoimmune Disease
- Joint Inflammation
- Disease-Modifying Antirheumatic Drugs
- Erythrocyte Sedimentation Rate (ESR)

CRITICAL THINKING QUESTIONS

1. **Which of the following is the most specific antibody for systemic lupus erythematosus (SLE)?**
   a. ANA (Antinuclear antibody)
   b. Anti-dsDNA
   c. Anti-Ro (SSA)
   d. Rheumatoid factor
2. **A 55-year-old woman has joint pain, dry mouth, and dry eyes. What is the most likely diagnosis?**
   a. Rheumatoid arthritis
   b. Sjögren's syndrome
   c. SLE
   d. Polymyalgia rheumatica
3. **Which of the following HLA alleles is strongly associated with ankylosing spondylitis?**
   a. HLA-DR4
   b. HLA-B27
   c. HLA-A2
   d. HLA-DR3
4. **Morning stiffness lasting more than 1 hour and symmetric joint involvement is most characteristic of:**
   a. Osteoarthritis
   b. Gout
   c. Rheumatoid arthritis
   d. Psoriatic arthritis
5. **Which of the following findings is most characteristic of gout on joint aspiration?**
   a. Positively birefringent crystals
   b. Negatively birefringent needle-shaped crystals
   c. Rhomboid-shaped calcium crystals
   d. Cloudy synovial fluid with low WBC

Short Answer Questions

1. What is rheumatoid arthritis?
2. What is osteoarthritis?
3. Which imaging modalities are most sensitive for early detection of joint erosion in rheumatoid arthritis (RA)?
4. What is the best treatment for rheumatology?
5. Describe the role of the rheumatologist.

Answers to Critical Thinking Questions

1. (b); 2. (b) ; 3. (b); 4. (c); 5. (b)

REFERENCES

1. Kumar, S., Singh, J., Rattan, S., DiMarino, A. J., Cohen, S., & Jimenez, S. A. (2017). Review article: pathogenesis and clinical manifestations of gastrointestinal involvement in systemic sclerosis. *Alimentary Pharmacology & Therapeutics*, *45*(7), 883–898. https://doi.org/10.1111/apt.13963Acharya, D., Barlow, J., Barry, A., Buhrman, B., Buzzard, C., Cour, P., Eckman, E., et al. (2014). A review of evidence about behavioral and psychological aspects of chronic joint pain among people with hemophilia. https://core.ac.uk/download/46171148.pdf (accessed on 16th July 2025).
2. Adams, J., Bakkers, M., Balážová, P., Baxter, D., et al. (2020). Prevention and management of osteoporotic fractures by non-physician health professionals: A systematic literature review to inform EULAR points to consider. https://core.ac.uk/download/322918822.pdf (accessed on 16th July 2025).
3. Adelchi, A., Croce, A., D'Aguanno, V., De Vincentiis, M., De Virgilio, A., et al. (2018). Audio-vestibular symptoms in systemic autoimmune diseases. https://core.ac.uk/download/188823057.pdf (accessed on 16th July 2025).
4. Ahmad, U., Bartels, C. M., Chang, I., Ezeh, N., et al. (2020). Investigating lupus retention in care to inform interventions for disparities reduction: An observational cohort study. https://core.ac.uk/download/288432759.pdf (accessed on 16th July 2025).
5. Alexander, R. V., Arriens, C., Collins, C. E., Dervieux, T., et al. (2020). Complement activation in patients with probable systemic lupus erythematosus and ability to predict progression to American College of Rheumatology-classified systemic lupus erythematosus. https://core.ac.uk/download/323065797.pdf (accessed on 16th July 2025).
6. Assar, M. F. A., Abd El Gayed, E. M., Ewis, A. S. A. E., Zaid, A. B., & Fouda, E. A. A. M. (2024). Biochemical study of ZNF76 rs10947540 and SCUBE3 rs1888822 single nucleotide polymorphisms in the Egyptian patients with systemic lupus erythematosus. Journal of Immunoassay and Immunochemistry, 45, 415–431. https://www.semanticscholar.org/paper/9b70e6df1f0de73c1883492c857713727061c405 (accessed on 16th July 2025).
7. Assassi, S., Fischbach, M., GENISOS Study Group, Gonzalez, E. B., et al. (2011). Predictors of fatigue severity in early systemic sclerosis: A prospective longitudinal study of the GENISOS cohort. https://core.ac.uk/download/323073807.pdf (accessed on 16th July 2025).
8. Astorri, D., Azzolina, D., Botsios, C., Done, L., et al. (2019). Adherence in rheumatoid arthritis patients assessed with a validated Italian version of the 5-item compliance questionnaire for rheumatology. https://core.ac.uk/download/287601309.pdf (accessed on 16th July 2025).
9. Atzeni, F., Bazzichi, L., Casale, R., Di Franco, M., et al. (2015). Pain in systemic connective tissue diseases. https://core.ac.uk/download/54524187.pdf (accessed on 16th July 2025).
10. Bagnall, A., Day, R., & Kime, N. H. (2013). *Systematic Review of Transition Models for Young People with Long-Term Conditions: A report for NHS Diabetes*. https://core.ac.uk/download/29018738.pdf (accessed on 16th July 2025).
11. Bashinskaya, B. (2016). *Effects of Obesity on Walking Patterns and Adaptability During Obstacle Crossing*. https://open.bu.edu/bitstream/2144/16125/1/Bashinskaya_bu_0017N_11114.pdf (accessed on 16th July 2025).

12. Beral, V., Berkel, J., Bullard, J., Coleman, M., Gulliford, M., Møller, H., Phekoo, K., et al. (2013). Cancer recording and mortality in the General Practice Research Database and linked cancer registries.

13. Boenink, M., & van der Laan, A. L. (2015). Beyond bench and bedside: Disentangling the concept of translational research. https://core.ac.uk/download/pdf/11486878.pdf (accessed on 16th July 2025).

14. Borg, A. A., Camilleri, L., & Magro, R. (2017). Translation and validation of the Fatigue Severity Scale, Pittsburgh Sleep Quality Index and Modified Health Assessment Questionnaire into the Maltese language, in a cohort of Maltese systemic lupus erythematosus patients. https://core.ac.uk/download/322748488.pdf (accessed on 16th July 2025).

15. Cartron, A. M., Chung, C., Osler, M., Trinidad, A., et al. (2020). Nuclear matrix protein 2 antibody-positive adult dermatomyositis: A case report and review of the literature. https://core.ac.uk/download/322493868.pdf (accessed on 16th July 2025).

16. Cutolo, M., Llado, A., Paolino, S., Pizzorni, C., et al. (2016). Capillaroscopy in 2016: New perspectives in systemic sclerosis. https://core.ac.uk/download/74613576.pdf (accessed on 16th July 2025).

17. Desjardins, C., Ehrenberg, R. G., & St. Clair, E. W. (2009). The scope and scale of clinical research accomplished by rheumatologists early in their careers. https://core.ac.uk/download/5131729.pdf (accessed on 16th July 2025).

18. Desjardins, C., Ehrenberg, R. G., & St. Clair, E. W. (2010). Analysis of the workforce and workplace for rheumatology, and the research activities of rheumatologists early in their careers. https://core.ac.uk/download/5131730.pdf (accessed on 16th July 2025).

19. Done, D. J., Hughes, L. D., & Young, A. (2013). A 5-item version of the Compliance Questionnaire for Rheumatology (CQR5) successfully identifies low adherence to DMARDs. https://core.ac.uk/download/29840355.pdf (accessed on 16th July 2025).

20. Faarvang, K. L., & Pereira da Silva, J. A. (2009). Competencies in rheumatology: A European framework. https://core.ac.uk/download/61494866.pdf (accessed on 16th July 2025).

21. Funk, J., Gay, S., Müller-Ladner, U., Straub, R. H., et al. (2017). Molecular imaging: Novel tools in visualizing rheumatoid arthritis. https://core.ac.uk/download/85212391.pdf (accessed on 16th July 2025).

22. Gensichen, J., Joos, S., Körner, T., Muth, C., et al. (2005). Rationale, design and conduct of a comprehensive evaluation of a primary care-based intervention to improve the quality of life of osteoarthritis patients. The PraxArt-project: A cluster randomized controlled trial [ISRCTN87252339]; study protocol. https://core.ac.uk/download/14504006.pdf (accessed on 16th July 2025).

23. Gilbody, S. M., House, A. O., & Sheldon, T. (2002). Routine administration of health-related quality of life (HRQoL) and needs assessment instruments to improve psychological outcome: A systematic review. https://core.ac.uk/download/57460.pdf (accessed on 16th July 2025).

24. Grange, S. (2011). Current Issues and Regulations in Tendon Regeneration and Musculoskeletal Repair with Mesenchymal Stem Cells.

25. Hannech, E., Boussetta, N., Guediche, N., Arfaoui, B., Ajili, F., Abdelhafidh, N., Sayhi, S., et al. (2021). P047 Musculoskeletal symptoms as first clinical presentation of juvenile-onset systemic

lupus erythematosus: Experience from a military internal medicine department. Rheumatology. https://www.semanticscholar.org/paper/e6f89bedfd02c3e2336d90402a7d28b090f486f1 (accessed on 16th July 2025).

26. Harmsen, E. J., Lyddiatt, A., Oostveen, J. C. M., Oostveen, A. C., et al. (2012). Translation and validation of the Dutch version of the Effective Consumer Scale (EC-17). https://core.ac.uk/download/pdf/11485631.pdf (accessed on 16th July 2025).

27. Iagnocco, A., Jain, A., Premkumar, A., Iagnocco, A., Fornage, B. D., Martinoli, C., Bong, D., et al. (2016). How does a cadaver model work for testing ultrasound diagnostic capability for rheumatic-like tendon damage? https://core.ac.uk/download/74318646.pdf (accessed on 16th July 2025).

28. Jalali, K., & Mandl, L. A. (2024). Rheumatology: What you may have missed in 2023. Annals of Internal Medicine, 177, S82–S90. https://doi.org/10.7326/m24-0678 (accessed on 16th July 2025).

29. Koreli, U. Y., Torun, E., & Adas, M. (2025). Role of positron emission tomography-computed tomography scan in reaching definite diagnosis in patients with fever of unknown origin and inflammation of unknown origin in rheumatology outpatient clinic. *Open Access Rheumatology: Research and Reviews, 17*, 25–32. https://www.semanticscholar.org/paper/431fc87e961b019cc941e0f44b05cf800627d6b0 (accessed on 16th July 2025).

30. Lehtsaar, T., & Meel, L. (2017). Interdisciplinary team-based pastoral care: A potentially adaptable model for Estonian healthcare. https://digitalcommons.georgefox.edu/cgi/viewcontent.cgi?article=2019&context=ree (accessed on 16th July 2025).

31. McBain, H. B., Newman, S. P., & Shipley, M. (2018). Clinician and patients' views about self-management support in arthritis: A cross-sectional UK survey. https://core.ac.uk/download/146487163.pdf (accessed on 16th July 2025).

32. Mendes, C. E. E., Chimeli, D., Albuquerque, M., Ferreira, T., Carvalho, S., Ribeiro, C. A., & Gomes, S. A. A. (2024). Implementation of a palliative care service in a tertiary hospital in a developing country: Methods, strategies and results. *Journal of Clinical Oncology*. https://www.semanticscholar.org/paper/f795099ed5035bda573fdd7cf3b4d063f3b7ba99 (accessed on 16th July 2025).

33. Millar, N. L., & Murrell, G. A. C. (2012). Heat shock proteins in tendinopathy: Novel molecular regulators. https://core.ac.uk/download/9651505.pdf (accessed on 16th July 2025).

34. Mohannad, N., Moaaz, M., & Shehata, R. M. (2021). AB0345 Th9 cells and their associated cytokines: The probable players in systemic lupus erythematosus (SLE) and type 1 diabetes mellitus (T1DM). Annals of the Rheumatic Diseases, 80. https://www.semanticscholar.org/paper/d55254e0f8f2c17790e8de66944e9e6c608cf39a (accessed on 16th July 2025).

35. Mustafa, M. H., Tony, E., Elgendi, S., Abdelkader, A. S., Salah, A. A., & Madkour, R. A. (2024). Urinary tissue factor (uTF), tissue factor pathway inhibitor (TFPI) and plasmin as novel biomarkers in early diagnosis of lupus nephritis. The Egyptian Journal of Immunology, 31(1), 143–154. https://www.semanticscholar.org/paper/cec4ea0fcab92e961381744bb4c9cdbe4eb96a91 (accessed on 16th July 2025).

36. N/A. (2025). Assessment of the Australian Rheumatology Association Database for National Population Health Monitoring: Working paper. https://core.ac.uk/download/pdf/30673534.pdf (accessed on 16th July 2025).

37. Sankoh, M. A., Bangura, B. C. Y., Jalloh, M. J., Pambu, D. M., Turay, M. L., & Koroma, J. D. (2024). Challenges and opportunities in combating infectious diseases in Sierra Leone: A narrative review of the role of community health and internal medicine. International Journal of Research and Scientific Innovation. https://www.semanticscholar.org/paper/083973968f8ff8dfc76c0415305acec1b14ff367 (accessed on 16th July 2025).

38. Sedighi, S., Aghaei, M., Musavi, S., Nomali, A., et al. (2014). Relationship between serum level of interleukin-2 in patients with systemic lupus erythematosus and disease activity in comparison with control group. https://core.ac.uk/download/52204560.pdf (accessed on 16th July 2025).

39. Shumway-Cook, A., Shumway-Cook, A., Qutubuddin, A. A., Newstead, A. H., Leddy, A. L., Leddy, A. L., Bayer, A., et al. (2015). Recommendations for a core outcome set for measuring standing balance in adult populations: A consensus-based approach. https://core.ac.uk/download/293879326.pdf (accessed on 16th July 2025).

40. Song, S. Y., Han, H. Y., Park, S. Y., Kim, J., Park, K. M., & Kyong, T. (2024). Current status of hospitalist practice and factors influencing job satisfaction in Korea. Journal of General Internal Medicine, 40, 302–308. https://www.semanticscholar.org/paper/98ee83f8b7dd6ba2579879c29d8144b438e14694 (accessed on 16th July 2025).

41. Talele, C., Gohil, D., Kumari, M., Shah, N., & Sadhu, P. (2024). Comprehensive review of rheumatoid arthritis: Insights, challenges, and prospects. https://core.ac.uk/download/603897628.pdf (accessed on 16th July 2025).

42. Williamson, P., Altman, D. G., Bagley, H., Barnes, K. L., Blazeby, J., Brookes, S., Clarke, M., et al. (2017). The COMET Handbook: Version 1.0. Trials, 18. https://doi.org/10.1186/s13063-017-1978-4 (accessed on 16th July 2025).

NEUROLOGY (MEDICAL)

10

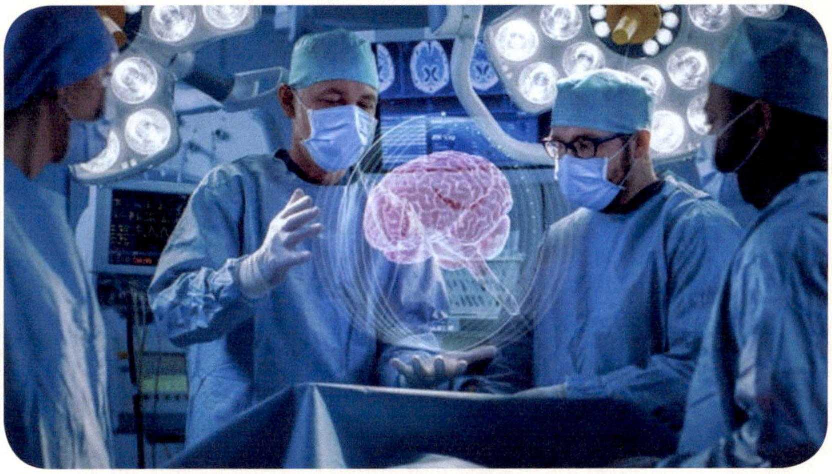

LEARNING OBJECTIVES

After studying this chapter, you will be able to:

1. Describe the anatomy of the nervous system
2. Describe the common neurological disorders
3. Understand the diagnostic techniques in neurology
4. Know the treatment approaches in neurology
5. Understand the role of neurologists
6. Describe the advances in neurological research

Introduction

Neurology is a branch of medicine that specializes in the diagnosis and treatment of conditions affecting the nervous system. This system consists of a vast network of the brain, spinal cord, and peripheral nerves, all of which play crucial roles in regulating body functions and facilitating communication within the body. Understanding the intricate workings of the nervous system is not just critical to the identification of a variety of neurological disorders, such as epilepsy, Parkinson's disease, and multiple sclerosis, but also for developing effective treatment protocols. Beyond that, advances in neurological science have underscored the importance of integrating neuropsychological understanding into patient care, particularly as clinical practice increasingly becomes multidisciplinary. By promoting a holistic understanding of neurological conditions, clinicians can deliver more comprehensive care, addressing the physical and psychological dimensions of patient well-being. The impact of environmental factors on neurological health warrants extensive research. The COVID-19 pandemic, for instance, has drastically altered the landscape of cognitive and mental health, creating a wave of anxiety, depression, and post-traumatic stress in vulnerable groups, including healthcare workers and children. These observations underscore the relevance of psychological health to neurology and demonstrate how sociocultural factors can influence the clinical presentation of neurological illness. In this context, technological developments in telepsychology and remote healthcare become pivotal, enabling practitioners to reach patients and provide care even with physical distancing. Such technological advancements point to the necessity for neurology to revamp in response to the challenges of the modern era, while continuing to maintain an educated perspective on mental health and its significance in neurologic disease management (Saladino et al., 2020). With the onset of wearable medical devices, the future of neurology appears increasingly intertwined with technology-driven healthcare interventions.

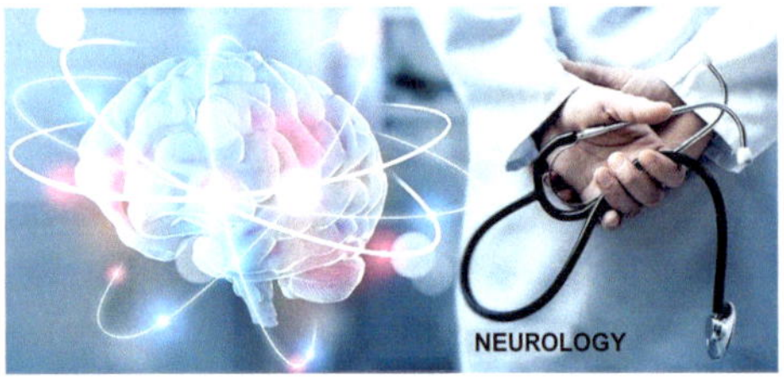

Figure 10.1. Neurology.

Source: https://careandcurehospital.co.in/wp-content/uploads/2022/02/neurology-manu-hospital.jpg.

These sensors enable continuous, real-time monitoring of physiological metrics, providing a rich pool of information for real-time clinical decision-making. This integration not only aids in the management of chronic conditions but also facilitates diagnostic processes and rehabilitation interventions for patients convalescing from neurological events, e.g., strokes. As this technology matures, the profession must address the current shortcomings in terms of user accessibility and issues regarding privacy. With these advancements, neurologists can optimize patient care and design individually tailored treatment protocols that meet patients' needs, with the long-term aim of transforming the clinical practice of neurology for decades to come (Lu et al., 2020) (Figure 10.1).

Definition and Scope of Neurology

Neurology, as a medical discipline, is the investigation and treatment of disorders of the nervous system, including the brain, spinal cord, and peripheral nerves. Not only does its definition hinge on the understanding of neurological disease, but it also extends to the physiological and structural mechanisms that produce the conditions. Neurologists deal with an enormous variety of disorders, varying from frequent conditions like migraines and epilepsy to more complicated diseases like multiple sclerosis and Parkinson's disease. In line with developmental knowledge of the nervous system, so too is the scope of neurology, requiring medical professionals to keep up to date with new research and treatments. One significant aspect of this specialty is not just diagnosis and treatment but also ongoing care to educate and rehabilitate the patient, highlighting the crucial role neurologists play in improving patients' quality of life. The field of neurology has expanded significantly over the years due to advances in technology and increased neurobiological knowledge. Neurologists frequently work with other medical specialists to provide a full spectrum of care, drawing on psychiatry, neurosurgery, and rehabilitation medicine. This interprofessional model is critical, given that many of the neurological conditions overlap with mental illnesses, requiring a treatment strategy that considers both neurological and psychological domains. Present developments, such as the development of the Neurohospitalist Core Competencies, aim to harmonize care across environments and ensure that trainees and practicing clinicians alike possess the knowledge needed to treat complex neuro cases (Gold et al., 2024). As neurology continues to grow and evolve, it is all the more crucial to define and refine its scope in response to emerging challenges and advancing technology. Moreover, the integration of innovative technologies into neurologic practice is essential for advancing diagnostic and treatment strategies.

Telemedicine and artificial intelligence, for instance, transform patient interactions through timely interventions and improved management of neurological disease. Notably, advances in communication technologies, particularly the introduction of 5G, have enhanced coordination of emergency medical services, which are critical for situations requiring immediate neurological assessment and intervention (Association Professional Committee Of Emergency Resuscitation et al., 2024). Improved development of these technologies will expand the scope of neurology to incorporate new solutions that meet patients' needs while preserving best practices. The commitment to continuous learning and adaptation in the vocation keeps neurologists one step ahead of medical science, thus addressing the complexities of the human nervous system (Figure 10.2).

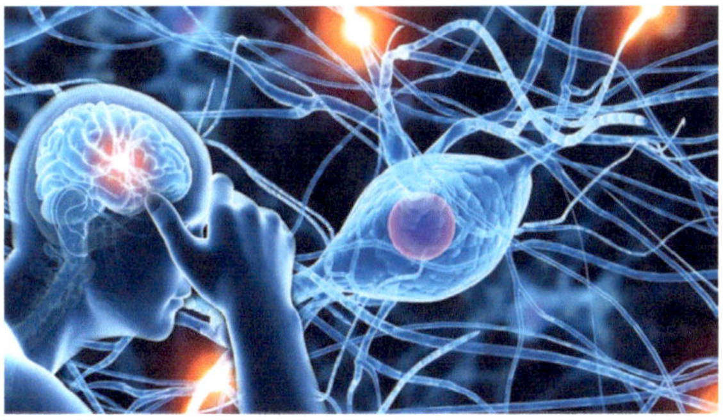

Figure 10.2. Definition of neurology.

Source: https://apollosage.in/assets/upload/blog/1695378468-blog.webp.

Importance of Studying the Nervous System

Learning about the nervous system is of utmost importance in the medical profession, as it forms the foundation for understanding human health and disease. Neurological illnesses are the leading causes of morbidity and mortality globally, with millions of patients suffering from these illnesses every year. As the nervous system regulates vital functions such as movement, cognition, and sensation, any disorder can lead to serious health consequences. As per recent studies, a high proportion of deaths and disability-adjusted life years (DALYs) results from neurological disorders, emphasizing the need for intensified research and education on medicine. An understanding of the complexities of the nervous system can allow for the development of targeted treatments and intervention methods that improve patients' quality of life and overall health outcomes (Murray et al., 2022)]. Apart from that, developments in neurobiological science are increasingly revealing intricate interactions between the nervous system and various physiological phenomena. The integration of knowledge from neurology with other medical disciplines, such as immunology, endocrinology, and gastroenterology, can provide deeper insight into comorbidities and the multicausality of disease. For instance, recent bibliometric analyses illustrate that studies in neurology are frequently published in high-impact general medicine journals, highlighting their universality across medical specialties (Wilson et al., 2021). This interdisciplinarity can lead to novel treatment approaches that consider not only the neurological aspects of disease but also its systemic implications, fostering a holistic understanding of patient care. Apart from the clinical and research importance, studying the nervous system is crucial to inform individuals about mental health and neuropsychiatric disorder pathophysiology. Depression, anxiety, and schizophrenia are increasingly rooted in neurobiological dysfunction and have extensive repercussions on individuals and society at large. By providing up-to-date knowledge of the nervous system to health professionals, we are better positioned to tackle the rising incidence of such disorders and facilitate integrated mental health services. The emergence of this topic is also underscored by the need to bring mental health issues into both health care and public policy discussions to ensure that neurological well-being receives the attention it deserves within the broader context of medical research and practice (Wilson et al., 2021).

Overview of Neurological Disorders

Neurological disorders encompass a broad range of conditions affecting the brain, spinal cord, and nerves. These conditions exert a severe influence on motor function, cognition, and emotional regulation, with the generation of a range of crippling symptoms that undermine the quality of life. The most prevalent neurological diseases are stroke, Alzheimer's disease, and traumatic brain injury. These conditions have some pathophysiological issues, each requiring dysfunction at more than one level of neuronal activity. For example, stroke produces acute cerebral ischemia, which leads to neuronal death and functional disruption. Alzheimer's disease, in contrast, is characterized by the insidious deposition of amyloid plaques and tau tangles that disrupt neuronal transmission and produce intellectual impairments. In general, these diseases add evidence to the intricate interactions among genetic, environmental, and lifestyle determinants of their development and course. Neurological research has increasingly focused on understanding the mechanisms behind neurological disorders and treating them. Advances in molecular biology revealed standard pathological mechanisms of disease, such as oxidative stress, neuroinflammation, and mitochondrial impairment. Interestingly, evidence suggests that the nuclear factor erythroid 2-related factor 2 (Nrf2) signaling pathway plays a significant role in modulating cellular stress responses. Increased Nrf2 expression has emerged as a promising therapeutic target, and the potential of new treatment strategies is being explored. Current studies on natural compounds, such as quercetin, show their neuroprotective action, and future alternatives for the management of neurological disorders are implied. Effective treatment strategies are needed to , address the rising incidence of these disorders, and improve patient outcomes (Zamanian et al., 2023). In addition to the common neurological diseases, recent evidence has also revealed the severe neurological consequences of post-viral syndromes, particularly following the COVID-19 pandemic. Survivors of COVID-19 have had a series of prolonged neurological symptoms, which have been referred to as long-COVID. These latter ones are presentations in the form of cognitive impairment, fatigue, and sensory disturbances, which necessitate a clear understanding of the brain's response to viral infection.

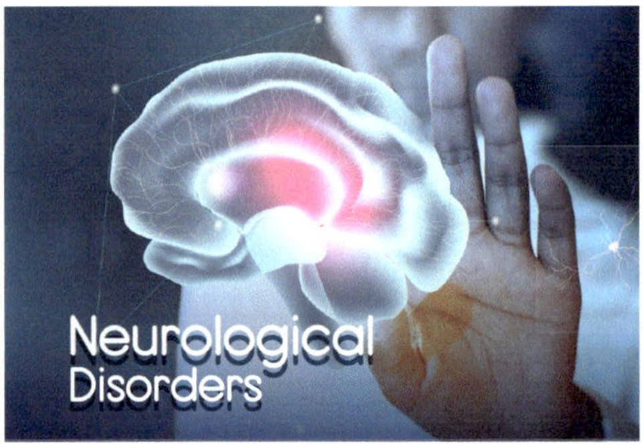

Figure 10.3. Neurological disorders.

Source: https://www.outsourcestrategies.com/wp-content/uploads/2023/07/five-common-neurological-disorders.jpg.

Current evidence suggests that neuroinflammatory mechanisms may underlie the neurological sequelae of long-COVID; therefore, more research into therapeutic strategies is required. Meanwhile, as the medical community works to address these complex problems, it is critical that meticulous diagnostic and treatment regimens be developed and adopted to assist in addressing the complexity of neurological disorders and their dynamic evolution (Maria-Stefanou et al., 2022) (Figure 10.3).

10.1. Anatomy of the Nervous System

Learning Outcome

1. Describe the central nervous system (CNS)
2. Define the peripheral nervous system (PNS)
3. Discuss the functional divisions of the nervous system

The nervous system, a highly developed system governing body functions, consists of the central nervous system (CNS) and the peripheral nervous system (PNS). The CNS, which consists of the brain and spinal cord, is the primary center for processing sensory information and coordinating responses. The various structures of the brain, such as the cerebrum, cerebellum, and brainstem, regulate functions ranging from voluntary movement to control functions like heartbeat and breathing. The spinal cord is a channel for nerve impulses between the brain and other parts of the body, enabling reflex action and voluntary movement. Such dynamic structuring is important for maintaining homeostasis and facilitating the complex interactions in the human body necessary for survival. The PNS extends the nervous system beyond the CNS, being composed of nerves that reach other parts of the body. It is categorized into the somatic and autonomic nervous systems that manage voluntary and involuntary actions, respectively. The somatic nervous system regulates activities, such as muscle movements and sensations, while the autonomic nervous system regulates involuntary actions, such as digestion and cardiopulmonary functions. Its subdivision into the sympathetic and parasympathetic systems regulates the body's response to stress and relaxation. It is essential to understand these subdivisions in the diagnosis and treatment of neurological disorders, as disruption of the PNS can lead to severe dysfunction, impairing an individual's quality of life. Neurological diseases are often triggered by traumatic injury, genetic predisposition, or environmental influences. Because the nervous system's anatomical structure is interconnected, interruptions can lead to complex symptoms.

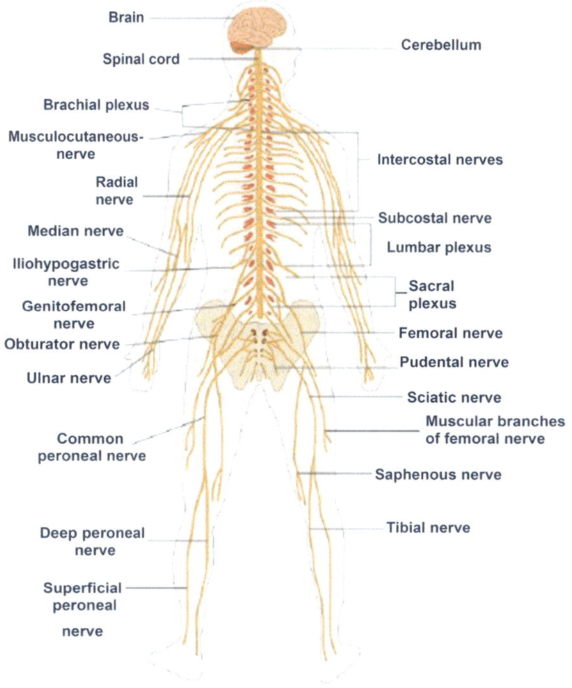

Figure 10.4. The human nervous system.

Source: https://upload.wikimedia.org/wikipedia/commons/b/b2/TE-Nervous_system_diagram.svg.

For example, neurogenic erectile dysfunction (ED), which was identified in a sample of 37 male patients with existing neurological disorders, highlights the importance of studying the nervous system's function in overall well-being. The condition, which appears in a significant percentage of patients with neurological disorders, highlights the necessity for neurologists and specialists related to the field to address sexual health, thereby addressing an essential aspect of patients' well-being. The findings suggest that a thorough appreciation of the nervous system's anatomy is critical to interventions and improved patient outcomes in neurological practice (Kirilenko et al., 2025). With the progress of contemporary medicine, integrating time-tested wisdom, such as Ayurvedic principles—specifically the effects of doshas, such as Vata—can create an integrated approach to treating neurological disorders (Sharma et al., 2024) (Figure 10.4).

10.1.1. Central Nervous System (CNS)

The CNS, comprising the brain and spinal cord, is a highly developed network that processes sensory information, coordinates motor activity, and supports cognitive functions. Through an extensive network of neurons and glial cells, this complex system maintains homeostasis within the body. Normal CNS functioning is required for integrating various body systems so that an organism can respond to internal and external stimuli. With advances in understanding CNS physiology, scientists have now begun to investigate cellular and molecular mechanisms underlying brain health and the effects of injury and disease on its functioning, e.g., intracranial hemorrhage (ICH) (Li et al., 2025). Recent findings have highlighted the involvement of the glymphatic system in CNS health, particularly following injury. The glymphatic pathway plays a role in brain waste clearancesuch that , enabling the removal of toxic metabolites accumulated due to various neurological diseases. For example, the evolution of hematomas following ICH may lead to secondary injury to the brain with accumulation of perihematomal edema and toxic metabolites. Research has shown that exosomes from reactive astrocytes can enhance recovery of the glymphatic system by suppressing toxic protein aggregation and neuronal apoptosis, thereby maintaining cognitive and motor function in patients with the condition (Li et al., 2025). This information underscores the importance of therapeutic interventions targeting the glymphatic clearance system to minimize damage and promote recovery after CNS injury. Further, the crosstalk between viral infections and CNS illnesses has attracted increasing attention since the COVID-19 pandemic.

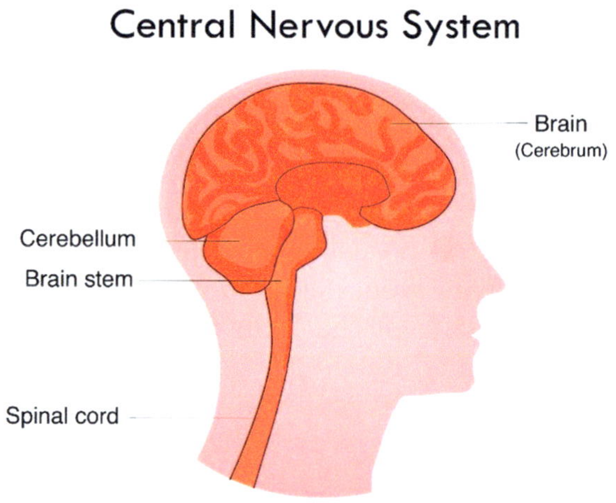

Figure 10.5. Central nervous system (CNS).

Source: https://www.simplypsychology.org/wp-content/uploads/what-is-cns.jpeg.

Evidence suggests that viruses can directly influence neurodegenerative processes through a multitude of mechanisms, including amyloid aggregation related to illnesses like Alzheimer's disease. Notably, studies confirm that neuroinvasive viruses such as SARS-CoV-2 can cause protein aggregation in cerebrospinal fluid, which may lead to long-term cognitive complications in infected individuals. This connection between viral infection and neurodegeneration underscores the multifaceted nature of CNS pathologies and implies that, to understand these interactions in depth, effective therapeutic strategies are needed, especially when dealing with emergent infectious diseases. As knowledge advances, understanding the relationships among the immune response, neuroinflammation, and viral mechanisms remains fundamental for disentangling the complexity of CNS diseases (Figure 10.5).

10.1.2. Peripheral Nervous System (PNS)

PNS links the CNS to the limbs and organs and serves as a communication relay through which the brain and spinal cord communicate with the body. Comprising sensory and motor neurons, the PNS transmits sensory information to the CNS and motor commands to the effector organs. This intricate system consists of cranial and spinal nerves and is subclassified further into the somatic and autonomic nervous systems. The somatic nervous system controls voluntary movement and sensory perception, while the autonomic nervous system controls involuntary functions such as heart rate and digestion. Proper function of the PNS is essential for maintaining homeostasis and facilitating easy interaction with the environment, underscoring its importance for overall neurological health. PNS dysfunction may lead to a variety of complex disorders, which significantly impact patients' quality of life. One such is polyneuropathy, whose feature is decreasing sensation and motor function, tending to develop due to complications such as diabetes or autoimmune illnesses. Specifically, polyneuropathy due to immunoglobulin M (IgM) monoclonal gammopathy is a unique clinical problem due to its heterogeneous manifestations, ranging from mild gait disturbance to severe sensory ataxia and impairment. The immunological factors involved, namely antibodies against myelin-associated glycoproteins, underscore the intricacy of PNS diseases. Evidence indicates that although treatment modalities such as rituximab hold promise, responses are not uniform, posing a challenge for clinicians seeking successful interventions (Dalakas et al., 2018). Research into the unpredictable expression of PNS disorders is necessary to improve diagnostic and treatment methods in neurology. Research on neurotoxicity highlights the PNS's vulnerability to chemicals that disrupt nerve function. Neurotoxicity encompasses a wide range of neurotoxic effects, which may be delayed or acute, representing the impact of the environment on neurological health. For instance, some chemicals can directly damage neural cells or interfere with essential metabolic processes sustaining nervous system function.

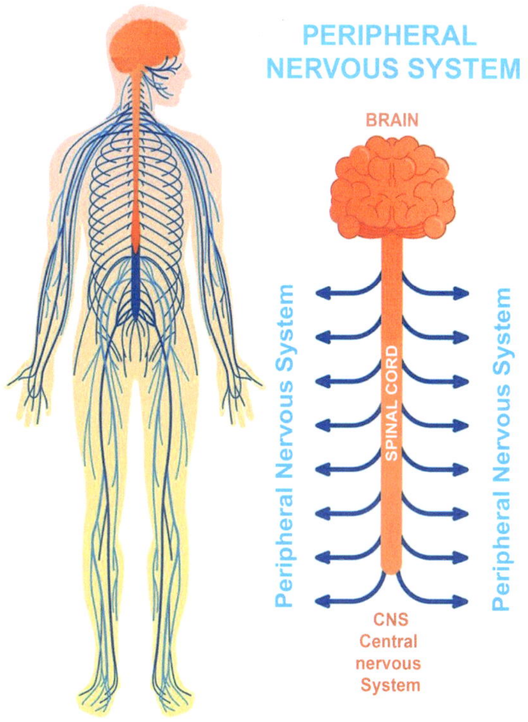

Figure 10.6. Peripheral nervous system (PNS).

Source: https://www.simplypsychology.org/wp-content/uploads/peripheral-nervous-system-1-796x1024.jpeg.

This two-edged quality of neurotoxicants poses enormous issues in the pathophysiology of PNS disorders, where exposure can lead to transient or long-lasting deficits in nerve function and conduction as a whole. Research on neurotoxicity requires rigorous controls and increased vigilance for potential neurotoxic substances in clinical and daily practice environments, ultimately leading to healthier outcomes for those afflicted with PNS-related conditions (Brust et al., 2014) (Figure 10.6).

10.1.3. Functional Divisions of the Nervous System

Functional divisions of the nervous system are the building blocks for understanding how various neurological processes regulate body function. The nervous system is generally separated into the central nervous system (CNS) and the peripheral nervous system (PNS). The CNS, which consists of the brain and spinal cord, serves as the processing center of information and the sending of responses to the entire body. Compared to the CNS, the PNS connects the CNS to the limbs and organs via sensory and motor pathways, thereby facilitating communication between the periphery and the brain. Both divisions play a crucial role in not only sensory perception but also motor performance and movement function, highlighting the sophistication of the nervous system's functional organization. Such sophisticated interplay enables the body to respond appropriately to internal and external stimuli, underscoring the importance of healthy neurological function. The other division of the nervous system's functions includes the somatic and autonomic divisions.

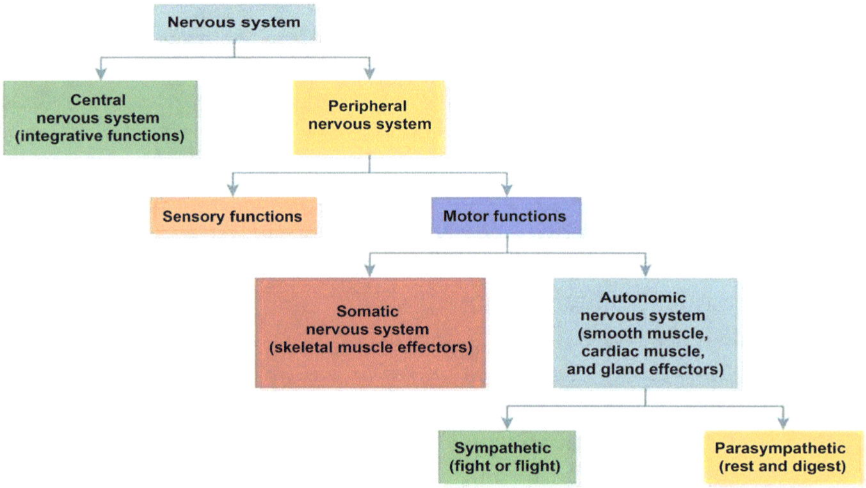

Figure 10.7. Major subdivisions of the nervous system.

Source: https://www.pharmacy180.com/media/article/article-Divisions-of-the-Ner-tWo.jpg.

The somatic nervous system regulates voluntary movement and conveys sensory data from the external environment to the CNS to enable motor responses to match conscious purpose. The system facilitates complex behavior and encompasses everything from basic reflexes to sophisticated motor abilities. The autonomic nervous system, in contrast, functions involuntarily and controls such body processes as heart rate, digestion, and respiratory rate without the effort of volition. This division goes even deeper into the sympathetic and parasympathetic divisions, which prepare the body to act or conserve energy, respectively. Understanding these divisions is crucial to understanding how many neurological diseases can affect both voluntary movement and automatic function, thereby complicating patient diagnosis and treatment plans in the clinical setting. The significance of functional divisions extends to the level of their applicability in medical research and treatment, particularly the process of drug development. As an illustration, studies performing drug safety experiments on juvenile animals have revealed the functional impact on neurological development in terms of how chemicals can affect CNS pathways like neurobehavioral consequences such as locomotor activity and ability to learn (Fisher et al., 2019). Further, recent studies highlight the association between gut microbiota and nervous system function and predict an implicated relationship in which dysbiosis may lead to neurological disorders (Rinninella et al., 2019). is that proper interventions, pharmacological or lifestyle, can restore balance between these functional sectors of the nervous system and ultimately offer new hope for the treatment of central and peripheral nervous system disorders. With the progressive growth of the discipline of neurology, understanding these divisions will remain imperative for advancing the science of medicine and for beneficial health care interventions (Figure 10.7).

Test Your Knowledge

1. What are the main structural divisions of the nervous system?
2. How do the central and peripheral nervous systems differ in function?

10.2. Common Neurological Disorders

Learning Outcome

1. Define the stroke and its types
2. Describe the neurodegenerative diseases (e.g., Alzheimer's, Parkinson's)
3. Discuss on epilepsy and seizure disorders

Neurological disorders are a broad range of conditions with their own presentations and modes of treatment. Of these, the acute hepatic porphyrias (AHPs) are a particularly compelling example since they have intermittent neurovisceral attacks that are typically inappropriately diagnosed as more prevalent disorders. The four AHPs—5-aminolevulinic acid dehydratase deficiency porphyria, acute intermittent porphyria, hereditary coproporphyria, and variegate porphyria—are potentially apt to produce a lot of patient misery if not correctly identified and treated. Notably, the most common and harmful form, acute intermittent porphyria, occurs in approximately 1 in 1600 Caucasians and has low penetrance clinically. Accurate diagnosis requires elevated levels of porphyrin precursors in urine, which demands greater awareness among healthcare workers to prevent potentially irreversible neurological sequelae in affected individuals (Wang et al., 2018). Another common neurological disorder is Parkinson's disease (PD), a motor disorder that poses considerable diagnostic as well as management problems. With multiple motor and non-motor features, clinical diagnosis of PD can be problematic, with significant overlap with other disorders. The most widely used drug in PD is levodopa; however, the occurrence of levodopa-induced dyskinesia (LID) complicates long-term treatment. LID occurs following extended treatment and results in unwanted movements that severely impair quality of life. Surgical interventions, such as unilateral pallidotomy and deep brain stimulation, have proved effective alternatives for non-responsive patients, underscoring the multidisciplinary approach required to manage PD successfully (Goyal et al., 2018). In addition to AHPs and Parkinson's disease, epilepsy is another common neurological disorder that significantly affects patients and their families. Characterized by frequent seizures, epilepsy possesses various titles based on seizure type and etiology, necessitating a particular approach to treatment. Antiepileptic drugs remain the cornerstone of therapy, yet there exists a concern with drug efficacy and side effects. More invasive therapies, including vagus nerve stimulation and surgical resection of the seizure focus, promise new hope for drug-resistant epilepsy sufferers. Familiarity with the spectrum of epilepsy is not only necessary for its proper management but also to reduce the stigma associated with the condition in the past. Continued research into the pathophysiology of epilepsy may provide increasingly innovative treatments that could enhance outcomes for individuals with this neurological condition (Figure 10.8).

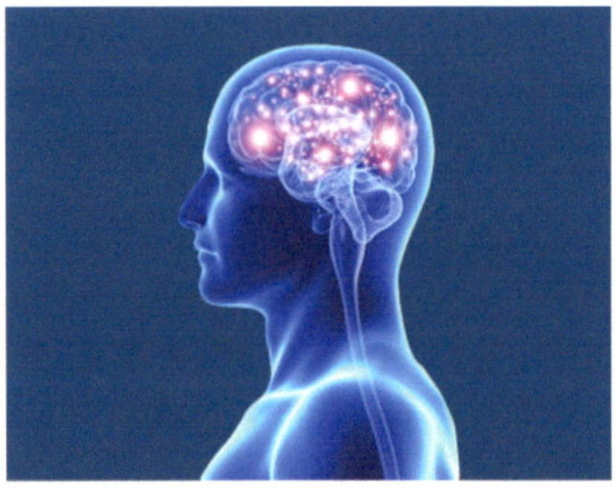

Figure 10.8. Understanding neurological disorders.

Source: https://omnihospitals.in/wp-content/uploads/2024/02/Neurological-disorders-700.jpg.

10.2.1. Stroke and Its Types

Stroke is a potentially dangerous medical condition resulting from a disruption in the blood supply to the brain, causing cell damage and possibly disabling consequences. Ischemic and hemorrhagic strokes are the two largest categories of stroke. Ischemic strokes are caused by a blood vessel that supplies blood to the brain becoming occluded, typically by a blood clot. It is the most prevalent stroke, accounting for approximately 87% of all strokes, and is subdivided into thrombotic and embolic strokes. Thrombotic strokes result from the accumulation of plaque in the arteries, thereby narrowing the blood vessels, while embolic strokes result from a clot breaking away from another part of the body and becoming lodged in the cerebral arteries. These must be accurately grasped for optimal management and treatment, since each requires unique medical interventions to restore cerebral perfusion and prevent further injury. Hemorrhagic strokes, however, are caused by the rupture of a blood vessel within the brain and intracranial hypertension and bleeding. Subarachnoid hemorrhage (SAH) and intracerebral hemorrhage (ICH) fall under this category. SAH occurs with bleeding between the brain and the covering layer, typically due to aneurysm rupture, and is an urgent medical condition with significant morbidity and mortality rates (Muehlschlegel, 2018). Intensive management of SAH is optimized by a multidisciplinary team, with immediate recognition of the bleeding site and specialized treatment regimens. Intracerebral hemorrhage refers to bleeding within the brain tissue itself, usually secondary to hypertension or vascular malformations. Both types of hemorrhagic strokes emphasize the importance of early intervention to prevent secondary injury to the brain, emphasizing the importance of awareness and prompt response in clinical settings. The impact of stroke extends far beyond the acute medical crisis to influence long-term health, rehabilitation, and quality of life for survivors. Treatment varies widely depending on the type of stroke. For example, ischemic stroke can be treated with the use of thrombolytics to break up clots, while hemorrhagic strokes can be treated with surgery to relieve the pressure on the brain and close damaged, leaking vessels. Besides, guidelines have been established to provide optimal stroke care and enhance patient outcomes, following field standards of practice (Williams et al., 2018). Long-term rehabilitation efforts focus on restoring lost functions through physical, speech, and occupational therapy, tailoring interventions to each patient's specific needs. Familiarity with the various types of strokes and their respective characteristics is important in successful treatment and rehabilitation plan formulation, with the eventual goal of improving the prognosis for the afflicted (Figure 10.9).

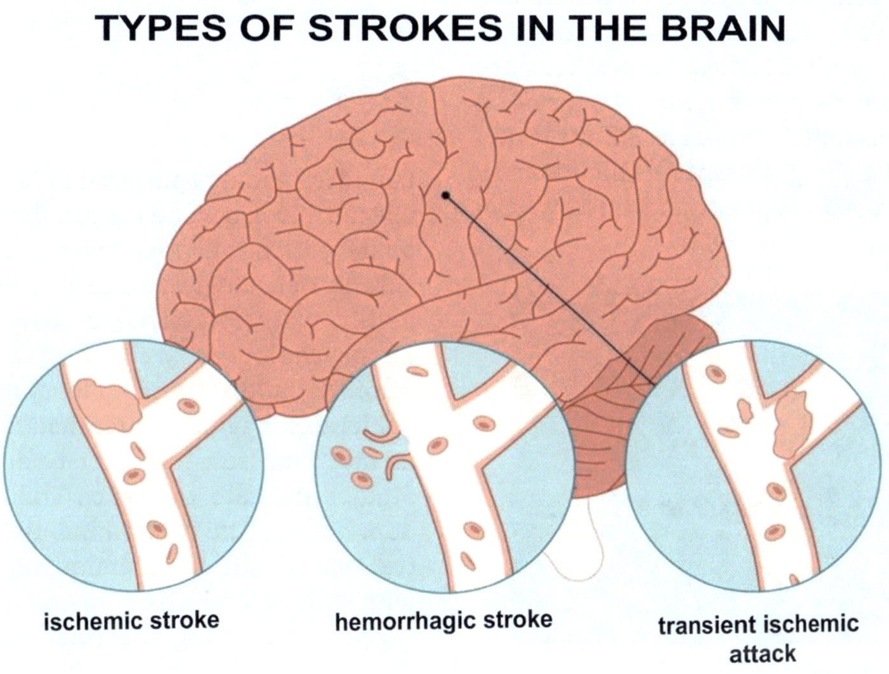

Figure 10.9. Types of strokes.

Source: https://i0.wp.com/post.healthline.com/wp-content/uploads/2021/11/1672630-Everything-You-Need-to-Know-About-Stroke_1296x1059-1.jpg?w=1155&h=2223.

10.2.2. Neurodegenerative Diseases (e.g., Alzheimer's, Parkinson's)

The prevalence of neurodegenerative diseases such as Alzheimer's and Parkinson's disease has risen exponentially, challenging medical science and the health system globally to an unprecedented extent. In the progression of these diseases, patients develop severe motor and cognitive impairment, which directly affects their quality of life. Alzheimer's disease is similarly best known for its eventual mental decline, first manifesting as forgetfulness and confusion, and eventually total amnesia and loss of bodily functions. Parkinson's disease, however, comes principally with motor skills and coordination, as characterized by tremors and stiffness. Both of these afflictions are typified by neuronal loss due to the buildup of misfolded proteins, as evidenced by amyloid protein deposition in Alzheimer's and alpha-synuclein aggregates in Parkinson's, reflecting the common pathological theme in these diseases. Current treatments for neurodegenerative diseases are limited, primarily symptom-focused rather than causative. This difference highlights the need for early detection methods and new treatment strategies to halt disease progression. The evidence indicates that the initial symptoms of these diseases, which become apparent only after substantial neuronal loss, make early intervention challenging. The lack of selective probes to identify toxic amyloid forms complicates the diagnosis of Alzheimer's and Parkinson's disease at a prodromal stage. Furthermore, current drug therapies are inadequate, and thus it is critical to focus on designing compounds capable of targeting early amyloid aggregates specifically, thereby enabling improved diagnosis and therapy (Cui et al., 2024).

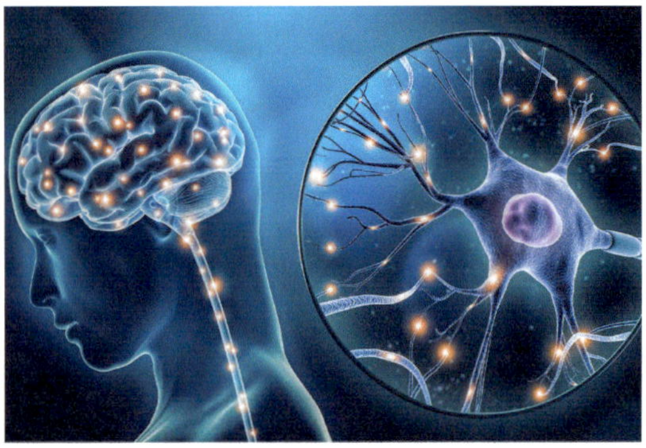

Figure 10.10. Neurodegenerative diseases.

Source: https://wpcdn.web.wsu.edu/news/uploads/sites/2797/2022/06/neurodiseases.jpg.

Advances in molecular and genetic therapy have emerged as viable means of managing the complexities of neurodegenerative disease. Techniques such as CRISPR/Cas9 have shown potential for gene editing to fix pathogenic mutations in such diseases. In Parkinson's disease, for instance, strategies to specifically target genes that are involved in mitochondrial function and synaptic transport have been explored. In Alzheimer's disease, research has been directed towards manipulating amyloid precursor protein mechanisms to avoid neurodegeneration and loss of cognitive functions. These advancements could revolutionize the management of neurodegenerative disorders, bringing hope for a more favorable outcome in the future. Breeding genetically manipulated model organisms, such as the Guangxi Bama miniature pig, also illustrates the potential for further understanding disease mechanisms and evaluation of novel therapeutic approaches (Cui et al., 2024) (Figure 10.10).

10.2.3. Epilepsy and Seizure Disorders

In understanding epilepsy and seizure disorders, one must look beyond their multifaceted impacts on the patient's life. With seizures recurring as a chronic neurological disease, it extends beyond bodily manifestations to leave deep marks on psychological well-being and emotional stability. Children with epilepsy are particularly vulnerable, having greater instances of multiple mental illnesses, like anxiety and depression. Studies indicate that such children are often deprived of the right kind of psychological treatment, and their families have to deal with stigma and stress without the required support. Detecting the relationship between mental health and epilepsy is essential in developing comprehensive treatment programs that treat both of them more effectively, which can enhance the overall quality of life of the affected (Pilarczyk et al., 2025). Furthermore, the cognitive impacts of epilepsy are often underappreciated in the clinical setting. Studies establish that the cognitive ability among epilepsy patients could be affected by numerous variables, including the age at onset, seizure frequency, and total disease duration. Of most concern is the existence of a high rate of epilepsy patients with cognitive impairment as seen using standardized testing. For instance, younger age at onset and longer seizure duration are robustly correlated with lower cognitive function. These results emphasize the importance of initiating treatments early and monitoring cognition regularly in epilepsy patients; neglecting these conditions may hinder attempts at giving holistic care (Malau et al., 2024). Besides, the management of seizure disorders and epilepsy as a whole requires an integrated treatment approach that addresses both the medical treatment and the psychosocial treatment. As noted in the recent findings, the relationship between seizure control and psychological well-being has to be recognized at the clinical level, whereby one-sided treatment of seizure control risks neglecting the overall effect of the disorder. There needs to be a multidisciplinary treatment team, including neurologists, psychologists, and social workers, to address the various challenges faced by patients and their families. Not only does this improve seizure control, but it also enhances resilience against the psychosocial consequences involved, thereby allowing patients to live a good quality of life despite having the condition (Malau et al., 2024; Pilarczyk et al., 2025) (Figure 10.11).

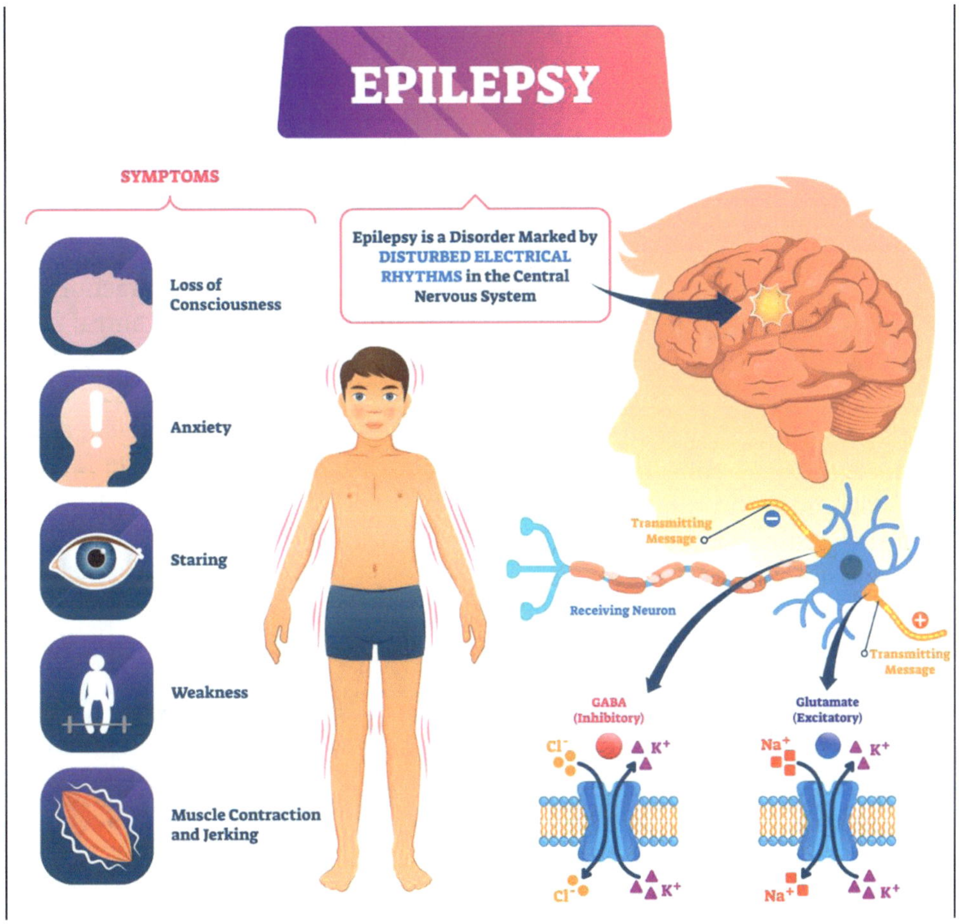

Figure 10.11. Epilepsy.

Source: https://continentalhospitals.com/uploads/mceu_70495666211700724034625.jpg.

Test Your Knowledge

1. What are the most common neurological disorders affecting adults?
2. How do acute neurological conditions differ from chronic neurological diseases?

10.3. Diagnostic Techniques in Neurology

Learning Outcome

1. Describe the neuroimaging methods (magnetic resonance imaging (MRI), computed tomography (CT) scans)
2. Understand the electrophysiological tests (electroencephalography (EEG) and electromyography (EMG))
3. Define the lumbar puncture (LP) and cerebrospinal fluid analysis (CSF)

In neurology, diagnosis is crucial to the point of being indispensable because neurologic diseases can have heterogeneous and multifarious manifestations. Among the diagnostic tools, neuroimaging modalities such as magnetic resonance imaging (MRI) and computed tomography (CT) are of utmost importance. Indeed, MRI offers superb resolution of the central nervous system, enabling visualization of structural and functional abnormalities of the brain. This technique targets pathology diagnosis such as brain tumors, vascular malformations, and demyelinating diseases. MRI enables the clinician to have excellent differentiation among various pathological processes with high-resolution images. CT scanning, by comparison, is usually reserved for emergency assessments, where immediate detection of hemorrhage or acute trauma is required. Thus, integration of these imaging techniques is key to effective clinical management and treatment in neurology. Electrophysiological investigations are equally valuable diagnostic tools in neurology, particularly for assessing the functional integrity of nerves and muscles. Techniques such as electromyography (EMG) and nerve conduction studies (NCS) enable assessment of neuromuscular diseases, including neuropathies and myopathies. The results of these tests can be used to characterize the type of nerve injury—axonal degeneration or demyelination. Secondly, the combination of EMG with clinical examination allows the clinician to form a comprehensive picture of the patient's condition and to deliver more targeted therapy. Of particular significance is the fact that electrophysiological tests are often combined with imaging studies, enriching the diagnostic process and enhancing clinical outcomes. Lastly, their role is more than mere diagnosis; they influence treatment and contribute to a more advanced understanding of neuromuscular pathology. In addition to imaging and electrophysiological techniques, more specialized diagnostic procedures, such as cerebrospinal fluid (CSF) examination, are also part of the diagnosis of neurological disease. Lumbar puncture allows CSF to be withdrawn for analysis of biomarkers, cells, and infectious pathogens. Such an approach has particular utility in rare cases of infection, inflammatory conditions, and certain central nervous system malignancies. Detection of oligoclonal bands within CSF, for instance, is diagnostic for multiple sclerosis, providing crucial diagnostic specificity. Moreover, autopsy-based research has unveiled the long-term usefulness of postmortem studies in forcing premortem diagnosis, particularly in cases of suspected nonneoplastic disease.

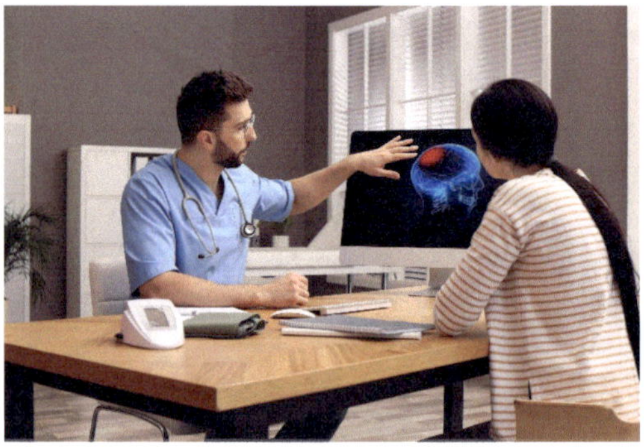

Figure 10.12. Understanding diagnostic procedures neurologists use.

Source: https://premierneurologycenter.com/wp-content/uploads/sites/436/2023/10/shutterstock_2154535477-min-scaled.jpg.optimal.jpg.

These results illustrate that combining CSF examination and autopsy findings can enhance diagnostic accuracy, reiterating the importance of utilising a multidimensional approach in neurology (Macrae et al., 2024; Das et al., 2025) (Figure 10.12).

10.3.1. Neuroimaging Methods (Magnetic Resonance Imaging (MRI), Computed Tomography (CT) Scans)

Neuroimaging modalities, i.e., MRI and CT scans, have revolutionized the practice of neurology since they provide valuable information on brain structure and function. MRI uses intense magnetic fields and radio waves to generate high-resolution images of brain tissues that allow the examination of both normal and disease states, such as tumors, stroke, and neurodegenerative conditions. One of MRI's greatest strengths is that it can produce high-resolution images without ionizing radiation, making it safer for patients who require repeated examinations. In addition, MRI technology has improved considerably, including several techniques such as functional MRI (fMRI), which measures changes in blood flow to assess brain function, thereby increasing our understanding of cognitive processes and illnesses. On the other hand, CT scans employ X-rays, providing quicker imaging findings at a lower cost, which is critical during emergencies. Although CT scans subject patients to ionizing radiation, their ability to supply rapid cross-sectional images of brain anatomy is crucial in diagnosing such acute pathologies as hemorrhage and fractures. Besides, the integration of sophisticated algorithms and reconstruction techniques enhances the quality of CT imaging, enabling clinicians to derive valuable information (Jessica, 2024). However, one must remain aware of the limitations of CT scans, e.g., far lower contrast resolution than MRI, which may affect the detectability of small brain lesions. Hence, it is essential to be aware of the pros and cons of these neuroimaging modalities to make optimal clinical decisions. Recent developments in neuroimaging emphasize the synergy between MRI and CT modalities, particularly for augmented and virtual reality applications. By combining MRI and CT data with immersive technologies, clinicians and researchers can create three-dimensional models that enhance visualization and support better surgical planning and medical training (Ziyad et al., 2024). This cross-disciplinary approach not only maximizes the interpretative power of neuroimaging but also holds the potential for future breakthroughs in personalized medicine. As accurate, fine-grained diagnostic tools become increasingly needed, the incremental march of neuroimaging technologies will increasingly drive neurological care forward, providing crucial insights into treatment efficacy and disease progression. Recurring investments in research, education, and technological innovation are required to maximize the application of these procedures in routine clinical practice.

10.3.2. Electrophysiological Tests (Electroencephalography (EEG) and Electromyography (EMG))

Electrophysiological tests such as EEG and EMG are essential tools in the clinical practice of neurology, yielding information on brain and muscle electrical activity. EEG, a minimally invasive test, records brain wave patterns via electrodes on the scalp. This technique is instrumental in diagnosing conditions like epilepsy, sleep disorders, and various neurological anomalies. By analyzing the frequency and amplitude of brain waves, clinicians can understand the brain's functional state, particularly in differentiating between drowsy and alert states. As illustrated in some studies, adequate identification of drowsiness from EEG signals can lead to enhanced safety measures in everyday life, such as driving, where states of mind directly impact performance (Arif et al., 2023). EMG, however, provides valuable information about muscle electrical activity. This test measures the electrical potentials generated by muscle cells when they are electrically or neurologically activated. EMG plays a critical role in the diagnosis of neuromuscular disease, in the assessment of nerve injury, and in the assessment of muscle function. Using surface electrodes or fine-wire techniques, practitioners obtain information about muscle activation and recruitment patterns during both voluntary and involuntary movements. As technology that brings EMG capabilities continues to advance, it opens the door to real-time feedback and monitoring for rehabilitating patients, further enhancing the quality of care for mobility-impaired patients (Powell et al., 2020). The combination of EEG and EMG technologies not only deepens one's understanding of neurological function but also enables the development of advanced therapeutic devices. With the presence of equipment to stream biosignals for analysis in multiple channels, researchers can prototype and create biomedical devices better. An instance is the NeuroDAC system, which can replicate EEG and EMG biosignals to test closed-loop algorithms in adaptive therapies. These advancements indicate the applicability of electrophysiological tests in clinical settings, enabling healthcare providers to obtain sufficient data to personalize treatments effectively. With progress in technology, the use and accessibility of these electrophysiological tests will become more prevalent, ultimately benefiting patient recovery in rehabilitation and neurotherapy (Powell et al., 2020).

10.3.3. Lumbar Puncture (LP) and Cerebrospinal Fluid Analysis (CSF)

LP is a procedure at the heart of neurology, both as a diagnostic and a treatment method. During this procedure, CSF is drawn for analysis, which may yield valuable information about several neurological diseases such as meningitis and encephalitis. Lumbar puncture provides direct access to CSF, allowing clinicians to analyze its constituents, including cell count, protein, and glucose. This test is required to distinguish meningitis into various forms, as the biochemical content of CSF indicates whether the cause is viral or bacterial. Additionally, the test itself is pretty harmless if conducted correctly, though proper technique must be employed so that complications are not produced. Thus, LP is an invaluable tool in paediatricians' and neurologists' diagnostic armamentarium, enabling early and appropriate intervention for patients with suspected central nervous system disease. The applicability of lumbar puncture extends beyond diagnosis as it sheds light on the causative infectious etiologies of neurological illness. In the present study, scientists noted that a large percentage of patients infected with CSF viruses also presented with clinical signs of encephalitis and a high prevalence of human herpesvirus 6 (HHV-6) and enteroviruses (Kuruma et al., 2025). This association suggests that although the mere determination of pathogen presence is not important, the determination of viral burden can be used as a prognostic factor. By establishing a correlation between viral load and illness severity, clinicians can make evidence-based decisions about treatment and follow-up care. Such information regarding the composition of the CSF and the potential pathogens it harbors plays a key role in the continued quest for enhanced diagnostic accuracy and therapeutic interventions in neurology. Nor should the clinical value of LP be overlooked in children, and especially in diagnosing meningitis. A study of pediatric patients revealed that among those who come in with seizure and fever, a large percentage have meningitis, indicating the utility of LP in such patients (Mehjabin et al., 2025). CSF interpretation provides an unambiguous way to distinguish meningitis from other potential causes of neurological presentations. Apart from that, specific meningeal signs observed during clinical evaluation have varying sensitivities and specificities, which enhance diagnostic accuracy. The statistical association between CSF findings and clinical presentations underscores the significant role of lumbar puncture as a diagnostic procedure, especially in young infants. It is thus a key procedure in neurology, allowing one to obtain precise diagnoses and customized treatment programs for the management of multiple neurological disorders.

Test Your Knowledge

1. What diagnostic tests are commonly used to assess neurological function?
2. Why is neuroimaging important in diagnosing nervous system disorders?

10.4. Treatment Approaches in Neurology

Learning Outcome

1. Discuss the pharmacological treatments in neurology
2. Define the surgical interventions in neurology
3. Understand the rehabilitation therapies

Treatment approaches in neurology have significantly evolved, particularly for paraneoplastic neurological disorders. These complex conditions are prone to occur in patients even before tumor detection, thereby posing greater challenges for diagnosis and treatment. The identification of anti-neuronal antibodies is a key decision-making factor because they may suggest the presence of an underlying malignancy even in the absence of apparent tumor symptoms. Concurrently, diagnostic methods such as MRI, cerebrospinal fluid tests, and electrophysiological tests enhance neurologists' ability to make early, accurate diagnoses. As tumor therapy is the pillar of treatment in these diseases, early immune therapy should also be initiated alongside it. Advances in understanding the autoimmune pathophysiology of these illnesses, particularly the role of cytotoxic T cells, could open new therapeutic opportunities (Graus et al., 2004). With neurodegenerative diseases like Parkinson's Disease (PD), interventions include both pharmacologic and non-pharmacologic choices. Among the heterogeneous symptoms of PD, postural instability (PI) has profound implications for the quality of life in patients through an elevated risk of falls and attendant disabilities. Traditional treatments with pharmacological agents, such as dopaminergic drugs, address the motor aspects of the disease but rarely regulate non-motor manifestations. Recent studies have examined novel non-drug treatments, such as dance therapy, which have been proven effective in enhancing gait performance and balance in PD patients. By integrating these treatment modalities, clinicians can offer a more cohesive strategy for the treatment of neurological diseases, addressing patients' multiple demands (Agnetti et al., 2012). The overlap of different treatment modalities underscores the need for an individualized treatment plan in neurology. Neurologists must consider the unique characteristics of each patient, including the specific nature of their illness, comorbid conditions, and individual responses to treatment. Individualized treatment is critical in treating complex diseases such as multiple sclerosis, where treatment efficacy can vary widely among patients. By implementing a regimen of combined disease-modifying therapies, symptomatic drug therapy, lifestyle changes, and adjunctive treatments such as cognitive-behavioral therapy, clinicians can create personalized management plans that optimize outcomes. Ongoing research projects and clinical trials continue to evolve the ever-changing range of treatment modalities, underscoring the necessity of flexibility and creativity in the practice of neurology. With the development of the field, the coordination among clinicians, researchers, and patients will be critical in streamlining treatment strategies in neurology (Figure 10.13).

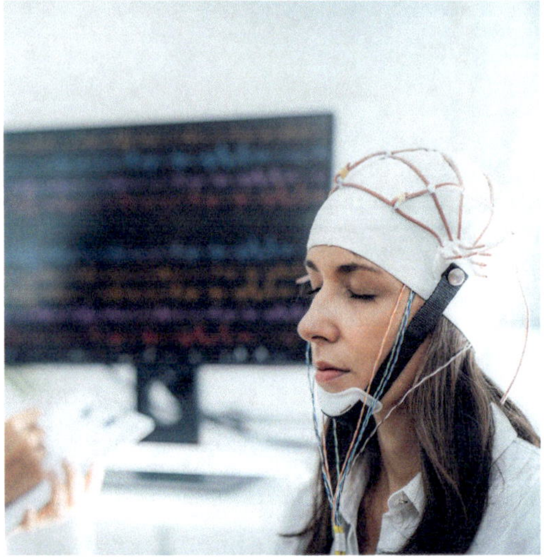

Figure 10.13. Innovative approaches in treating neurological conditions.

Source: https://atlneuroinstitute.org/wp-content/uploads/2023/09/Innovative-Approaches-in-Treating-Neurological-Conditions-image2.jpg.

10.4.1. Pharmacological Treatments

Pharmacological management of neurological conditions encompasses a broad range of treatments for the symptoms of numerous neurological diseases. The variability of neurological illnesses, ranging from epilepsy to multiple sclerosis, calls for an individualized medication approach. Antiepileptic medication, for example, can be prescribed as a means of seizure control, while other medicines like muscle relaxants can be administered for spasticity in multiple sclerosis patients. The efficacy of these pharmacologic interventions depends not only on the underlying pathophysiology but also on the patient's individual response, necessitating careful monitoring and dose adjustments. Furthermore, recent advances in pharmacotherapy have introduced novel agents that target individual pathways implicated in neurological conditions, offering promise for more targeted symptom management and improved quality of life. In addition to traditional pharmacological management, recent literature supports the inclusion of psychological therapies in neurological practice. The Italian Consensus Conference was particularly insistent on the efficacy of psychological therapy for managing pain secondary to neurological illness and emphasized the benefit of treatment by a multidisciplinary team. Interventions such as Cognitive-Behavioral Therapy and Acceptance and Commitment Therapy have been proven to significantly reduce pain severity among patients affected by conditions such as fibromyalgia and post-stroke pain. This framework posits that, alongside pharmacological interventions, psychological treatments can also contribute to the management of emotional and psychological symptoms of neurological diseases, ultimately supporting a more holistic approach to patient care (Agostini et al., 2016). In kids, particularly with headache treatment, behavioral interventions are a practical addition, or alternative, to pharmacological ones. Psychosocial factors are identified as having a considerable effect on headache prevalence and severity in both children and adolescents, making behavioral interventions particularly suitable. Techniques such as biofeedback and relaxation training not only enhance the effectiveness of pharmacotherapy but also reduce the amount of medication required, which often has the potential for side effects (Arruda et al., 2016). By reducing the intensity and recurrence of headaches through behavioral control, medical professionals can increase the overall quality of life for young patients. Accordingly, a multimodal treatment protocol using both pharmacological and non-pharmacological methods could be the answer to effectively treating neurological manifestations, particularly in vulnerable people.

10.4.2. Surgical Interventions

Surgical therapies in neurology are typically undertaken as emergency measures to alleviate disabling conditions that significantly impact patients' lives. For instance, thoracic outlet syndrome (TOS) is a condition that is most often surgically treated due to its incapacitating presentations of intense pain and paralysis of the upper limbs. TOS arises when the neurovascular bundle in the thoracic outlet is compressed, typically due to anatomic defects. Patients presenting with TOS along with cervicothoracic scoliosis have been revealed through literature to have particular clinical and radiographic features that warrant treatment. The procedures commonly utilized—such as anterior scalenectomy, pectoralis minor release, or resection of the first rib—have been highly effective, with the majority of the patients showing a great deal of functional improvement following the procedure, thereby enhancing their quality of life as has been illustrated in current studies (Bowman et al., 2025). The field of neurosurgery has also been further transformed by advances in anesthesiology, including the development of muscle relaxants. These medications have shifted procedures beyond routine anaesthetic practice, particularly in neural procedures that demand precise regulation of muscular functions. Muscle relaxants facilitate safer, more effective interventions by enabling enhanced coordination between surgical maneuvers and patient physiology. They are also crucial in intensive care situations, where their use supports numerous emergency interventions, including tracheal intubation and invasive procedures such as lumbar punctures and tracheostomies. The significance of muscle relaxants in ensuring maximal surgical success underscores the vibrant development of neurology, where cross-disciplinary collaboration ensures optimal therapeutic outcomes (Chyngyshova et al., 2023). By considering the broader context of neurosurgical interventions, it is essential to recognize the multidisciplinary nature of modern medical practice. The coordination of surgical procedures with rehabilitation and physiotherapy supports the best patient care, as it collectively ensures maximum effectiveness of surgical success. Coordinated care for not only acute neurological deficits but also later rehabilitation needs underscores the necessity of an integrated model of care. With continued improvements in surgical equipment and understanding of neurological disease, opportunities for improved patient outcomes in neurosurgery are more clearly evident. As has been shown in many case studies, including those on TOS, ongoing evaluation and progress in surgery will continue to shape neurology, making surgery more effective and improving the overall quality of life for patients.

10.4.3. Rehabilitation Therapies

Rehabilitation therapy is a significant aspect of the healing and management of neurological disorders, with the aim of restoring function and improving the patient's quality of life. As patients most often get through multiple impairments following neurological events such as stroke, traumatic brain damage, or neurodegenerative conditions, tailored rehabilitation protocols are essential. Typically, physical, occupational, speech, and cognitive therapies are integrated into plans to support multidimensional recovery. Especially with technological developments, new methods such as virtual reality are potent forces that complement traditional rehabilitation methods. Those therapies that are patient interaction-based and tailored interventions have shown promise, particularly in encouraging neuroplasticity, something crucial to rehabilitating injured brain areas. The integration of heterogeneous treatment modalities ensures comprehensive care and meets the multifaceted demands of patients navigating rehab. Among the various models of rehabilitation, virtual reality (VR) has been one of the spotlighted advanced therapy methods in neurology. With multisensory stimulation in virtual environments, VR enhances patient motivation, participation, and involvement in rehabilitation therapy. Studies have shown that VR treatment can achieve high rates of improvement in both motor and cognitive function, particularly beneficial for individuals with moderate to severe impairment (Golota et al., 2025). By enabling the users to practice movements and cognitive tasks within a safe and controlled setting, VR also decreases pain and anxiety and facilitates making it more straightforward to provide a more therapeutic setting for therapy. The potential of VR technology lies in its ability to create realistic simulations that allow patients to practice daily activities and acquire knowledge effectively, thereby enhancing their skills and confidence. This novel approach to rehabilitation exemplifies the intersection of technology and biomedical sciences to improve patient outcomes in neurology. More specifically, the establishment of specialized journals, such as the Journal of Medical Rehabilitation Sciences, reflects a marked interest in advancing research and practice in rehabilitation therapy (Al-Otaibi, 2025). Such publications establish essential channels for disseminating first-class, peer-reviewed research that has the potential to influence clinical guidelines and treatment approaches. Through interdisciplinary collaboration, these journals encourage the crossing of rehabilitation paradigms among disciplines such as physical therapy, speech therapy, and occupational therapy. Through the collaborative process, the singular pursuit aims to address fundamental challenges for the field and eventually culminate in improved patient care and outcomes. With advances in rehabilitation research, emphasis on evidence-based practice will ensure that interventions are not only innovative but also underpinned with scientifically validated methods. This motivation will undoubtedly push the advancement of effective rehabilitation treatments, shaping the future of medical rehabilitation in neurology.

Test Your Knowledge

1. What are the common treatment options for neurological disorders?
2. How do medications and rehabilitation therapies work together in managing nervous system diseases?

10.5. The Role of Neurologists

Learning Outcome

1. Define the education and training requirements in neurologists
2. Describe the specializations within neurology
3. Understand the collaboration with other medical professionals

Neurologists play an important role in the field, with expertise in diagnosing and treating conditions affecting the central and peripheral nervous systems. Their professional function comprises a wide variety of neurological diseases, including epilepsy, multiple sclerosis, Parkinson's disease, and neurodegenerative diseases. Neurologists conduct thorough neurological exams, employ advanced imaging techniques, and perform electrodiagnostic tests to arrive at precise diagnoses. Through this thorough methodology, they can formulate customized treatment programs that meet each patient's specific requirements. Neurologists can also collaborate with other medical specialists, such as primary care physicians, physical therapists, and psychologists, to deliver comprehensive treatment that integrates medical and rehabilitation techniques. Their role is not only crucial in the management of neurological disease, but also in improving patients' quality of life when faced with chronic neurological illness. The contribution of a neurologist extends beyond treatment and diagnosis; they are involved in an integral contribution of patient education and advocacy. The complexity of neurological disease demands a multidimensional understanding of the disorders, which can be frustrating for patients and families. Thus, neurologists take charge of explaining diagnoses and delineating treatment options, enabling informed decision-making. They guide patients through the nuances of their conditions and the potential impact on daily living. In disorders such as autism spectrum disorder (ASD), where early detection is crucial, neurologists work with multi-disciplinary teams to provide holistic care, as highlighted in research demanding early intervention services (and et al., 2023). Not only does such patient empowerment inspire the patients, but it also enhances treatment compliance, ultimately leading to better health outcomes. In addition, technological advances have similarly transformed the roles of neurologists in contemporary medicine. Advances in telemedicine, for example, have boosted access to specialist consultations, particularly for patients who are far away or based in rural areas. Neurologists use such technologies to stay in touch with their patients, monitor their conditions, and adjust treatment plans in real time. This is especially useful for treating chronic neurological diseases, where constant patient interaction is imperative. In addition, decision tools in computer applications have become key assets for their role in improving patient and neurologist shared decision-making so that patients participate actively in their treatment decisions (Alan Research In Implementation Science And EHealth, 2021). As the nature of neurological disorders becomes increasingly complex, neurologists are well positioned to leverage these technologies to enhance patient care, enabling them to remain at the vanguard of medical advancement and patient advocacy (Figure 10.14).

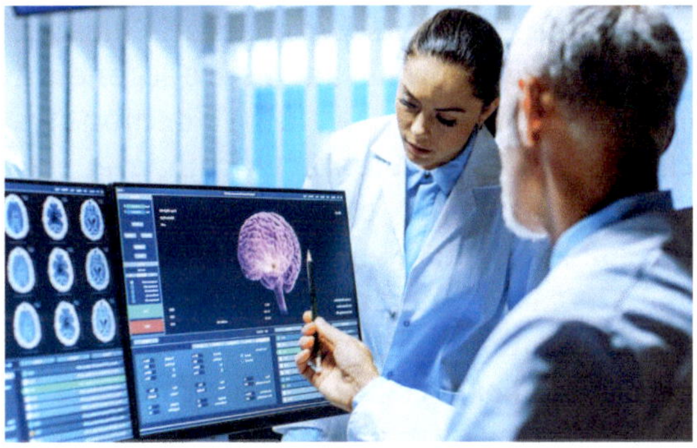

Figure 10.14. The role of neurologists.

Source: https://neuromedpa.com/wp-content/uploads/2024/08/general-brain-studies-2-1024x626.jpg.

10.5.1. Education and Training Requirements

The field of neurology, with its sophisticated understanding of the nervous system, requires rigorous education and training for would-be medical practitioners. Typically, this begins with a four-year undergraduate degree, followed by a medical degree from an accredited institution, also taking around four years. During medical school, students are exposed to a broad curriculum in basic medical sciences, clinical rotations, and neurology to build a sound foundation. The initial part of education is important because it lays the groundwork for sound medical principles that will come in handy during subsequent specialized training in neurology. In addition, early exposure to formal research is advantageous for most students and is positively correlated with residency research productivity (Michael O'Shea et al., 2025). This indicates a key aspect of preparation because research skills enhance clinical practice and patient care in neurology. Following medical school, candidates must complete a neurology residency program for approximately 4 years. The residency is pivotal to developing clinical competencies necessary to evaluate and treat various neurological disorders. Training involves practical experience in the diagnosis and treatment of patients with severe disorders such as epilepsy, stroke, and neurodegenerative conditions. Residents must demonstrate technical and non-technical competency, as contemporary approaches to neurology highly value communication and decision-making skills in patient care. Systematized residency training programs integrate observation, mentorship, and hands-on experience, but residents identify barriers such as time constraints and inadequate mentorship. Overcoming these barriers requires a designed residency training program that accords prioritized, supported learning models and ongoing mentorship to facilitate professional growth in neurology (Michael O'Shea et al., 2025).

Apart from traditional educational pathways, the incorporation of cutting-edge technology and modern learning styles is increasingly mandatory in the training and education of neurologists. Traditional approaches are gradually being augmented by newer learning methods that use virtual reality (VR) simulation and serious games to enhance clinical training, particularly for procedural and diagnostic skills. For instance, the application of simulation-based tools promotes experiential education and can significantly enhance the cognitive and psychomotor skills of healthcare practitioners. Such new training models can efficiently simulate realistic neurological exams, thereby optimizing the learning process for clinicians and learners alike. By facilitating an interactive learning environment, these advancements not only enhance the acquisition of required skill sets but also aim to increase patient safety and the quality of care. Hence, integrating modern learning technologies into neurology education can close existing gaps and best equip future neurologists for their critical roles in the clinical environment.

10.5.2. Specializations Within Neurology

Neurology possesses an enormous array of specializations to match the diverse and intricate nature of neurological diseases. Every specialization addresses the unique characteristics of nervous system illnesses and involves particular diagnostic and therapeutic interventions. For example, neurophysiology is concerned with understanding the electrical functions of the brain, spinal cord, and peripheral nerves, which aid in diagnosing disorders such as epilepsy and neuropathies.

In contrast, vascular neurology revolves around cerebrovascular diseases, i.e., stroke and transient ischemic attacks, where early treatment is essential for maximizing patient outcomes. These specialized branches enable neurologists to meet specific patient needs and optimize the overall efficacy of treatments, ultimately redefining the future of neurological medicine. A second significant neurology specialty is neuropsychology, which investigates the interface between brain function and behavior. Neuropsychologists use several tests to ascertain cognitive impairments caused by brain injury, developmental disorders, or neurodegenerative diseases. Their skills play a central role in designing individualized rehabilitation programs for patients suffering from loss of memory, attention deficit, or executive functioning impairment. Neuropsychology also sets the stage for interdisciplinary collaboration by combining findings with psychiatry and rehabilitation sciences to unravel the complex emotional and psychological dimensions of patients. With neurodegenerative diseases on the rise, this specialization plays an increasingly important role in formulating holistic strategies that support emotional and cognitive well-being, ensuring support for patients who undergo these intricate processes. Further, technological developments have fueled the emergence of new specializations in neurology, particularly with the use of artificial intelligence (AI) in the clinical environment. Artificial intelligence-powered expert systems are beginning to revolutionize neurology treatment protocols and diagnostics, mimicking human decision-making processes in order to maximize patient results (Ramirez et al., 2025).

As AI technology becomes more prominent, AI application experts in neurology have the mandate to harness it to improve diagnostic accuracy and maximize patient care. Meanwhile, the intersection of physiotherapy and neurology is emerging. By using advanced technologies such as nanotechnology in therapeutic procedures, neurologists can better treat conditions such as stroke rehabilitation and traumatic brain injury (Cardoza et al., 2024). With such specialized practice, neurology is evolving into a more effective, patient-centered field, underscoring the importance of specialization in managing the complexities of neurological health.

10.5.3. Collaboration with Other Medical Professionals

Multidisciplinary practice is a critical component of effective neurology practice, as it facilitates a team approach to patient care. Neurologists tend to collaborate with other healthcare providers, such as primary care physicians, rehabilitation therapists, and nurses, to facilitate comprehensive management of neurological illness. Collaborative practice offers improved insight into a patient's situation, facilitating timely intervention and decision-making.

Regular interdisciplinary meetings, case conferences, and shared care planning ensure that all team members contribute their specialist expertise, ultimately enhancing patient outcomes. Not only does this improve continuity of care, but it also enables professional relationships to form that can foster improved clinical practice and research endeavors. Furthermore, co-posing different medical perspectives alongside one another is paramount in addressing the multidisciplinary approach of neurological conditions. For instance, neuropsychologists often collaborate with neurologists to evaluate cognitive impairment secondary to various diseases, including Alzheimer's or traumatic brain injury. The two, in consultation, can guide individualized rehabilitative treatment, taking into account both the neurological and psychological processes. Additionally, cooperation with physical and occupational therapists is essential for designing rehabilitation plans that take into account motor skills and activities of daily living. These interdisciplinary ventures demonstrate the value of cross-disciplinary collaboration in developing comprehensive treatment plans tailored to the unique needs of patients with neurologic disorders. Furthermore, collaboration in neurology also encompasses research and education. Neurologists often work with academic institutions and professional organizations to develop practice guidelines and conduct high-quality research on contemporary issues in neurology. For example, through collaborative networks, neurologists can participate in multicenter studies that provide valuable information on disease prevalence and treatment efficacy, ultimately informing evidence-based guidelines. Such initiatives not only develop the profession's shared knowledge but also strengthen coalitions with collaborating professionals, generating innovation and promoting enhanced health outcomes. As seen in recent discussions regarding potential conflicts of interest with industry collaborators, ensuring the integrity and ethical basis of these collaborations is critical to building trust and advancing neurology as a health science (Robbins, 2018; Whelton et al., 2017).

Test Your Knowledge

1. How do neurologists diagnose and manage complex nervous system disorders?
2. What role do neurologists play in coordinating long-term care for patients with chronic neurological diseases?

10.6. Advances in Neurological Research

Learning Outcome

1. Define the emerging technologies in neurology
2. Describe the genetic research and its implications
3. Identify the future directions in neurological studies

Recent developments in neurological research have greatly expanded our understanding of many nervous system disorders. Advances in imaging technologies, including functional MRI and PET scans, enable greater precision in visualizing brain activity. These methods enable scientists to detect biomarkers for conditions such as Alzheimer's disease and Parkinson's disease, which result in earlier diagnosis and personalized treatment programs. Furthermore, breakthroughs in gene therapy and pharmacotherapy have opened new avenues for treating previously incurable neurological conditions. Ongoing advancements now give researchers the potential to de-mystify the complexity of neurodegeneration and eventually transform patient treatment and outcomes. The ongoing research into the molecular mechanisms underlying such conditions has serious implications for the planning of effective treatments and underscores the necessity of a multidisciplinary approach to neurological health. In addition to classical neurological disease, advanced research technologies are also shedding light on the intricacies of nervous system trauma and neuroinflammation.

Researchers are increasingly investigating the immune system's role in neurological diseases, which has led to the emergence of a field of study called neuroimmunology. This cross-disciplinary field of research has demonstrated that neuroinflammatory mechanisms may aggravate underlying neurological diseases and accelerate disease progression. Current developments indicate that modulating immune responses may offer new therapeutic interventions for clinical treatment. Furthermore, research into stem cell therapy and neurogenesis is promising, particularly for nerve regeneration following injury or trauma. Neuroimmunology, stem cell research, and advanced imaging offer a thrilling frontier where ancient boundaries of neurology are being recharted, bringing promise to patients with disabling illnesses. Ethics are also fundamental to contemporary neurological research, particularly as treatments such as deep brain stimulation (DBS) increasingly come to the fore. With the power to modify neurological functioning comes fundamental ethical issues regarding consent, identity, and the nature of cognition. As researchers progress along the potential implications of manipulating brain function to treat everything from depression to obsessive-compulsive disorder, the union of neuroethics and practical application only gains greater significance. Stressing the imperative to maintain patient autonomy while encouraging innovation, researchers examine the ethical considerations of developing therapies and their implications for society. The current debate in the field emphasizes the need for an overall system that balances ethical responsibility with the pressure for revolutionary therapies, ensuring that advances in neurological science benefit society as a whole. Current developments in these fields are an integration of science, ethics, and humanity and have the potential to redefine our conception of neurological health and wellness.

10.6.1. Emerging Technologies in Neurology

The integration of genomic medicine into neurology practice is an essential advancement in the study and management of neurological illnesses. Advances in new technologies, including next-generation sequencing, have fundamentally revolutionized the practice by improving the precision of risk tests and enabling the early identification of diseases like Alzheimer's and Parkinson's. By examining an individual's genetic profile, medical practitioners can tailor treatment to their genetic susceptibility, thereby increasing treatment efficacy. The applications of genomic medicine extend beyond diagnostics; they can even include gene-editing tools such as CRISPR-Cas9 to correct genetic defects at the molecular level. As understanding of the human genome deepens, such technology cannot only maximize treatment modalities but also drive a revolution in personalized practice in neurology, leading to improved patient outcomes and targeted prevention (Patel et al., 2025). Furthermore, advances in imaging technology are transforming the process of diagnosis in neurology. Techniques such as functional Magnetic Resonance Imaging (fMRI) and Positron Emission Tomography (PET) enable real-time visualization of brain activity and structure, enabling more precise diagnoses of neurological disease. Non-invasive techniques allow doctors to observe the changes that accompany conditions such as multiple sclerosis and epilepsy, which results in better treatment strategies. In addition, the advent of machine learning algorithms has enhanced the interpretation of imaging data, resulting in earlier detection of previously unsuspected neurological disorders. The integration of advanced imaging modalities with artificial intelligence not only enhances diagnostic accuracy but also increases the likelihood of timely intervention, which is essential for disorders that may respond to early treatment (Maitra et al., 2025). In addition, the application of neuromodulation techniques is under development as a pillar of treatment of a variety of neurological diseases. Techniques like transcranial magnetic stimulation (TMS) and deep brain stimulation (DBS) have achieved promising evidence for the treatment of disorders from depression and chronic pain to movement disorders. These methods regulate neurophysiological function to enhance brain function or alleviate symptoms, thereby creating new treatment options in cases where traditional medications are ineffective. The continued innovation of minimally invasive neuromodulation techniques, supported by robust clinical trials, underscores the potential for these technologies to improve the well-being of patients with debilitating neurological diseases. With advancing science, the understanding of the mechanisms by which these technologies function will undoubtedly deepen, paving the way for improved applications in neurology (Patel et al., 2025).

10.6.2. Genetic Research and its Implications

The merger of genetic studies and neurology has profound implications for the etiology and treatment of neurological diseases. Genetic investigations have illuminated the hereditary causes of conditions such as autism spectrum disorder (ASD) and epilepsy, emphasizing the value of correct genetic diagnosis for the direction of medical care. Nonetheless, despite these seminal findings, the majority of patients remain undiagnosed or under-tested, undermining effective treatment protocols. Neurologists, genetic counselors, and geneticists play key roles in advancing diagnostic practice, but their distinct practices can contribute to inconsistent patient treatment. The call for uniform guidelines underscores the urgent need for interdisciplinary coordination in neurology to achieve optimal outcomes for patients with such disorders, reflecting the overall trend of integrating genetic discoveries into clinical practice (Wofford et al., 2018). Besides, the uses of genetic research extend beyond the diagnostic context to also encompass bioethical issues. With increased use of neurointerventions for treating neurological diseases through genetic research, ethical concerns are raised about the form of consent and the alteration of cognitive processes.

The ability to interfere with neurological processes raises controversy about the boundaries of such interventions that are acceptable, particularly in the criminal justice system, where biological factors can change the mental conditions of criminals. The public perception of these technologies has a significant influence on policy and clinical practice and therefore warrants a reflective debate on the ethical use of neurointerventions to advance treatment while safeguarding individual rights (Whitaker et al., 2018). Lastly, integrating genetic research into neurology requires an integrated education system for professionals. Many pediatric neurologists, for example, report a lack of self-efficacy in ordering genetic testing, and there is a need for genetics training as part of neurology curricula. This information gap can lead to misdiagnosis and delayed treatment, and thus educating healthcare professionals about the changing face of genetic diagnostics is crucial. By leveraging the skills of genetic counselors in pediatric neurology clinics, neurologists' workload can be reduced through a more streamlined, well-informed approach to patient care. By this paradigm, not only is diagnostic accuracy enhanced but the general knowledge of the genetic basis of neurological illnesses is also better understood, which ultimately benefits the patient and his/her family.

10.6.3. Future Directions in Neurological Studies

With advances in neurology, future neurological research is increasingly defined by the application of artificial intelligence (AI) and newer imaging techniques. One key trend is the application of deep learning algorithms to diagnose and treat neurological disorders. Research has shown that applying AI to MRI data analysis can greatly improve the precision of diagnosing conditions such as brain tumors, Alzheimer's disease, and Parkinson's disease. This not only simplifies the diagnostic process but also opens the door to customized treatment regimens tailored to each patient. This explainable nature of such AI models, enabled by explainable AI (XAI) techniques, is essential for building clinicians' and patients' confidence and ensuring smoother adoption in clinical settings. These advancements are crucial for addressing existing diagnostic challenges in neurology, offering a promising avenue for future research (Ratnakar et al., 2025). Another emerging direction is a bibliometric assessment to shed light on the neurological research environment. The systematic review uses quantitative methods to compare trends, estimate the impact of benchmark studies, and identify collaboration networks within the discipline. Recent studies report a significant increase in publications on AI applications in neuroscience, particularly from leading countries such as the United States, China, and the United Kingdom. This surge, particularly from the mid-2010s onward, marks a turning point in the integration of interdisciplinary approaches and innovation in neurological imaging and brain-computer interfaces (BCI). With bibliometric methods, researchers can identify future research of interest and streamline it to address issues in the field. Thus, these analyses will determine the course of neurological research, helping formulate revised research agendas in response to technological advancements and societal needs (Uğur Tekin and Murat Dener, 2025).

The future of neurological research ultimately depends on ethical issues related to AI and data privacy. With machine learning and AI being widely integrated into neurological studies, it is essential to ensure these technologies are used responsibly and ethically. Data protection, patient confidentiality, and the explainability of AI models are issues that need to be addressed in an organized manner to maximize their potential benefits. Researchers must unite across disciplines to develop ethical frameworks and procedures that govern the use of AI in clinical and research settings. By doing so, the neurology community can minimize the negative effects of new technologies while maximizing the benefits to patient care and to advancing knowledge of neurological disorders. The conduct of these ethics talks will not only ensure adequate research protocols but also solidify individuals' confidence in the emerging field of AI-based neurotechnology, which will serve as a basis for future neurological studies (Uğur Tekin and Murat Dener, 2025).

Test Your Knowledge

1. What recent research has improved the diagnosis of neurological disorders?
2. How are emerging therapies shaping the future treatment of neurological diseases?

SUMMARY

In summary, advances in neurology, particularly through treatments such as transcranial magnetic stimulation (TMS), highlight the dynamic nature of research and treatment methodologies in this field. TMS has evolved significantly over the years to refine its uses in various neurological and psychiatric conditions. As recent literature confirms, the vast database of over 500 studies has examined the efficacy of TMS in altering seizure activity and regulating disorders. This is a vital milestone toward greater insight into brain function and therapeutic capacity (Afifi, 2024). However, despite these advances, there is still a need for additional research to address current uncertainties in most TMS protocols and to determine whether outcomes are better established on empirical rather than experimental evidence. The results have broader implications beyond TMS itself, echoing the general trends in medical neurology. The current deluge of serological studies, particularly in infected children with COVID-19, mirrors the multifaceted interaction between infectious and neurological manifestations. For example, Omicron-infected children presented higher inflammatory markers, such as interleukin-6 to correlate with seizures (Lee et al., 2024). These findings not only cast light on the need for interdisciplinary practice involving neurology, immunology, and infectious disease specialties but also underscore the need to reassess how new global health threats affect neurological well-being across populations. Consequently, the trajectory of neurology continues to be challenged at unprecedented levels, necessitating that practitioners and researchers remain alert and active. As the field matures, there is a duty to translate collective experience into effective therapeutic interventions that optimally benefit patients. An area of future work in the neurology field must be the development of formal, evidence-based guidelines for broad-spectrum treatment and ensuring that all evidence contributes to a more robust foundation for understanding neurological diseases. The interplay between research, clinical practice, and patient treatment will ultimately define the next generation of neurological advances, driving the field toward enhanced control over neurological conditions today and tomorrow.

The complex specialty of neurology encompasses numerous neurological disorders that pose significant challenges for patients and healthcare systems. Central nervous system diseases, such as Multiple Sclerosis (MS) and stroke, illustrate these challenges through their complex symptomology and the profound impact they have on activities of daily living. MS, for instance, is characterized by a range of disabling symptoms that affect not only physical function but also emotional and social functioning, placing an endless adjustment process on individuals afflicted with it (Bogosian et al., 2009). The disease has taken an unpredictable path, which has led to difficulty in preserving work, interpersonal relationships, and life goals. With rising incidences of such disorders, identifying their impact on quality of life is required to enable effective interventions and adequate support systems for patients suffering from them. Recent clinical trials have aimed to enhance adjustment among MS-diagnosed patients through various therapeutic approaches. One of the larger-scale trials compares the efficacy of Cognitive Behavior Therapy (CBT) versus supportive listening in decreasing distress and improving social functioning in MS patients in the earlier stages of the disease (Bogosian et al., 2009). The new approach focuses on the integration of psychosocial care provided by skilled nurses, potentially making it more accessible and feasible for healthcare systems. By collecting data through self-report questionnaires and interviews, researchers can learn a lot from participants' experiences and how mechanisms facilitate psychosocial adjustment. This trial helps understand the psychological aspects of MS and develop effective treatment models that can be replicated in the medical setting. Stroke care has also progressed significantly in the field by the development of data-sharing programs, which aim to optimize clinical trial design and implementation. The Virtual International Stroke Trials Archive is a single platform that houses large amounts of data from numerous trials performed on thousands of stroke patients. Researchers can conduct exploratory analyses of patient data using this platform, which inform hypotheses and enhance clinical trial designs. By collating data from a diverse patient population, the archive enables research on disparate outcome measures, such as the Barthel Index and the National Institutes of Health Stroke Scale, thereby enabling a focused research endeavor. The provision of such an instrument is a milestone for the field of neurology with the promise to enhance stroke care protocols and ultimately stroke patient outcomes in this special public health space.

KEY TERMS FROM THIS CHAPTER

- Neuron
- Peripheral Nervous System (PNS)
- Epilepsy
- Multiple Sclerosis (MS)
- Neuropathy
- Headache
- Dementia
- Electroencephalogram (EEG)
- Central Nervous System (CNS)
- Stroke
- Parkinson's Disease
- Alzheimer's Disease
- Seizure
- Migraine
- Neurotransmitters

CRITICAL THINKING QUESTIONS

1. **A patient presents with sudden onset right-sided weakness and aphasia. CT head is normal. What is the most likely diagnosis?**
   a. Subarachnoid hemorrhage
   b. Ischemic stroke
   c. Intracerebral hemorrhage
   d. Transient ischemic attack (TIA)
2. **The most common cause of intracerebral hemorrhage in adults is:**
   a. Trauma
   b. Amyloid angiopathy
   c. Hypertension
   d. Arteriovenous malformation
3. **Which of the following is the first-line treatment for status epilepticus?**
   a. Carbamazepine
   b. Phenytoin
   c. Diazepam or Lorazepam
   d. Levetiracetam
4. **A 30-year-old woman has sudden visual loss in one eye and pain on eye movement. What is the most likely diagnosis?**
   a. Acute angle-closure glaucoma
   b. Optic neuritis
   c. Retinal detachment
   d. Cataract
5. **Which of the following features are not typical of Parkinson's disease?**
   a. Bradykinesia
   b. Rigidity
   c. Rest tremor
   d. Hyperreflexia

Short Answer Questions

1. What are the 3 regions of the brain?
2. What is the central nervous system?
3. What is the peripheral nervous system?
4. Name the two types of strokes.
5. What diagnostic techniques do neurologists use to diagnose patients?

Answers to Critical Thinking Questions

1. (b); 2. (c) ; 3. (c); 4. (b); 5. (d)

REFERENCES

1. Afifi, S. Y. (2024). A new era of current and future treatment applications of transcranial magnetic stimulation. *The Egyptian Journal of Neurology Psychiatry and Neurosurgery, 60*(1). https://doi.org/10.1186/s41983-024-00825-9
2. Agnetti, V., Aiello, E., De Natale, E., Deriu, R., et al. (2012). Effects of dance therapy on balance, gait and neuro-psychological performances in patients with Parkinson's disease and postural instability. https://core.ac.uk/download/16749566.pdf (accessed on 16th July 2025).
3. Agostini, M., Alfonsi, E., Aloisi, A. M., Alvisi, L., et al. (2016). Psychological treatments and psychotherapies in the neurorehabilitation of pain: Evidences and recommendations from the Italian Consensus Conference on Pain in Neurorehabilitation. https://core.ac.uk/download/54538696.pdf (accessed on 16th July 2025).
4. Al-Otaibi, H. M. (2025). Charting a new course in medical rehabilitation sciences. Medical Rehabilitation Sciences. https://www.semanticscholar.org/paper/c287727faf00883e3360c4cc9a0d7c24d058a495 (accessed on 16th July 2025).
5. Alan Research in Implementation Science and eHealth. (2021). Computer-based decision tools for shared therapeutic decision making in oncology: A systematic review (Preprint). https://www.semanticscholar.org/paper/927ee4f29eacc593ca61501b2e67918ee99670ec (accessed on 16th July 2025).
6. Ali, M., Bath, P. M. W., Curram, J., Davis, S., et al. (2007). The Virtual International Stroke Trials Archive. https://core.ac.uk/download/110682.pdf (accessed on 16th July 2025).
7. Arif, S., Munawar, S., & Ali, H. (2023). Driving drowsiness detection using spectral signatures of EEG-based neurophysiology. Frontiers in Physiology, 14. https://www.semanticscholar.org/paper/15eaa8fc6ae8dca35e4d888edfd50f763ad1597c (accessed on 16th July 2025).
8. Arruda, M., Cerutti, R., Faedda, N., Guidetti, V., et al. (2016). Behavioral management of headache in children and adolescents. https://core.ac.uk/download/74325348.pdf (accessed on 16th July 2025).
9. Association Professional Committee of Emergency Resuscitation, Medicine Rescue and Protection Branch of China Medical Rescue. (2024). [Chinese expert consensus on the process of 5G+ helicopter aviation medical rescue (2024 edition)]. *Zhonghua Wei Zhong Bing Ji Jiu Yi Xue, 36*(3), 225–230. https://www.semanticscholar.org/paper/b17870380d30cc951092eb11aa1c718e2a0a687e (accessed on 16th July 2025).
10. Bisi, N., Pinzi, L., Rastelli, G., & Tonali, N. (2024). Early diagnosis of neurodegenerative diseases: What has been undertaken to promote the transition from PET to fluorescence tracers. Molecules, 29. https://www.semanticscholar.org/paper/d66369440a650d198529dcc3af79e9383f19b5d0 (accessed on 16th July 2025).
11. Bogosian, A., Janssens, A., Stuifbergen, A. K., Williams, A., Wearden, A. J., Stuifbergen, A. K., Beck, A. T., et al. (2009). Protocol for the saMS trial (supportive adjustment for multiple sclerosis): A randomized controlled trial comparing cognitive behavioral therapy to supportive listening for adjustment to multiple sclerosis. https://core.ac.uk/download/pdf/8648829.pdf (accessed on 16th July 2025).
12. Bowman, K. M., Ansari, D. S., & Hanna, A. S. (2025). Thoracic outlet syndrome associated with cervicothoracic scoliosis. Surgical Neurology International, 16. https://www.semanticscholar.

org/paper/3bc6820d463a5261d6cff0021e36cddc55b6bef2 (accessed on 16th July 2025).

13. Brust, J. C. M., Creeley, C., Feldman, R., Grandjean, P., Herken, H., Panzica, G., Parent, M., et al. (2014). Neurotoxicity. https://core.ac.uk/download/286729125.pdf (accessed on 16th July 2025).
14. Cardoza, J. V., Ali, Z., Simon, S., Thakkar, D., George, S. S., & Isaac, S. P. (2024). The role of nanoparticles in accelerating tissue recovery and inflammation control in physiotherapy practices. Cureus, 16. https://www.semanticscholar.org/paper/8499be7b537420c8a2671bc1667fed13bdfc8fc5 (accessed on 16th July 2025).
15. Christ, W., Kapell, S., Sobkowiak, M. J., Mermelekas, G., Evertsson, B., Sork, H., Saher, O., et al. (2024). SARS-CoV-2 and HSV-1 induce amyloid aggregation in human CSF resulting in drastic soluble protein depletion. bioRxiv. https://www.semanticscholar.org/paper/2b87b042c742ade46174e4f22d0d6a2b84b504c7 (accessed on 16th July 2025).
16. Chyngyshova, Z., Raimbekov, Zh., Turdusheva, D., Turdiev, U., & Nazarbekov, D. (2023). Historical and physiological aspects of muscle relaxation and application in medical practice. Bulletin of Science and Practice. https://www.semanticscholar.org/paper/69a86bf94e666219c391fd703010fc2cd73041d6 (accessed on 16th July 2025).
17. Cui, H., & Zhong, Z. (2024). Neurodegenerative diseases treatment based on CRISPR. Highlights in Science, Engineering and Technology. https://www.semanticscholar.org/paper/a1b0a8ccbdf6f75fb72e57f1e691fd913fafbb29 (accessed on 16th July 2025).
18. Dalakas, M. (2018). Advances in the diagnosis, immunopathogenesis and therapies of IgM-anti-MAG antibody-mediated neuropathies. https://core.ac.uk/download/155271624.pdf (accessed on 16th July 2025).
19. Das, N., Chandana, P., Chhabra, M., & Basanagoudar, P. L. (2025). Quadrangular space schwannoma affecting the axillary nerve. Surgical Neurology International, 16. https://www.semanticscholar.org/paper/68d180784a7352dcaf8eb32dcfd0edfff15c3b55 (accessed on 16th July 2025).
20. Deoliveira, D. C., Rekik, Y., & Malandain, S. (2024). GlasgowSim–Glasgow Coma Scale simulation. *Human Interaction and Emerging Technologies (IHIET 2024)*. https://www.semanticscholar.org/paper/cfb63f3fda77ab8fb80b955cf5b90db2a4d5ed8b (accessed on 16th July 2025).
21. Fisher, J. E., Ravindran, A., & Elayan, I. (2019). CDER experience with juvenile animal studies for CNS drugs. International Journal of Toxicology, 38, 88–95. https://doi.org/10.1177/1091581818824313 (accessed on 16th July 2025).
22. Gold, C. A., Klein, J. P., Richie, M. B., Morris, J. G., & Wold, J. J. (2024). Neurohospitalist core competencies: Development and methodology. *The Neurohospitalist, 15*, 5–12. https://www.semanticscholar.org/paper/3a0c3d3c2f0fa107e5067f5987a82d3dea9d81c2 (accessed on 16th July 2025).
23. Golota, A., Shcherbak, S., Vologzhanin, D. A., Makarenko, S. V., & Kamilova, T. A. (2025). Virtual reality in medical rehabilitation. *Physical and Rehabilitation Medicine, Medical Rehabilitation*. https://www.semanticscholar.org/paper/8f9ceda8abbfd011af56bcc236d1b59d362f508b (accessed on 16th July 2025).
24. Goyal, V., & Radhakrishnan, D. M. (2018). Parkinson's disease: A review. Neurology India, 66, 26–26. https://doi.org/10.4103/0028-3886.226451 (accessed on 16th July 2025).

25. Graus, F., & Voltz, R. (2004). Diagnosis and treatment of paraneoplastic neurological disorders. https://core.ac.uk/download/16432364.pdf (accessed on 16th July 2025).

26. Jessica, E. C. (2024). Advancements and challenges in algebraic techniques for medical imaging: A comprehensive review of MRI and CT scan applications in Nigeria. Newport International Journal of Biological and Applied Sciences. https://www.semanticscholar.org/paper/91654d34182d72675a759d337f27056f54aa2170 (accessed on 16th July 2025).

27. Kirilenko, E. A., Byvaltsev, V., Sysin, S. A., Sereda, E. V., Koval, Y. A., & Stasiv, O. V. (2025). Screening for erectile dysfunction in patients with nervous system pathology as an interdisciplinary problem. Sibirskij Medicinskij Vestnik. https://www.semanticscholar.org/paper/e9c9a935426f7f551130e29e8516520083847b0b (accessed on 16th July 2025).

28. Kuruma, K., Funakoshi, H., Shibata, M., Kinoshita, K., & Horikoshi, Y. (2025). Association of encephalitis with viruses in cerebrospinal fluid in children: A case series. Cureus, 17. https://www.semanticscholar.org/paper/91240d413b9fe16f921a340a7741e1f08539999a (accessed on 16th July 2025).

29. Lee, S., Kim, K. R., & Koo, C. (2024). Analysis of inflammatory markers and electroencephalogram findings in pediatric patients with COVID-19: A single-center study in Korea. Annals of Child Neurology. https://www.semanticscholar.org/paper/8c4e88949437845bec35409a3599d0ca1c7ebb56 (accessed on 16th July 2025).

30. Li, K., Liu, Y., Gong, J., Li, J., Zhao, M., Hong, C., Zhang, Y., et al. (2025). Reactive astrocyte-derived exosomes enhance intracranial lymphatic drainage in mice after intracranial hemorrhage. Fluids and Barriers of the CNS, 22. https://www.semanticscholar.org/paper/ed13e00fc25fd9ed24644beb3fab1112f285a47c (accessed on 16th July 2025).

31. Lu, L., Zhang, J., Xie, Y., Gao, F., Xu, S., Wu, X., & Ye, Z. (2020). Wearable health devices in health care: Narrative systematic review. JMIR mHealth and uHealth, 8, e18907–e18907. https://doi.org/10.2196/18907 (accessed on 16th July 2025).

32. Macrae, C. B., Grieco, K. C., & Solomon, I. H. (2024). Diagnostic yield of postmortem brain examination following premortem brain biopsy for neoplastic and nonneoplastic disease. *Journal of Neuropathology and Experimental Neurology, 83*, 331–337. https://www.semanticscholar.org/paper/f6d01f6df67ad7bf2b6ab35aae2cacb588d839d4 (accessed on 16th July 2025).

33. Maitra, S., Das, S., Sinha, D., Mukherjee, M., Kumari, L., & Roy, T. (2025). Recent advancements and future perspectives in diacerein delivery systems for rheumatoid arthritis: Novel strategies and emerging technologies. Palestinian Medical and Pharmaceutical Journal. https://www.semanticscholar.org/paper/0211549b8005f077f359ccff08de4e92d484674a (accessed on 16th July 2025).

34. Malau, T. B., Ritarwan, K., Muzasti, R., Sari, M. D., & Anggreiny. (2024). Relationships between age of onset, seizure frequency, and disease duration with cognitive function in epilepsy patients at the neurology clinic of H. Adam Malik Central Hospital, Medan. Journal of Endocrinology, Tropical Medicine, and Infectious Disease (JETROMI). https://www.semanticscholar.org/paper/28ae99d5508ba0d20d5c7233eb493697486969c1 (accessed on 16th July 2025).

35. Marder, E., DeLong, M. R., Gazzaniga, M. S., & Wichmann, T. (2008). 2008 progress report on brain research. https://core.ac.uk/download/71349141.pdf (accessed on 16th July 2025).

36. Mehjabin, S., Joseph, S., & Ravi, A. (2025). Epidemiology of lumbar puncture and the validity of meningeal signs in predicting meningitis in children: A cross-sectional study. Journal of Clinical and Diagnostic Research. https://www.semanticscholar.org/paper/3cab1d4c23ed2

d1358ef964fc644c0e3bebbd06f (accessed on 16th July 2025).

37. Muehlschlegel, S. (2018). Subarachnoid hemorrhage. CONTINUUM Lifelong Learning in Neurology, 24, 1623–1657. https://doi.org/10.1212/con.0000000000000679 (accessed on 16th July 2025).

38. Murray, C. J. L., Ikuta, K. S., Sharara, F., Swetschinski, L. R., Robles Aguilar, G., Gray, A. P., Han, C., et al. (2022). Global burden of bacterial antimicrobial resistance in 2019: A systematic analysis. *The Lancet, 399*, 629–655. https://doi.org/10.1016/s0140-6736(21)02724-0 (accessed on 16th July 2025).

39. N/A. (2000). Focal Spot, Spring 2000. https://core.ac.uk/download/129069317.pdf (accessed on 16th July 2025).

40. O'Shea, M., Ashcherkin, N., Karikalan, S. A., Biondi, M., Chaffin, H., Umar, S., Delafield, N., et al. (2025). A mixed methods survey of research education requirements for residents in internal medicine, neurology and transitional programs. Medical Education Online, 30. https://www.semanticscholar.org/paper/6b513a63a08cc6f2a17b6213b736d143030e5002 (accessed on 16th July 2025).

41. Patel, H. N., Patel, N. H., Mathukiya, S., Parekh, B., Purohit, K. A., Patel, S. P., & Patel, J. (2025). Genomic medicine: Applications in disease prevention and treatment. Journal of Pharmacy and Bioallied Sciences. https://www.semanticscholar.org/paper/e98c0815154a22e46c2f2fd78b42efc3a5175c47 (accessed on 16th July 2025).

42. Pilarczyk, K., Grzesik, K., Rabęda, A., Klepacz, N., Adamska, H., Sawczuk, H., Nowak, W., et al. (2025). Epilepsy in children: Coexistence of mental disorders and the impact of social factors. Medical Science Pulse. https://www.semanticscholar.org/paper/b8b11c70bc30ced6d388ecac0b024e0c5fc93337 (accessed on 16th July 2025).

43. Powell, M., Anso, J., Gilron, R., Provenza, N., Allawala, A., Silva, D., Bijanki, K., et al. (2020). NeuroDAC: An open-source arbitrary bio signal waveform generator. Journal of Neural Engineering, 18. https://www.semanticscholar.org/paper/7c4f1082c470b429b5aa87ab6f787e667f2d9e6a (accessed on 16th July 2025).

44. Ramirez, J. E. G., Valerio, M. K. A., Layug, J. R., Santiago, C. S., Ulanday, M. L. P., & Alabanza, J. E. (2025). Application of expert systems with artificial intelligence in the medical field: A literature review. ASEAN Journal of Scientific and Technological Reports. https://www.semanticscholar.org/paper/917e4463111ce27871c0cb655ca2f2e8af2a4c28 (accessed on 16th July 2025).

45. Ratnakar, A., Sawant, S., & Karajagikar, J. (2025). Explainable AI-driven deep learning for neurological disease diagnosis using MRI: A systematic review and future directions. *International Journal of Science and Research Archive*. https://www.semanticscholar.org/paper/51d853faf99d88a88de13325534c46e99ed10f42 (accessed on 16th July 2025).

46. Rinninella, E., Raoul, P., Cintoni, M., Franceschi, F., Miggiano, G. A. D., Gasbarrini, A., & Mele, M. C. (2019). What is the healthy gut microbiota composition? A changing ecosystem across age, environment, diet, and diseases. Microorganisms, 7, 14–14. https://doi.org/10.3390/microorganisms7010014 (accessed on 16th July 2025).

47. Robbins, N. M. (2018). Ethical issues pertaining to conflicts of interest between neurologists and the pharmaceutical and medical device industries. Seminars in Neurology, 38, 589–598. https://doi.org/10.1055/s-0038-1668081 (accessed on 16th July 2025).

48. Saladino, V., Algeri, D., & Auriemma, V. (2020). The psychological and social impact of COVID-19: New perspectives of well-being. Frontiers in Psychology, 11. https://doi.org/10.3389/fpsyg.2020.577684 (accessed on 16th July 2025).

49. Sharma, T., Meghwal, C. R., Prajapat, M., & Sharma, A. K. (2024). Conceptual study of Vata Dosha w.s.r. to nervous system. Journal of Ayurveda and Integrated Medical Sciences. https://www.semanticscholar.org/paper/0b9c8d0031e72cbf1829406481e7264e72307717 (accessed on 16th July 2025).

50. Stefanou, M. I., Palaiodimou, L., Bakola, E., Smyrnis, N., Papadopoulou, M., Paraskevas, G. P., Rizos, E., et al. (2022). Neurological manifestations of long-COVID syndrome: A narrative review. Therapeutic Advances in Chronic Disease, 13. https://doi.org/10.1177/20406223221076890 (accessed on 16th July 2025).

51. Tanese, M. A., Local Health Authority, Kazakhstan Parents Perspective, et al. (2023). Intersectoral care for children with autism spectrum disorder in Kazakhstan: Parents perspective. *The European Journal of Public Health, 33*. https://www.semanticscholar.org/paper/e33390d072cef7808ca965a6ca6b6a72311aae17 (accessed on 16th July 2025).

52. Tekin, U., & Dener, M. (2025). A bibliometric analysis of studies on artificial intelligence in neuroscience. Frontiers in Neurology, 16. https://www.semanticscholar.org/paper/401a9172d5db79b59501b164afe993449bcf9b89 (accessed on 16th July 2025).

53. Wang, B., Rudnick, S., Cengia, B. T., & Bonkovsky, H. L. (2018). Acute hepatic porphyrias: Review and recent progress. *Hepatology Communications, 3*, 193–206. https://doi.org/10.1002/hep4.1297 (accessed on 16th July 2025).

54. Whelton, P. K., Carey, R. M., Aronow, W. S., Casey, D. E., Collins, K. J., Himmelfarb, C. D., DePalma, S. M., et al. (2017). 2017 ACC/AHA/AAPA/ABC/ACPM/AGS/APhA/ASH/ASPC/NMA/PCNA guideline for the prevention, detection, evaluation, and management of high blood pressure in adults: A report of the American College of Cardiology/American Heart Association Task Force on Clinical Practice Guidelines. Hypertension, 71. https://doi.org/10.1161/hyp.0000000000000065 (accessed on 16th July 2025).

55. Whitaker, H. N. (2018). Attitudes on Medical Ethics of Criminal Neurointerventional Treatment. https://core.ac.uk/download/213462108.pdf (accessed on 16th July 2025).

56. Williams, B., Mancia, G., Spiering, W., Rosei, E. A., Azizi, M., Burnier, M., Clement, D. L., et al. (2018). 2018 ESC/ESH guidelines for the management of arterial hypertension. *European Heart Journal, 39*, 3021–3104. https://doi.org/10.1093/eurheartj/ehy339 (accessed on 16th July 2025).

57. Wilson, M., Sampson, M., Barrowman, N., & Doja, A. (2021). Bibliometric analysis of neurology articles published in general medicine journals. JAMA Network Open, 4, e215840–e215840. https://doi.org/10.1001/jamanetworkopen.2021.5840 (accessed on 16th July 2025).

58. Wofford, S. (2018). Genetic Testing Practices of Genetic Counselors, Geneticists, And Pediatric Neurologists with Regard to Childhood-Onset Neurogenetic Conditions. https://core.ac.uk/download/212897114.pdf (accessed on 16th July 2025).

59. Zamanian, M. Y., Soltani, A., Khodarahmi, Z., Alameri, A. A., Alwan, A. M. R., Ramírez-Coronel, A. A., Obaid, R. F., et al. (2023). Targeting Nrf2 signaling pathway by quercetin in the prevention and treatment of neurological disorders: An overview and update on new developments. Fundamental and Clinical Pharmacology, 37, 1050–1064. https://doi.org/10.1111/fcp.12926 (accessed on 16th July 2025).

CLINICAL PHARMACOLOGY AND THERAPEUTICS

11

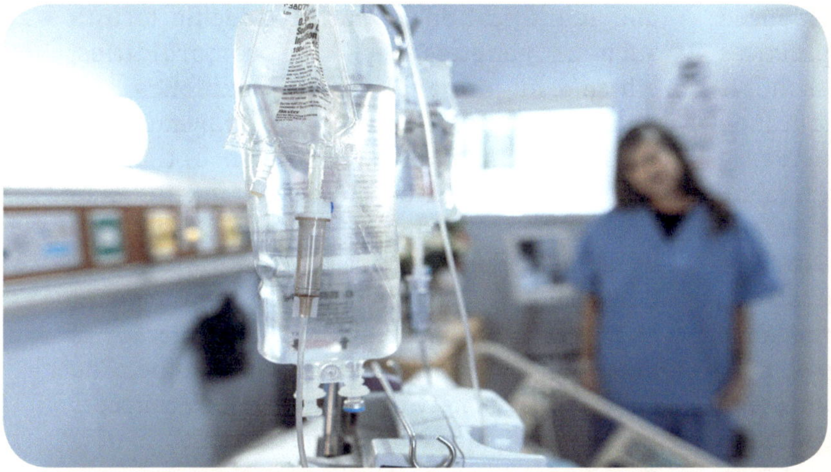

LEARNING OBJECTIVES

After studying this chapter, you will be able to:

1. Understand Pharmacokinetics
2. Explain Pharmacodynamics
3. Describe Drug Development Process
4. Focus on Therapeutic Drug Monitoring
5. Know Adverse Drug Reactions
6. Describe Emerging Trends in Clinical Pharmacology

Introduction

Clinical pharmacology is a critical interface between therapeutic practice and pharmacological principles in patient treatment. As an academic subject, clinical pharmacology education lies at the center of equipping medical students with the understanding necessary for therapeutic decision-making. The emphasis on the pharmacodynamics and pharmacokinetics of groups of drugs is grounded in comprehension of how drugs function in the human organism. This primary understanding is typically supplemented by educational reforms, such as Problem-Based Learning (PBL), that promote active learning through difficult case studies. With a focus on general drug categories and collaborative learning, educators can enhance students' knowledge and application of pharmacological principles, ultimately preparing them for real-world clinical environments, as suggested by recent pedagogical effectiveness trends in pharmacology education (Garetto et al., 2010). Moving still further in pedagogic approaches adopted for teaching pharmacology, interactive and integrative styles of learning are preferred. Students eagerly demand instruction integrating theoretical foundations with clinical application, an indicator of the shift towards practice and case-based learning environments. Research suggests that students find a variety of teaching approaches, including the use of audiovisual aids and group discussion, conducive to active learning and better recall of pharmacologic material. Moreover, integrating clinical pharmacology into the curriculum not only develops core knowledge but also increases students' confidence in prescribing and monitoring complex medication regimens, as evidenced by assessments of new educational practices (Bhargava et al., 2017). This pedagogical shift is part of an overall movement in medical education that reflects the need to build a more interactive and clinically relevant pharmacology curriculum for future healthcare professionals. The peak of these changes in clinical pharmacology teaching is reflected in students' increased preparedness for clinical practice. By employing innovative pedagogies and integrating pharmacology courses with a therapeutic focus, educators can equip future medical practitioners with the preparation needed to address the challenges of patient care. A strong introduction to clinical pharmacology not only enhances students' knowledge of drugs but also stimulates problem-solving and critical thinking abilities, which are fundamental to clinical practice. This repetition of pharmacology principles becomes essential, particularly when medical students are in their clinical years, where they have to apply theoretical principles to real-world patient scenarios. Lastly, integrating effective pedagogical strategies into the design of the clinical pharmacology course enhances student performance and prepares them to handle the intricacies of therapeutics in real-world practice (Bhargava et al., 2017; Garetto et al., 2010).

Definition and Scope of Clinical Pharmacology

Clinical pharmacology is the science of drugs and their application to clinical medicine, with an emphasis on explaining how these chemicals affect human physiology. This discipline integrates drug science with clinical practice to maximize the optimization of drug therapy for patients. By examining the actions, efficacy, and safety profiles of drugs, clinical pharmacology empowers clinicians with information to make evidence-based decisions in choosing treatment interventions. Moreover, its use comprises the evaluation of drug therapy's therapeutic impact, exploration of drug-drug interaction, and identification of patient-specific factors such as genetics, age, and comorbidities, which can influence pharmacokinetics and pharmacodynamics. Clinical pharmacology thus plays an important role in optimizing the treatment efficacy while minimizing side effects, leading to improved patient care and outcomes. Furthermore, the importance of clinical pharmacology is increasingly evident in personalized medicine, in which therapy is tailored to the individual patient profile. The convergence of network pharmacology concepts with personalized medicine provides a new paradigm in drug discovery and application. By focusing on the complex interactions among several biological pathways and drug agents, clinical pharmacologists can design more effective treatment regimens that are precisely counterpoised to the patient's particular profiles. This paradigm shift results in a better understanding of how medicines operate in biological systems, beyond the one-size-fits-all conceptions. Consequently, clinical pharmacology not only enhances therapeutic performance but also paves the way for new methodologies that prioritize patient safety, therefore revolutionizing contemporary medical practices and therapy research (Marsh et al., 2010). Finally, the general scope of clinical pharmacology within the healthcare system underscores its adaptability and forward-looking application. The field plays a central role in drug development, with clinical pharmacologists conducting trials to assess the safety and effectiveness of new medications prior to market release. Regulatory bodies rely on this valuable information to ensure that treatments adhere to planned safety standards and achieve therapeutic outcomes. Furthermore, clinical pharmacology research continues to yield new therapeutic compounds and repurposed drug administration concepts. The complexities of treatment regimens require a robust understanding of the pharmacotherapy's implications, again highlighting the need for expert education in this field. As the future of modern medicine proceeds, the role of clinical pharmacology will continue to assume an increasingly pivotal position in offering safe, effective, and customized therapeutic interventions in a vast range of clinical settings (Schenk et al., 1959) (Figure 11.1).

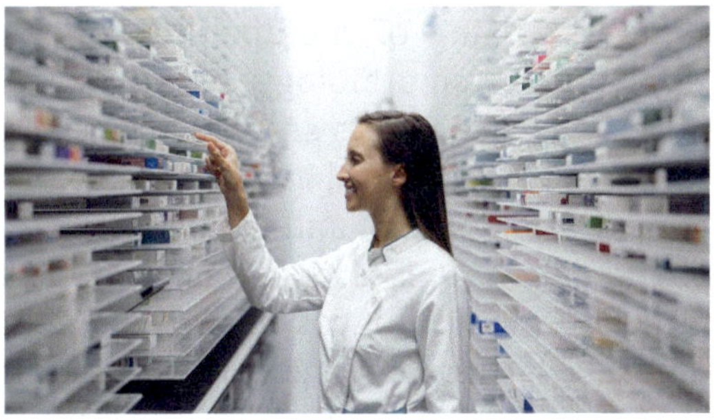

Figure 11.1. The field of clinical pharmacology encompasses the study of drugs and their clinical applications, focusing on understanding how these substances affect human physiology.

Source: https://www.totaljobs.com/advice/wp-content/uploads/what-jobs-can-you-get-with-a-pharmacology-degree-in-the-uk_6214931.jpg.

Importance in Modern Medicine

Clinical pharmacology, as the new science, has greatly revolutionized modern medicine with an enhanced understanding of drug mechanisms and therapeutic applications. This science not only provides a general framework for prescribing drugs safely but also supports individualized therapy tailored to the patient's profile. Personalization is the hallmark in an age when polypharmacy and chronic disease care are the norm. Clinicians rely on the understanding that clinical pharmacology provides for the prevention of adverse drug effects, optimization of therapeutic benefits, and promotion of compliance with treatment regimens. Therefore, the application of pharmacological concepts into clinical practice is a landmark change that supports enhanced health gains and patient safety, a need whose importance deeply resonates in today's medical practice. Furthermore, the integration of clinical evidence and pharmacology continues to drive the development of drugs and therapeutic approaches, substantiating its value in protecting public health and well-being (Terzic et al., 2017). Besides, clinical pharmacology is a core field that is engaged in regulations that direct drug approval and monitoring, to the level of making medications effective and safe to be employed on a mass level. Science incorporates drug effectiveness assessment, safety profiles, and side effects, thereby informing regulatory agencies such as the Food and Drug Administration (FDA) about the potential of new therapeutic drugs. This critical analysis is even more essential in the case of new treatments, such as biologics and personalized medicine, where stringent clinical trials and data analyses are the norm. Without rigorous clinical pharmacological reviews, risks outweighing the benefits of new drugs may threaten patient safety. In addition, the clinical pharmacology practice of encouraging interdisciplinary collaboration among healthcare professionals facilitates widespread strategies in treating patients, enhancing the total capacity to treat numerous medical ailments (Reynolds et al., 2008). With the healthcare environment evolving rapidly, the role of clinical pharmacology extends beyond medicine development and drug safety regulation to encompass education, policy-making, and public health. With the complexity of drug therapies, integration of clinical pharmacology into medical training becomes crucial. Such medical professionals with a strong pharmacological foundation are better equipped to handle the complexities of drug regimens and further improve evidence-based practice. Besides that, engagement of clinical pharmacologists in health care policy can shape regulatory frameworks that favor patient-focused care for medicines. This synoptic view of pharmacotherapy not only informs clinical practice but also directly influences public health policy aimed at maximizing medication adherence and outcomes in populations. Clinical pharmacology is therefore still the cornerstone pillar of modern medicine, the basis on which the therapeutic revolution's power can be realized to maximize health systems globally (Terzic et al., 2017).

Historical Development of the Field

The evolution of clinical pharmacology and therapeutics throughout history is a multifaceted tale that traces the development from herbal remedies in ancient times to sophisticated pharmacologic interventions. Prehistoric human use of natural substances for disease treatment began before written history, much of which was embedded in cultural mores and anecdotal practice. A shift towards a more scientific, systematic approach began in the 19th century with the development of the scientific method, which laid the groundwork for the investigation of drug action and interactions. Pharmacodynamics and pharmacokinetic studies heralded the emergence of pharmacology as an independent discipline. This revolutionary shift laid the foundation for the development of more specific therapeutics, the separation from the mysticism of earlier healing practices, and the establishment of a foundation for today's clinical pharmacology. In the 20th century, rapid progress in biochemistry and molecular biology further developed the field of clinical pharmacology and therapeutics. The discovery of man-made drugs and the development of regulatory principles ushered in a new era of drug development, with a focus on safety and efficacy. The period witnessed key milestones, including the discovery of antibiotics and the development of vaccines, which had significant effects on public health. The synergy between clinicians and pharmacologists increased understanding of drugs' effects on human physiology, enabling personalized medicine approaches. Also, the establishment of pharmacogenomics—how genetic variations affect drug response—has underscored the importance of tailoring treatments to patient profiles, marking yet another milestone in the evolution of the science. In the past decade, the convergence of omics technologies has yielded revolutionary insights into the nature of disease and health and has become a standard tool in clinical pharmacology. The integration of big data analytics and traditional pharmacological research enables the merging of large biological datasets to enhance our understanding of therapeutic processes. By applying systems biology, researchers can identify new drug targets and optimize existing therapies to refine clinical interventions further. This integration of data and medicine is not an epiphenomenon; it is a paradigm shift in the identification and application of therapeutics. As clinical pharmacology advances to address these groundbreaking alterations, it remains committed to advancing therapeutic innovation and maximising patient care in a more complex healthcare context, as attested by the ongoing advances outlined in Alfirevic et al. (2016) and Terzic et al. (2017).

11.1. Pharmacokinetics

Learning Outcome

1. Understand the absorption and bioavailability
2. Define distribution and protein binding
3. Describe the metabolism and excretion

Pharmacokinetics, or what happens to drugs once they have been absorbed into the body, is a core concept in clinical pharmacology and therapeutics. It is essential to know how drugs function within the body to achieve maximum therapeutic benefit while minimizing toxicity. For instance, the rate of drug absorption significantly influences its bioavailability, with direct consequences for its effectiveness in treating various conditions. Other variables, such as drug formulation, route of administration, and the patient's unique characteristics—age, weight, and comorbidities—must be considered to personalize pharmacotherapy. Knowledge of these pharmacokinetic principles allows clinicians to design evidence-based, individualized treatment regimens that deliver the best possible therapy to patients based on their condition. Treatment of conditions like neonatal abstinence syndrome (NAS) is an example of how pharmacokinetics is utilized in clinical practice. For NAS, newborns exposed to opioids in the neonatal period can receive pharmacologic therapy for withdrawal symptoms. The pharmacokinetics of medications such as morphine and methadone are relevant in establishing dosing regimens that provide adequate symptom control. The latest studies on the pharmacokinetics and pharmacodynamics of buprenorphine have been encouraging for use in NAS treatment, demonstrating continued efforts to enhance therapeutic interventions in at-risk groups (Adeniyi-Jones et al., 2017). This ongoing investigation underscores the need to understand how drugs are metabolized by the body to realize clinical benefits better and inform future pharmacological development for children. Moreover, the importance of population heterogeneity cannot be overstated in pharmacokinetics. Variations among patients based on genetics, body status, and environment may considerably influence drug metabolism and effect. During conversations at the American Academy of Veterinary Pharmacology and Therapeutics, researchers highlighted how modeling and simulation methods aid in identifying such variabilities and in using existing pharmacokinetic data to optimize dosing regimens (Bailey et al., 2018). Researchers and clinicians can better predict how various populations will respond to therapies through the investigation of the determinants of dose-exposure-response relationships. This results in more individualized and effective therapies in clinical pharmacology. Understanding such complexities is required to advance therapeutic methods and ensure safe and effective drug use across different patient groups (Figure 11.2).

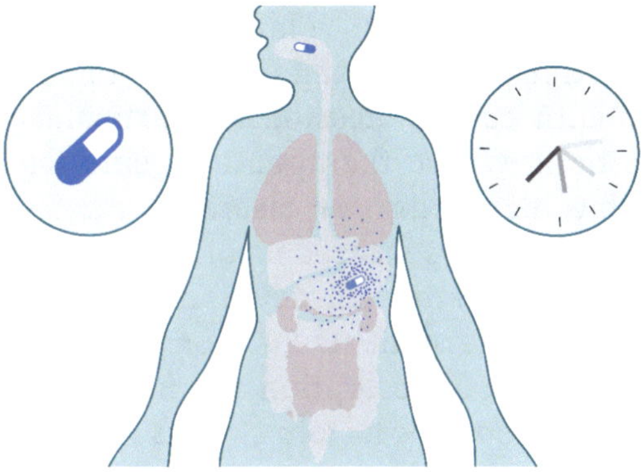

Figure 11.2. Pharmacokinetics.

Source: https://mrctcenter.org/wp-content/uploads/2024/03/pharmacokinetics-Study-PK-study-2023-08-09-1.png.

11.1.1. Absorption and Bioavailability

The processes of absorption and bioavailability are core in clinical pharmacology and are crucial for the success of therapy. Absorption is the movement of drugs from the site of administration to the blood, where they will exert their pharmacological effects. A number of factors affect this process, including the drug's physicochemical properties, formulation, and route of administration. Oral drugs, for instance, must cross the gastrointestinal tract, where pH, food intake, and gastrointestinal motility can significantly affect absorption efficiency. This variability makes it challenging for physicians to account for absorption nuances when prescribing drugs, ensuring patients receive efficacious dosages tailored to their unique physiological conditions. Bioavailability, on the other hand, refers to the proportion of the drug that is presented and enters systemic circulation in unchanged form. It is an predictor of therapeutic action, guiding calculations of dosage and treatment regimens (Kraft et al., 2020). For instance, extensively first-pass metabolized drugs may possess considerably lower bioavailability after oral administration than through parenteral administration. Understanding the relationship between absorption and bioavailability is important for health care professionals, particularly in conditions where therapeutic agents exhibit variable metabolism or clearance rates. This data enables personalized medicine approaches that lead to better efficacy and reduced side effects for the patient. Further complicating the problems of absorption and bioavailability are patient-specific factors such as age, gender, genetics, and disease states.

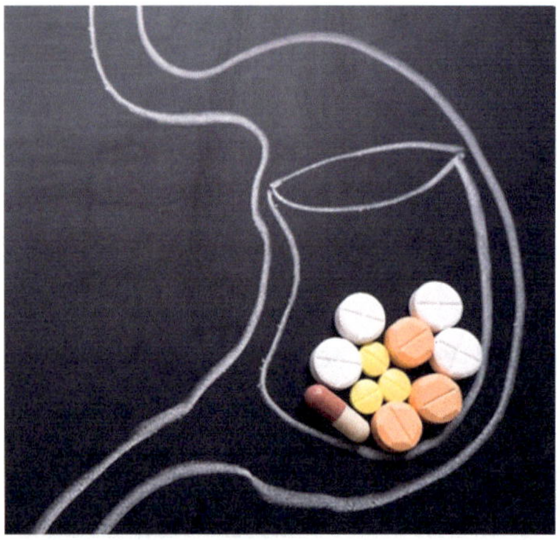

Figure 11.3. Drug absorption is crucial to the effective design and administration of pharmaceuticals, as it directly influences the therapeutic outcomes of medications.

Source: https://d2jx2rerrg6sh3.cloudfront.net/image-handler/picture/2019/6/shutterstock_1185054181.jpg.

These individual differences can significantly impact pharmacokinetics, affecting drug absorption and bioavailability and, as such, its therapeutic effectiveness (Bailey et al., 2018). The pharmacokinetic properties of geriatric patients, for example, may differ significantly from those of young patients, as their physiological functions are altered. Clinicians should thus be keenly aware of these variables and consider them when selecting a drug and prescribing dosages. The combination of absorption processes and subject variability underscores the need for ongoing research and development in pharmacology to maximize therapeutic efficacy in light of the heterogeneity of the patient population in the clinical environment (Figure 11.3).

11.1.2. Distribution and Protein Binding

The distribution of drugs in the body is an important aspect of pharmacokinetics that dictates their therapeutic effect and toxicity. It involves the spreading of drugs among various compartments in the body, e.g., blood, tissues, and organs. Distribution is influenced by the drug's lipophilicity, molecular size, and ability to penetrate biological membranes. In addition, the volume of distribution (Vd) quantifies how much a drug redistributes from the plasma into body tissues. Increased distribution may enhance therapeutic effects; however, excessive side effects or toxicity may occur if concentrations in target tissues exceed therapeutically safe levels. Protein binding contribution to drug distribution should not be overstated because it has a very significant influence on the free (unbound) fraction of a drug, which can cause its pharmacological effects. Protein binding refers to the reversible binding of a drug to plasma proteins, predominantly albumin and alpha-1-acid glycoprotein. This binding has a dual role, often extending the drug's half-life while simultaneously reducing its bioavailability, as the bound drug cannot be measured to exert therapeutic effect. The proportion of serum protein binding dictates the extent to which the drug is available to act on target cells, and this is a significant consideration in determining the drug's efficacy. For instance, in marbofloxacin investigations, an association with 49% protein binding was reported; this altered the unbound serum minimum inhibitory concentrations (MIC) relative to predictions based on total concentration alone (Dorey et al., 2017). Understanding these mechanisms allows clinicians to individualize drug dosages to deliver effective therapy while reducing adverse effects. The clinical importance of protein binding is also exemplified in pharmacodynamic studies linking drug concentrations to their effects. For example, the pharmacodynamics and pharmacokinetics of oxytetracycline highlighted the impact of serum concentrations on bactericidal activity against pathogens such as *Mannheimia haemolytica* and *Pasteurella multocida*. In light of area under the concentration-time curve (AUC) to MIC ratios, evidence indicated that although effective serum concentrations were significantly higher than those derived from broth data under in vivo settings (Aliabadi et al., 2018), this points to the necessity of dependence on serum data for therapeutic dose prediction and necessity for calibration of these with respect to individual patient parameters, including protein binding. Lastly, drug distribution and protein binding must be well understood in order to justify therapeutic strategies in clinical pharmacology and therapeutics.

11.1.3. Metabolism and Excretion

Metabolism and excretion both contribute significantly to the field of clinical pharmacology and therapeutics because they directly influence the pharmacokinetics of drugs. Metabolism is the biochemical transformation of pharmaceuticals within the body, predominantly in the liver by enzymatic mechanisms. These reactions may involve mechanisms such as oxidation, reduction, hydrolysis, and conjugation, forming metabolites that are generally water-soluble and easier to excrete. Variability among individuals in metabolic pathways, particularly those catalyzed by the cytochrome P450 enzyme system, can significantly affect drug efficacy and safety. For example, cytochrome P450 enzyme polymorphisms, such as CYP2C9 and CYP2C19, were found to be implicated in variability in people's metabolism of nonsteroidal anti-inflammatory drugs (NSAIDs), an action that can cause side effects such as NSAID-gastropathy (Balabanseva et al., 2016). Excretion is the second step after metabolism, focusing on the elimination of drugs and metabolites from the body, primarily via the kidneys. Renal excretion includes glomerular filtration, tubular secretion, and reabsorption, and is thus crucial for maintaining therapeutic drug levels. Clinicians need to accurately understand the excretory mechanisms, as compromised renal function can lead to drug accumulation with the potential for toxicity.

This is particularly relevant in drugs with narrow therapeutic windows, where small changes in drug concentration have significant clinical effects. Additionally, renal function plays a significant role in certain drugs, such as aminoglycosides, which require specific monitoring. Further, factors such as age, hydration status, and comorbidities may complicate excretion and necessitate individualized patient assessment for optimal therapeutic effect. Metabolic and excretory interplay is very strongly clinically relevant, primarily in drug interactions and adverse drug reactions. As noted in recent critiques, a deeper understanding of the involved pathways could identify potential biomarkers for predicting nausea and other side effects of drug treatments. Underlying mechanisms for complex symptoms like nausea remain poorly understood, making treatment challenging. Nonetheless, developments in pharmacogenomics may help provide personalized pharmacologic interventions tailored to individual patients based on their metabolic profiles. This emphasizes the importance of continuous clinical pharmacology research, as increased insight into metabolism and excretion can lead to the use of more effective and safer therapeutic regimens (Aapro et al., 2015) (Figure 11.4).

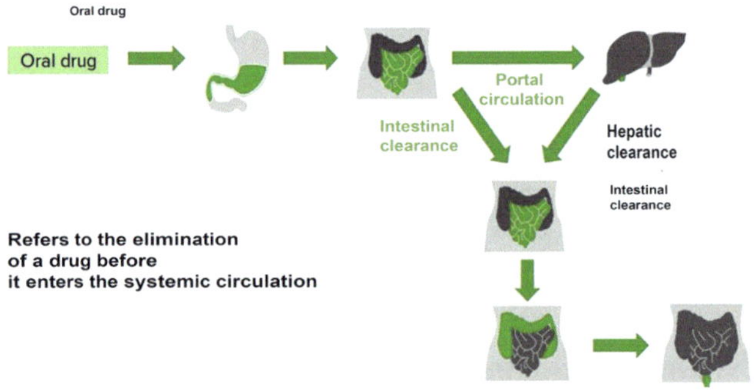

Figure 11.4. The phenomenon of first-pass metabolism plays a pivotal role in pharmacokinetics, primarily affecting the bioavailability of orally administered drugs.

Source: https://cdn.lecturio.com/assets/drug-undergoing-the-first-pass-metabolism.jpg.

Test Your Knowledge

1. What is pharmacokinetics and why is it important in drug therapy?
2. What are the main processes involved in pharmacokinetics? (ADME)

11.2. Pharmacodynamics

Learning Outcome

1. Define the mechanisms of drug action
2. Know the dose-response relationships
3. Describe the therapeutic index and safety

Pharmacodynamics is a fundamental principle of clinical pharmacology that explores the relationship between drug concentrations and their pharmacologic actions. Pharmacodynamics essentially seeks to establish how drugs exert their actions at the site of action to cause their desired therapeutic effects, including drug-receptor interactions and the consequent biological response. An understanding of such principles is essential for clinicians in optimizing treatment regimens, particularly in the management of complex conditions like neonatal abstinence syndrome (NAS). In NAS, a neonate exposed to opioids in utero may present with symptoms requiring pharmacologic intervention. Morphine and methadone are examples of first-line pharmacological treatments, with consideration given to the need for knowledge of their pharmacodynamics to optimally reduce the horrific symptoms of affected neonates (Adeniyi-Jones et al., 2017). Thus, this information has direct application in decision-making in the clinical setting, enhancing the overall treatment of infected babies. Pharmacodynamics also plays a critical role in effective infection treatment, particularly in patients receiving peritoneal dialysis. Peritoneal dialysis-associated peritonitis patients require strict application of the pharmacodynamic principles to ensure significant therapy outcomes. Intraperitoneal vancomycin is administered as first-line treatment regularly, but dosing regimens in patients on automated peritoneal dialysis (APD) are usually empiric in nature with less strong clinical evidence. It is also essential to understand the pharmacodynamic interactions because it help to achieve drug concentrations that result in desired antimicrobial action with the minimum amount of adverse effects. Recent studies have attempted to fill knowledge gaps in vancomycin dosing among patients with CAPD and APD, underscoring the urgent need to correlate pharmacokinetic information with pharmacodynamic effects to develop more effective dosing algorithms in clinical practice (Kraft et al., 2020). With advances in pharmacodynamics, ongoing clinical research remains significant in developing successful treatment regimens.

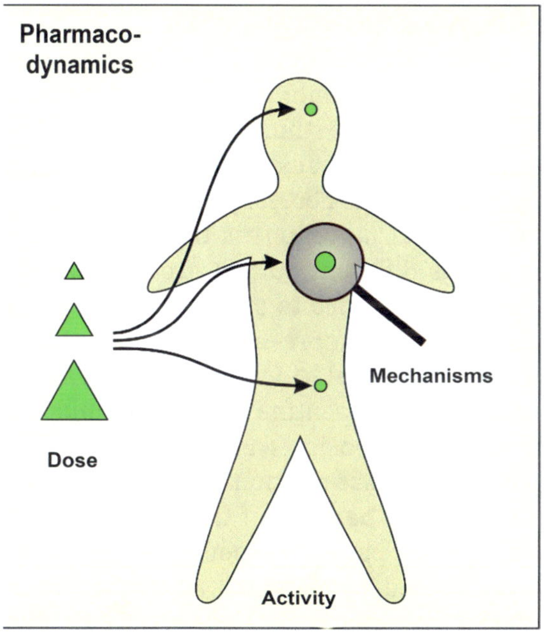

Figure 11.5. Pharmacodynamics.

Source: https://upload.wikimedia.org/wikipedia/commons/thumb/c/c5/Pharmacodynamics.svg/1200px-Pharmacodynamics.svg.png.

The nuanced interaction of drug effects with patient physiology and disease states demands an integrated pharmacotherapy strategy. For instance, as practitioners seek to maximize therapeutic outcomes, they must also consider the heterogeneity of drug response driven by genetic, environmental, or pathological factors. For the management of NAS and peritoneal dialysis-related infections, the successful application of pharmacodynamic concepts can provide a platform for customized therapies providing maximal efficacy with minimal risk. In sum, a strong understanding of pharmacodynamics enables healthcare providers to make appropriate choices in drug selection, dosing, and monitoring, and it is part of the larger scheme of clinical pharmacology and therapeutics (Figure 11.5).

11.2.1. Mechanisms of Drug Action

Understanding mechanisms of drug action is essential in clinical pharmacology in designing effective therapeutic interventions. Drugs can act by binding to their intended biological targets, predominantly proteins such as receptors, enzymes, and ion channels. Agonists, for instance, bind to receptors and activate them, mimicking the effects of endogenous molecules within the body, whereas antagonists block receptors, thereby inhibiting their activation. This dynamic interaction is central to facilitating physiological responses and therapeutic action. By studying such mechanisms, scientists can uncover the pharmacodynamics of drugs, thereby significantly influencing drug formulation and administration routes. Robust mechanistic insight enables clinicians to make optimally informed decisions regarding treatment regimens, dose titration, and potential drug interactions, thereby optimizing patient care in numerous therapeutic situations. In addition to receptor interaction, metabolic activities that regulate drug effects are also crucial in pharmacology. Drugs are biotransformed mainly in the liver, in particular by enzymes that activate or deactivate pharmacologic entities. Metabolic activation can affect drug efficacy and toxicity, underscoring the importance of understanding individual drug metabolic heterogeneity. Genetic polymorphisms in drug-metabolizing enzymes can lead to differences in drug response among patients, necessitating the use of personalized medicine and therapies. Also, research into adverse drug reactions determines how unanticipated alterations in these metabolic pathways can lead to toxic outcomes. Knowledge of such metabolic mechanisms is essential for formulating safe and effective treatment regimens, thereby developing an integrated approach to patient safety in clinical therapeutics. Despite the advancements in understanding drug mechanisms, certain areas remain less clear, especially concerning complex phenomena such as nausea. Nausea can arise from numerous stimuli and is often a side effect of medications. Current research highlights the multifaceted neural pathways associated with nausea, which remain poorly understood. Synthesizing animal model and human evidence, researchers continue to investigate the mechanisms underlying this side effect, with an eye towards identifying potential therapeutic targets to prevent it. As highlighted in recent literature, improved understanding of these mechanisms could lead to the development of clinically useful biomarkers for nausea, providing enhanced management options in human and veterinary medicine (Aapro et al., 2015). Therefore, further study of such mechanisms is vital to maximize therapeutic efficacy and patient quality of life (Beeh et al., 2015).

11.2.2. Dose-response Relationships

The investigation of dose-response relationships is at the heart of clinical pharmacology and therapeutics practice since it illustrates how the response of the drug is associated with its concentration in the body. Accurate interpretation of such relationships enables clinicians to determine the optimal drug dose that balances efficacy and safety, minimizing toxicity and maximizing benefits. Such relationships are complex primarily because of factors such as differences between individual patients, including genetic differences, age, and pre-existing health conditions. Such differences complicate the formulation of generic dosing recommendations and, as such, highlight the necessity for patient-specific therapy plans founded on characteristics unique to patients and influencing drug metabolism and response. In addition, advances in pharmacokinetic and pharmacodynamic modeling techniques enhance our understanding of dose-response relationships. This allows researchers to forecast patient-specific responses based on available pharmacokinetic information, thereby enhancing recommendations for various populations. An example is veterinary pharmacology, where population heterogeneity was examined at a recent meeting of the American Academy of Veterinary Pharmacology and Therapeutics. Here, the significance of simulation and modelling was recognized in determining sources of variability that influence the therapeutic use of drugs across different species and, by implication, proposed the same necessity in human medicine: establishing drug regimens that work but are safe across different patient groups (Bailey et al., 2018). Reference to specific drug examples could illuminate more on the implications of dose-response relationships in therapeutic contexts. The rifapentine case, an antibiotic for treating tuberculosis, is used to illustrate that exposure-response relationships are essential in optimizing the benefits of treatment. Evidence indicates that patient responses to rifapentine are influenced by patients' demographic and clinical characteristics, such as co-infection with HIV and the size of lung cavities. The findings suggest that a maximal treatment effect may require higher doses of rifapentine, especially in patients with extensive lung cavities and reduced response even at high doses (Dooley et al., 2017). This situation attests to the necessity of tailoring drug dosing to a patient's specific conditions and underscores ongoing challenges in delineating consistent exposure-response models across varied populations in the clinical environment.

11.2.3. Therapeutic Index and Safety

In therapeutics and clinical pharmacology, the therapeutic index (TI) is an important metric for assessing a drug's safety and efficacy. It is a ratio measure of the toxic dose to the effective dose and is used to indicate a larger margin between therapeutic and toxic effects, thereby enhancing the drug's safety profile. In the management of conditions such as psoriatic arthritis (PsA), the intricacies of the therapeutic index become more apparent. The introduction of tumor necrosis factor inhibitors (TNFi) has greatly improved clinical outcomes for many patients, but their associated safety concerns underscore the importance of determining their TI in practice. Understanding of drug pharmacokinetics and immunogenicity enables clinicians to tailor therapeutic regimens for effectiveness, a safeguard for patients who are not well responsive to therapy or who experience worsening efficacy over time, as the literature currently indicates (Kraft et al., 2017). Drug stereochemistry research contributes to ongoing discussions of therapeutic indices and safety. Because many synthetic chiral drugs are marketed as racemic mixtures, the individual enantiomers often exhibit significant differences in pharmacology and toxicology. Awareness of stereochemistry's role in drug action underscores the potential benefits of developing enantiomerically pure drugs, which could improve therapeutic ratios while reducing side effects. Through racemic decoupling, the pharmacologist can create drugs that are not only more effective but also offer a greater margin of safety. This consideration requires a critical re-examination of regulatory policy in drug registration, and the specific need to examine the implications of chirality in assessing a drug's overall safety profile and therapeutic utility (Mifsud et al., 1994). Lastly, the therapeutic index is an essential measure in the interaction of clinical pharmacology and patient safety. While the therapeutic effects of such agents like TNFi in the management of PsA are compelling, they also indicate the immediate need for continuous monitoring and evaluation of the patient. An elevated TI is a promising therapeutic approach; however, clinicians remain cautious about the potential side effects that can arise from pharmacologic interventions. Therapeutic conditions evolve with the addition of novel biologics and chiral drugs, yet the fine balance between efficacy and safety remains a greater concern. Thus, future research must focus on maximizing the therapeutic index through pharmacogenomics and personalized medicine approaches to enhance safety and therapeutic benefit and to develop more effective health interventions (Figure 11.6).

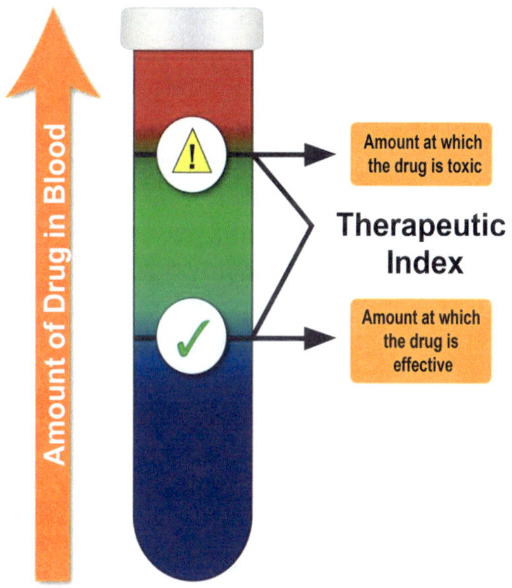

Figure 11.6. Therapeutic index (TI) serves as a crucial metric in evaluating the safety and efficacy of a drug.

Source: https://clinicalinfo.hiv.gov/sites/default/files/glossaries/images/Therapeutic-Index-800.jpg.

Test Your Knowledge

1. What is pharmacodynamics and how does it affect drug action in the body?
2. How do drug-receptor interactions influence therapeutic and adverse effects?

11.3. Drug Development Process

Learning Outcome

1. Define the preclinical research and testing
2. Discuss on clinical trial phases
3. Understand the regulatory approval and post-marketing surveillance

The drug development process is a multi-aspect and well-regimented process through which a new substance is transformed into an approved drug product. In preclinical studies, the process involves laboratory-based research and animal experiments to assess the safety, efficacy, and pharmacokinetic properties of the compounds. Scientists examine how the drug interacts with biological systems, specifically absorption, distribution, metabolism, and excretion (ADME). Clarification of these factors is crucial for forecasting human responses and detecting potential adverse effects. Furthermore, lessons learned from such studies inform the subsequent design of clinical trials. For this reason, the preclinical stage is critical for safeguarding the development of a drug rationale and dosage regimen determination as it progresses to human trials, which can be riddled with heterogeneity in patient responses to interventions (Bailey et al., 2018). Whereas, in clinical trials, the drug development is rigorously conducted through phases I to III to assess the compound's safety and efficacy in human patients. Phase I recruits small cohorts of healthy volunteers, primarily focusing on safety, pharmacokinetics, and determining the appropriate dosage. Phase II expands the participant pool to include subjects with the target condition, with a focus on efficacy and additional safety testing. Finally, Phase III trials are conducted in large populations across multiple sites to provide comprehensive information on the drug's efficacy and any unusual side effects that may not have appeared in earlier stages. All these phases require thoughtful planning and ethical considerations, with patient safety as the highest priority. Efficient performance in these trials is paramount for regulatory authorization and ensuring that the drug is effective enough to meet medical demands (Reynolds et al., 2008). Once the clinical trials are complete, regulatory bodies such as the FDA comprehensively examine the evidence gathered before approving market entry.

This rigorous testing includes taking into consideration the evidence strength on the drug's efficacy and safety, together with the procedures employed in manufacturing to ensure quality. Upon approval, the drug enters the post-marketing surveillance phase, also known as Phase IV, where real-world experience regarding its long-term effects, performance across different populations, and any side effects is documented. The post-marketing surveillance phase is crucial in continuously assessing the drug's risk-benefit ratio among the general population. In addition, post-marketing surveillance evidence can lead to recommendations for label changes or restrictions to keep clinical pharmacology abreast of continually emerging evidence (Bailey et al., 2018). The drug development process thus demonstrates a commitment not only to scientific advancement but also to patient safety and public health (Figure 11.7).

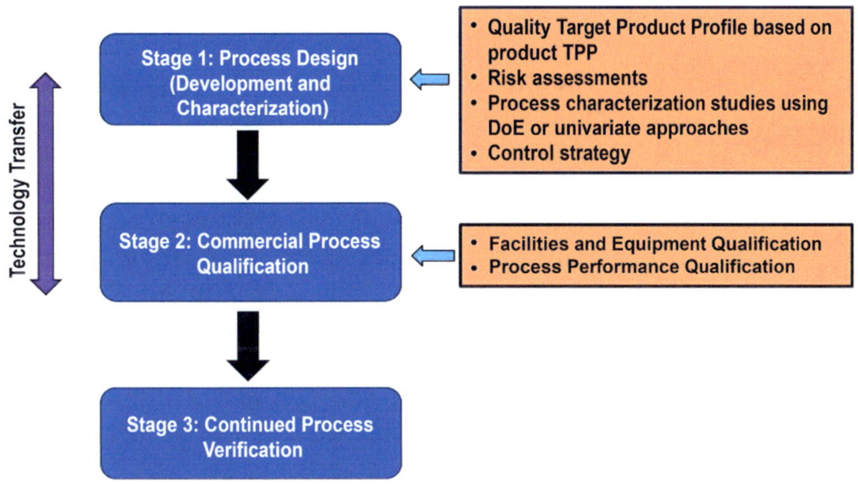

Figure 11.7. The stages of drug development are critical in ensuring the safety and efficacy of pharmaceutical interventions before they reach the market.

Source: https://jpharmsci.org/cms/10.1016/j.xphs.2023.11.004/asset/1e6275ff-b79d-4fc9-a5d8-8d14364c4606/main.assets/gr2_lrg.jpg.

11.3.1. Preclinical Research and Testing

Preclinical research and testing represent the critical interface between basic scientific discovery and clinical application in clinical pharmacology and therapeutics. The research phase primarily consists of animal studies and in vitro experiments to assess the pharmacokinetics, efficacy, and safety of new drugs before they are exposed to human trials. The value of preclinical assessment, for instance, is that it can identify toxicological impacts and suitable dosing regimens, thereby safeguarding patients' health during the transition to the clinical setting. Aside from this, the stage allows researchers to evaluate new drug candidates in relevant biological systems and provide information on mechanisms of action and therapeutic utility. Reliable preclinical models are necessary in cardiovascular medicine, where the complexity of human disease mandates rigorous testing paradigms that can accurately predict clinical outcomes. A growing area of research in preclinical science is the application of human induced pluripotent stem cells (iPSCs) to drug discovery and disease modeling. iPSCs are increasingly sought after for their ability to differentiate into various cardiovascular cell types and to enable personalized medicine approaches in drug development and screening. The ease of iPSC malleability allows researchers to generate patient-specific models that reproduce individual genetic backgrounds without the limitations commonly associated with animal models. Although traditional drug discovery efforts have relied heavily on such animal models, their inherent interspecies heterogeneity can lead to misleading results in humans. Increasingly, iPSCs are a sophisticated platform that can enhance the reproducibility of preclinical studies and the translational potency of cardiovascular therapeutics – a field that has historically lagged behind oncology (Chandy et al., 2020). Preclinical efficacy is evidenced by studies of the pharmacological actions of compounds such as levo-tetrahydropalmatine (l-THP), with therapeutic promise for addiction treatment. Studies have demonstrated that l-THP potently inhibits the cocaine-reinforcing effect in model animals, providing a rationale for its possible application in the clinic. The transition from the bench to the bedside entails rigorous testing of compounds at preclinical levels to assess efficacy, determine dosing recommendations, and characterize safety profiles. The studies help map the therapeutic benefits and identify potential side effects in formulating the drug. As studies progress, l-THP illustrates the challenges of winning regulatory approval, illustrating the inexorably required preclinical validation to support clinical trials and finally assist addicted patients (Mantsch et al., 2012).

11.3.2. Clinical Trial Phases

The journey of clinical trials is important in safe and effective drug development. Typically divided into four phases, clinical trials begin with Phase I, which is generally focused on assessing the safety and side effects of an experimental drug in a small group of healthy volunteers. It determines the drug's pharmacokinetics and pharmacodynamics, ensuring safe dosage levels. As was noted at the American Academy of Veterinary Pharmacology and Therapeutics meeting, between-population variation can be important at this stage in guiding dosing regimens (Bailey et al., 2018). By considering variation among individuals in response to the drug, scientists can begin to understand how the drug behaves in a heterogeneous group of patients, including what may be driving therapeutic effects. Following the critical safety testing of Phase I, Phase II trials increase the number of patients to a larger population that may have the diseases the drugs will treat. It not only tests the effectiveness of the drug but also closely monitors its safety profile in great detail. The data obtained from Phase II are pivotal, as they provide a foundation for optimizing dose and calculating risk-benefit in advance of translating results into larger populations. The learning obtained can be applied to pharmacometric model-based approaches that combine different data sources, as discussed in veterinary pharmacology settings (Bailey et al., 2018). These models enable scientists to predict therapeutic efficacy and optimize dosing, bringing us closer to the era of personalized medicine. Finally, please, Phase III trials are conducted on even larger groups of patients to confirm the therapeutic activity discovered in earlier phases, while still assessing how well the drug performs and monitoring for long-term side effects. This phase cannot be stressed enough in terms of relevance, because favorable outcomes lead to regulatory submissions and, eventually, product approval. In addition, Phase III findings are translated into practical application, particularly in terms of the evaluation of diseases like neonatal abstinence syndrome (NAS), where the accurate dosing of medications like buprenorphine can be calculated based on trial data. As the process of clinical trial development continues to evolve, these phases are an integral component of the broader practice of clinical pharmacology and therapeutics, ensuring that novel treatments are both safe and effective for the broader patient population.

11.3.3. Regulatory Approval and Post-marketing Surveillance

Regulatory approval is a significant clinical pharmacology and therapeutics practice because it certifies the safety and effectiveness of drug products before they go on the market. Governments and regulatory agencies, such as the Food and Drug Administration (FDA) in the USA, are the authorities responsible for scrutinizing data presented by manufacturers, such as outcomes of clinical trials and post-marketing requirements. This thorough assessment seeks to ensure that a drug's benefits outweigh its risks. However, due to pressure to speed up approval processes, there is often apprehension about compromising safety standards, as one can observe an overdose of conflicting global regulatory approaches. The recent launch of the South African Health Products Regulatory Authority (SAHPRA) is a case in point of efforts to centralize regulatory systems and address issues such as application backlogs and long product registration timelines, in a bid to harmonize regulatory processes (Antrobus et al., 2018). Post-marketing surveillance is a required complement to the initial regulatory approval process, serving as a tool of ongoing monitoring of drugs when they are in widespread use. While pre-approval testing subjects its subjects to controlled conditions, post-marketing surveillance extends its scope to a broader, more diverse population and thus identifies possible adverse effects that did not appear in clinical trials. Monitoring is needed, since in certain instances risk factors or side effects may only arise in specific populations or after prolonged use. The FDA and other regulatory bodies are working diligently to collect information from healthcare providers and patients so that any safety concerns can be addressed promptly. By enhancing pharmacovigilance activities, regulators can further ensure public health and establish trust in the therapeutic use of drugs (Abbott et al., 2014). The interaction between post-marketing surveillance and regulatory approval indicates a dynamic balance between safeguarding public health and facilitating access to new therapies. While enhanced regulation can improve drug safety, it can also delay patient access to otherwise therapeutic drugs. The regulatory landscape must balance on a risk-based system, weighing the needs of extensive investigations against patient demand pressures. Increased requirements for off-label reporting and strengthening of post-market surveillance programs are central to maintaining balance. Moreover, a more refined system of categories of drug use could distinguish safer therapeutic options from those of less evidentiary support. Eventually, proactive approaches in regulatory licensure and surveillance are necessary to create an effective pharmaceutical environment that honors patient safety while encouraging therapeutic advancement (Abbott et al., 2014; Antrobus et al., 2018).

Test Your Knowledge

1. What are the main stages involved in the development of a new drug?
2. Why is clinical testing essential before a drug is approved for use?

11.4. Therapeutic Drug Monitoring (TDM)

Learning Outcome

1. Understand the importance of monitoring drug levels
2. Describe the factors affecting drug response
3. Identify the case studies in therapeutic drug monitoring (TDM)

Effective TDM is essential in clinical pharmacology and therapeutics because it ensures the optimal drug dosage tailored to an individual's pharmacokinetic features. TDM relies on measurement of drug levels in body fluids to ascertain whether a patient is receiving an adequate dose for therapeutic effect with minimal toxicity. Variability in patient response generally requires monitoring; age, weight, organ function, and concomitant medications all contribute to considerable interpatient variation in drug clearance and metabolism. Such variation is particularly pertinent in populations with established variability. As described in reports from a recent pharmacology conference, variability influences dose-exposure-response relationships. It requires modeling and simulation techniques to optimize drug therapy in heterogeneous patient populations (Bailey et al., 2018). Thus, TDM is very valuable, especially with drugs having a narrow therapeutic index, where dosing with known precision can make all the difference in patient outcomes. In the critically ill patient, however, the issue with TDM is further compounded. Conditions requiring sophisticated therapeutic interventions, such as extracorporeal membrane oxygenation (ECMO), have a significant effect on the pharmacokinetics of various drugs. In these situations, TDM is necessary to make sure that drug exposures are appropriately controlled despite physiological changes induced by interventions like ECMO. Because ECMO can alter pharmacokinetic profiles, reducing efficacy or increasing side effects, continuous monitoring is a key part of patient management. Research has established that drug-specific changes in pharmacokinetics remain poorly characterized, highlighting the imperative to continue research aimed at providing guidelines for TDM in such populations (Aebi et al., 2017). Such monitoring protocols not only improve therapeutic outcomes but also enhance patient safety by enabling clinicians to make informed decisions. Furthermore, the integration of TDM into routine clinical practice is evolving as advances in technology improve measurement accuracy and timeliness. The evolution of point-of-care testing and pharmacogenomic genotyping is enabling more tailored approaches to drug management. By identifying genetic factors that affect drug metabolism, clinicians can adjust dosing strategies and thereby enhance the utility of TDM. Tailored disease management is particularly relevant in disease conditions where chronic disease is being managed through prolonged drug use. As the field advances, the role of TDM will remain integral to clinical pharmacology and therapeutics, as it continues to provide personalized patient care optimized for therapeutic efficacy while minimizing adverse drug reactions. The technologies and methods that underpin TDM will increasingly be at the center of defining clinical outcomes as we enhance our understanding of pharmacotherapy (Figure 11.8).

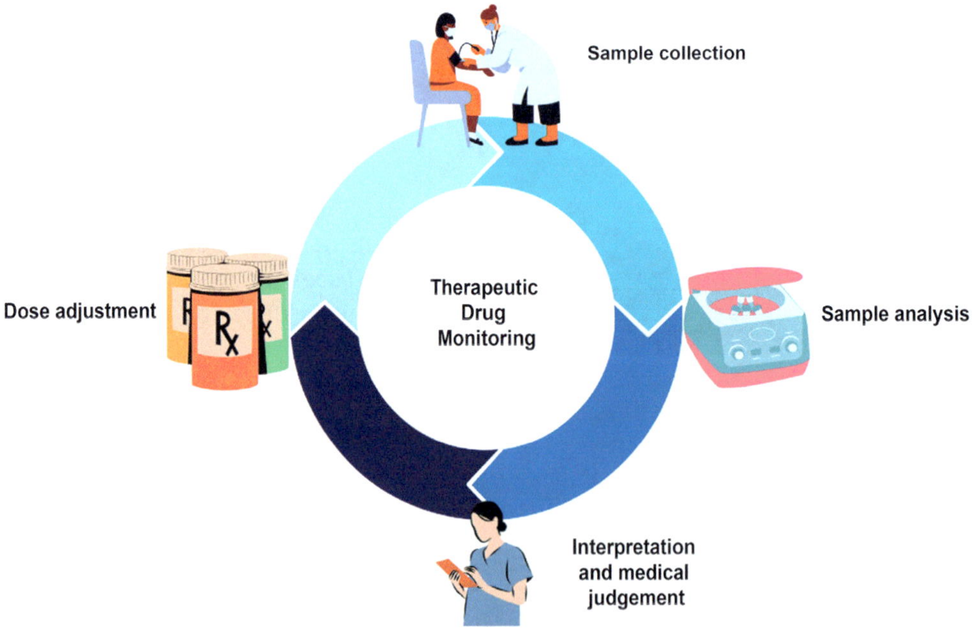

Figure 11.8. Therapeutic drug monitoring (TDM).

Source: https://www.mdpi.com/pharmaceuticals/pharmaceuticals-17-00642/article_deploy/html/images/pharmaceuticals-17-00642-g001.png.

11.4.1. Importance of Monitoring Drug Levels

Monitoring drug levels is important for enhancing the safety and efficacy of pharmacotherapy. The rationale of TDM ensures that the drug is at a concentration within a predetermined therapeutic range, thereby reducing the risk of side effects and treatment failure. The method becomes increasingly important for drugs with a narrow therapeutic index, where the margin between therapeutic and toxic concentrations is narrow. Maintenance of proper drug levels is essential in the treatment of chronic illnesses, like epilepsy or cardiovascular disorders, where sustained exposure to drugs can profoundly affect patient outcomes. Regular monitoring, therefore, enables timely adjustment of dosing regimens so that clinicians can tailor treatments to the unique needs of individual patients. Personalized treatment through this method increases the efficacy of drugs while minimizing the risk of adverse effects due to suboptimal drug administration. In veterinary pharmacology, the role of drug level monitoring is also expressed in terms of the population variability concept, as argued by recent controversies in pharmacologic symposia. Population variability may significantly influence dose-exposure-response relationships, and therefore, a profound understanding of how different physiological characteristics interact with drug pharmacokinetics is imperative. Such diversity is particularly relevant when one considers the role that up-to-date pharmacokinetic data and modeling software can play in streamlining dosing regimens across various species. By incorporating both observed and predicted outcomes, clinicians can better cope with the complexities of veterinary medicine. This justification aligns with a broader trend in clinical pharmacology, emphasizing the importance of tailoring treatments to systematic evidence and modeling, as evidenced by the outcomes of the 2017 Biennial meeting of the American Academy of Veterinary Pharmacology and Therapeutics (Bailey et al., 2018). Similarly, monitoring of drug levels is an essential component of specialist treatment settings such as peritoneal dialysis (PD), where empirical dosing strategies often prevail due to insufficient data. For instance, vancomycin, employed in the treatment of PD-related peritonitis, requires accurate determination of dosing regimens that can significantly differ between CAPD and APD patients. Given the complexity of pharmacokinetic profiles in these populations, using available data to guide dosing and avoid underdosing or toxicity is required. A proposed dosing algorithm for PD patients aims to address knowledge gaps while accounting for patient variability and drug disposition, underscoring the importance of individualized pharmacotherapy. Therefore, ongoing monitoring and adjustments according to monitoring drug levels is all inclusive to optimizing clinical outcomes in patients on specialized treatment regimens (Kraft et al., 2020).

11.4.2. Factors Affecting Drug Response

It is essential in clinical pharmacology and therapeutics practice to understand the several determinants of drug response. Genetic patient differences are a significant factor in how patients metabolize and respond to drugs. Genetic polymorphisms may affect drug-target pathways, enhancing or diminishing the efficacy of pharmacological agents. For instance, alterations in drug-metabolizing enzymes, such as cytochrome P450, can profoundly affect drug pharmacokinetics. As a result, personalized medicine, i.e., the individualization of therapeutic strategies based on an individual's genetic susceptibility, has emerged as a key intervention to achieve optimal drug effectiveness with minimal risk of adverse effects. This focus on genetic factors enables the optimization of treatment protocols so that patients are treated with the most appropriate drugs for their personalized biochemical contexts. Environmental factors also greatly impact drug response, such as diet, lifestyle, and co-existing medical illnesses. Dietary influences are particularly significant, as the consumption of certain foods can augment or decrease drug metabolism. For instance, grapefruit juice is said to be a cytochrome P450 enzyme inhibitor, leading to elevated plasma concentrations of some drugs and thereby enhancing the risk of toxicity. Additionally, environmental factors like alcohol consumption and smoking can also interact against drug metabolism and action, necessitating dosing regimen modification. Furthermore, the presence of co-existing medical conditions can modify pharmacotherapeutic effects. For example, chronic kidney disease will reduce drug clearance and require careful dose adjustment to avoid accumulation and toxicity. Such an interaction emphasizes the value of proper patient evaluation in daily practice to implement more subtle prescribing strategies that consider environmental variation. Pharmacological issues also contribute significantly to the factors involved in the response to drugs. Route of administration, dosage form, and dosage will have considerable effects on therapeutic effects. For instance, the absorption rates of orally administered medications can differ based on the gastrointestinal pH, presence of food, and the integrity of the gastrointestinal tract. Furthermore, the choice of drug formulation—whether immediate-release versus extended-release—can affect the duration and intensity of therapeutic effects. The pharmacodynamics of drug interaction with target receptors also differ from person to person, based on receptor density, affinity, and downstream signaling. In certain situations, such as the case of opioid analgesic use in pregnant patients, pharmacokinetic and pharmacodynamic considerations become even more complicated, as evidenced by the treatment of neonatal abstinence syndrome after prenatal opioid exposure (Davis et al., 2016). Therefore, a full understanding of these intricate factors is essential for the pursuit of effective and safe therapeutic regimens (Figure 11.9).

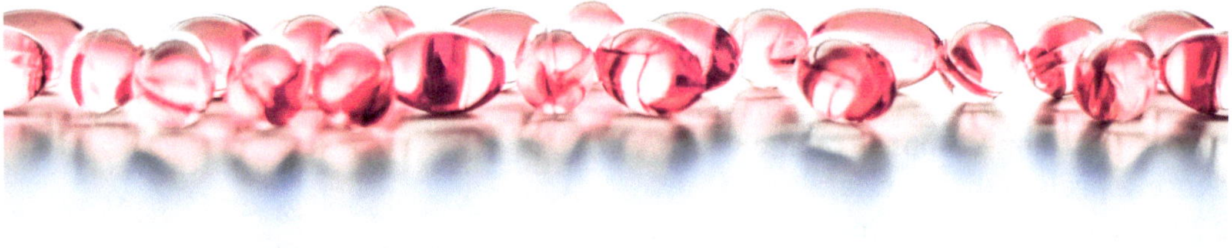

Figure 11.9. A drugs therapeutic range is the concentration within which it yields the desired therapeutic effect without producing toxicity.

Source: https://www.allucent.com/wp-content/uploads/2020/04/What-is-Toxicokinetics-TK_.webp.

11.4.3. Case Studies in Therapeutic Drug Monitoring (TDM)

TDM significantly contributes to optimizing pharmacotherapy and minimizing adverse effects, especially with drugs of narrow therapeutic index. TDM case studies illustrate how variability among individual patients, due to genetic, physiologic, and environmental factors, affects drug metabolism and response. Variability in liver enzymes, for instance, can create significant differences in drug clearance rates between patients. Such measurement allows clinicians to titrate the dosage based on instantaneous levels, thereby enhancing therapeutic effect while reducing toxicity. The applicability of such monitoring practice is highlighted under discussion on population heterogeneity and model simulation tool usage to forecast dose-exposure-response relationships, as at the American Academy of Veterinary Pharmacology and Therapeutics conference (Bailey et al., 2018). A patient case history of ECMO treatment highlights the subtleties of TDM during treatment-induced physiological alterations. ECMO is responsible for modulating pharmacokinetic parameters, thereby altering drug absorption, distribution, metabolism, and excretion. As a result, clinicians frequently encounter difficulties achieving optimal drug levels and therapeutic efficacy.

For instance, drugs with high protein binding are found to experience changes in efficacy when plasma volume and the proteins' binding capacity are changed during ECMO. The need for customized dosing regimens based on continuous drug concentration monitoring arises, as one needs to minimize the risk of dangerous drug interactions and ensure optimal therapeutic effects. It underscores the importance of developing specific regulations for drug administration in specialized patients, given the complexity of pharmacotherapy (Aebi et al., 2017). Moreover, the inclusion of case studies in TDM can enhance our understanding of how some drugs respond to specific patient circumstances. When these studies are published, they provide helpful information about best practices for medication management, particularly for those medications that must be accurately dosed. By documenting patient responses and drug concentrations, clinicians can identify trends and develop improved monitoring regimens. The clinical application of these observations transcends numerous patient groups, for instance, patients with comorbidities or on intensive regimens, where drug interactions and shifts in pharmacokinetics may be the rule. Ultimately, optimizing TDM practice through ongoing case studies will lead to enhanced patient safety and more personalized therapeutic control, in turn facilitating the key role of pharmacokinetic information in clinical pharmacology and therapeutics.

Test Your Knowledge

1. What is the purpose of therapeutic drug monitoring in patient care?
2. Which types of drugs commonly require monitoring to ensure safety and efficacy?

11.5. Adverse Drug Reactions (ADRs)

Learning Outcome

1. Describe the types of adverse drug reactions (ADRS)
2. Define the risk factors and patient demographics
3. Identify the strategies for prevention and management

ADRs are a significant challenge in therapeutics and clinical pharmacology and influence treatment effectiveness as well as patient safety. ADRs are unintended or adverse effects resulting from the administration of medication. They may be mild, such as nausea, or lethal, such as anaphylaxis or organ failure. Increased complexity of patient care and polypharmacy, where patients are prescribed several drugs, increases the risk of ADR exposure. Moreover, individual characteristics such as genetics, age, and comorbidities contribute to susceptibility to ADRs. Clinicians play a significant role in the understanding of the reactions since it inform risk evaluation and management during drug prescription. The post-thalidomide historical backdrop highlighted the need for rigorous testing and monitoring of drugs, which has affected the current pharmaceutical regulatory landscape, as noted in accounts of the evolution of clinical pharmacology during the mid-20th century (Reynolds et al., 2008). The development and severity of ADRs necessitate thorough pharmacovigilance—an integral component of clinical pharmacology. This ongoing process encompasses detection, assessment, and prevention of adverse effects resulting from the consumption of drugs. Establishing comprehensive databases and reporting systems has enabled the detection of patterns and trends in ADR events, providing valuable information for healthcare professionals. Advances in technology, including the integration of electronic health records, have further enhanced the ability to monitor ADRs in real time, enabling early intervention. Despite these limitations, underreporting remains the most significant hindrance, typically due to a lack of awareness among patients and healthcare providers regarding the importance of reporting such reactions. With efforts to increase ADR reporting and publicity, clinical pharmacology can enhance patient protection in healthcare and maximize therapeutic modalities (Marsh et al., 2010). Moreover, the introduction of personalized medicine has the potential to significantly reduce the incidence of ADRs. By utilizing genetic and metabolic profiles, clinicians can tailor pharmacotherapy to the individual patient, increasing efficacy at the expense of side effects. It is consistent with the principles of network pharmacology that more integrative drug development and drug optimization will yield therapeutic benefits and optimize outcomes. Personalized medicine not only addresses the issue of variability in drug responses but also emphasizes understanding ADR mechanisms. With the advancement of this field, integrating concepts from both personalized medicine and network pharmacology is likely to revolutionize drug development, rendering therapies safer and more efficient for different patient populations (Marsh et al., 2010) (Figure 11.10).

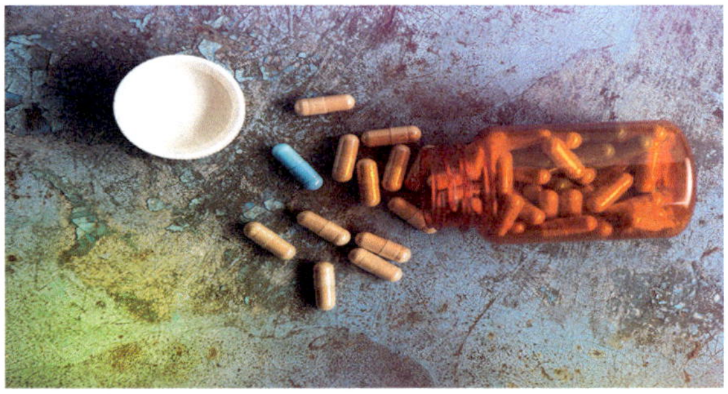

Figure 11.10. Adverse drug reactions (ADRs).

Source: https://hospitalpharmacyeurope.com/wp-content/uploads/2004/03/ADR-1.jpg.

11.5.1. Types of Adverse Drug Reactions (ADRs)

The classification of ADRs is critical for understanding their role in therapeutics and clinical pharmacology. ADRs can be divided into two general categories: Type A (augmented) and Type B (bizarre) reactions. Type A reactions are dose-related and predictable; they occur most commonly due to the drug's pharmacologic action. Such reactions, for example, side effects of nausea with antibiotics or sedation with opioids, are likely to be expected based on the drug's known characteristics. Type B, on the other hand, is idiosyncratic, unpredictable, and nondose-related, due to patient-specific sensitivities or genetic predisposition. Awareness of these types enables healthcare professionals to anticipate possible reactions, leading to improved patient management and safety, and thus further advocating the need for ongoing ADR monitoring and reporting by professionals to prevent drug therapy-related risks. A survey of ADRs reveals their heterogeneity in severity and clinical effects, which significantly affects patient outcomes. In a study on admission to medical wards, it was observed that 76.8% of ADRs were mild, yet 66% were severe enough to necessitate immediate medical intervention.

This accentuates the danger of ADRs to hospitalized patients and, in worst cases, to death since reports indicate that at most three patients in this category died of ADR-related complications. Of most significant concern were reactions to commonly used substitutes for antimicrobials and central nervous system (CNS) drugs, which accounted for a large percentage of adverse events recorded. The study shows that a significant proportion of ADRs could be due to drug interaction and mutual play of certain drugs, and hence the need for vigilant monitoring to prevent morbidity and mortality caused by adverse drug reactions in therapeutic settings (Adhikari et al., 2009). As the field of personalized medicine evolves, the role of pharmacogenetics in preventing and managing ADRs cannot be overemphasized. Genetic polymorphisms have a significant bearing on the drug response of individuals, usually producing varying amounts of therapeutic effects or side effects. Pharmacogenetic testing has proven to be a fascinating field, enabling targeted drug treatment based on an individual's genetic variation and thereby optimizing therapeutic potential while minimizing risk. By being able to identify patients at risk of certain ADRs based on their genetic makeup, clinicians can make more informed decisions about medications and dosages, resulting in a better benefit-to-risk ratio for pharmacologic therapy. Furthermore, the use of pharmacogenetic information in clinical practice is a significant step towards more tailored and effective therapeutic practices, with greater safety and improved disease management, in accordance with the principles of clinical pharmacology and therapeutics (Fenech et al., 2014) (Figure 11.11).

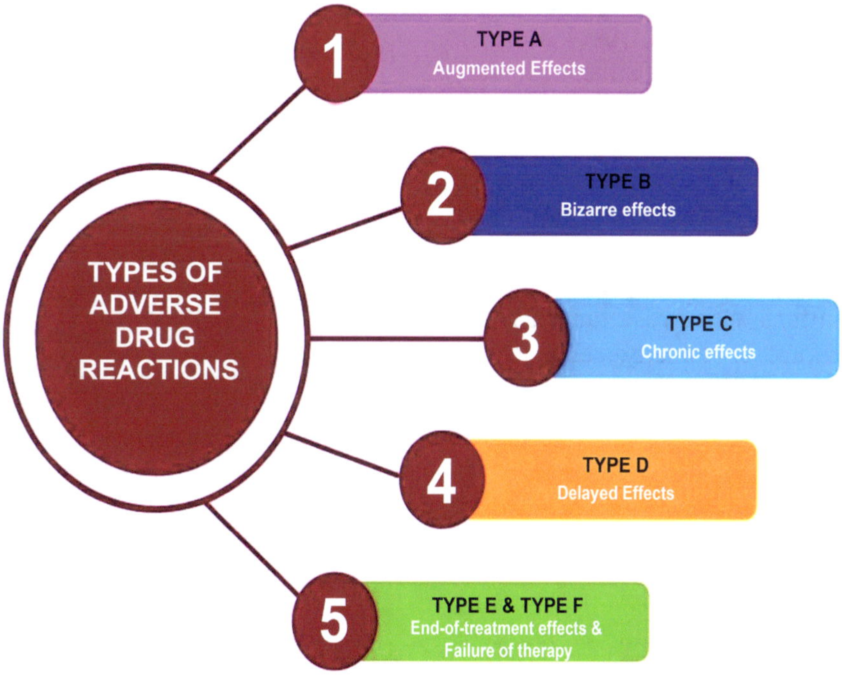

Figure 11.11. Various types of adverse drug reactions (ADRs).

Source: https://lh5.googleusercontent.com/u_xvKgpYqMmEyFb4Oi0T_13-mz-keUHVyVxpwKCvos4GU2Z71I6FsddZ8v73as--86rzjEuYKCzKtAAYJtpQyF0PMZUhxIhLmKnAn9J2gK5zn8yoxvRoW1gW0Jnn_9s1R2LB4j_8gGR9Ue0R-w=s1600-rw.

11.5.2. Risk Factors and Patient Demographics

In clinical pharmacology and therapeutics, it is essential to understand risk factors and patient demographics to determine maximal drug efficacy and minimize adverse effects. Physiological variations due to age, sex, genetic factors, and comorbidities may significantly affect a patient's response to drugs. For example, older patients often manifest altered pharmacokinetics due to physiological changes with age and hence are at risk of both under- and over-medication. Similarly, some patient populations, like those with chronic illnesses such as CKD, present special challenges. Managing these patients poses such challenges that they require individualized therapeutic regimens tailored to their specific risk profiles to maximize treatment efficacy while minimizing side effects. CKD patients are particularly characteristic of the interaction between risk factors and drug dosing. Evidence indicates that these patients are under considerable risk stemming from both the disease condition and the pharmacotherapy employed, more so with drugs such as vancomycin. Overestimation or underestimation of drug dosage in CKD patients can lead to subtherapeutic or supratherapeutic plasma concentrations with a resultant increase in the risk of failure or toxicity, respectively. A recent study developed a population pharmacokinetic model for vancomycin dosing in CKD patients, highlighting the need for individualized dosing regimens based on each patient's unique physiological parameters and pharmacokinetics (Chae et al., 2019). This model is a good demonstration of how integrating patient demographics and clinical features can significantly improve treatment effects, highlighting the use of more individualized pharmacotherapy. Besides, the relationship between patient demographics and treatment outcomes is emphasized in the context of antiepileptic drug (AED) treatment. It was in a matched cohort study that highlighted the fact that seizure-free patients with a switch of AEDs were more likely to have a recurrence of seizures compared to those who maintained their present drug regimen, demonstrating the determinative role of demographic factors such as seizure status and previous treatment histories (Finamore et al., 2016). Understanding nuances in patient profiles, including past responses to medications, helps the clinician make informed decisions when treating epilepsy.

11.5.3. Strategies for Prevention and Management

The therapeutic and clinical pharmacology environment is increasingly embracing preventative strategies, shifting the focus from reactive to proactive medical interventions. This is exemplified by an acute understanding of disease mechanisms at the molecular level, enabling the development of targeted interventions. Preventive interventions may include pharmacological interventions, such as vaccines and prophylactic drugs, aimed at preventing disease before its symptoms appear. By leveraging knowledge from genomics and molecular biology, clinicians can tailor these therapies to individual patients or even populations, thereby maximizing their impact. As newer studies continue to delineate pathways of health, clinical practice must also catch up and include prevention as a fundamental concept in therapeutic management, rather than a secondary process. This paradigm supports the general goals of modern medicine, which increasingly emphasize the role of prevention in disease control and health promotion (Cirino et al., 2017). Alongside medication, combined behavioral measures are determinative for disease control and prevention. These strategies include lifestyle modifications, such as promoting physical activity, good nutrition, and mental health treatment, that are crucial in lowering the risk of chronic diseases. By addressing these behavioral factors, health care practitioners can comprehensively support patients' well-being, thereby enhancing adherence to pharmacologic therapy. For instance, patient education initiatives that enlighten individuals about the need for early diagnosis and preventive interventions can empower them to take proactive steps towards their own health. Guided by behavioral science, these programs can exert a strong influence on disease pathways, ultimately leading to improved health outcomes.

Accordingly, successful prevention strategies must incorporate therapeutic and behavioral aspects to construct an integrated plan of health management in clinical pharmacology (Terzic et al., 2019). Beyond that, the difficulty of incorporating research evidence into clinical practice calls for novel strategies for prevention and management in pharmacology. The successful application of preventive practices requires multidisciplinary collaboration among healthcare practitioners, researchers, and policymakers. All this synergy is crucial to optimize public health programs and providing preventive therapies to different segments of society. Protection programs and outreach efforts can further complement these protective effects by generating awareness and encouraging people for preventive health screenings and immunization campaigns. By strengthening collaborations across sectors, the healthcare system can establish a robust system of disease prevention that not only meets the needs of individual patients but also advances public health. The adoption of preventive approaches in pharmacology can significantly contribute to society by extending healthy lifespans and advancing a healthy future for everyone (Cirino et al., 2017).

Test Your Knowledge

1. What are adverse drug reactions and how do they differ from side effects?
2. Which factors increase the risk of experiencing an adverse drug reaction?

11.6. Emerging Trends in Clinical Pharmacology

Learning Outcome

1. Define the personalized medicine and pharmacogenomics
2. Discuss the advances in drug delivery systems
3. Understand the role of technology in pharmacology

Advancing trends in clinical pharmacology support a paradigm shift that includes emerging techniques and technologies to improve drug therapy and discovery. The advent of personalized medicine signals a clear paradigm shift, in which treatments are tailored to each patient's individual parameters, e.g., genetic basis, lifestyle, and environment. It not only improves therapeutic efficacy but also minimizes side effects by optimizing drug selection based on the patient's individual profile. All this is possible because of platforms like Clinical Pharmacology & Therapeutics (CPT), which are worth more than gold as sources of the information required at the interface between drug discovery and clinical application, thereby fueling the progress of clinical pharmacology and enhancing patients' well-being (Terzic et al., 2017). Additionally, the advent of omics technologies, such as genomics, proteomics, and metabolomics, has changed our understanding of health and disease at the molecular level. Omic technologies generate large, high-dimensional biological data sets, enabling scientists to analyze complex interactions in biological systems. The combination of these data with clinical, demographic, and environmental datasets enables systems-level understanding of disease processes and treatment responses. As such data-driven approaches evolve, they provide a gateway to new therapeutic protocols and better drugs tailored for heterogeneous patient groups. The marriage of large-scale data analysis with clinical pharmacology is transforming the landscape of modern therapeutics, making it more adaptive and potent in the treatment of complex health issues (Alfirevic et al., 2016). Also, big data analytics has emerged as a critical component of the evolution of clinical pharmacology, enabling greater capacity to process and analyze large datasets generated by omics technologies and other clinical research endeavors. Clinical pharmacology is designed to optimize the storage, transmission, and analysis processes required to efficiently combine multidimensional datasets, enabling clinicians and scientists to derive meaningful insights that drive therapeutic discovery. This also facilitates a more pragmatic presentation of actionable information. Through the use of sophisticated machine learning techniques and statistical modeling, scientists can identify patterns, make predictions about patient responses, and uncover newly identified drug interactions to support better clinical decision-making. Thus, big data not only increases the utility of clinical pharmacology but also solidifies its role in closing the gap between scientific discovery and applied therapeutic use, towards a more efficient healthcare system (Alfirevic et al., 2016).

11.6.1. Personalized Medicine and Pharmacogenomics

The development of personalized medicine and pharmacogenomics is a pivotal step in clinical pharmacology and therapeutics. Personalized medicine differs from traditional medicine, which uses a one-size-fits-all approach, by tailoring treatment regimens to an individual's genetic profile, lifestyle, and environmental experiences. This precise treatment can enhance therapeutic efficacy and reduce drug-induced adverse effects, thereby improving patient outcomes. The intersection of personalized medicine and pharmacogenomics heightens sensitivity to how patients metabolize and respond to medication. By utilizing genetic information, clinicians are better positioned to select medicines and dosing regimens, thereby maximizing a course of therapy based on the patient's individualized biochemical profile. Personalized medicine is thus not so much a new method of drug delivery as an entirely new paradigm for patient care. Pharmacogenomic investigations yield crucial insights into the interaction between genetics and drug action, enabling the development of customized therapies. Pharmacogenomics is interested in identifying genetic variation that impacts pharmacokinetics and pharmacodynamics and in providing a scientific basis for individualized treatment strategies. For instance, genetic variability of drug-metabolizing enzyme genes can significantly impact drug efficacy and toxicity. As envisioned in recent discussions, such as those at the Golden Helix Pharmacogenomics Days, it is essential to foster global collaborations among researchers, clinicians, and industry members to expand the domain of individualized medicine. Collaboration with experts from various multidisciplinary fields enables a broad analysis of the implications of pharmacogenomics, enriching the therapeutic possibilities in the hands of healthcare providers. This intersection can ultimately lead to more naturalistic drug discovery strategies and improved drugs that are better aligned with patient profiles, thereby enhancing patient compliance and satisfaction. Furthermore, the notion of network pharmacology as an interesting supplement to personalized medicine holds promise for the development of novel therapeutic modalities. By combining system biology and pharmacogenomics, researchers can study the multifactorial nature of diseases and how they interact within biological networks. What network pharmacology uncovers may provide insight into developing personalized therapies that interact best with these networks and become more effective. As noted in the relevant literature, advancement toward personalized medicine necessitates a critical reorientation of thought in which drug discovery and development processes are informed by the interconnectedness of biological systems. These approaches can not only enhance the precision of therapeutics but also pave the way to an era of safer, more effective treatments that harmonize with the complexities of human physiology, ultimately revolutionizing clinical pharmacology and therapeutic practice (Marsh et al., 2010; Borg et al., 2012).

11.6.2. Advances in Drug Delivery Systems

Drug delivery systems have come a long way in changing clinical pharmacology and therapeutic practice with more effective treatment regimens and improved patient outcomes. Traditional drug delivery systems were typically restricted by poor bioavailability, dosing variability, and side effects due to uncontrolled release mechanisms. Recent advances, particularly nanotechnology, have enabled the production of targeted drug delivery systems that can enhance the pharmacokinetics of therapeutic molecules. These new methods allow targeted delivery of diseased cells, reducing systemic exposure and resulting in fewer side effects. The addition of innovative materials that respond to physiological conditions also offers a paradigm shift in drug delivery, where therapeutics can be released in response to specific stimuli, i.e., medicines can be delivered at the right time and dosage, ultimately making patient care and treatment compliance even better. Among the striking trends in drug discovery is the convergence of network pharmacology with personalized medicine. The approach aims to consider the complex interplay among biological pathways that leads to disease onset, rather than targeting a single therapeutic target. By conceiving drug action in light of network pharmacology, researchers can develop more nuanced treatments tailored to individual patient profiles. This paradigm release makes the entry open to global drug-delivery systems, enabling the exploitation of multimodal therapeutic methods and thereby increasing efficacy while constraining the risk of resistance. As personalized medicine gains momentum, its interface with network pharmacology offers a promising line of research that may lead to safer, more efficient treatments that address the individual needs of heterogeneous patient populations (Marsh et al., 2010). Besides, emerging manufacturing technologies such as 3D printing and microfluidics are further transforming drug delivery systems. They allow the rapid manufacture of complex drug formulations and devices that can be engineered precisely to match individual patient requirements. For instance, 3D printing enables the manufacture of pills with varied release profiles and dosages, facilitating more personalized treatment. Similarly, microfluidic systems make nanoparticle and other delivery vehicle formulation easier, with better control over particle size, shape, and drug-loading capacity. As these technologies continue to evolve, they are expected to spur the development of more advanced drug-delivery vehicles that achieve maximum therapeutic effects while ensuring maximum patient compliance. Overall, the evolution of drug delivery systems is part of the broader movement in clinical pharmacology towards precision medicine, a paradigm shift in our approach to managing complex disease (Terzic et al., 2017).

11.6.3. Role of Technology in Pharmacology

Technology has been applied to the practice of pharmacology in a critical way, shaping contemporary clinical pharmacology and therapeutic practice. Innovations such as high-throughput screening and computer-aided drug design enable scientists to identify potential drug candidates more rapidly and accurately. The technologies not only speed up the early stages of drug development but also reduce reliance on manpower-intensive, time-consuming traditional approaches. Using sophisticated algorithms and simulations, pharmacologists can better predict how new chemicals will behave within living organisms, thereby offering greater hope of successful treatment. This groundbreaking process highlights the central role of technology in accelerating drug discovery and optimizing treatment modalities, ultimately resulting in improved patient outcomes and reduced healthcare costs, as seen in the innovations presented in Clinical Pharmacology & Therapeutics (CPT) (Terzic et al., 2017). Technology also plays a central role in personalized medicine and pharmacogenomics beyond drug discovery. Using genetic testing and large genomic databases, clinicians can individualize treatments for each patient based on their genetics, thereby improving efficacy and safety. The shift toward individualized treatment regimens marks a departure from the one-size-fits-all approach. Next-generation sequencing is one of the tools that can empower physicians to make evidence-based choices, leading to outstanding improvements in patient outcomes while reducing the adverse effects of standard treatments. This preventive strategy aligns with the vision of expanding not just survival but overall wellness across populations, thereby enabling a paradigm shift in how therapeutic interventions are developed and delivered (Terzic et al., 2019). Moreover, the advancement of digital health technologies, including mobile health applications and telemedicine platforms, has revolutionized patient activation and compliance with pharmacological therapy. They allow the patient to control their health by providing immediate access to information on drug timing and potential side effects. They also foster greater cooperation between healthcare professionals and patients by facilitating immediate realignment of treatment whenever necessary. As such, technology is not only helpful in monitoring and maximizing drug compliance but also as a means for the propagation of vital drug-related information on a large scale. With the application of these innovations, clinical pharmacology can respond effectively to diverse patient needs, enhancing therapeutic strategies and optimizing healthcare delivery systems to meet modern demands (Terzic et al., 2017) (Figure 11.12).

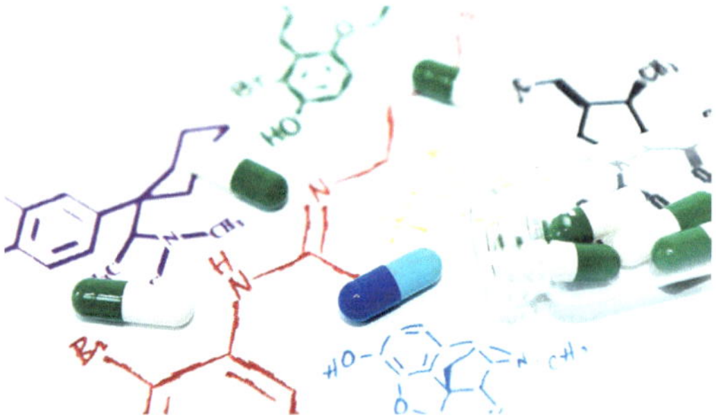

Figure 11.12. Advances such as high-throughput screening and computational drug design allow researchers to identify potential drug candidates more efficiently and accurately.

Source: https://cdn.sanity.io/images/0vv8moc6/pharmtech/580d696e6779c421e7d7e721880a1587961e7cfb-1280x720.jpg?fit=crop&auto=format.

Test Your Knowledge

1. How is personalized medicine influencing clinical pharmacology today?
2. What role do digital health tools and AI play in advancing drug therapy and monitoring?

SUMMARY

In a voyage through clinical pharmacology and therapeutics, it is crucial to highlight the contribution of personalized medicine to optimizing drug treatment outcomes. As research unmasks the genetic determinants underpinning variable drug responses, such as cytochrome P450 enzyme polymorphisms, clinicians must integrate such data into prescribing. This affords the potential to individualize treatment more effectively and safely. The relationship between drug metabolism and genetics accounts for why specific genotypes, e.g., CYP 2C19*17, place patients at risk for responses such as NSAID-induced peptic ulcers. Thus, knowledge of such genetic variations not only facilitates risk assessment but also represents a major step towards precision medicine in clinical pharmacology (Balabanseva et al., 2016). Secondly, the findings of pharmacokinetic studies emphasize the importance of understanding drug distribution and concentration in target tissues to inform practice. For instance, the pharmacokinetic profile of tulathromycin, which has established efficacy for treating respiratory infections in calves, illustrates how drug effect can vary greatly depending on the biological matrix in which it operates. They highlight the need to develop practical therapeutic guidelines that include pharmacokinetic/pharmacodynamic (PK/PD) measures to facilitate appropriate dosing regimens for different patient populations. Their creation is required to ensure that desired pharmacological effects are achieved without risking patient safety, thereby capitalizing on the landmark contribution of clinical pharmacology to drug therapy decision-making (Aliabadi et al., 2016). In conclusion, the future of clinical therapeutics and pharmacology lies in the seamless integration of biological, genetic, and pharmacodynamic concepts into everyday clinical practice. As the science continues to unfold, enabling a collaborative link among researchers and clinicians remains the most significant objective. Innovation in drug development and the dissection of drug-drug interactions and therapeutic endpoints can be sourced from this interaction. Additionally, the prospects of ongoing research underscore the need for ongoing professional education among health care providers to ensure effective management in the complex world of pharmacotherapy. The shared goal must be to enhance patient management through rational, evidence-based decisions that take into account individual variability in drug response and metabolism, ultimately transforming therapeutic approaches in clinical pharmacology.

In clinical therapeutics and pharmacology, understanding drug response variability is an intrinsic challenge. Patient-to-patient variability can occur because of genetic variation, environmental reasons, and related medical illnesses, which makes it difficult for the successful implementation of pharmacotherapy. The American Academy of Veterinary Pharmacology and Therapeutics focuses on population variability, illustrating the effect on dose-exposure-response relationships. By isolating and simulating such variables, medical professionals can better predict how patients will respond to specific medications, enabling more individualized treatment protocols. Such a precise approach promotes the safe and efficient use of medications, ultimately aiming for optimal therapeutic outcomes across different patient groups (Bailey et al., 2018). Enhanced simulation and modeling technology has significantly improved the understanding of pharmacokinetic data for clinical practice. These new methodologies allow the inclusion of drug physicochemical properties and species-specific physiologic parameters. Using both measured and predicted in vitro data, clinicians are able to explore better sources of variability influencing drug efficacy and safety. This comprehensive examination of factors that control pharmacotherapy provides essential information regarding the optimization of drug regimens for individual patients. Since these computer programs will continue to evolve, their application may further refine dosing regimens, ensuring interventions remain balanced with specific patient requirements (Bailey et al., 2018). Moreover, the evolution of therapeutic drug monitoring (TDM) has emphasized the value of incorporating a patient's historical data and pharmacokinetic models to achieve optimal therapeutic outcomes. Classic Bayesian predictive methods, in turn, rely primarily on maximum a posteriori estimates and fall short when quantifying treatment outcomes and assessing corresponding risks. The incorporation of Bayesian data assimilation methods addresses these limitations by providing a more probabilistic understanding of treatment outcomes, enabling healthcare practitioners to make informed decisions under uncertainty. By analyzing interoccasion variability and integrating TDM data more effectively, practitioners can be confident they are providing improved patient care across all therapeutic categories, especially in complex areas such as oncology, where optimal dosing is critical to achieving maximum treatment outcomes.

KEY TERMS FROM THIS CHAPTER

- Pharmacokinetics
- Bioavailability
- Therapeutic Index
- Drug Interaction
- Dose-Response Curve
- Receptor Binding
- Antagonist
- Personalized Medicine
- Pharmacodynamics
- Half-life
- Drug Metabolism
- Adverse Drug Reaction (ADR)
- First-pass Effect
- Agonist
- Therapeutic Drug Monitoring (TDM)

CRITICAL THINKING QUESTIONS

1. **Which of the following best defines "bioavailability"?**
   a. The degree to which a drug binds to plasma proteins
   b. The rate and extent to which a drug reaches systemic circulation
   c. The proportion of drug excreted unchanged in urine
   d. The amount of drug distributed to the tissues
2. **A drug that binds to a receptor and activates it to produce a response is called:**
   a. Antagonist
   b. Inhibitor
   c. Agonist
   d. Modulator
3. **Which of the following is an example of a drug with a narrow therapeutic index?**
   a. Paracetamol
   b. Warfarin
   c. Amoxicillin
   d. Ibuprofen
4. **The volume of distribution (Vd) of a drug is influenced by:**
   a. Route of administration only
   b. Renal excretion rate
   c. Lipid solubility and protein binding
   d. The patient's height only
5. **Which phase of a clinical trial primarily assesses drug safety in humans?**
   a. Phase I
   b. Phase II
   c. Phase III
   d. Phase IV

Short Answer Questions

1. What is clinical pharmacology, and how does it differ from basic pharmacology?
2. Define pharmacokinetics and pharmacodynamics.
3. What are the primary routes of drug administration, and what are the advantages of each?
4. Explain the concept of the therapeutic index.
5. What factors affect drug absorption and bioavailability?

Answers to Critical Thinking Questions

1. (b); 2. (c); 3. (b); 4. (c); 5. (a)

REFERENCES

1. Kenward, H., Pelligand, L., Savary-Bataille, K., & Elliott, J. (2014). Nausea: Current knowledge of mechanisms, measurement and clinical impact. *The Veterinary Journal, 203*(1), 36–43. https://doi.org/10.1016/j.tvjl.2014.10.007Abbott, R., & Ayres, I. (2014). Evidence and extrapolation: Mechanisms for regulating off-label uses of drugs and devices. https://core.ac.uk/download/62566275.pdf (accessed on 16th July 2025).
2. Adeniyi-Jones, S. C., Gastonguay, M., Kraft, M. D., et al. (2017). Population pharmacokinetic and pharmacodynamic analysis of buprenorphine for the treatment of neonatal abstinence syndrome. https://core.ac.uk/download/83049668.pdf (accessed on 16th July 2025).
3. Adhikari, P., Padmaja, U., & Pereira, P. (2009). A prospective analysis of adverse drug reactions in a South Indian hospital. https://core.ac.uk/download/pdf/87416.pdf (accessed on 16th July 2025).
4. Aebi, S., Shah, A. G., Anderson, R., Arlt, W., Barr, M., Barthelemy, J., Beiderlinden, M., et al. (2017). Medication complications in extracorporeal membrane oxygenation. https://core.ac.uk/download/129191716.pdf (accessed on 16th July 2025).
5. Alfirevic, A., Ball, A., Chen, Y., Costa, C., Driest, S. L., Fang, H., Harpaz, R., et al. (2016). Big data transforms discovery-utilization therapeutics continuum. https://core.ac.uk/download/46976098.pdf (accessed on 16th July 2025).
6. Aliabadi, F. S., Aliabadi, M. H., Aliabadi, M. A., Brentnall, J., Craig, D., Davey, P., de Jong, A., et al. (2018). Pharmacokinetic–pharmacodynamic integration and modelling of oxytetracycline for the calf pathogens *Mannheimia haemolytica* and *Pasteurella multocida*. https://core.ac.uk/download/132194056.pdf (accessed on 16th July 2025).
7. Aliabadi, F. S., Anonymous, Bosnar, M., Committee for Medicinal Products for Human Use (CHMP), Committee for Medicinal Products for Veterinary Use (CVMP), Evans, J., Gladue, D., et al. (2016). Standard PK/PD concepts can be applied to determine a dosage regimen for a macrolide: The case of tulathromycin in the calf. https://core.ac.uk/download/76980779.pdf (accessed on 16th July 2025).
8. Antrobus, R., Bujar, M., Crisp, N., Dukes, G., Gouws, J., Gouws, J., Green Thompson, L., et al. (2018). The South African regulatory system: Past, present, and future. https://core.ac.uk/download/287581368.pdf (accessed on 16th July 2025).
9. Bailey, J., Bon, C., Cox, E., Darwich, A., Dorey, L., Duwal, S., Ette, E. I., et al. (2018). Population variability in animal health: Influence on dose-exposure-response relationships: Part II: Modelling and simulation. https://core.ac.uk/download/159992803.pdf (accessed on 16th July 2025).
10. Balabanseva, A., Onischuk, L., & Tkach, S. (2016). *CYP2C19*17 polymorphism as a risk-factor for NSAIDs-induced ulcers. https://core.ac.uk/download/322516268.pdf (accessed on 16th July 2025).
11. Beeh, K. M., Cazzola, M., Price, D., Roche, N., et al. (2015). Assessing the clinical value of fast onset and sustained duration of action of long-acting bronchodilators for COPD. https://core.ac.uk/download/30435639.pdf (accessed on 16th July 2025).
12. Bhargava, V. K., Dhami, D. B., Neupane, G., Rathor, M., et al. (2017). Student's perceptions and feedback about teaching-learning pharmacology in Nepalgunj Medical College of Chisapani, Nepal. https://core.ac.uk/download/539895930.pdf (accessed on 16th July 2025).

13. Borg, J. J., Fenech, A. G., Grech, G., Patrinos, G. P., et al. (2012). Conference scene: Golden Helix Pharmacogenomics Days: Educational activities on pharmacogenomics and personalized medicine. https://core.ac.uk/download/46603880.pdf (accessed on 16th July 2025).
14. Chae, J. W., Chan, A., Dorajoo, S. R., Goh, K. L., et al. (2019). Optimizing vancomycin dosing in chronic kidney disease by deriving and implementing a web-based tool using a population pharmacokinetics analysis. https://core.ac.uk/download/323066264.pdf (accessed on 16th July 2025).
15. Chandy, M., Paik, D. T., & Wu, J. C. (2020). Patient and disease-specific induced pluripotent stem cells for discovery of personalized cardiovascular drugs and therapeutics. https://core.ac.uk/download/323062894.pdf (accessed on 16th July 2025).
16. Cirino, G., & Maffia, P. (2017). Targeting inflammation to reduce cardiovascular disease risk. https://core.ac.uk/download/96884613.pdf (accessed on 16th July 2025).
17. Davis, J. M., Kraft, W. K., & Stover, M. W. (2016). Neonatal abstinence syndrome: Pharmacologic strategies for the mother and infant. https://core.ac.uk/download/46976212.pdf (accessed on 16th July 2025).
18. de Wiljes, J., Hartung, N., Huisinga, W., Kloft, C., et al. (2020). Bayesian data assimilation to support informed decision-making in individualized chemotherapy. https://core.ac.uk/download/286352833.pdf (accessed on 16th July 2025).
19. Dooley, K. E., Dorman, S. E., Engle, M., Johnson, J. L., et al. (2017). Defining the optimal dose of rifapentine for pulmonary tuberculosis: Exposure-response relations from two phase II clinical trials. https://core.ac.uk/download/323074013.pdf (accessed on 16th July 2025).
20. Dorey, L., Hobson, S., & Lees, P. (2017). Potency of marbofloxacin for pig pneumonia pathogens *Actinobacillus pleuropneumoniae* and *Pasteurella multocida*: Comparison of growth media. https://core.ac.uk/download/76980948.pdf (accessed on 16th July 2025).
21. Fenech, A. G., & Grech, G. (2014). Pharmacogenetics: The science of predictive clinical pharmacology. https://core.ac.uk/download/46602555.pdf (accessed on 16th July 2025).
22. Finamore, J. M., Mintzer, S., Nei, M., Skidmore, C., et al. (2016). Seizure outcome after switching antiepileptic drugs: A matched, prospective study. https://core.ac.uk/download/46976197.pdf (accessed on 16th July 2025).
23. Garetto, L. P., Gregson, K. S., & Romito, L. M. (2010). Integration of pharmacology into a dental school's problem-based learning curriculum. https://core.ac.uk/download/46964833.pdf (accessed on 16th July 2025).
24. Kraft, W. K. (2018). Buprenorphine in neonatal abstinence syndrome. https://core.ac.uk/download/155271558.pdf (accessed on 16th July 2025).
25. Kraft, W. K., Lam, E., Lien, Y. T. K., Piraino, D., et al. (2020). Vancomycin in peritoneal dialysis: Clinical pharmacology considerations in therapy. https://core.ac.uk/download/322850154.pdf (accessed on 16th July 2025).
26. Kraft, W. K., Mantravadi, S., & Ogdie, A. (2017). Tumor necrosis factor inhibitors in psoriatic arthritis. https://core.ac.uk/download/83049994.pdf (accessed on 16th July 2025).
27. Mantsch, J. R., & Wang, J. B. (2012). L-tetrahydropalamatine: A potential new medication for the treatment of cocaine addiction. https://core.ac.uk/download/213079126.pdf (accessed on 16th July 2025).

28. Marsh, A., Singer, D. R. J., Taylor, P. C., Watkins, C., et al. (2010). Personalized medicine: The impact on chemistry. https://core.ac.uk/download/45676.pdf (accessed on 16th July 2025).

29. Mifsud, J. (1994). Chiral drugs: One drug or two? Clinical pharmacology through the looking glass: Reflections on the racemate vs enantiomer debate. https://core.ac.uk/download/46601970.pdf (accessed on 16th July 2025).

30. Reynolds, L. A., & Tansey, E. M. (2008). *Clinical Pharmacology in the UK, c.1950–2000: Industry and Regulation*. https://core.ac.uk/download/30696180.pdf (accessed on 16th July 2025).

31. Schenk, K. (1959). A study to determine if facts about drugs and drug therapy can be learned as effectively by a patient-centered approach as by classroom presentation. https://open.bu.edu/bitstream/2144/21940/1/Schenk_Katharine_1959_web.pdf (accessed on 16th July 2025).

32. Terzic, A., & Waldman, S. A. (2017). Clinical pharmacology & therapeutics: Past, present, and future. https://core.ac.uk/download/83049656.pdf (accessed on 16th July 2025).

33. Terzic, A., & Waldman, S. A. (2019). Health care evolves from reactive to proactive. https://core.ac.uk/download/213444739.pdf (accessed on 16th July 2025).

ENVIRONMENTAL AND OCCUPATIONAL MEDICINE

12

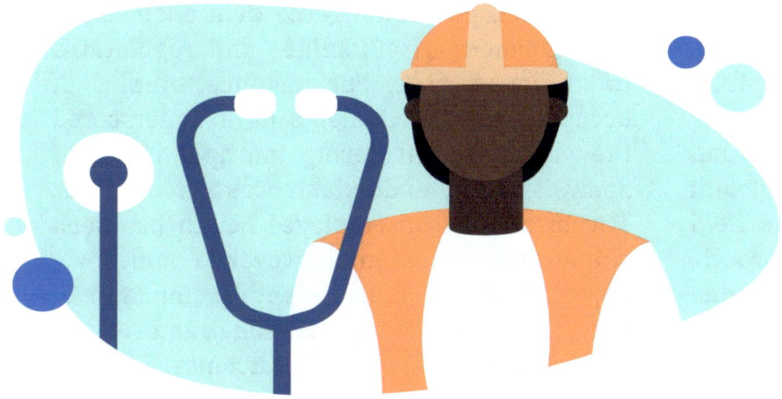

LEARNING OBJECTIVES

After studying this chapter, you will be able to:

1. Understand Historical Background
2. Explain Major Environmental Health Hazards
3. Describe Occupational Health Risks
4. Focus on Assessment and Diagnosis
5. Learn Prevention Strategies

Introduction

Occupational and environmental medicine is a vital intersection of public and occupational health, encompassing the mechanisms by which environmental and occupational exposures can affect health. It is a highly varied field encompassing such issues as toxic agent exposure, the psychosocial work environment, and the impact of workplace design and function on workers' well-being. With evolving industries and new technologies, an understanding of the trends in this dynamic sector becomes increasingly important. Moreover, because health outcomes are determined by a range of social, economic, and environmental factors, an integrated approach is necessary in occupational and environmental medicine. Occupational and environmental medicine, therefore, aims not only to prevent workers' injury but also to foster an integrated perception of health based on different environmental determinants. The search to examine workplace quality of life also underscores the need for occupational and environmental medicine. As further confirmed by recent studies, many psychosocial risks in the work setting profoundly affect the quality of life and mental health of employees. For instance, it has been shown through evidence that work stress and inadequate support systems are the causes of diminished well-being, especially if gendered differences in work experience are included (Cedrone et al., 2017). Understanding these determinants is necessary to create tailored interventions that can minimize risks and facilitate welfare among workers. integrate conventional medical evaluation with an understanding of the broader sociocultural forces at play, so as to foster a more multidimensional conception of health in occupational settings. A multilevel approach is required to fully understand the multifaceted interactions among individual behaviors, workplace dynamics, and broader societal influences on employee health outcomes. Surprisingly, research in the field has largely adopted a unidimensional approach, neglecting the many layers that affect mental health and overall well-being (Arnetz et al., 2014). Recognizing the multilayered impacts is feasible to develop more robust organizational interventions. By applying methods that assess and improve the workplace psychosocial climate at multiple levels, health practitioners can strengthen responsive, inclusive practice tailored to the needs of diverse worker populations. In the process, environmental and occupational medicine not only mitigates existing hazards but also lays the foundation for healthier, more supportive workplaces in the future.

Definition of Environmental Medicine

Environmental medicine is a multidisciplinary field that addresses the role of environmental determinants in human health. It attempts to describe how environmental exposures—such as chemicals, contaminants, and biological agents—affect health outcomes. The field is essential because it transcends the traditional boundaries of medicine, drawing on the fields of epidemiology, toxicology, and public health. The impact of environmental factors on health is significant, affecting the prevalence of chronic disease, respiratory conditions, and even mental illness. As familiarity with these relationships grows, it becomes clear that medical professionals must be familiar with environmental medicine, which underscores the need for research that demystifies the risks and prevention options associated with environmental exposure. Of special relevance to environmental medicine is emphasis on preventive health measures and public policy measures. By identifying harmful environmental agents and assessing their effects on affected populations, the field enables the establishment of guidelines and regulations to minimize risks. For instance, studies of occupational environments have underscored the value of considering multiple levels of analysis to fully understand occupational risks. The discussion on employee health has been single-topic oriented; however, a multilevel approach allows for an in-depth examination of how the individual, organizational, and societal levels are related to health outcomes. Findings from these studies inform organizational-level interventions for improving employees' mental well-being and health, further confirming the relevance of environmental medicine in the workplace (Arnetz et al., 2014). Furthermore, the intersection between social and environmental problems in occupational medicine demands responsiveness and regard to the narratives of the affected communities. The adult film industry is one such case in point where controls, such as the mandate on condom use following HIV outbreaks, are shaped by broader societal opinion regarding sexual health and workplace safety. Regulatory measures would often overlook the voice of performers, leaving policies and decisions that may not match their actual circumstances or work needs. Hearing these stories is important for understanding the industry's complexity and for creating health policies that effectively address workers' unique issues. By understanding these dimensions, environmental medicine can facilitate integrative approaches aimed at health outcomes and empower and foster flourishing individuals in precarious occupational niches (Gooya et al., 2020) (Figure 12.1).

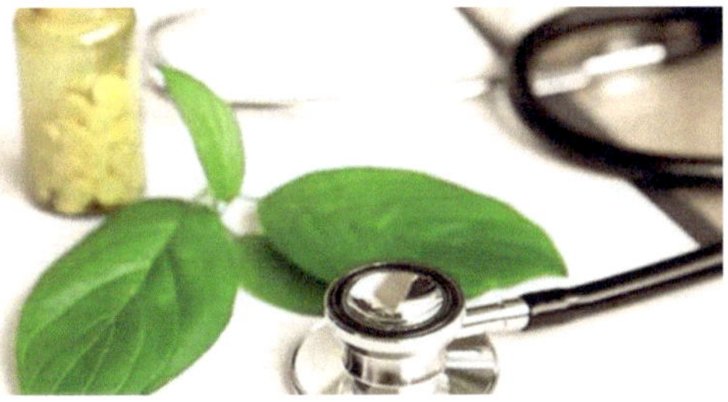

Figure 12.1. Environmental medicine encompasses a multidisciplinary field that addresses the interactions between environmental factors and human health.

Source: https://insightdermaclinic.com/wp-content/uploads/2020/11/Environmental-Medicine-inner-555x250.jpg.

Definition of Occupational Medicine

Occupational medicine is a medical specialty that focuses on the health and safety of workers, including occupational hazards and environmental exposures. It encompasses prevention, evaluation, diagnosis, and management of work-related illness and injury. As workplaces become more diverse and understanding of workplace environments improves, the field has expanded to include chronic workplace diseases, including musculoskeletal disorders, respiratory diseases, and mental disorders. Occupational medicine also focuses extensively on job design and ergonomics, which enhance worker health, productivity, and safety. The primary objectives of this practice are not only to treat workplace illnesses but also to implement preventive interventions that protect workers, resulting in a healthier workforce across various industrial environments. Occupational health assessment calls for collecting and analyzing evidence for workplace exposures. This is particularly relevant in identifying hazards in some occupations, as evidenced by the use of job exposure matrices (JEMs) in research. For example, evidence indicates strong associations between work exposures, such as repetitive motion, and the development of carpal tunnel syndrome (CTS) among workers, underscoring the significance of occupational factors in health outcomes. The knowledge obtained from JEMs can contribute to better understanding of how differing physical conditions affect the incidence of work-related disorders. Moreover, such matrices would also be valuable tools in epidemiological research, as they help establish associations between occupational exposure and resulting health conditions, even with potential limitations from exposure misclassification (Dale et al., 2014). In addition to examining physical health, occupational medicine also offers ways to counter the effects of occupational exposure on the psyche, particularly in workplaces where hazardous materials, including pesticides, are frequently used. Research has indicated that subjects with past low-level organophosphate pesticide exposure self-report increased levels of psychological distress compared to their unexposed peers. This correlation suggests the value of screening for mental health in occupational medicine due to workplace stressors having the potential to exacerbate pre-existing psychological illnesses or cause new ones. By facilitating comprehensive health assessments that span physical and psychological aspects, occupational medicine can effectively address the complexity of workers' well-being and promote improved workplaces and a reduction in the overall incidence of occupational diseases (Ahmed et al., 2016).

Importance of the Field in Public Health

The contribution of occupational and environmental medicine to public health cannot be overstated, as it plays a crucial role in averting dangers arising from various work environments and workplaces. Occupational and environmental medicine is the study of how environmental factors, such as harmful substances and physical agents, affect human health. When these determinants are linked to health outcomes, public health professionals can develop interventions to reduce exposure and address health disparities. Additionally, integrating occupational health into public health models optimizes workers' overall health, further enhancing community health outcomes. The emphasis in this field on prevention is not only for the protection of personal well-being but for the promotion of economic productivity through the reduction of workplace sickness and injury, highlighting the interdependency of health and financial security. Further, identifying occupational stress as a key area of concern in occupational health underscores the need for specialist public health interventions. Research indicates that work stress is prevalent across industries and negatively impacts health, as shown in a descriptive study of occupational stress among mine workers in Burkina Faso, where 26.23% exhibited occupational stress signs (Hinson et al., 2021). The above facts suggest that public health professionals need to assess the mental health outcomes in workplaces. Incorporating supportive workplace policies, such as stress-reduction programs and valuing workers' contributions, can significantly boost job satisfaction and overall workplace morale. Thus, understanding the health implications of work-related stress is of utmost importance in planning integrated public health programs that protect against not only physical but also mental health in the workplace. In addition to addressing occupational and environmental risks and stress, environmental and occupational medicine practice is important for developing public policy grounded in evidence-based research. Evidence resulting from this practice is important in assisting policy decisions to improve environmental and occupational levels of health, ensuring they are grounded in scientific research. For instance, studies on the sociological determinants of health portray the intricate relationships between socio-economic factors and health outcomes, promoting a public health approach that acknowledges these intricacies (Nettleton, 2009). Such analysis, when integrated, helps policies to be guided by the intricacy of health and provide equal access to care and resources. As public health itself develops and expands, the wisdom gained from environmental and occupational medicine will be at the core of planning for impending health issues and creating resilient communities that can manage the nuances of modern health challenges (Figure 12.2).

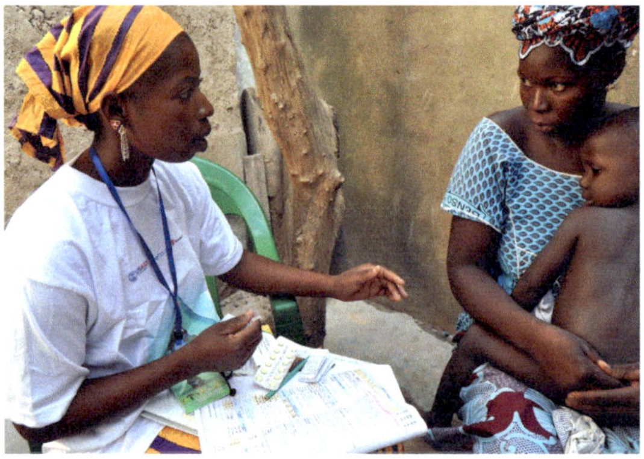

Figure 12.2. The integration of occupational health into public health frameworks enhances the overall health of workers, which, in turn, contributes to improved community health outcomes.

Source: https://upload.wikimedia.org/wikipedia/commons/f/f1/Community_Health_Worker_treats_child_%2819165929668%29.jpg.

12.1. Historical Background

Learning Outcome

1. Understand the evolution of environmental medicine
2. Define the development of occupational medicine
3. Describe the key milestones in the integration of both fields

The history of environmental and occupational medicine stems from industrial advancement in the 19th and 20th centuries. As societies transitioned from agrarian to industrial economies, the onset of injurious working conditions came into the open. This prompted the initial academic investigation of the health consequences of occupational exposure to a broad spectrum of agents, such as chemicals and physical agents. In Japan and Korea, for instance, the rising incidence of work-related musculoskeletal disorders (WMSD) highlighted the necessity of organized worker health strategies. Historical analyses show that the two countries developed parallel compensation schemes for these disorders as they evolved alongside their respective socio-cultural developments and industrial transitions, thereby sparking innovations in occupational health policies in response to an all-pervasive issue in the workforce (Kim et al., 2014). In environmental medicine, the historical context of chemical toxic exposure has significantly influenced public health policy. The most representative example is benzene exposure, which is well known to be related to hematologic neoplasia like leukemia. The consequences of benzene on occupational health were revealed through massive cohort studies since the 1970s, mainly in industrial areas. These studies showed a clear link between greater exposure to benzene and increased risk of leukemia and related diseases in workers. These regulations began to affect industrial practice, broadening our understanding of the importance of chemical exposure monitoring and control. These environmental studies have established a foundation for synthesizing toxicological, epidemiological, and clinical data into meaningful health practice, emphasizing the essential interfaces among occupational exposure and general environmental health topics (Hayes et al., 1997). Throughout history, this knowledge has been used to develop policies and preventive programs in environmental and occupational medicine. As more individuals became exposed to the detrimental effects of unhealthy working conditions, there was a need for a comprehensive management approach that would directly aim to minimize exposure risk and maximize worker safety. In countries like Japan and Korea, policy has transcended injury reimbursement to encompass active measures for identifying and preventing workplace hazards. Despite differences in enforcement practices, both nations have attempted to promulgate guidelines and instructional materials to promote healthier workplaces. The developmental history of such legislation points to the need for a concerted effort to consolidate medical, environmental, and occupational knowledge for worker health protection in a changing industrial context (Kim et al., 2014).

12.1.1. Evolution of Environmental Medicine

The evolution of environmental medicine has followed a significant path over time, in step with shifts in social perceptions and scientific advances in understanding the environment's role in the causation of illness. Having originated in public health initiatives during the mid-20th century, the field sought to understand and prevent the impact of environmental hazards on individuals' health. As industrialization progressed, concerns about occupational exposure to hazardous substances led to the creation of regulatory frameworks to protect worker health. This early model laid the foundation for environmental medicine and the need to assess risk and formulate preventive measures. The discovery of diseases caused by environmental factors led to a more organized effort, which eventually became a specialty within medical practice and public health policy. With greater scientific understanding, environmental medicine played a central role in solving diseases caused by environmental exposure. By integrating findings from other fields, including toxicology, epidemiology, and environmental science, professionals would be better able to assess the interactions between environmental factors and health outcomes. The Global Burden of Diseases, Injuries, and Risk Factors Study 2015 examined this interaction in depth, finding that environmental and occupational hazards accounted for a large proportion of global morbidity and mortality. Specifically, results indicated that more than half of global mortality and a significant share of disability-adjusted life-years (DALYs) may be due to environmental factors, underscoring the pressing need for ongoing research and intervention in this area (Forouzanfar et al., 2016). These findings shed light on the crucial role that environmental medicine plays in health policy and resource allocation, directing efforts toward optimal disease prevention measures. The discipline of environmental medicine is today faced and challenged by modern environmental issues such as climate change, pollution, and infectious diseases. The emerging tidal wave of metabolic and chronic diseases, often paired with escalating environmental risks, underscores the importance and urgency of an interdisciplinary model integrating environmental health and occupational medicine. The past few decades have witnessed increased literature on the health implications of environmental alterations, and pioneering journals have expanded on these topics. The bibliometric study in this case shows diversification and expansion of health research domains, mirroring emerging public health concerns, and warns of paradigm shifts in understanding the intricate interrelationship between the environment and resultant health outcomes (Merigó et al., 2016). With the advancements in the discipline, it is still necessary to adapt to emerging risks and create new strategies that favorably react to the impact of environmental factors on health.

12.1.2. Development of Occupational Medicine

The growth of occupational medicine has primarily been influenced by growing awareness of occupational health as an integral part of public health. The field first expanded from the accelerated levels of on-the-job injury and sickness that defined the industrial revolution. Over the years, occupational medicine has evolved from mere management of acute injuries to a multifaceted practice encompassing chronic conditions, mental health, and the psychosocial factors affecting workplace environments. This progress attests to a more substantial value placed on knowing how workplace conditions contribute to health and productivity. Besides, industrial modernization and new technologies pose constant challenges for practitioners, underscoring the necessity of continuous education and research in occupational health. With a better understanding of these interconnected phenomena, occupational medicine is increasingly being considered not only as a clinical specialty but also as part of environmental and occupational health practice. The convergence of various cultural perspectives, particularly in regions rich in traditional medicine, has also contributed to shaping occupational medicine. For instance, individuals in South Africa often rely on traditional herbal medicine for myriad conditions and approach it as mainstream healthcare. Their integration and inclusion in occupational health frameworks are critical, especially given their significant role in the lives of so many. Recent evidence points to a critical gap in health sciences training in herbal and indigenous medicines, underscoring that their inclusion would enable future healthcare providers, including occupational medicine professionals, to be more culturally responsive. Recognizing the potential benefits of supplementing traditional medicine with complementary remedies would improve patient education and foster a more integrated practice of occupational health, ultimately improving workers' outcomes (Mashigo et al., 2024). Furthermore, as occupational medicine evolves, systemic changes in educational and mentorship practices are essential to more accurately represent and understand diverse populations. The 2030 vision centres on the necessity of robust mentorship systems that incorporate underrepresented groups into STEM fields, similar to occupational medicine practice diversity. By creating mentorship programs that address the structural barriers faced by these groups, there is potential for drastic shifts in understanding and approach to occupational health issues. Training and mentorship programs can cultivate a responsive workforce attuned to cultural identities and capable of recognizing the complexities of occupational health in diverse contexts. By embracing such practices, not only will healthcare professionals' skills be enhanced, but also inclusive models will be promoted, which are required to address various challenges in occupational medicine today (2030Collaboration S et al., 2023) (Figure 12.3).

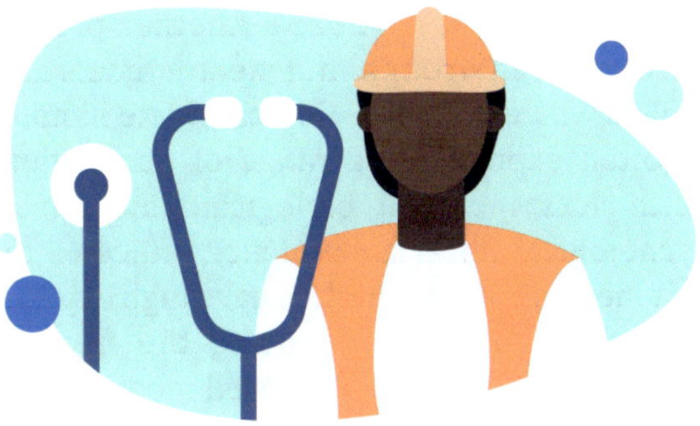

Figure 12.3. The evolution of occupational medicine has been significantly influenced by the growing recognition of occupational health as a critical component of public health.

Source: https://www.bmj.com/careers/getasset/d93f59b9-7b6c-408b-8519-244c0791657c/.

12.1.3. Key Milestones in the Integration of Both Fields

Synthesis between occupational and environmental medicine has been marked by significant milestones in recent decades, inspired by the growing recognition of the interdependence between workplace settings and broader ecological influences. Among the most significant milestones for such synthesis has been the development of occupational health standards, with environmental hazards taken into account. For example, regulatory frameworks began requiring assessments of how environmental factors may affect workplace exposures to produce holistic health and safety solutions. The shift does not just highlight the need to protect workers but also considers the broader societal aspect, where environmental degradation can increase occupational risks. The intersection of these fields has thus culminated in a more expansive view of health, relating individual wellbeing to environmental and community health (Negri et al., 2021). Another significant accomplishment is tracing the evolution back to the study methods created to investigate the overlap between environmental and occupational health. The evolution of interdisciplinary research has facilitated the identification of common risk factors, enabling researchers to analyze how exposure to environmental factors, such as water and air quality, influences workforce health. This is supplemented by augmented literature on the significance of sustainable practices within industries that hitherto prioritized worker productivity over worker safety. Initiatives for sustainable supply chains have also been undertaken, highlighting the interconnectivities between occupational health and environmental sustainability. These innovations indicate the necessity of measures to address not only short-term urgent health issues but also long-term environmental issues, thereby establishing resilience in both spheres (Negri et al., 2021). The COVID-19 pandemic is a milestone in the convergence of occupational and environmental medicine, best exemplified by the lens of telework as a precautionary measure. Telework was readily adopted by companies not just as a health-driven reaction but also as a strategy for business continuity while maintaining employee health. This new practice also highlighted the significant intersection of safety and environmental sustainability, as teleworking reduces the environmental footprint of commuting and office use. Hence, the pandemic catalyzed a re-examination of work habits, and there is a paradigm shift in which safety factors, including environmental concerns, are integral to occupational health discourse. This integrative approach is set to deliver fresh research agendas that explore the interactions among safety, environmental impact, and organizational policy, further solidifying bridges for comprehensive occupational and environmental health practice.

Test Your Knowledge

1. How did industrialization influence the development of environmental and occupational medicine?
2. What were some early milestones in recognizing workplace-related health hazards?

12.2. Major Environmental Health Hazards

Learning Outcome

1. Describe the air pollution and its effects
2. Define the water contamination and health risks
3. Discuss the chemical exposures in the environment

Knowledge of significant environmental health risks is crucial for effective mitigation and prevention measures in environmental and occupational medicine. Exposure to harmful agents in the workplace and environmentally contaminated areas has severe public health implications, leading to acute conditions and chronic diseases. Forensic and mortuary workplaces are particularly important for highlighting the importance of workplace risk assessment, as workers in these settings come into contact with various hazards, including chemical exposure and ergonomic risks. For example, exposure to formaldehyde and ergonomic overload as a result of manual handling and twisted postures can result in debilitating conditions, including nasopharyngeal carcinoma and low back pain. Overall health risk assessment, for example, as utilized by the Forensic Medicine and Mortuary Unit of Persahabatan General Hospital, is responsible for identifying these risks and developing proper interventions to safeguard worker health and safety (Ratman et al., 2025). Another pressing concern in environmental health hazards is medical waste disposal. Medical waste handlers are often exposed to a range of occupational health risks, including biological, physical, and psychological hazards. Evidence indicates that most medical waste handlers have high exposure to these hazards, highlighting the need for greater knowledge and improved medical waste handling practices. The most recent assessment concluded that over 83% of employees were exposed to biological hazards and approximately 95% to physical hazards. Alarming enough, the majority of workers lacked sufficient information about the dangers of their occupation and about poor practices in handling medical waste. The bridge of knowledge and practice implies that continuous training and education can go a considerable distance towards minimizing such risks and increasing overall worker protection (Amin et al., 2024). Finally, the management of high-level environmental health hazards transcends local industries; it requires an integrated strategy that calls for legislative frameworks and public involvement. Effective interventions must be rooted in a detailed understanding of the particular risks involved across different working conditions. Government agency coordination, health facilities, and schools can assist in developing comprehensive training programs and public campaigns. These programs aim to reduce workers' exposure to environmental risk factors, improve workers' health literacy, and promote safe working practices across industries. Through safety and health in the work environment, environmental and occupational medicine practitioners can be positive contributors to healthier surroundings and, ultimately, more favorable public health results for the community as a whole.

12.2.1. Air Pollution and Its Effects

Air pollution poses an immense threat to public health, with its effects extending to numerous non-communicable diseases. A comprehensive bibliometric analysis of air pollution studies published from 1960 to 2022 indicated a significant focus on particulate matter (PM), particularly PM2.5. The study found that respiratory health effects were most frequently cited, highlighting the concern about the ill effects of long-term exposure to air pollution. With 22.3% of the papers reviewed focusing on PM2.5, a significant amount of the literature highlights its negative impact on lung and cardiac conditions, showing a clear relationship between exposure to pollution and patient morbidity. Thus, information on air pollution's pervasiveness is necessary to craft effective public health interventions and policies to reduce exposure and promote improved environments in urban and rural settings (Bochenek et al., 2025). In an unexpected turn, future studies have begun to examine the less well-known effects of air pollution on the eyes, particularly in relation to PM2.5. As one example, research has found that long-term exposure to greater levels of PM2.5 is associated with a significant increase in the prevalence of myopia among adults aged between 40 and 69. The research used binary logistic regression to examine how various PM2.5 levels were associated with myopia prevalence, finding a significant correlation above healthy guideline levels. Such findings highlight the need for further research into air pollution's broader implications for ocular health, thereby providing novel areas of investigation in environmental and occupational medicine. Control strategies for PM2.5 levels are not only aimed at promoting pulmonary well-being but will also be equally important for preserving ocular well-being, underscoring the multifaceted risks of air pollution (Jung et al., 2025). The intersection of environmental exposures, such as air pollution, and occupational health cannot be overstressed. Workers in industries with higher exposure to air pollutants commonly experience compounded health hazards, hence necessitating stringent regulation and monitoring. The interaction between occupational air quality and health outcomes underscores the need for interprofessional practices that merge environmental considerations with occupational health policy.

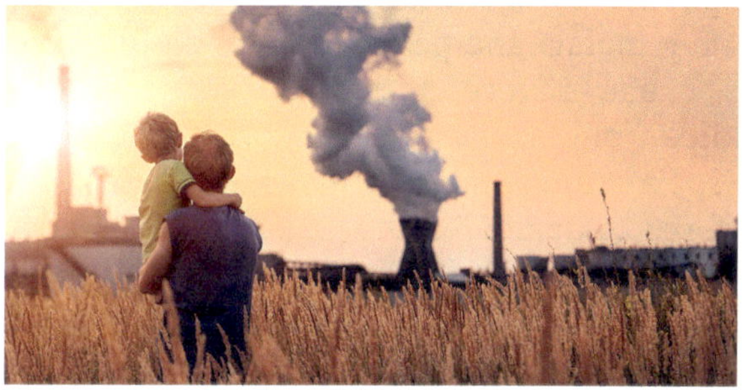

Figure 12.4. Air pollution presents a significant challenge to public health, with its ramifications extending to various non-communicable diseases.

Source: https://www.niehs.nih.gov/sites/default/files/health/assets/images/air_pollution_og.jpg.

Counteraction to air pollution's differential impacts, especially on vulnerable populations like industrial workers, necessitates collaborative action by public health professionals, policymakers, and industries. Efficacious measures must be developed to not only stop exposure to hazardous pollutants in the environment but also keep workers in such conditions healthy. Ultimately, research development on air pollution and its health consequences will play a vital role in developing effective interventions as well as promoting safer workplaces across the globe (Bochenek et al., 2025) (Figure 12.4).

12.2.2. Water Contamination and Health Risks

Water pollution is a critical public health issue, often linked to other health risks that greatly affect vulnerable populations. Contaminated water sources can cause acute and chronic diseases, particularly in regions with inadequate sanitation and waste management systems. Bacteria, viruses, and parasites, common in contaminated environments, can cause gastrointestinal disease, which is most harmful to children and the elderly. Moreover, long-term exposure to chemical contaminants such as heavy metals and pesticides has the potential to cause severe health effects, including cancer and neurodegenerative illness. The association between water quality and health effects underscores the importance of strict regulation and quality control of water sources to protect community health. The geographical characteristics of environmental exposure, as described in medical geology, highlight the importance of considering geographical history in evaluating health to accurately estimate health hazards (Boulos et al., 2016). It is also necessary to understand the human-induced causes of water contamination to plan effective interventions. Agricultural runoff, industrial discharges, and urban activities are among the significant sources of pollutants in water. In most developing countries, such as Malawi, limited resources and infrastructure exacerbate these issues, perpetuating a cycle of poor health and pollution. Research has highlighted extensive disparities in the environmental health sector, which further make it increasingly challenging to produce actionable health policies. Prioritizing research outlined in consultancy reports can guide targeted action to reduce risks from contaminated water supplies (Lungu et al., 2010). By facilitating interdisciplinary collaboration, public health practitioners can effectively tackle environmental and occupational health challenges and help build healthier communities. Ultimately, confronting water contamination must be an integrative process that reconciles environmental science and public health action. Strategies must not only include enhancing water quality by technological innovations but also educating the community about sustainable practices to avoid pollution. The education could include encouraging best agriculture practices to reduce fertilizer runoff or convincing the treatment of wastewater before releasing it. Further, enhancing health literacy about the risks posed by polluted water and cost-effective testing enables the community to take early action. As evident in the cross-disciplinary investigation of medical geology, effective solutions to waterborne health issues are achieved through coordination among scientists, healthcare workers, and policy-makers (Boulos et al., 2016). Hence, resolving the issue of water pollution is a critical element of providing overall health in the context of Environmental and Occupational Medicine.

12.2.3. Chemical Exposures in the Environment

Exposure to environmental chemicals plays a significant role in occupational safety and public health, and therefore, gaining a good understanding of their implications is necessary. A variety of harmful chemicals, ranging from heavy metals to anthropogenic chemicals, enter the air, water, and land and can potentially harm human health. These exposures tend to manifest their impact through adverse health effects, ranging from instantaneous responses to chronic disease, and it is therefore imperative that health practitioners evaluate the scale of such exposures. Effective monitoring and evaluation of environmental contamination can serve as the platform for planning prevention strategies that counteract health risks. Regulatory bodies can enhance public safety by setting standards that specify acceptable exposure levels and compelling industries to adopt safer methods, thereby implementing a preventive strategy for environmental health within the framework of Occupational Medicine. The working environment is not immune to environmental chemical exposure, as most workers are exposed to harmful substances daily. These sectors involve manufacturing, agriculture, and construction, which put the workers at risk of toxic chemicals, now and in the future. In response to these hazards, health professionals need to identify potential risks and administer proper interventions. A convergence of data from various case studies suggests the importance of regulatory strategies to protect workers and the effectiveness of product and design strategies in mitigating exposure (Kriebel et al., 2011).

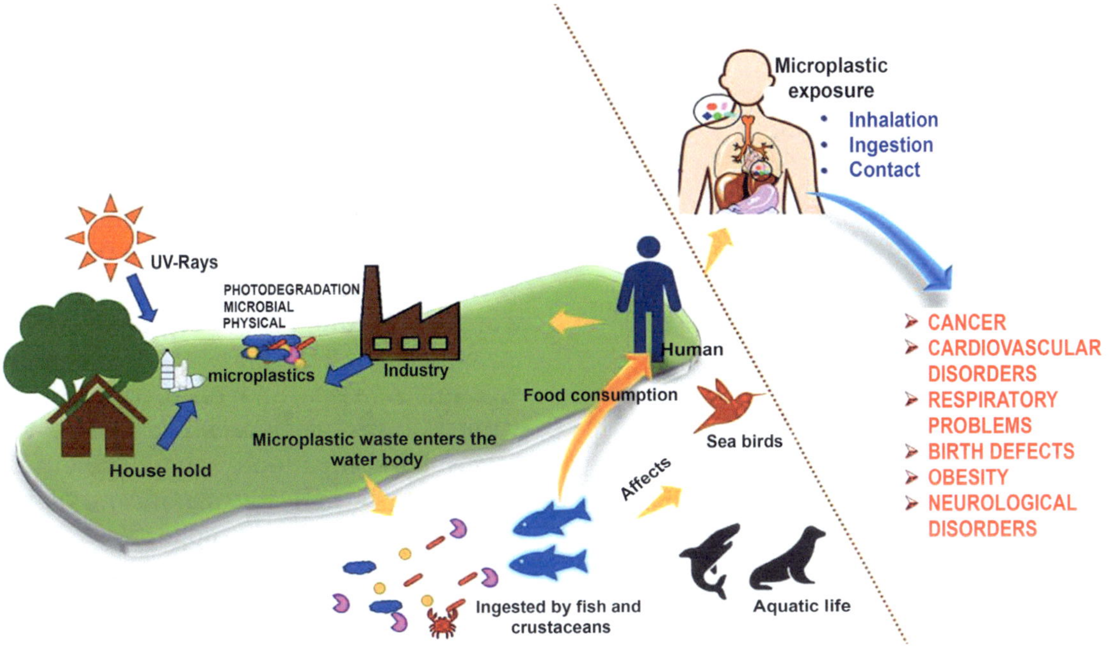

Figure 12.5. Chemical exposures in the environment play a significant role in shaping public health and occupational safety, necessitating a robust understanding of their implications.

Source: https://www.tandfonline.com/action/showGraphicalAbstractImage?doi=10.1080%2F07388551.2024.2344572&id=ibty_a_2344572_uf0001_c.jpg.

Through the use of strict safety measures, including practical training, adequate personal protective equipment, and frequent health screenings, the workforce benefits from less exposure to harmful chemicals, ultimately contributing to improved working conditions. Further, ensuring employees' health in the face of environmental chemical exposure risks requires systematic approaches, such as comprehensive medical examinations and the establishment of effective working procedures. Analysis of biomedical data sheets, particularly in large organizations such as NASA, indicates that quality medical histories and toxicity data gathering are necessary for effectively monitoring employee health. Such increased vigilance not only facilitates early detection of occupational irregularities but also facilitates long-term health upkeep habits. By prioritizing regular health monitoring and developing a culture of safety, institutions can actively reduce the prevalence of diseases linked to chemical exposures, underscoring the importance of integrating environmental considerations into occupational health policies. These actions are important in ensuring that both workplace and environmental health hazards are properly controlled, leading to a healthier population as a whole (Figure 12.5).

Test Your Knowledge

1. What are the most common environmental hazards that impact human health?
2. How do chemical, physical, and biological hazards differ in their effects on health?

12.3. Occupational Health Risks

Learning Outcome

1. Describe the common workplace hazards
2. Discuss how to impact of ergonomics on worker health
3. Define the role of safety regulations in mitigating risks

Occupational health risks are framed in terms of the dynamic relationship between employee and workplace health, particularly in the context of the complexity and uncertainty of an ageing population. The COVID-19 pandemic showed how rapidly changing circumstances can accelerate physical and mental health risks at work. One example was the shift from traditional office layouts to remote work from home, which created significant ergonomic problems and a spike in musculoskeletal disorder case rates. Secondly, the psychological consequences of telecommuting combined with isolation and job insecurity have been linked to rising levels of anxiety and stress for employees. This dual exposure to physical and psychological risks underscores the urgent need for proactive occupational health services that address these emerging threats and adapt to the evolving workplace landscape, as outlined by Mansyur et al. (2023). In regulating occupational health risks, law plays a central role in giving the definitions of safety standards and measures that protect workers. A comprehensive review of health-affecting legislation, particularly in nations such as Latin America and the Caribbean, reveals strengths and weaknesses in the regulations governing occupational safety. The outcome of such scrutiny indicates significant gaps in the regulatory mechanisms supporting occupational health and safety in countries. These constraints can hinder efforts to prevent environmental pollution and occupational hazards, potentially endangering workers' health. Through legislation enactment and its consolidation, nations achieve a better workplace that not only complies with international standards but also takes an extra step to mitigate risks, thereby enhancing public health, as seen in Mónica Bolis (2025). With the evolution of the workplace, similarly, the measures to effectively manage occupational health risks must evolve. The measures put in place during the pandemic constitute a bedrock for future improvement of occupational health services. It is critical to enhance these services since not only does it address immediate health concerns, but also ensures long-term productivity and health for employees. Ongoing enhancement of best practices in occupational medicine is essential to overcoming emerging health challenges, especially given how quickly working conditions are changing. Moreover, institutional collaboration, such as demonstrated by initiatives such as the Occupational & Environmental Journal of Indonesia, is essential in disseminating research and establishing effective health interventions. This collective publication is capable of making a significant contribution to occupational health risk awareness and management in an increasingly complicated world of work, as reflected in Mansyur et al. (2023).

12.3.1. Common Workplace Hazards

In environmental and occupational medicine, recognizing and managing common workplace hazards is of utmost importance. Occupational hazards can be grouped into physical, chemical, biological, ergonomic, and psychosocial categories. Physical risks include noise, radiation, and poor lighting and can cause health issues such as hearing loss and eye strain. Chemical risks, such as exposure to harmful chemicals, have been linked to respiratory disease as well as neurological disease. Further, the majority of workplaces are not addressing issues of ergonomics properly, which could lead to musculoskeletal disorders and chronic pain in the workers. Understanding such hazards is crucial, as it informs the development of preventive measures to minimize risks and enhance workers' safety across sectors. New work arrangements, particularly necessitated by the COVID-19 pandemic, have exacerbated existing hazards while introducing new ones. With remote work becoming widespread, many workers faced ergonomic issues due to poor-quality home office equipment. Indications show increased work-related musculoskeletal disorders attributed to inappropriate sitting and organization of desks when working from home, which requires combined health interventions in occupational health care. Moreover, the psychosocial climate was significantly altered during this period, leading to increased stress, anxiety, and emotional disorders among workers. As organizations try to keep pace with this ever-evolving environment, it becomes important to recognize the need for continuous monitoring and effective occupational health programs to address emerging health risks promptly (Mansyur et al., 2023). Even occupational health risks that are ubiquitous in the workplace affect demographic factors such as ethnicity and socioeconomic status, revealing disparities in occupational health.

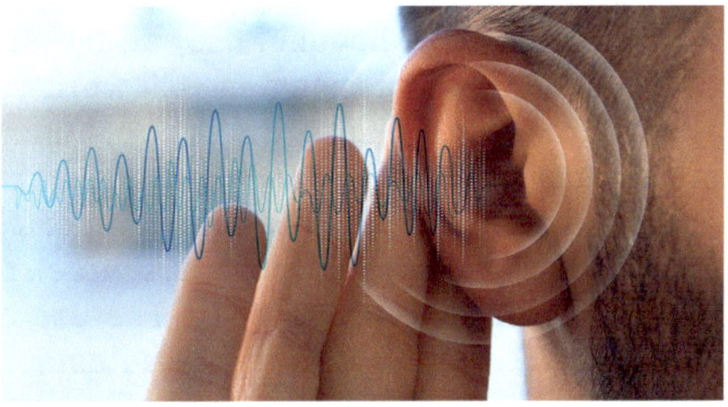

Figure 12.6. Physical hazards encompass issues such as noise, radiation, and poor lighting, which can contribute to various health complications, including hearing loss and eye strain.

Source: https://www.apexhospitals.com/_next/image?url=https%3A%2F%2Fbed.apexhospitals.com%2Fuploads%2Fhearing_loss2_83f8031121.jpg&w=1920&q=75.

Black and minority ethnic groups are found to experience particular disadvantages at the workplace, despite being represented in dangerous occupations less frequently overall. UK South Asians, for instance, experience higher rates of poor health and long-term illness, ultimately leading to withdrawal from the workplace at higher rates compared to their white counterparts (Clay et al., 2004). This highlights the necessity for individually tailored occupational health promotion interventions that address the specific vulnerabilities of ethnic minority employees. By guaranteeing equal access to health resources and maximizing surveillance and data collection, the field of environmental and occupational medicine can contribute even more to addressing these disparities, thereby improving the welfare and productivity of employees in general (Figure 12.6).

12.3.2. Impact of Ergonomics on Worker Health

The application of ergonomic principles in the workplace has a wide-ranging impact on worker health, primarily by preventing musculoskeletal disorders (MSDs). Ergonomics addresses workstation and task design to match workers' physical abilities, reducing the risk of injury from repetitive motions, strained postures, and overexertion. Notably, MSDs have been reported to contribute to occupational absenteeism significantly and lost productivity. The use of ergonomic interventions, such as adjustable workstations and appropriate tools, can reduce physical stress, thereby enhancing employees' welfare. By planning the workplace in a way that considers employees' physical strain, organizations not only optimize productivity but also cut health care costs related to work-related ailments, thereby building a healthier workforce. Increased ergonomic vigilance and adherence to ergonomic guidelines are crucial for minimizing risk, underscoring the straightforward correlation between ergonomic design and overall health benefits in the workplace. Incorporating ergonomics also goes beyond the physical dimension; it encompasses psychological well-being, which has been accorded increased importance in recent years. The COVID-19 pandemic illustrated the importance of mental well-being at work as problems such as employment insecurity and forced isolation have had lasting impacts on workers' psychological state. Ergonomics at the workplace can mitigate such stressors by ensuring that work environments are not only physically but also psychologically conducive. For instance, ergonomically designed shared workspaces enable collaboration while reducing tension related to physical discomfort. Improving organizational architecture and resilience training may also help employees adapt to shifting environments, particularly in stressful occupations. Emphasis on the holistic aspect of ergonomics encompasses the psychological factors affecting workers' well-being, thus further establishing its merit in the lexicon of Environmental and Occupational Medicine (Giorgi et al., 2020). Also, the link between ergonomics and globalization must be considered, especially in low- and middle-income countries, where labor regulations are typically weak. While industries aim to reduce costs, they may do so at the expense of ergonomic factors, exposing workers to hazardous working conditions. The offshoring of labor-intensive production to less-regulated environments elevates the demand for robust ergonomics to prevent workplace accidents. Studies have indicated that migrant workers, who are usually subjected to below-standard ergonomic practices, exhibit heightened incidences of occupational injury and illness (Abdalla et al., 2017). Therefore, implementing ergonomic training programs specifically for these vulnerable worker segments is important for reducing injuries and improving health outcomes. Generally, recognition of the multidimensional impact of ergonomics on workers' health is crucial in policy formulation and best practice within the dynamic framework of global employment.

12.3.3. Role of Safety Regulations in Mitigating Risks

In policymaking within the framework of environmental and occupational medicine, safety legislations play a critical role in minimizing risks associated with unsafe working conditions. These regulations aim to safeguard employees' health and the environment by imposing safety practices and procedures. For instance, in the floriculture industry, where employees directly interact with pesticides daily, strict safety measures must be implemented to prevent acute and long-term health issues. Studies conducted by Vázquez-Venegas et al. observe that a lack of effective safety protocols encourages the risks workers are exposed to, necessitating strong regulatory systems to enable compliance with best practices. With serious regulatory enforcement, instances of pesticide-induced health issues can be significantly reduced, evincing the important intersection of effective safety regulation and better occupational health outcomes (Narvaez et al., 2025). Moreover, safety regulations not only protect individual workers against immediate hazards but also have long-term implications for public health and environmental sustainability. Employees in forensic and mortuary settings are exposed to several occupational hazards, including chemical hazards and ergonomic hazards, which, if unregulated, can have serious adverse health effects. It is an important study that recently highlighted the need to apply a structured Health Risk Assessment model to quantify and effectively regulate these risks. The findings highlight such significant hazards as low back strain and exposure to harmful chemicals, which recognize the necessity for general controls needed by safety legislation. With the promotion of ergonomically designed tools and better operational processes, legislation can promote smoother workspaces, ultimately promoting productivity and worker health (Ratman et al., 2025). Regular training and education are also integral components of safety legislation that reduce occupational risks even further. Educated employees about safety protocols and occupational risks are also more equipped to look after themselves and others. For the floriculture sector, for instance, supplementary training on the proper use of personal protective equipment (PPE) and safe handling of pesticides can significantly reduce health risks. Through an education-promoted safety culture, employees are more likely to take care of their own health and follow safety guidelines. In addition, cooperation between governments, industries, and workers is central to the effective regulation of these rules. Through this cooperation, safety standards are not only applied but also routinely revised to reflect the changing nature of workplace dangers, thereby underscoring the importance of safety regulations in protecting worker health and maintaining environmental integrity (Narvaez et al., 2025) (Figure 12.7).

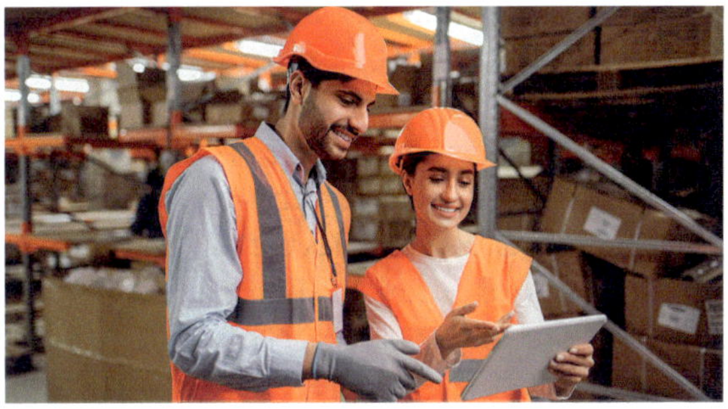

Figure 12.7. Safety regulations play a pivotal role in mitigating risks associated with hazardous work environments.

Source: https://exeedcollege.com/wp-content/uploads/2023/11/safe-work-place-sustainable-features.jpg.

Test Your Knowledge

1. What are the common health risks faced by workers in different industries?
2. How do ergonomic and chemical exposures contribute to occupational illnesses?

12.4. Assessment and Diagnosis

Learning Outcome

1. Understand the methods for evaluating environmental exposures
2. Describe the techniques for assessing occupational health
3. Identify the importance of interdisciplinary approaches

Environmental and occupational medicine-related health conditions require diagnosis and assessment, which is a multidimensional approach, most commonly a mix of subjective feedback and objective clinical evaluation. The complexity of this is further highlighted by research on the psychological impact of exposure to hazardous materials. For instance, research discovers that individuals with a history of exposure to pesticides, like sheep farmers, exhibit elevated rates of psychological distress compared to their non-exposed counterparts. This inference is made from the research outcome, where self-report questionnaires showed high incidence levels of anxiety and depression in exposed individuals. The above illustrates the importance of including a range of assessment tools—subjective and structured clinical interviews—to quantify the multifaceted effects of environmental toxins on mental health. The implications for diagnosis are profound, as psychological symptoms may manifest independently of physical health evaluations, thereby limiting a complete understanding of the individual's overall health status (Ahmed et al., 2016). Early diagnosis remains crucial in working environments, most importantly regarding occupational stressors leading to chronic conditions such as cardiovascular disease (CVD). Working conditions also present particular issues that might increase health risks, as different aspects of job stress can influence vascular health in variable ways. Combining clinical examination, such as conventional echocardiography, with more recent imaging techniques, such as three-dimensional echocardiography, provides a more comprehensive evaluation of cardiovascular health in workers. These advanced diagnostic techniques reveal complexities in assessing myocardial function and contribute to the earliest possible identification of potential health issues. Nevertheless, despite improvements in diagnostic equipment technology, such trends in health indicators can limit accurate clinical assessment, and accordingly, an ethical and balanced interpretation of results based on occupational exposure is necessary (Capotosto et al., 2018). Furthermore, the interactive relationship between environmental exposure and health outcomes highlights the importance of continuous surveillance and monitoring in occupational medicine. The rise in the use of subjective symptom questionnaires and the latest imaging technologies can facilitate improved overall evaluation of a patient's health trajectory in the workplace. The demand of multidisciplinary assessment also stems from consideration of more universal psychosocial determinants that may influence health outcomes, such as stress, lifestyle, and supportive networks. Through holistic evaluation and diagnosis, healthcare practitioners can develop targeted interventions to minimize the risks of specific workplace exposures. The end goal remains to enhance the well-being and health of workers, alongside fulfilling the psychological and physical health needs arising from exposure to the workplace environment (Ahmed et al., 2016; Capotosto et al., 2018).

12.4.1. Methods for Evaluating Environmental Exposures

Environmental exposure evaluation is an important aspect of environmental and occupational medicine because it directly impacts public health interventions and regulations. Several methods have been employed to assess these exposures, including epidemiology, biomonitoring, and geographic information systems (GIS). Epidemiology, for instance, helps link environmental hazards and health status, allowing investigators to track patterns and trends over time. This can be complemented by biomonitoring, in which chemicals or their metabolites are measured in biological samples from a person, thereby providing a more direct measure of exposure levels. An integration of these strategies can offer an integrative understanding of how environmental factors impact health and, in turn, guide policy reforms necessary to prevent and protect vulnerable populations. As the context of environmental health continues to evolve, these strategies must be continuously refined to monitor and intervene effectively. The Centers for Disease Control and Prevention (CDC) identified the importance of robust tracking systems to measure environmental exposures more accurately. By developing a national environmental public health tracking system, the CDC aims to enhance surveillance capacity for environmental hazards and their associated health impacts (Balmes et al., 2006). This initiative aims to integrate federal, state, and local data into a single database to inform community disease prevention efforts. The strategy employed is the development of a technology infrastructure that enables the electronic linking of environmental exposure data with related health outcomes. With these systems applied at the state level, effective scrutiny of exposure risk can enable evidence-based policy-making for environmental health, ultimately leading to improved public health outcomes and responses. In addition to traditional and technological methods, psychiatric evaluation is increasingly being recognized as a key component in the evaluation of the impact of environmental exposures on mental health. Evidence has shown that individuals exposed to certain pesticides, for example, report higher levels of psychological distress than those who are not exposed (Ahmed et al., 2016). These findings highlight the need to include mental health assessments in large-scale environmental health screenings. By using standardized clinical interviews and self-report instruments, researchers can capture the nuances of how environmental exposures lead to psychological disorders. The correlation between mental outcomes and physical health effects demonstrates the interconnectedness of environmental exposure and general well-being, and the relevance of detailed evaluations involving both physical and psychological health perspectives in environmental and occupational medicine.

12.4.2. Techniques for Assessing Occupational Health

Occupational health assessment is essential to ensure the work setting remains safe and productive. A critical way to measure health outcomes is through a multilevel approach that considers many determinants of worker well-being. By considering individual, workgroup, organizational, and societal factors, researchers can examine how intricately these levels are interwoven and how they impact mental health outcomes. This multilevel perspective is typically underappreciated in occupational health studies but offers greater insight into outcomes and the path to more successful interventions. Since it has been recognized, a significant need has emerged for periodic multilevel assessment of the psychosocial work environment, which can lead to specific measures to lower risks and improve overall employee health outcomes (Arnetz et al., 2014). Lastly, adopting this comprehensive methodology can enhance the design of organizational interventions and policymaking towards healthier workplaces. Tracking exposure to harmful substances, particularly in sectors that utilize advanced technologies such as nanotechnology, is an essential component of occupational health assessment. Engineered nanomaterials introduce new workplace challenges that necessitate rigorous health and environmental hazard assessments. Techniques such as air monitoring and biological sampling are used to assess exposure levels, but there remains a significant gap in best practices for effectively monitoring these hazards. Occupational safety and health management must transform to encompass materials that were recently developed and may pose a health risk to employees, especially regarding the effects of nanoparticles. Evidence indicates that without proper monitoring processes in workspaces, workers may expose themselves to unforeseen health hazards that could have significant impacts on their health (Adamec et al., 2019).

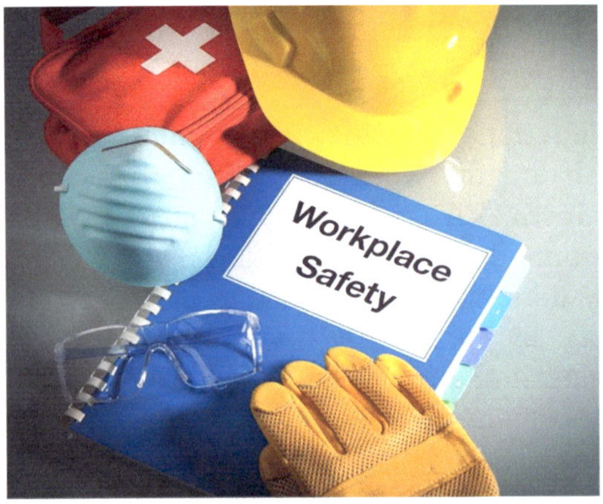

Figure 12.8. Assessing occupational health is crucial for maintaining a safe and productive work environment.

Source: https://d8it4huxumps7.cloudfront.net/uploads/images/65fac27c5c471_2.jpg?d=2000x2000.

Thus, it is crucial to develop practical evaluation tools for this purpose. Employee input and involvement in occupational health examinations can generate tremendous value. By employing focus groups and surveys, organizations can obtain first-hand information about workplace hazards and health problems directly from employees. This participatory approach not only enhances the quality of data that is being collected but also instills a safety and well-being culture within the organization. Moreover, these approaches foster openness and trust, allowing employees to actively engage in the identification and resolution of health problems. As organizations implement multilevel measurements and worker-centered approaches, they can build a more adaptive occupational health system. This will lead to more effective interventions and a healthier workplace overall, further underscoring the need for continual change in testing methods and practices in environmental and occupational medicine (Arnetz et al., 2014) (Figure 12.8).

12.4.3. Importance of Interdisciplinary Approaches

The interdisciplinary programs' role in environmental and occupational medicine is increasingly recognized as a critical factor to address complex health issues. Environmental health situations often overlap with occupational risk exposure, requiring interdisciplinary collaboration among fields such as epidemiology, toxicology, and public health. By combining expertise from these fields, health practitioners can develop a comprehensive understanding of the determinants of disease expression. An example would be combining the biomedical approach and the social model of disability to increase knowledge of how environmental and workplace hazards contribute to human function. All these approaches not only offer an integrative view towards health but also enable one to develop specific interventions to minimize risks as well as improve overall well-being, for example, in the models of the International Classification of Functioning, Disability and Health (ICF) (Grimby et al., 2007). Interdisciplinary collaboration also enables one to have a thorough investigation of the long-term effects of environmental exposure on health. Special care must be taken of an individual's place history, as it yields vital background information for chronic disease diagnosis and treatment. The intricate interplay between geographic history and outcome underscores the importance of considering an individual's environmental exposure history in clinical evaluation.

Extensive analysis of this kind can detect patterns and potential risk factors that inform individualized treatment strategies. As embodied in the connections made in medical geology, an interdisciplinary approach that unifies geoscience, epidemiology, and biomedicine is critical. By appreciating the spatial and environmental determinants of health, practitioners can enhance the predictability, prevention, and control of disease manifestations arising from the interaction between intricate mixtures of environments and human biology (Boulos et al., 2016). Moreover, effective interdisciplinary communication propels innovation in occupational and environmental medicine, paving the way for future research and application. Specialist expertise across various disciplines not only improves communication but also facilitates a reflection of diverse perspectives. For example, cooperative interaction among environmental scientists, occupational health experts, and healthcare providers can yield sound policy recommendations and public health programs that reduce the risk of unsafe environments. The establishment of collaborative networks and research training programs promoting such interdisciplinarity is central to building research capacity in rehabilitation and human functioning. By integrating perspectives across disciplines, environmental and occupational medicine can become responsive to the multifaceted challenges posed by the health problems of the day and ultimately alleviate the suffering these populations endure (Grimby et al., 2007).

Test Your Knowledge

1. What methods are used to assess health risks in occupational and environmental settings?
2. Why is early diagnosis important in preventing work-related and environmental diseases?

12.5. Prevention Strategies

Learning Outcome

1. Define the public health initiatives for environmental protection
2. Discuss on workplace safety programs and training
3. Focus on role of legislation in promoting health

Effective prevention in environmental and occupational medicine requires a sensitive understanding of the unique stressors workers face. An individualized approach becomes a necessity, particularly when dealing with psychological distress among healthcare workers. Studies indicate the importance of tailoring these approaches to account for healthcare workers' personal values and experiences rather than relying solely on expert knowledge. This congruence not only amplifies workers' involvement in protecting their own well-being but also makes intervention programs aimed at mitigating psychological stress more effective. By cultivating organizational support and specifying responsibilities in the context of mental health prevention, healthcare organizations can significantly improve their employees' overall well-being, which, in turn, can lead to better patient care outcomes and reduced stress-related absenteeism (Emal et al., 2024). In addition to psychological determinants, the plan should also encompass physical and psychosocial determinants influencing occupational health and safety (OHS). A review of the literature indicates that organizational determinants, such as corporate culture, management style, and worker attributes, significantly influence workplace conditions. Such complexity can be addressed by developing composite prevention strategies that address multiple determinants. For instance, developing mental health-friendly policies, offering ergonomic working conditions, and instituting strict training programs can significantly lower occupational hazards. Consequently, these methods together foster a safety and health culture, which benefits employees and employers alike by reducing healthcare costs and increasing productivity through better health (El Kholti et al., 2024).

In addition, it is necessary to emphasize that effective prevention measures must be evidence-based, supported by an in-depth review of current and historical trends in workplace health risks. By applying an evidence-based, integrated approach grounded in empirical studies, policymakers can inform their interventions with a clear appreciation of the unique health risks posed by varied work situations. Involving both management and employees in the formulation of these plans through participatory structures can help ensure diverse viewpoints are incorporated and foster greater acceptance and compliance with health plans. Finally, the successful implementation of targeted prevention strategies relies on continuous monitoring and adaptation, affirming the commitment to encouraging safer and more sustainable working environments in the field of environmental and occupational medicine (El kholti et al., 2024; Emal et al., 2024).

12.5.1. Public Health Initiatives for Environmental Protection

Public health interventions to protect the environment must be implemented to prevent the harmful health impacts of environmental degradation. These initiatives generally target specific pollutants, and air quality management is most prominent because it is directly related to respiratory health. In Poland, for instance, a sequence of interventions aimed at reducing particulate matter (PM10) has led to statistically significant reductions in concentrations from 2014 to 2019 across several cities. Despite this encouraging trend, the relationship between improved air quality and decreased hospitalization for chronic conditions like asthma and chronic obstructive pulmonary disease (COPD) is complex, as air pollution is only one of many factors that affect health outcomes. This necessitates an interdisciplinary approach involving investments in health care infrastructure and community awareness, resulting in a stronger, combined strategy for environmental conservation and public health (Ścibor et al., 2024). Public health programs' interdisciplinary nature also makes them more effective in environmental conservation by integrating results from fields such as epidemiology, sociology, and environmental science. This cooperative effort promotes a better understanding of the multifaceted determinants of health. For example, blending new technologies and techniques—e.g., real-time air quality monitoring systems—can yield rich data that can guide both policy and public education strategies. Sound data analysis supports targeted interventions that are essential in managing particular environmental health threats. Moreover, new concepts, such as the application of nanotechnology to reduce industrial emissions, can significantly redefine public health outcomes by eliminating exposure to harmful pollutants (Bawab et al., 2024). In that view, implementing an interdisciplinary approach not only optimizes protective measures but also builds an effective public health system that supports environmental sustainability. Communities are central in ensuring the success of public health measures for environmental protection because their engagement is paramount in carrying out and sustaining such practices. Health awareness campaigns that develop sensitization to environmental health risks are vital for ensuring community participation and sparking grassroots movements.

By engaging citizens in monitoring local air quality or encouraging sustainable practices, public health programs can instill a sense of ownership and responsibility towards environmental health. Additionally, collaboration among governmental agencies, non-profit organizations, and community groups can provide access to shared resources and collective efforts toward advocating for cleaner environments. Such initiatives, premised on community involvement, are more likely to achieve long-term success by ensuring that public health and environmental protection are made mutual goals, ultimately resulting in healthier communities and sustainable environments (Bawab et al., 2024; Ścibor et al., 2024) (Figure 12.9).

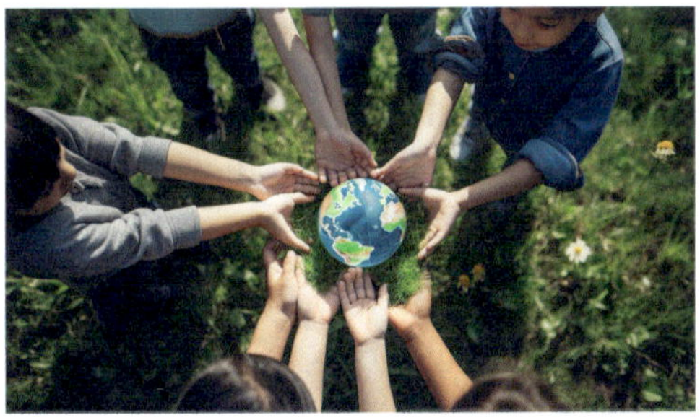

Figure 12.9. Public health initiatives designed to protect the environment play a critical role in mitigating the adverse health outcomes associated with environmental degradation.

Source: https://one-more-tree.org/wp-content/uploads/2024/04/599323.jpg.

12.5.2. Workplace Safety Programs and Training

In the discipline of Environmental and Occupational Medicine, workplace safety programs and training serve as the fundamental support pillars for protecting workers' health and well-being. They are designed to anticipate and respond to potential dangers, enhance safety features, and foster a culture of organizational health. Effective training programs can improve employees' awareness of workplace risks and equip them with skills to identify and avoid risks. For instance, formal training not only familiarizes employees with safety processes but also equips them to proactively prevent accidents. By integrating extensive safety training into the employee onboarding process, organizations do more than meet regulatory compliance; they create a safe work environment, which can reduce the prevalence of occupational hazards and the illnesses they cause. Moreover, the effectiveness of workplace safety programs is significantly enhanced by a participatory approach that involves employees at all levels. Engaging employees to contribute to safety talks and provide their input, it creates ownership and accountability towards safety cultures. This has worked in other industries, where specific hazards were identified and personalized interventions developed. By receiving ongoing feedback and participating in safety seminars, employees become more engaged with their environment. Moreover, team-based training and communication reinforce workplace relationships, thereby promoting a safety culture. Such teamwork, in turn, reduces the risk of accidents, underscoring the pivotal role of safety programs in occupational health management (Abdalla et al., 2017). Furthermore, checking and modifying safety programs is essential to maintaining their effectiveness over time. Regular monitoring enables organizations to assess the effectiveness of their training programme, identify areas for improvement, and adapt to emerging threats. Businesses can determine the usefulness of their safety regimes through measurements like reporting incidents and employee feedback, ensuring training remains effective and adaptable to new workplace challenges. Additionally, integrating technological advances, such as virtual reality simulations for training, can enhance learning sessions and retention. As industries advance and face increasingly novel challenges, a commitment to ongoing evaluation and improvement of workplace safety initiatives will be essential to protecting worker health and preventing occupational accidents.

12.5.3. Role of Legislation in Promoting Health

Legislation will play an essential role in protecting public health by making and enforcing rules that protect people from a wide range of environmental and work-related risks. Regulations and laws are intended to address risks in work environments, such as exposure to toxins, noise, and ergonomic stressors. By mandating safety standards and healthcare, legislation can significantly improve workers' overall health. Additionally, such policies ensure that employers not just provide a safe working place but also the mental and emotional well-being of the workers. For instance, work-life policies and access to mental health support can enhance employee productivity and reduce absence, ultimately leading to a healthier society overall. Thus, the intersection of legislative action and occupational health is essential so that diseases are prevented and health benefits are maximized in numerous sectors. In addition, good laws help mitigate health issues caused by environmental conditions, including air and water quality, which significantly influence community health. Stringent regulatory measures can limit the release of contaminants, thereby making living conditions safer. The law governing the application of hazardous chemicals in industry is particularly important for protecting workers and the general public from exposure to chemicals that cause long-term and acute diseases. For instance, legislation requiring the use of protective equipment and procedures in hazardous workplaces is very important for preserving employees' health and reducing occupational accidents. All the while, more detailed environmental legislation enforces sustainable action, which, in turn, contributes to better population well-being in the long run. Thus, legislation is a foundation point for reconciling environmental integrity with public health aspirations (Groneberg et al., 2012). Furthermore, legislation not only averts widespread diseases but also provides opportunities for ongoing public health advancements through persistent research and proactive initiatives.

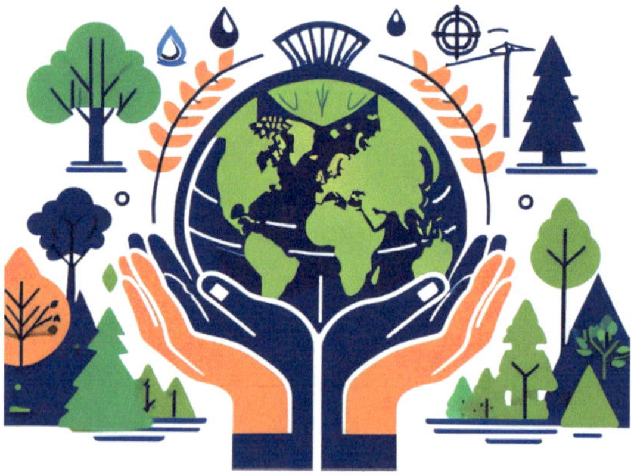

Figure 12.10. Legislation plays a crucial role in safeguarding public health by establishing and enforcing regulations that address various environmental and occupational hazards.

Source: https://cdn.prod.website-files.com/6583722c166f0828cd927558/6632ea1fe8d98e308c6ffb78_JHb9AngmqYYfNq50xYfXgyMhis7iseyg0DqYyux192QNemALB-out-0.png.

Policies that support funding for health programs, education, and technology development are essential to developing new prevention strategies. For example, comprehensive bicycle safety legislation, with regulations governing mandatory helmet use, has a direct influence on health outcomes by lowering the incidence of severe head injuries among bicyclists (Groneberg et al., 2012). These regulations bring together various stakeholders, from policymakers to urban planners, who all contribute to an integrated response in health promotion. Therefore, responsive legislative frameworks addressing emerging health issues, coupled with public education and awareness, are important in sustaining health gains and improving the quality of life in communities (Figure 12.10).

Test Your Knowledge

1. What strategies are used to prevent occupational and environmental diseases?
2. How does workplace safety and regulation reduce health risks for workers?

SUMMARY

Environmental and Occupational Medicine stands at the crossroads, reflecting the complex interdependence of human and environmental factors. As demonstrated by a series of studies and bibliometric analyses, the United States has consistently been a research productivity leader in this field, contributing significantly to the broader domains of Preventive Medicine and Public Health. The classic study of research trends demonstrates that USA researchers accounted for a significant share of research in these areas, a testament as much to a robust institutional framework as to a commitment to developing scientific evidence that will ultimately guide policy and practice. This leadership role is important because it underscores the need for ongoing research on occupational and environmental hazards, ultimately informing public health policies that aim to minimize risks and enhance community health (Falagas et al., 2010). Additionally, the shifting nature of authorship in Occupational Medicine journals reflects broader trends within the academic community. The prevalence of multi-author articles in the specialty is consistent with other medical journal research. It suggests the collective approach to resolving complex health issues involving combinations of environmental exposures and occupational hazards. As has been observed, progress toward more authors per article portends a collaborative movement to bring together a diversity of expertise and multidisciplinary perspectives, which are essential to addressing the complexities of occupational and environmental health. Notably, the higher impact factors of such journals are positively correlated with collaborative research, underscoring the need for researchers to collaborate across disciplines to boost innovation and health outcomes (Aw et al., 2009). In conclusion, the field of Environmental and Occupational Medicine is essential in the maintenance of public health in the context of ongoing environmental exposures and occupational risks. The assertive guidance of American researchers in the field, together with the growing trend towards collaborative research, underscores the need for ongoing investment in this field. Less developed nations must cultivate their scientific capabilities to deliver wholesome health advancement to the world. By fostering environments conducive to cross-disciplinary collaboration and by funding scientific endeavors, nations can enhance their contributions to this critical mission. Lastly, empowering researchers worldwide will not only strengthen the overall pool of knowledge but also ensure that appropriate interventions are implemented to protect vulnerable populations from environmental and occupational health hazards.

In environmental and occupational medicine, several factors underlie both workers' health and the environment in which they work. The identification of fever in intensive care unit (ICU) patients underscores the complexity of diagnosing and managing emerging conditions influenced by both healthcare practice and environmental stressors. New recommendations from a task force comprising representatives from several critical care fields emphasize the need to recognize normal variation in body temperature across populations, underscoring the convergence of occupational health and environmental factors. Such legislation provides excellent recommendations to practitioners, which guide the control of fevered patients by considering both clinical and environmental factors, as well as underlying reasons that might not be immediately apparent on standard examinations (Stegall et al., 2025). Collaboration is also a primary element in promoting occupational health development, particularly within academic settings. Moroccan universities are at the forefront of developing novel solutions to occupational health through multidisciplinary task forces that represent all disciplines. The task forces are responsible for reviewing existing practices and facilitating the development of policies and guidelines specifically for students and staff. Stakeholder involvement is essential in formulating an all-inclusive framework that addresses shared occupational health problems and adheres to local legislation and international standards. This strategic approach not only enhances the workplace but also prepares higher institutions to embark on significant world-class projects safely (Azeddoug, 2024). Moreover, integrating occupational health education into curricula is essential to creating a workforce that values and prioritizes safety and health across professional settings. By integrating occupational health principles into academic programs, universities can equip students with the necessary skills and sensitization to address the changing issues in the field. Such initiatives as health campaigns and training courses can also further prepare students and faculty to adopt healthy lifestyle practices and stress management strategies. The anticipated outcomes of these training programs are two-pronged in that they not only enhance the learning environment but also create a culture of wellness and safety that permeates the work environment and contributes positively to the overall health of the community (Azeddoug, 2024).

KEY TERMS FROM THIS CHAPTER

Occupational Exposure
Toxicology
Noise-Induced Hearing Loss
Ergonomics
Personal Protective Equipment (PPE)
Risk Assessment
Repetitive Strain Injury (RSI)
Environmental Health
Industrial Hygiene
Air Pollution
Hazardous Substances
Respiratory Hazards
Occupational Health Surveillance
Heat Stress
Work-Related Stress

CRITICAL THINKING QUESTIONS

1. **Which of the following is the most common route of exposure to environmental toxins in the general population?**
   a. Intravenous
   b. Inhalation
   c. Ingestion
   d. Dermal contact
2. **What is the primary occupational disease caused by chronic exposure to asbestos?**
   a. Asthma
   b. Mesothelioma
   c. Chronic bronchitis
   d. Emphysema
3. **The concept of "Threshold Limit Value" (TLV) is used to describe:**
   a. The maximum safe drug dose in medicine
   b. The concentration of a chemical that causes immediate death
   c. The level of a substance a worker can be exposed to daily without adverse effects
   d. The environmental concentration at which a pollutant is visible
4. **Lead poisoning in children can cause which of the following?**
   a. Improved attention span
   b. Irreversible neurological damage
   c. Decreased bone density
   d. Hypoglycemia
5. **Which of the following is a primary prevention strategy in occupational health?**
   a. Early detection of disease
   b. Rehabilitation after injury
   c. Use of personal protective equipment (PPE)
   d. Symptom management

Short Answer Questions

1. What is environmental medicine, and how does it differ from occupational medicine?
2. How do environmental exposures impact human health?
3. What is the exposome, and why is it essential in environmental health?
4. What are the common respiratory diseases caused by occupational exposures?
5. What are the main routes of toxic substance exposure?
6. How does ozone differ in the upper and lower atmosphere in terms of health impacts?

Answers to Critical Thinking Questions

1. (c); 2. (b); 3. (c); 4. (b); 5. (c)

REFERENCES

1. Abdalla, S., Apramian, S. S., Cantley, L. F., & Cullen, M. R. (2017). Occupation and risk for injuries. In *The World Bank eBooks* (pp. 97–132). https://doi.org/10.1596/978-1-4648-0522-6_ch6Abdalla, S., Apramian, S. S., Cantley, L. F., & Cullen, M. R. (2017). Occupation and risk for injuries. In *The World Bank eBooks* (pp. 97–132). https://doi.org/10.1596/978-1-4648-0522-6_ch6Adamec, V., Köbölová, K., Pavlíková, S., Procházková, K., et al. (2019). Current approaches of occupational and safety health management in work environments containing nanoparticles. https://core.ac.uk/download/287648860.pdf (accessed on 16th July 2025).
2. Ahmed, A., Aldridge, T., Ames, C., Amr, M., Bazylewicz-Walczak, B., Beach, J., Beard, J., et al. (2016). Anxiety and depression following cumulative low-level exposure to organophosphate pesticides. https://core.ac.uk/download/82983113.pdf (accessed on 16th July 2025).
3. Amin, E. A., Hussien, H. M. M., & Hassan, M. M. (2024). Occupational health hazards among workers dealing with medical waste disposal in outpatient clinics. *Egyptian Journal of Health Care*. https://www.semanticscholar.org/paper/660b0354380247c0b6dbc760803c0684976e6a47 (accessed on 16th July 2025).
4. Arnetz, B., Bacharach, S., Bamberger, P., Biron, M., Biron, C., Biron, D., Biron, R., et al. (2014). The psychosocial work environment, employee mental health and organizational interventions: Improving research and practice by taking a multilevel approach. https://core.ac.uk/download/30650323.pdf (accessed on 16th July 2025).
5. Aw, T. C., & Shaban, S. (2009). Trend towards multiple authorship in occupational medicine journals. https://core.ac.uk/download/pdf/8261435.pdf (accessed on 16th July 2025).
6. Azeddoug, H. (2024). SPL09 Leading innovation for excellence in occupational health in Moroccan universities on the eve of major world-class projects. Occupational Medicine. https://www.semanticscholar.org/paper/7487799e6f65c7d1d005246c79e00d5c521b36ea (accessed on 16th July 2025).
7. Bader, M., De Cremer, K., De Paepe, P., De Smedt, D., et al. (2016). Short-term health effects in the general population following a major train accident with acrylonitrile in Belgium. https://core.ac.uk/download/84041781.pdf (accessed on 16th July 2025).
8. Balmes, J. R., Buffler, P. A., Kyle, A. D., Lee, S., et al. (2006). Integrating research, surveillance, and practice in environmental public health tracking. https://core.ac.uk/download/323082246.pdf (accessed on 16th July 2025).
9. Bawab, T., Al-Shariah, M., Majed, H., Alshammri, H., Naytah, T., Aseeri, S. M., & Al Julaih, A. (2024). A multidisciplinary perspective on public health: The role of fuel cells and nanotechnology in advancing epidemiology, occupational health, emergency services, nursing, and laboratory operations. Fuel Cells Bulletin. https://www.semanticscholar.org/paper/6a4566506ca08202914112ebb677df0fce3acb13 (accessed on 16th July 2025).
10. Beamer, P. I., Brody, J. G., Brown, P., Loh, M., et al. (2016). Reporting back environmental exposure data and free choice learning. https://core.ac.uk/download/323063135.pdf (accessed on 16th July 2025).
11. Belzunegui Eraso, Á. G., & Erro-Garcés, A. (2020). Teleworking in the context of the COVID-19 crisis. *Sustainability, 12*, 3662–3662. https://doi.org/10.3390/su12093662 (accessed on 16th July 2025).

12. Bochenek, B., Jankowski, M., Wieczorek, J., Gruszczyńska, M., Pinkas, J., & Figurski, M. (2025). A bibliometric analysis with data OpenAlex and mining methods of 41,525 abstracts of papers on the health impact of air pollution published between 1960 and 2022. *International Journal of Occupational Medicine and Environmental Health*. https://www.semanticscholar.org/paper/9a8e7f3d919e8de5cf7aa2bc9d0468ef5e6b9df2 (accessed on 16th July 2025).

13. Bolis, M. (2025). Legislation and control of health risks in Latin America and the Caribbean. https://core.ac.uk/download/pdf/6442042.pdf (accessed on 16th July 2025).

14. Boulos, M. N. K., & Le Blond, J. S. (2016). On the road to personalized and precision geomedicine: Medical geology and a renewed call for interdisciplinarity. https://core.ac.uk/download/77008358.pdf (accessed on 16th July 2025).

15. Capotosto, L., De Sio, S., Massoni, F., Ricci, F., et al. (2018). Early diagnosis of cardiovascular diseases in workers: Role of standard and advanced echocardiography. https://core.ac.uk/download/141696274.pdf (accessed on 16th July 2025).

16. Cedrone, F., Corbosiero, P., De Sio, S., Di Traglia, M., et al. (2017). Quality of life in workers and stress: Gender differences in exposure to psychosocial risks and perceived well-being. https://core.ac.uk/download/141696237.pdf (accessed on 16th July 2025).

17. Clay, D., Davies, R., Elias, P., Gumber, A., et al. (2004). Review of the occupational health and safety of Britain's ethnic minorities. https://core.ac.uk/download/105299.pdf (accessed on 16th July 2025).

18. Dale, A. M., Evanoff, B. A., Franzblau, A., Zeringue, A., et al. (2014). Using job-title-based physical exposures from O*NET in an epidemiological study of carpal tunnel syndrome. https://core.ac.uk/download/80494858.pdf (accessed on 16th July 2025).

19. El Kholti, R., Soltani, S., Durand, P., & El Kholti, A. (2024). P-405 Understanding the role of determinants in improving occupational health and safety. Occupational Medicine. https://www.semanticscholar.org/paper/817e29ed74e4888ba38fc8846ecec4907b1effe0 (accessed on 16th July 2025).

20. Emal, L. M., Tamminga, S., Beumer, A., Kezic, S., Timmermans, D. R. M., Schaafsma, F., & van der Molen, H. F. (2024). Risk perceptions of health care workers and occupational health experts on psychological distress. Journal of Occupational and Environmental Medicine, 66, 1066–1071. https://www.semanticscholar.org/paper/c3026a46f78701a08778bff7bc2691ccc247f0da (accessed on 16th July 2025).

21. Falagas, M. E., & Soteriades, E. S. (2010). A bibliometric analysis in the fields of preventive medicine, occupational and environmental medicine, epidemiology, and public health. https://core.ac.uk/download/28934732.pdf (accessed on 16th July 2025).

22. Forouzanfar, M. H., Alexander, L., Anderson, H. R., Bachman, V. F., Biryukov, S., Bräuer, M., Burnett, R., et al. (2016). Global, regional, and national comparative risk assessment of 79 behavioral, environmental and occupational, and metabolic risks or clusters of risks, 1990–2015: A systematic analysis for the Global Burden of Disease Study 2015. The Lancet, 388, 1659–1724. https://doi.org/10.1016/s0140-6736(16)31679-8 (accessed on 16th July 2025).

23. Giorgi, G., Lecca, L. I., Alessio, F., Finstad, G. L., Bondanini, G., Lulli, L. G., Arcangeli, G., et al. (2020). COVID-19-related mental health effects in the workplace: A narrative review. *International Journal of Environmental Research and Public Health, 17*, 7857–7857. https://doi.org/10.3390/ijerph17217857 (accessed on 16th July 2025).

24. Gooya, N. C. (2020). The contemporary porn debate–Perceptions of sexual health of porn actors, the 2013 HIV crisis, and recognizing the complexities of the porn industry. https://core.ac.uk/download/322983186.pdf (accessed on 16th July 2025).

25. Grimby, G., Melvin, J., Reinhardt, J. D., & Stucki, G., et al. (2007). Developing human functioning and rehabilitation research from the comprehensive perspective. https://core.ac.uk/download/46967987.pdf (accessed on 16th July 2025).

26. Groneberg, J. D. A., Klingelhöfer, D., Müller, D., Uibel, S., et al. (2012). Bicycle helmet use and non-use–Recently published research. https://core.ac.uk/download/14524386.pdf (accessed on 16th July 2025).

27. Hayes, R., Yin, S., Dosemeci, M., Li, G., Wacholder, S., Travis, L., Li, C. Y., et al. (1997). Benzene and the dose-related incidence of hematologic neoplasms in China. Chinese Academy of Preventive Medicine–National Cancer Institute Benzene Study Group. Journal of the National Cancer Institute, 89(14), 1065–1071. https://www.semanticscholar.org/paper/cd274811873597dfd25d1acee4d2df0bced09397 (accessed on 16th July 2025).

28. Hinson, A., Aguèmon, B., Adjobimey, M., Damien, G., Ouili, I., Mikponhoue, R., Cissé, I., et al. (2021). Prevalence and associated factors of occupational stress in the mining sector: The case study of the Youga Mine at Zabre in Burkina Faso. *Occupational Diseases and Environmental Medicine*. https://www.semanticscholar.org/paper/5f3942f09a03cfc516ac07353d9feb3c308b8aeb (accessed on 16th July 2025).

29. Jung, M., Kim, H., Kim, J. H., Seo, D. J., Leem, J., Park, S., Lee, D. W., et al. (2025). Relationship between long-term PM2.5 exposure and myopia prevalence in adults: Analysis of the Korea National Health and Nutrition Examination Survey-Air Pollution Linked Data, 2020. Annals of Occupational and Environmental Medicine, 37, e8. https://www.semanticscholar.org/paper/0e7a876308585235ac4a135afd019ae0efdf53bc (accessed on 16th July 2025).

30. Kim, E. A., & Nakata, M. (2014). Work-related musculoskeletal disorders in Korea and Japan: A comparative description. *Annals of Occupational and Environmental Medicine, 26*, 17–17. https://www.semanticscholar.org/paper/8491b5b5d087af9e5fe34f141d2ba07fb49b760e (accessed on 16th July 2025).

31. Kriebel, D., Tickner, J., Jacobs, M., & Markkanen, P. (2011). Lessons learned: Solutions for workplace safety and health. https://core.ac.uk/download/71352756.pdf (accessed on 16th July 2025).

32. Lungu, K., Morse, T., & Taulo, S. (2010). Gap analysis of environmental health research in Malawi: Report to the National Commission of Science and Technology. https://core.ac.uk/download/19610167.pdf (accessed on 16th July 2025).

33. Mansyur, M. (2023). The importance of occupational health service in the era of VUCA and the dissemination of related research results. https://core.ac.uk/download/639382356.pdf (accessed on 16th July 2025).

34. Mashigo, M., Risenga, I., & Dukhan, S. (2024). First-year health sciences students' perspectives on indigenous knowledge and medical practices. African Journal of Research in Mathematics, Science and Technology Education, 28, 422–436. https://www.semanticscholar.org/paper/64b61d8118e4f5810793bf1350c2a56365b51b77 (accessed on 16th July 2025).

35. Merigó, J. M., & Núñez, A. (2016). Influential journals in health research: A bibliometric study. Globalization and Health, 12. https://doi.org/10.1186/s12992-016-0186-4 (accessed on 16th July 2025).

36. Naweed, A., & Chapman, J. (2015). Health initiatives to target obesity in surface transport industries: Review and implications for action. https://core.ac.uk/download/pdf/30671333.pdf (accessed on 16th July 2025).

37. Negri, M., Cagno, E., Colicchia, C., & Sarkis, J. (2021). Integrating sustainability and resilience in the supply chain: A systematic literature review and a research agenda. Business Strategy and the Environment, 30, 2858–2886. https://doi.org/10.1002/bse.2776 (accessed on 16th July 2025).

38. Nettleton, S. (2009). Commentary: The appearance of new medical cosmologies and the re-appearance of sick and healthy men and women: A comment on the merits of social theorizing. International Journal of Epidemiology, 38(3), 633–636. https://www.semanticscholar.org/paper/ada069509c84157afc4d71c7da8f93c7479fdcbe (accessed on 16th July 2025).

39. Orr, R. M., Pope, R., Rigby, T., Schram, B., et al. (2018). An analysis of reported dangerous incidents, exposures, and near misses amongst army soldiers. https://core.ac.uk/download/196606488.pdf (accessed on 16th July 2025).

40. Ratman, M. F., Meilia, P. D. I., Ariningsih, A., & Mubin, M. (2025). Health risk assessment in forensic and mortuary services at Persahabatan General Hospital: Identifying and mitigating occupational hazards. JMMR (Jurnal Medicoeticolegal dan Manajemen Rumah Sakit). https://www.semanticscholar.org/paper/3534b7ddfacb277b0085e9ad26883e8612899b8d (accessed on 16th July 2025).

41. Ścibor, M., Leoszkiewicz, K., Micek, A., Chomoncik, K., Dubas-Jakóbczyk, K., Kocot, E., Bąk, A., et al. (2024). The association between air pollutions and emergency hospitalizations due to COPD and asthma across 16 Polish cities: Population-based study. International Journal of Occupational Medicine and Environmental Health, 37, 110–127. https://www.semanticscholar.org/paper/06d8439f89f767a5dad8e65d23c3c30435b591f7 (accessed on 16th July 2025).

42. Stegall, C. J., Dao, T. H., & Jackson, C. D. (2025). Know your guidelines series: Key recommendations from the SCCM/IDSA guideline on evaluating new fever in the adult intensive care unit patient. *Southern Medical Journal, 118*, 338–340. https://www.semanticscholar.org/paper/bdfe287c4cc6c92844c1b10f3306cdc22088732a (accessed on 16th July 2025).

43. Villegas Narvaez, L. M., & Montero Reyes, Y. (2025). Occupational safety in floriculture: Challenges and solutions to the use of pesticides. SCT Proceedings in Interdisciplinary Insights and Innovations. https://www.semanticscholar.org/paper/9b6e6dcde9f93a0c7ac224660346d3630e7afc22 (accessed on 16th July 2025).

INDEX

A

Absorption, distribution, metabolism, and excretion (ADME). 354
Acid-suppressive therapy 119
Acute kidney injury (AKI) 135, 138, 142, 145, 151, 157, 163, 165
Acute lymphoblastic leukemia (ALL) 217
Acute myeloid leukemia (AML) 212, 217, 218, 224, 229
Adjunct treatment 118
Adrenal disease 180, 182, 199
Age/sex/gene expression score (ASGES) 39, 47, 60
Albumin-to-creatinine ratio (ACR) 148
Alcohol consumption 54, 59, 68, 360
Alloimmunization 210, 236
Angioplasty 52, 55, 165
Animal husbandry practices 252, 263
Ankle-brachial index (ABI) 20
Antibiotic misuse 260
Antibiotic resistance 82, 241, 244, 249, 250, 260, 261, 263, 266
Antibiotic treatment 82, 257
Anticoagulant treatments 88
Antiepileptic drug (AED) treatment 364
Anti-inflammatory medications 286
Antimicrobial guidelines 244, 270
Antimicrobial resistance (AMR) 90
Antimicrobial spectrum 257
Antimicrobial stewardship (AMS) programs 260
Antimicrobial therapy 82
Antineutrophil cytoplasmic antibody (ANCA) 136
Arthritis Self-Management Programs (ASMPs) 280
Artificial intelligence (AI) 17, 62, 84, 126, 161, 183, 191, 192, 228, 229, 231, 235, 284, 329, 332
Atrial fibrillation (AF) 43, 53
Attitudes about Complex Therapy Scale (ACTS) 25, 31
Audiological manifestations 282
Autism spectrum disorder (ASD) 327, 331
Autofluorescence (AF) 149
Autoimmune diseases 9, 120, 282, 285, 289, 293, 302
Autoimmune reaction 286
Automated peritoneal dialysis (APD) 351
Autosomal dominant polycystic kidney disease (ADPKD) 150

B

Bacterial infections 249
Bibliometric analysis 131, 341, 383, 402
Biological challenges 259
Biological mechanisms 227, 243
Biological variability 219
Blood diseases 211, 218, 229, 230
Blood transfusion therapy 223

Brain abnormalities 19
Broad-spectrum antibiotics 256
Bronchial thermoplasty (BT), 85
Bronchodilators 81, 82, 86, 87, 372
Bronchoscopy 85, 86
Bronchus-associated lymphoid tissue (BALT) 77, 95

C

Calcium nephrolithiasis 159, 160, 166
Cardiac magnetic resonance imaging (CMR) 59
Cardiac resynchronization therapy (CRT) 63
Cardiology 1, 3, 37, 38, 39, 40, 41, 42, 43, 44, 45, 47, 48, 49, 50, 51, 52, 53, 54, 55, 56, 57, 58, 59, 60, 61, 62, 63, 64, 67, 68, 100, 104, 129, 172, 191, 341
Cardiovascular conditions 16, 39, 43, 48, 54, 55, 61, 62, 136, 191
Cardiovascular disease 6, 13, 14, 16, 21, 31, 38, 40, 41, 42, 44, 49, 54, 55, 56, 57, 58, 59, 63, 91, 142, 153, 155, 179, 195, 203, 209, 278, 373, 390
Causation based 213
Cell-bound complement activation products (CB-CAPs) 274, 283
Cell reconstitution 224
Central nervous system (CNS) 311, 314, 363
Cerebrospinal fluid 312, 320, 323, 339
Chemotherapy 210, 217, 221, 222, 224, 227, 373
Chronic blood disorders 212, 213
Chronic disease 2, 4, 11, 12, 14, 18, 22, 29, 35, 40, 57, 58, 73, 144, 175, 192, 193, 209, 214, 215, 216, 226, 262, 289, 295, 345, 358, 376, 385, 393
Chronic endocrine diseases 188, 195, 196
Chronic illnesses 13, 21, 90, 171, 192, 199, 216, 291, 299, 359, 364
Chronic kidney disease (CKD) 29, 30, 135, 136, 137, 138, 142, 147, 152, 155, 156, 157, 159, 163, 165, 166
Chronic myeloid leukemia (CML) 217
Chronic obstructive pulmonary disease (COPD) 71, 79, 80, 87, 90, 92, 95, 394
Chronic pain 22, 274, 277, 286, 296, 331, 387
Clinical characteristics 277, 352
Clinical correlation 282
Clinical effects 349, 362
Clinical endeavors 136
Clinical evaluation 147, 181, 199, 221, 255, 256, 283, 289, 322, 390, 393
Clinical evaluations 283, 293
Clinical guidelines 23, 59, 60, 143, 153, 159, 279, 326
Clinical outcomes 10, 11, 42, 80, 81, 85, 119, 122, 124, 127, 151, 196, 213, 214, 245, 258, 281, 298, 299, 320, 353, 355, 358, 359, 364
Clinical pharmacology 343, 344, 345, 346, 347, 349, 350, 351, 352, 353, 354, 355, 356, 357, 358, 359, 361, 362, 363, 364, 365, 366, 367, 368, 369, 371, 373, 374
Clinical practice 2, 5, 6, 7, 8, 9, 15, 17, 18, 23, 28, 34, 38, 39, 47, 50, 51, 54, 55, 59, 60, 64, 66, 73, 75, 82, 85, 86, 104, 113, 117, 119, 125, 126, 127, 146, 154, 160, 165, 167, 168, 191, 194, 198, 199, 209, 212, 218, 219, 223, 229, 230, 232, 233, 236, 242, 247, 254, 256, 257, 259, 260, 263, 266, 267, 268, 275, 276, 277, 283, 285, 287, 288, 290, 294, 295, 296, 297, 299, 307, 308, 321, 327, 329, 332, 334, 344, 345, 346, 347, 351, 358, 363, 364, 365, 369
Clinical syndrome 47, 215
Clinical treatment 243, 330
Clostridium difficile 129, 132, 244, 245, 257, 270
Clostridium Difficile infection (CDI) 105
Cognitive Behavioral Therapy (CBT) 22
Collaborative platforms 247
Colorectal cancer (CRC) 105, 126
Colorectal cancer screening (CRCS) 126
Common pathological theme 317
Community-acquired pneumonia (CAP), 81
Comorbidities management 42
Competency levels 8
Complete blood counts (CBC) 18, 218
Complex clinical challenge 108
Complex diseases 125, 225, 277, 323
Complex rare genetic syndromes (CRGS) 172
Comprehensive methodology 391
Comprehensive treatment 1, 116, 127, 255, 274, 277, 286, 288, 290, 318, 326, 329
Computed tomography (CT) 17, 19, 112, 148, 149,

254, 284, 320
Continuous glucose monitoring (CGM) 188
Contraindications 220
Coronary cardiac tomography (CCT) 59
Coronary heart disease 44, 45, 54
Current developments 330
Customized treatment programs 323, 326
Cystic fibrosis-associated liver disease (CFLD) 112, 113

D

Dazzling complexity 182
Deaths and disability-adjusted life years (DALYs) 309
Depersonalization 27
Diagnostic accuracy 9, 15, 17, 20, 39, 50, 60, 62, 76, 83, 109, 110, 114, 117, 125, 183, 191, 251, 254, 283, 284, 293, 321, 322, 323, 329, 331, 332
Diagnostic equipment technology 390
Diagnostic process 60, 192, 253, 282, 284, 320, 332
Diagnostic skills 3, 328
Diagnostic yields 109
Dialysis procedures 153
Differentiated thyroid cancer (DTC) 185
Direct oral anticoagulants (DOACs) 53
Disability-adjusted life-years (DALYs) 380
Disease-modifying antirheumatic drugs (DMARDs) 289
Disease progression 16, 54, 87, 112, 124, 136, 143, 146, 150, 159, 161, 195, 212, 213, 231, 275, 294, 318, 321, 330
Disease Surveillance Networks (DSN) 15, 246, 261, 265, 267
Disease transmission 245, 252, 253, 255, 265
Disproportionately 245, 247, 262, 294
Drug Advisory Committee (DAC) 41
Drug resistance 227, 244, 253, 259

E

ECG tracing 50
Echocardiographic technology 50
Echocardiography 37, 42, 48, 49, 50, 51, 59, 192, 390, 402
Economic constraints 47
Economic sustainability 264
Electrocardiography (ECG) 49
Electrolyte balance 136, 138, 139, 140, 141
Electromyography (EMG) 320
Electronic health records 11, 17, 23, 206, 362
Embolic strokes 316
Emotional stability 318
Endocrine system 173, 174, 175, 176, 177, 178, 179, 201
Endocrinology 129, 173, 174, 175, 176, 183, 187, 190, 193, 194, 199, 204, 205, 206, 339
Endoscopic procedures 110
End-stage kidney disease (ESKD) 161, 165
End-stage renal disease (ESRD) 138, 151, 152, 153, 155, 160
Enforcement practices 379
Environmental medicine 375, 376, 377, 379, 380, 381, 393, 400, 402
Environmental risk 92, 383
Environmental sustainability 381, 382, 389, 395
Epidemiologic environments 264
Erectile dysfunction (ED) 311
Erythropoietin (EPO) 142
European Rheumatology 289
Evidence-based guidelines 2, 7, 43, 112, 118, 143, 155, 175, 223, 298, 329, 334

F

Fatigue Severity Scale (FSS) 275
Feature evaluation 185
Febrile neutropenia 210, 218, 258, 271
Fibrotic responses 152
Follicle-stimulating hormone (FSH) 184
Food and Drug Administration (FDA) 345, 356
Forced oscillation technique (FOT) 76
Fracture liaison 287
Framework of Occupational Medicine 385
Functional Magnetic Resonance Imaging (fMRI) 331
Fundamental components 7, 18, 231
Fundamentally revolutionized 331

G

Gastroenterology 1, 103, 104, 105, 106, 107, 108, 109, 110, 111, 112, 113, 114, 115, 116, 117, 119, 121, 122, 123, 124, 125, 126, 127, 128, 129, 130, 172, 309
Gastroesophageal reflux disease (GERD) 105, 106, 107, 114, 120
Gastrointestinal anatomy 104, 112
Gastrointestinal disease 104, 105, 106, 110, 112, 114, 116, 123, 124, 125, 126, 129, 384
Gastrointestinal disorders 103, 107, 113, 114, 115, 117, 118, 123, 124, 125, 126, 131
Gastrointestinal (GI) 105, 108, 130
Gastrointestinal Ultrasound (GIUS) 117
Genome-wide association studies (GWAS) 298
Genomic medicine 127, 340
Geographic information systems (GIS) 391
Gestational diabetes mellitus (GDM) 180
Global management 81
Glomerulonephritis 136, 144, 146, 149
Glucocorticoids 182, 278, 285
Growth hormone (GH) 177

H

Harmful chemicals 384, 385, 387, 389
Harmonize care 308
Health care environment 28, 209
Healthcare institutions 8
Healthcare model 155
Healthcare sector 5, 26
Healthcare services 14, 26, 249, 262
Healthcare workers 14, 27, 34, 46, 168, 197, 217, 229, 267, 308, 315, 384, 393
Healthier lifestyles 72, 180, 263
Health issues 4, 5, 6, 11, 18, 58, 73, 156, 175, 189, 310, 366, 378, 381, 384, 387, 389, 390, 392, 396, 397, 398
Health practitioners 23, 42, 136, 261, 274, 279, 376, 384, 385, 392
Health Risk Assessment 389
Heat shock proteins (HSPs) 277
Hematological illnesses 225
Hematological malignancies 225, 228, 229
Hematologic disease 211, 218, 232
Hematologic malignancies, 217, 221, 222, 228, 232
Hematology 207, 209, 210, 211, 213, 218, 221, 226, 228, 230, 232, 235, 236, 237, 238, 239
Hematology-oncology 207, 238
Hematopoietic stem cells (HSCs) 230
Hemodialysis (HD) 152
Hepatocellular carcinoma (HCC) 120
Hereditary hemorrhagic telangiectasia (HHT) 216
High-deductible health plans (HDHPs) 57
High-flow nasal therapy (HFNT) 78
High-resolution computed tomography (HRCT) 72
Hippocratic Corpus 6
HIV-associated neurocognitive disorder (HAND) 15
Holistic health 107, 258, 381
Holistic response 242
Hormonal control 178
Hormonal pathways 118, 178, 194
Hormone replacement therapies (HRTs) 174
Hormone replacement treatments (HRTs) 193
Horrific complications 108
Hospitalization 21, 81, 82, 89, 91, 122, 125, 156, 186, 394
Human health 5, 6, 176, 264, 265, 267, 309, 376, 377, 378, 384, 400
Hypertension 4, 13, 14, 16, 20, 23, 25, 30, 35, 40, 42, 44, 45, 46, 47, 48, 52, 54, 55, 56, 57, 59, 66, 67, 68, 69, 72, 97, 105, 111, 135, 136, 137, 138, 140, 142, 145, 147, 154, 155, 165, 179, 182, 187, 191, 316, 341
Hyperthyroidism 177, 179, 180, 181, 183, 189
Hypothyroidism 179, 180, 181, 184, 187

I

Idiopathic thrombocytopenic purpura (ITP) 214
Immunization campaigns 73, 365
Immunocompromised 79, 250, 251, 253, 254
Immunosuppression 255
Impairment screening 11
Inappropriate sitting 387
Induced pluripotent stem cells (iPSCs) 216, 355
Infectious diseases 3, 4, 6, 7, 13, 15, 16, 24, 35, 72, 82, 105, 136, 225, 241, 242, 243, 244, 245, 246, 247,

248, 249, 250, 251, 252, 253, 254, 255, 256, 257, 258, 259, 260, 261, 262, 263, 264, 265, 266, 267, 269, 271, 277, 305, 313, 380
Infectious etiologies 145, 322
Inflammatory bowel disease 104, 105, 106, 108, 109, 112, 114, 115, 116, 123, 124, 125, 131, 132, 270
Instantaneous levels 360
Institutional machinery 295
Integrative therapies 81
Interconnectedness 6, 92, 104, 155, 159, 175, 367, 391
Interdisciplinary approach 94, 136, 144, 172, 195, 393, 394
Interdisciplinary collaboration 47, 163, 210, 247, 291, 296, 326, 328, 345
Interdisciplinary model 245, 290, 380
Interdisciplinary practices 187
Internal medicine 1, 2, 3, 4, 6, 7, 9, 11, 13, 24, 25, 26, 28, 39, 40, 103, 104, 105, 155, 171, 172, 175, 176, 208, 210, 211, 242, 244, 249, 267, 274, 275, 277, 279, 299
Internal organ 103, 171
Internists 1, 2, 3, 4, 5, 9, 12, 28, 29, 40, 104, 105, 115, 155, 165, 166, 171, 172, 173, 197, 208, 209, 232, 242, 243, 244, 245, 274, 275
Interprofessional collaboration 15, 40, 53, 214, 287
Interstitial lung disease (ILD) 86
Invasive pulmonary aspergillosis (IPA) 250
Irritable bowel syndrome (IBS) 106, 115, 124
Ischemia-modified albumin (IMA) 220, 238

J

Job exposure matrices (JEMs) 377

K

Kidney transplantation 153

L

Laboratory examinations 211, 293
Laboratory techniques 82, 232
Laboratory workup 284
Left ventricular assist devices (LVADs) 39, 43, 57
Legislation 396, 402
Levodopa-induced dyskinesia (LID) 315
Lifestyle medicine 23
Lifestyle modification 13, 21, 40, 43, 47, 52, 56, 58, 106, 108, 116, 117, 119, 144, 146, 152, 189, 198, 211, 263, 273, 278, 286
Long-term implications 124, 389
Lower esophageal sphincter (LES) 119
Lymphoid development 77

M

Magnetic resonance cholangiopancreatography (MRCP) 109
Magnetic resonance imaging (MRI) 17, 19, 127, 149, 254, 282, 284, 320
Malabsorption disorders 216
Medical disorders 1
Medical Knowledge 8
Medical professionals 23, 42, 61, 62, 64, 78, 158, 172, 192, 219, 225, 261, 308, 324, 345, 369, 376
Medical science 173, 176, 277, 309, 317
Medicine community 244
Medicine information 173
Medicine professionals 26, 40, 242, 247, 274, 279, 380
Medicine residency 3, 222
Mentorship 220, 225, 226, 297, 328, 380, 381
Metabolic comorbidities 157
Metabolic waste 76, 77, 138, 139
Metagenomic next-generation sequencing (mNGS) 82, 246, 249, 250, 251, 260
Misdiagnosis 150, 187, 189, 225, 253, 282, 293, 332
Mucous membranes 74
Multichannel intraluminal impedance (MII) 119
Multidimensional paradigm 19
Multidisciplinary approach 15, 16, 42, 104, 175, 182, 184, 211, 213, 214, 216, 218, 243, 252, 255, 277, 290, 293, 316, 330
Multidisciplinary collaboration 7, 9, 108, 245, 365
Multidisciplinary practice 40, 290
Multidisciplinary teams 5, 55, 58, 136, 156, 159, 213, 214, 287
Multidisciplinary treatment 72, 145, 275, 319
Multifaceted needs 11, 280

Multifactorial problems 290
Multilevel measurements 392
Multimodal interventions 105, 257
Multiple sclerosis (MS). 21
Multisectoral AMS programs 265
Myocardial infarction 46, 62, 66, 69

N

Nanotechnology 99, 329, 367, 391, 394, 401
National Cholesterol Education Program (NCEP) 57
National Spanish Registry (RICA) 64
Necessitating stringent 383
Neonatal abstinence syndrome (NAS) 347, 350, 356
Nephrologist coordination 160
Nephrology 8, 26, 34, 35, 135, 136, 137, 138, 139, 140, 141, 143, 144, 145, 147, 148, 149, 150, 151, 152, 153, 154, 155, 156, 157, 158, 159, 160, 161, 162, 163, 164, 165, 166, 167, 168, 169, 203, 235
Nervous systems 311, 313, 326
Network pharmacology 344, 362, 366, 367
Neurodegeneration 312, 318, 330
Neurodegenerative 19, 312, 317, 318, 321, 323, 325, 326, 328, 337, 384
Neuroimaging modalities 321
Neurological anomalies 321
Neurological disease 308, 309, 318, 320, 325, 327, 330, 331, 340, 387
Neurological diseases 310, 312, 315, 322, 323, 324, 326, 327, 328, 330, 331, 332, 334
Neurological disorders 310, 315
Neurological function 314, 322
Neurological health 307, 313, 329, 330, 331
Neurological research environment 332
Neurologists 307, 308, 309, 312, 319, 320, 322, 327, 328, 329, 332, 336, 340
Neurology 307, 308, 320, 323, 328, 331, 337, 338, 339, 340, 341
Next-generation sequencing (NGS) 19, 229
Non-alcoholic fatty liver disease (NAFLD) 112, 188
Non-pharmacological treatments 88
Nonspecific symptoms 39, 279
Non-steroidal anti-inflammatory drug (NSAIDs) 108
Nurse practitioners (NPs) 37, 49

O

Obesity 197, 203, 302
Occupational absenteeism 388
Occupational exposure 377, 379, 390
Occupational health and safety (OHS) 394
Occupational health frameworks 380
Occupational medicine 236, 376, 377, 378, 379, 380, 381, 382, 383, 387, 388, 390, 391, 392, 393, 394, 398, 400, 401
Organizational interventions 376, 391, 401
Organ systems 2, 3, 15, 104, 138, 155, 274, 279
Overcoming disparities 196
Over-the-counter (OTC) 242, 243

P

Pancreatic disease 122, 123, 124
Parenteral administration 348
Parkinson's disease (PD) 315
Paroxysmal nocturnal hemoglobinuria (PNH) 220
Particularly endocrinology 171
Pathophysiological changes 74
Pathophysiology 16, 30, 46, 71, 72, 78, 79, 81, 103, 104, 105, 106, 117, 119, 120, 136, 150, 160, 178, 179, 209, 212, 215, 232, 242, 279, 309, 313, 316, 323, 324
Patient care 2, 3, 4, 5, 6, 7, 8, 9, 13, 14, 17, 19, 22, 26, 27, 28, 29, 33, 38, 39, 40, 41, 48, 50, 51, 52, 55, 56, 57, 58, 59, 62, 64, 72, 92, 94, 95, 103, 106, 108, 109, 113, 115, 124, 125, 126, 129, 136, 137, 147, 151, 159, 161, 163, 171, 173, 174, 176, 184, 186, 188, 189, 191, 192, 195, 199, 207, 210, 211, 213, 219, 221, 222, 223, 227, 229, 230, 231, 232, 233, 242, 245, 250, 254, 257, 258, 260, 267, 268, 277, 279, 284, 289, 290, 291, 293, 297, 298, 299, 307, 308, 309, 324, 325, 326, 327, 328, 329, 332, 333, 344, 346, 351, 358, 361, 364, 366, 367, 370, 394
Patient compliance 61, 62, 104, 106, 109, 124, 187, 193, 297, 366, 367

Patient morbidity 111, 122, 383
Patient populations 3, 5, 54, 59, 174, 186, 223, 229, 249, 253, 254, 256, 266, 357, 362, 364, 367, 369
Pedagogical effectiveness 343
Penicillin 246
Peptic ulcer disease (PUD) 107
Percutaneous coronary interventions (PCI) 55
Peripheral blood mononuclear cells (PBMCs) 216
Peritoneal dialysis (PD) 152, 359
Personalized medicine 2, 17, 51, 95, 114, 129, 150, 162, 184, 216, 217, 219, 222, 228, 230, 239, 298, 321, 344, 345, 346, 348, 352, 353, 355, 356, 359, 362, 363, 365, 366, 367, 368, 369, 373
Personalized treatment 86, 137, 153, 190, 211, 254, 280, 284, 289, 298, 330, 367
Personal protective equipment (PPE) 389, 400
Pharmaceutical industry's 250
Pharmacodynamics 343, 344, 347, 349, 350, 351, 356, 360, 366, 371
Pharmacokinetics 343, 344, 346, 347, 348, 349, 350, 353, 354, 355, 356, 358, 359, 361, 364, 366, 367, 370, 371, 373
Pharmacokinetic studies 346, 369
Pharmacological 16, 21, 22, 32, 41, 47, 53, 54, 81, 87, 88, 100, 115, 152, 165, 187, 188, 286, 287, 315, 323, 324, 343, 345, 346, 347, 348, 350, 355, 359, 364, 368, 369
Pharmacological interventions 21, 22, 32, 53, 81, 88, 115, 287, 324, 364
Pharmacological issues 360
Pharmacological management 152, 324
Pharmacological therapy 114
Pharmacologic treatment 52, 114, 146, 188
Pharmacologist 353
Pharmacology principles 344
Pharmacotherapy 20, 45, 54, 60, 72, 79, 115, 152, 157, 175, 187, 188, 221, 222, 256, 280, 324, 330, 345, 346, 347, 358, 359, 360, 361, 362, 364, 369
Pharmacotherapy's implications 345
Pheochromocytoma 190
Physical ability 73
Physical exercise 14, 58, 155, 175, 180, 197
Physical health 377, 390, 391
Physical recovery 56
Physician assistants (PAs) 37, 42, 49, 191
Physicians 21, 47, 50, 59, 105, 166, 174, 185, 208, 242
Physiological 2, 18, 25, 59, 74, 80, 86, 124, 139, 141, 142, 151, 154, 174, 176, 177, 178, 179, 182, 191, 216, 279, 308, 309, 338, 348, 351, 358, 359, 361, 364, 367
Physiological action 191
Physiological stability 141
Physiology 5, 6, 71, 74, 78, 96, 112, 135, 141, 159, 182, 312, 325, 344, 345, 346, 351, 367
Pioneering surgery 116
Point-of-care ultrasound (PoCUS) 186
Policymakers 48, 189, 243, 267, 365, 384, 394, 397
Polycystic ovary syndrome (PCOS) 187, 194, 197
Porcine Reproductive and Respiratory Syndrome (PRRS) 264
Positron Emission Tomography (PET) 185, 331
Postmenopausal women 181
Preclinical research 355
Preclinical studies 354, 355
preventive maintenance 175
Primary care physicians 5, 40, 155, 158, 163, 182, 254, 326, 329
Principal pathological 81
Psychological benefits 287
Psychological distress 274, 377, 390, 391, 393, 402
Psychological hazards 382
Psychologically conducive. 388
Psychological problems 259
Public awareness 180
Public health 4, 6, 14, 15, 16, 25, 28, 44, 45, 46, 47, 55, 56, 58, 71, 72, 73, 90, 91, 92, 93, 99, 104, 109, 136, 156, 180, 188, 189, 197, 209, 233, 241, 242, 243, 244, 245, 247, 248, 249, 250, 251, 252, 260, 261, 263, 264, 265, 267, 277, 335, 345, 346, 354, 357, 365, 376, 377, 378, 379, 380, 381, 382, 383, 384, 385, 386, 389, 390, 391, 392, 393, 394, 395, 396, 398, 401, 402
Public health interventions 265, 394
Pulmonary emphysema 83, 97
Pulmonary involvement 254
Pulmonary rehabilitation 72, 79, 81, 88

Q

Quality of life (QoL) 151

R

Reference change values (RCV) 219
Regenerative medicine therapies (RMTs) 151
Regulatory frameworks 90, 233, 346, 379, 381
Rehabilitation therapy 325
Renal function 42, 136, 137, 138, 139, 140, 142, 144, 145, 146, 147, 149, 150, 151, 155, 157, 159, 283, 349
Renin-angiotensin-aldosterone system (RAAS) 140, 141
Resource allocation 10, 380
Respiratory diseases 64, 71, 73, 74, 76, 78, 83, 85, 86, 87, 88, 90, 91, 92, 93, 95, 96, 99, 256, 377, 400
Respiratory medicine 71, 72, 82, 95
Retrospective evaluations 222
Rheumatic illnesses 277, 286
Rheumatoid arthritis (RA) 278, 294, 299, 301
Rheumatological conditions 273, 277, 282, 284, 286, 293, 300
Rheumatological disorders 277
Rheumatologists 276, 280, 283, 284, 286, 287, 288, 289, 290, 292, 294, 295, 296, 297, 299, 303
Rheumatology 273, 274, 275, 276, 277, 278, 279, 281, 282, 283, 284, 285, 287, 288, 290, 291, 292, 293, 294, 295, 296, 297, 298, 299, 300, 301, 302, 303, 304

S

Scientific knowledge 6, 7
Scientific principles 6, 104
Seizure control 319, 324
Self-management 11, 21, 47, 48, 58, 80, 151, 163, 188, 273, 274, 277, 278, 280, 287, 289, 291, 296, 298, 304
Sensory perception 313, 314
Sexual health 175, 312, 376, 403
Sickle cell disease (SCD) 226
Simple steatosis (SS) 112
Socioeconomic status 13, 29, 61, 262, 387
Sophisticated 3, 6, 9, 19, 29, 39, 43, 50, 54, 62, 86, 95, 139, 147, 155, 174, 184, 191, 209, 222, 230, 246, 249, 256, 264, 314, 321, 327, 346, 355, 358, 366, 368
Sophistication 90, 233, 242, 292, 314
South African Health Products Regulatory Authority (SAHPRA) 356
Southern African Centre for Infectious Disease Surveillance (SACIDS) 243, 261
Standardized mechanisms 44
Stethoscope 6
Strengthening community 61
Streptococcus 30, 81, 96, 97, 249
Supportive treatment 79, 123
Surgical planning 55, 321
Surgical therapies 325
Sustainable Development Goals (SDGs) 9, 83
Symbiotic patient-caregiver 291
Systematic approaches 385
Systemic lupus erythematosus 30, 274, 282, 283, 286, 289, 290, 294, 301, 302, 303, 304, 305

T

Tailored medicine 200, 231
Takayasu arteritis 284
Technological progress 62, 228, 233
Telemedicine 2, 20, 62, 106, 160, 173, 190, 191, 192, 193, 197, 203, 212, 296, 298, 327, 368
Telemonitoring schemes 193
Tendinopathies 277
Terminal patients 24
Therapeutic advances 229
Therapeutic approaches 9, 106, 125, 127, 136, 141, 146, 169, 177, 211, 220, 236, 245, 277, 318, 334, 345, 369
Therapeutic index 353, 358, 359, 360, 371
Therapeutic interventions 10, 15, 19, 41, 47, 52, 57, 75, 114, 143, 150, 151, 159, 175, 182, 184, 214, 221, 225, 229, 251, 274, 289, 312, 322, 328, 330, 334, 345, 347, 351, 358, 368
Therapeutic landscape 7
Therapeutic potential 151, 363
Therapeutic protocols 256, 366
Therapeutic regimens 42, 76, 155, 190, 191, 284, 350, 353, 360, 364
Therapeutics conference 361
Therapeutic strategies 19, 142, 150, 161, 178, 200,

221, 227, 252, 288, 292, 310, 313, 349, 359, 368
Therapeutic technique 51
Thrombocytopenia 128, 214, 222, 226, 238
Thrombocytopenic patients 231
Thromboembolism 176, 185, 203, 214, 226, 237
Thyroid-stimulating hormone (TSH) 181
Tissue factor pathway inhibitor (TFPI) 283, 304
Trans-boundary collaboration 15, 261
Transcranial magnetic stimulation (TMS) 331, 334
Translational research (TR) 126
Transplant systems 127
Treatment methodologies 3, 334
Treatment modifications 285
Treatment protocols 21, 23, 47, 94, 116, 123, 127, 147, 153, 160, 173, 182, 186, 188, 191, 194, 200, 211, 216, 218, 225, 226, 229, 250, 251, 254, 276, 284, 286, 288, 298, 307, 308, 329, 331, 359, 369
Treatment regimen 123, 127, 227, 228, 294
Treatment strategies 55, 110, 127, 136, 138, 139, 143, 146, 161, 163, 174, 180, 184, 199, 244, 246, 267, 285, 287, 292, 294, 309, 310, 318, 324, 331, 366, 393
Tricarboxylic acid (TCA) 143
Tyrosine kinase inhibitors (TKIs) 217

V

Vaccination programs 93, 248
Vascular network 74, 76
Veterans Affairs (VA) 249
Video-assisted thoracoscopic surgery (VATS) 89
Viral respiratory infections 79
Virtual reality (VR) 326, 328
Visceral hypersensitivity 115
Vulnerabilities 90, 262, 388

W

Water pollution 384
Work-related musculoskeletal disorders (WMSD) 379
World Federation of Hemophilia (WFH) 5, 7
World Health Organization (WHO) 92
Worsening symptoms 90

X

X-linked hypophosphatemia (XLH) 189